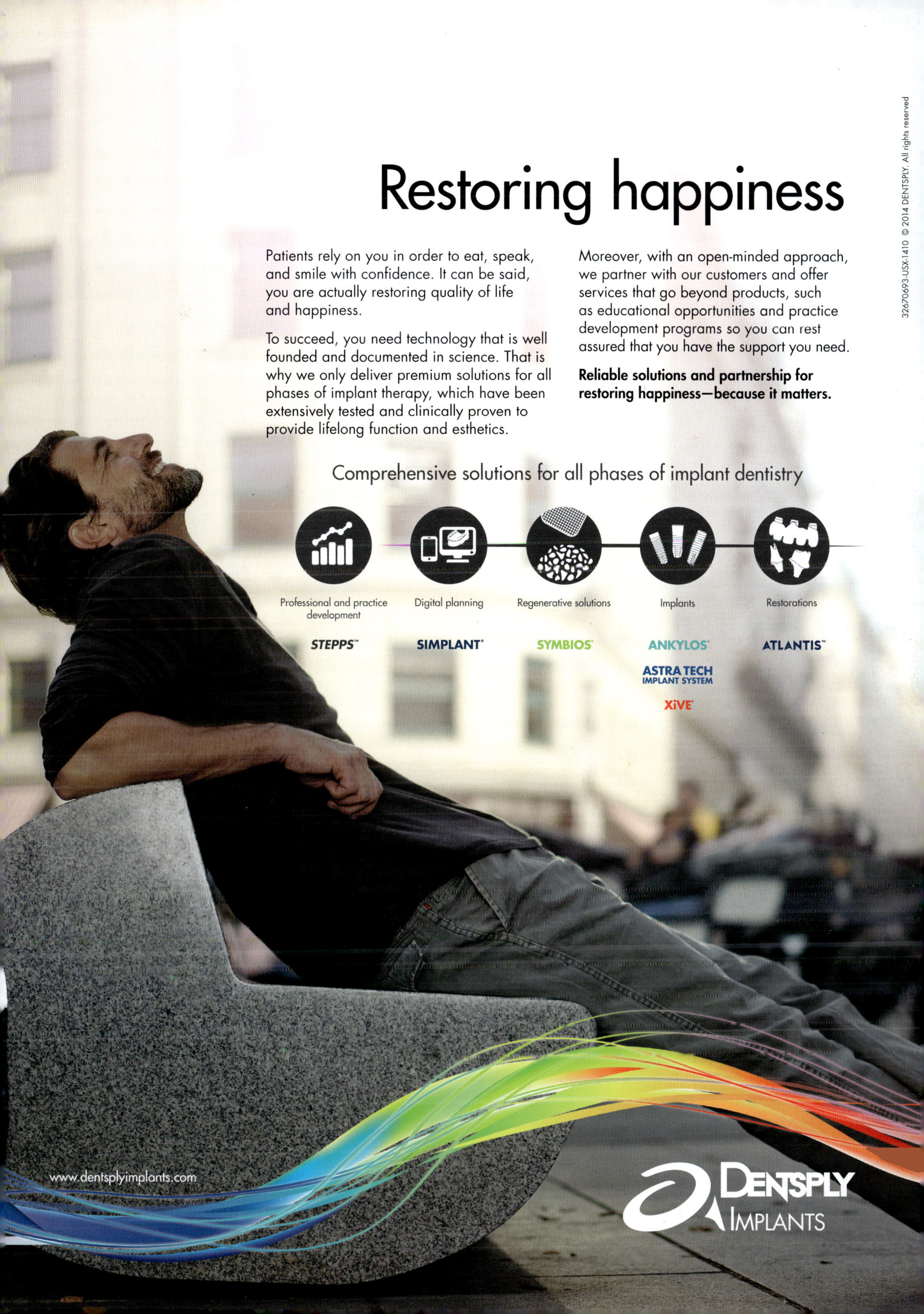
Restoring happiness
Patients rely on you in order to eat, speak, and smile with confidence. It can be said, you are actually restoring quality of life and happiness.
To succeed, you need technology that is well founded and documented in science. That is why we only deliver premium solutions for all phases of implant therapy, which have been extensively tested and clinically proven to provide lifelong function and esthetics.
Moreover, with an open-minded approach, we partner with our customers and offer services that go beyond products, such as educational opportunities and practice development programs so you can rest assured that you have the support you need.
Reliable solutions and partnership for restoring happiness—because it matters.
Comprehensive solutions for all phases of implant dentistry
Professional and practice development
Digital planning
Regenerative solutions
Implants
Restorations
STEPPS™
SIMPLANT®
SYMBIOS®
ANKYLOS®
ATLANTIS™
ASTRA TECH IMPLANT SYSTEM
XiVE®
www.dentsplyimplants.com
DENTSPLY IMPLANTS
32670693-USX-1410 © 2014 DENTSPLY. All rights reserved

Editorial

Success, Survival, or Failure Rates: Why They *Do* Matter

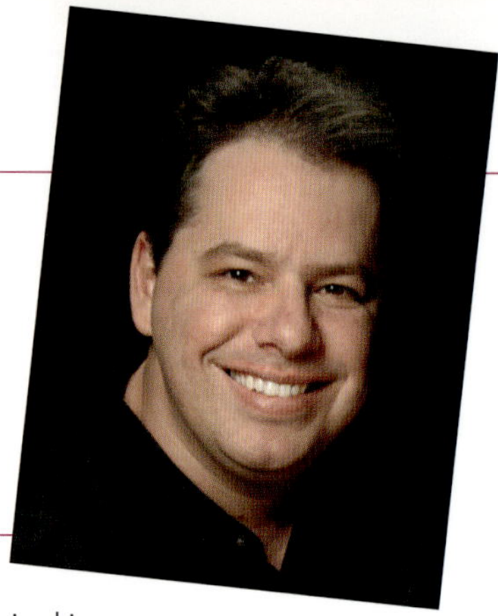

Independent scientific investigations are, unquestionably, one of the most important sources for understanding the behavior of biomaterials or techniques in our field. A modest web-based search reveals tens of thousands of articles focusing on different aspects of dental biomaterials published in peer-reviewed journals. However, when the search is narrowed to clinical trials, the amount of available literature drops significantly, to thousands of articles, and once success rate or survival rate is included in the search, the information drops to only a few hundred peer-reviewed articles. The difficulty of conducting an independent clinical investigation is titanic: developing a hypothesis; performing in vitro laboratory tests prior to the in vivo testing; obtaining and evaluating these results; assessing which laboratorial aspects (or techniques) could be clinically translated and truly important to be investigated; designing a research protocol that accurately leads to coherent results; preparing, submitting, and obtaining approval of an independent review board (IRB, also known as an independent ethics committee); being awarded financial support; and finding a group of individuals who agree to volunteer for the investigation. These are only the initial stages of the process required to perform a clinical trial.

Finally, when all of the above is accomplished, the actual testing can begin. But first, an investigator or group of investigators (researchers, clinicians, professionals, residents, and/or students) will undergo a calibration series to prevent one of the most undesirable problems in research: bias. Bias may occur unintentionally during trial planning, implementation, and/or data analysis. Rigorous criteria for case selection are essential to avoid confounding results. Only cases that perfectly satisfy the criteria can be used. During the surgical/restorative procedures, personal preferences and situations beyond the control of the investigators may arise that can jeopardize the final outcome of the investigation. Performance bias may obscure efforts to establish a cause-effect relationship between procedures and outcomes. Thus, in addition to undergoing calibration, investigators must remain impartial and dispassionate to achieve reliable results in clinical trials.

All the excitement of clinical investigations is realized only at the end, when after many months or years of work—and frustration—the results come to fruition. Inevitably, success, survival, and failure rates become the focus of many clinical investigations. Needless to say, failure rate is easy to define, whereas success and survival can be more complicated. Success may be validated by the absence of any biologic, technical, and esthetic complications, but identical parameters can be used for survival rate with some variation. Therefore, an unemotional, impersonal, and meticulously well-defined range for success is the most appropriate form of evaluation of a given work.

Clinical variables (such as technique, area to be restored, type of restoration, complexity of occlusion, periodontal health, and patient demographic, socioeconomic, and behavioral variables) as well as operator skill and knowledge no doubt play important roles in success, survival, and failure rates. Nonetheless, candid and unbiased retrospective analyses of treatments rendered are sine qua non for our own understanding of our limitations and successes.

This year, I invite you to celebrate our successes and the clinical investigations and retrospective analyses that have led to them. In the articles presented herein, discover how concepts explained in previous editions of *Quintessence of Dental Technology* are used with a different approach to elucidate and restore complex clinical cases. A special series of articles on treatment of the worn dentition plus gingival framework are worth your time and consideration; they will continue in future editions of QDT. Join me in exploring how CAD/CAM technologies, allied with human creativity, can reach impressive levels of natural beauty, or how ultraconservative esthetic surgical methods can grant highly predictable results. And the many exquisite techniques presented for delivering lifelike restorations—all are successes to be appreciated.

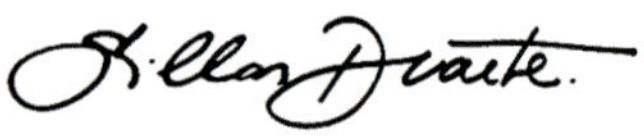

Sillas Duarte, Jr, DDS, MS, PhD
Editor-in-Chief
sillas.duarte@usc.edu

QDT 2015

Volume 38

QUINTESSENCE OF DENTAL TECHNOLOGY

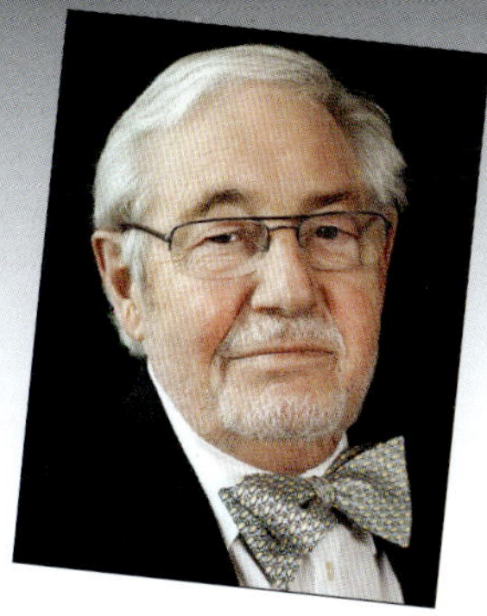

QDT 2015 is dedicated to Per-Ingvar Brånemark in celebration of his life.

Cover photo by Naoki Hayashi

PUBLISHER
H.W. Haase

EXECUTIVE VICE-PRESIDENT
William G. Hartman

JOURNAL DIRECTOR
Lori A. Bateman

PRODUCTION
Sue Robinson

ADVERTISING/EDITORIAL/SUBSCRIPTION OFFICE
Quintessence Publishing Co, Inc
4350 Chandler Drive
Hanover Park, Illinois 60133
Phone: (630) 736-3600
Toll-free: (800) 621-0387
Fax: (630) 736-3633
E-mail: service@quintbook.com
Website: http://www.quintpub.com

QDT is published once a year by Quintessence Publishing Co, Inc, 4350 Chandler Drive, Hanover Park, Illinois, 60133. Price per copy: $132.

MANUSCRIPT SUBMISSION
QDT publishes original articles covering dental laboratory techniques and methods. For submission information, contact Lori Bateman (lbateman@quintbook.com).

Printed in China
ISSN 1060-1341 / ISBN 978-0-86715-689-8

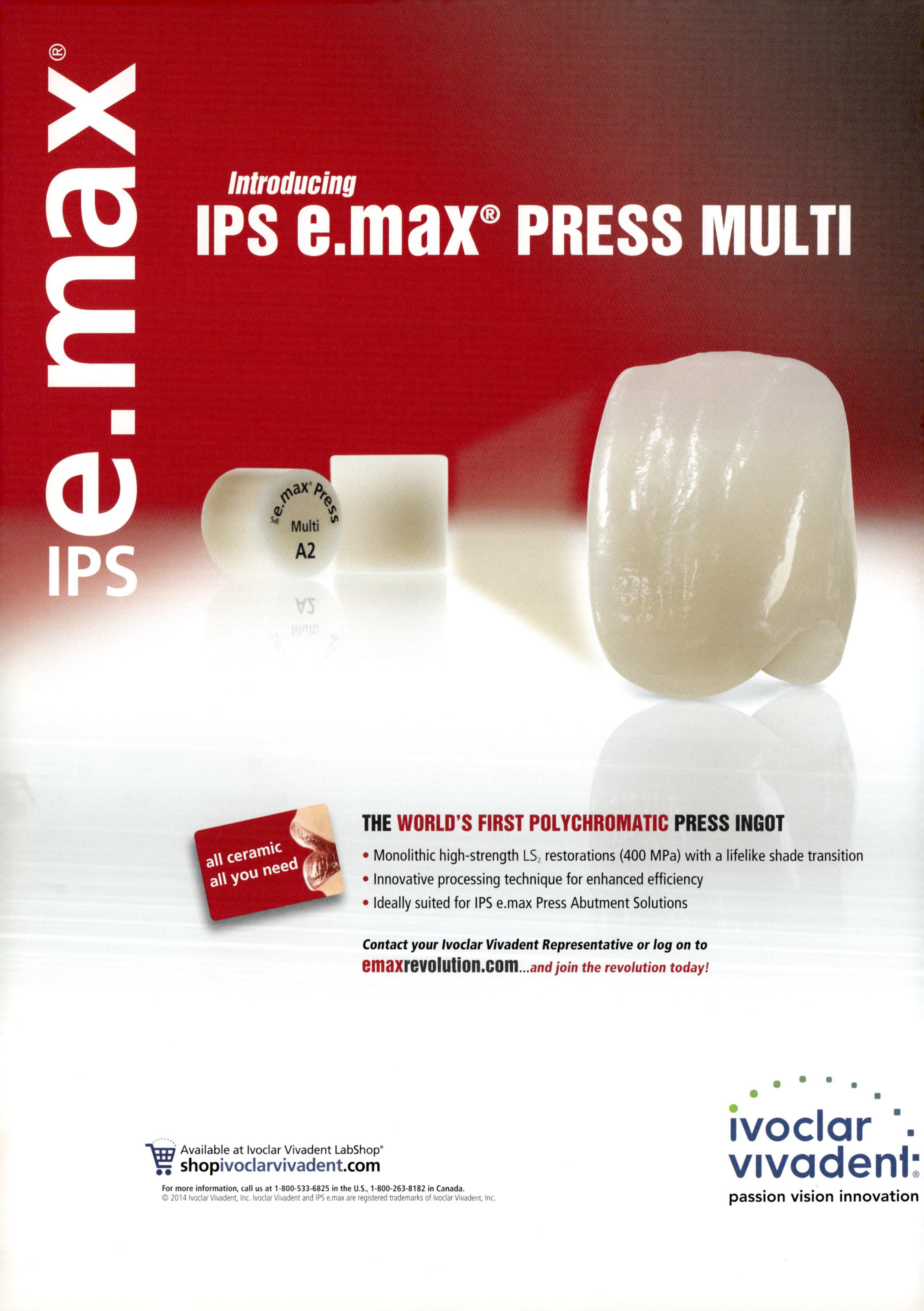
IPS e.max®
Introducing
IPS e.max® PRESS MULTI
e.max® Press
Multi
A2
all ceramic
all you need
THE WORLD'S FIRST POLYCHROMATIC PRESS INGOT
• Monolithic high-strength LS_2 restorations (400 MPa) with a lifelike shade transition
• Innovative processing technique for enhanced efficiency
• Ideally suited for IPS e.max Press Abutment Solutions
Contact your Ivoclar Vivadent Representative or log on to
emaxrevolution.com...and join the revolution today!
Available at Ivoclar Vivadent LabShop®
shopivoclarvivadent.com
For more information, call us at 1-800-533-6825 in the U.S., 1-800-263-8182 in Canada.
© 2014 Ivoclar Vivadent, Inc. Ivoclar Vivadent and IPS e.max are registered trademarks of Ivoclar Vivadent, Inc.
ivoclar vivadent®
passion vision innovation

Taking Control Over Challenging Esthetic Cases Using the Power Trio:

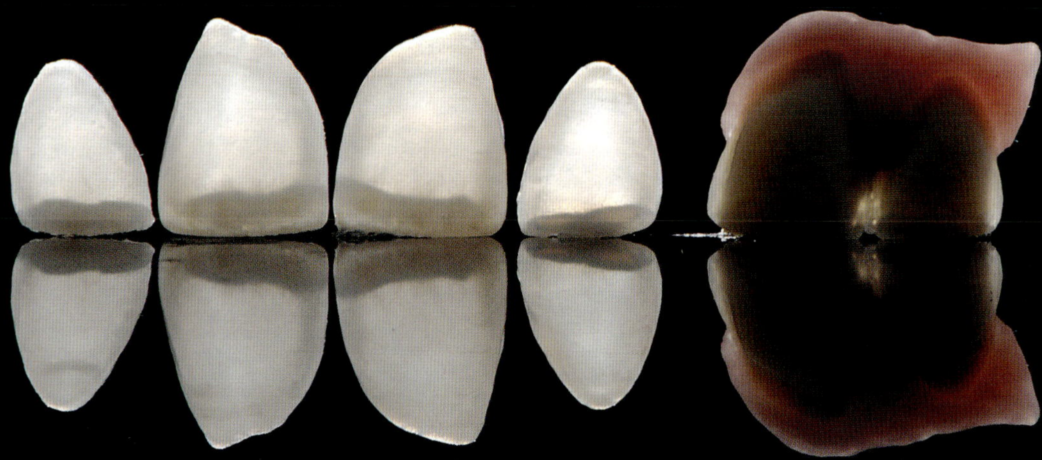

Pink Ceramics, Implants, and Veneers

Victor Clavijo, DDS, MS, PhD[1]
Leonardo Bocabella, CDT[2]
Paulo Fernando Mesquita de Carvalho, DDS, MS[3]

With the popularization of dental implants for single to complex restorations, the importance of treatment planning has been emphasized. If professionals who perform implant surgery neglect the necessary backwards planning, especially in terms of three-dimensional positioning, they are fostering future problems. The problems most frequently encountered with malpositioned implants are gingival recession, loss of the interdental papilla, grayish discoloration at the gingival margin, and complex prosthesis fabrication.[1,2] When patients present with malpositioned implants, dentists and dental technicians need to find solutions for improving their biologic, mechanical, and esthetic conditions. This article describes a technique that combines gingival and dental restorations on malpositioned implants with minimally invasive restorations on the adjacent contralateral teeth.

[1]Professor, Advanced Program in Implantology and Restorative Dentistry, ImplantePerio Institute, São Paulo, Brazil.
[2]Dental Technician, Campinas, Brazil.
[3]Director, Advanced Program in Implantology and Restorative Dentistry, ImplantePerio Institute, São Paulo, Brazil.

Correspondence to: Dr Victor Clavijo, Rua Cerqueira Cesar, 1078 Indaiatuba, São Paulo, Brazil 13330-005.
Email: clavijovictor@yahoo.com.br

CASE REPORT

A 42-year-old man presented with a chief complaint of unsatisfactory smile esthetics. Intraoral examination revealed the presence of dental disharmony, malpositioned implants (at the maxillary left central and lateral incisor sites), gingival recession, papilla loss, and dental and gingival discrepancy compared to the contralateral situation (Fig 1). To perform an effective evaluation of the implants, the cemented restorations were removed. Upon so doing, two metal abutments were found with the vestibular head of the screw emerging. This confirmed the poor position of the implants, and immediately afterward, the abutments were removed to verify the intrasulcular depth of the implants as well as the periodontal condition. Radiography and tomography were also performed to better evaluate the patient's condition.

Treatment Plan

After the diagnosis was made, and taking into account that the patient did not wish to have the implants removed, the following treatment plan and clinical sequence were suggested (Fig 2):

1. Transfer of implants to a new provisional implant prosthesis, with a pontic on the maxillary left lateral implant and a screw-retained crown on the left central implant to create a concave profile (subcontour).
2. After 3 months, flapless crown length to be increased on the contralateral teeth (right central and lateral incisors) and a connective tissue graft performed at the position of the implants to improve the gingival volume in this area, so avoiding overcontour of the prosthetic gingival restorations.
3. Minimally invasive preparation for veneers on the right central and lateral, and transfer to a dentogingival prosthesis of the left central and lateral incisors on the central incisor implant.
4. Bonded porcelain veneers and delivery of the dentogingival prosthesis.

Clinical Phases

Phase I: Provisional Implants

First the transfer of the central incisor implant was performed by using a transfer coping (Fig 3), and then a splinted provisional of the left central and lateral incisors was fabricated in polyvinyl siloxane (Virtual, Ivoclar Vivadent) and screwed in (Fig 4a). Also, in an attempt to make the gingival tissue migrate incisally, a more concave intrasulcular profile was included.[3] Finally, the left lateral incisor implant was buried to improve the interproximal appearance of the left central and lateral incisor restorations.

Phase II: Reshaping Gingival Contours, Tooth Preparation, and Impression

Three months after the provisional placement (considering the aforementioned modifications), the patient presented a small incisal "migration" of the gingival tissue. Thus, flapless[4] crown lengthening was performed on the right central and lateral incisors. A connective tissue graft (palate donor site) was used to increase the volume in the gingival area of the implants, which would reduce the prosthesis contour and facilitate its hygiene.

Two months after these procedures were performed, a significant improvement was observed in the anterior gingival discrepancy (Fig 4b); however, the papilla loss in the implant area remained, which modified the tooth form in this area. In order to adjust and improve the shape of the anterior segment, the right central and lateral incisors were minimally invasively prepared for veneer placement (Fig 5a), thus correcting the incisal contours and returning the labial anatomy that had been lost over the years. A mock-up was designed, following the technique described by Magne and Belser[5] and Gürel,[6] preserving all remaining enamel. Then a new impression of the preparation and the implant transfer was performed in order to fabricate the final ceramic restorations (Fig 5b). The prepared teeth as well as the gingival tissues were photographed to ensure accurate shade selection and harmony with the adjacent hard and soft tissues.

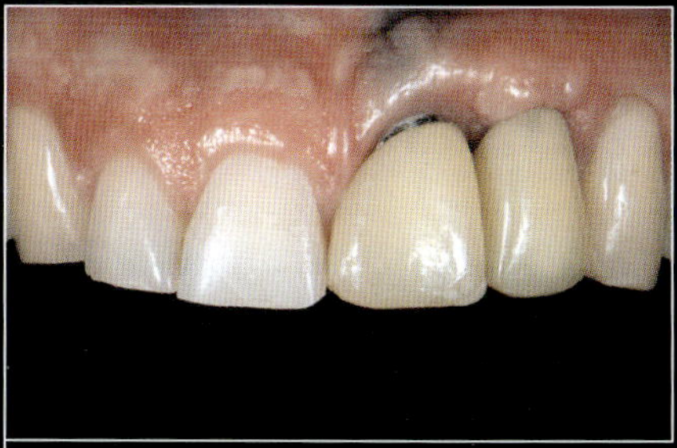
1a

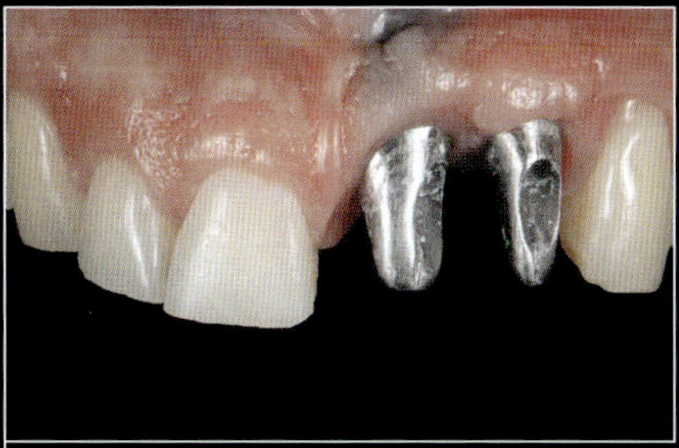
1b

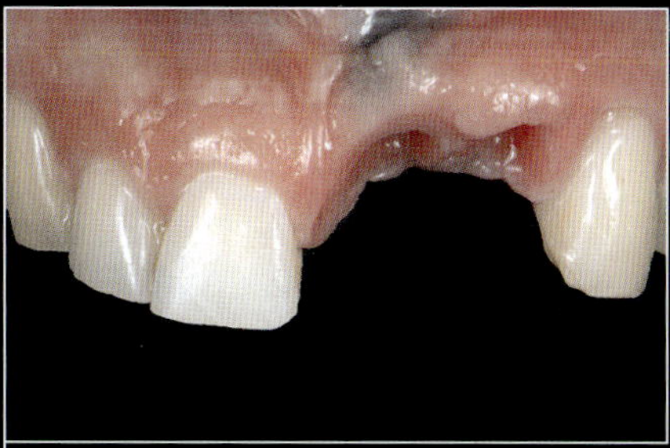
1c

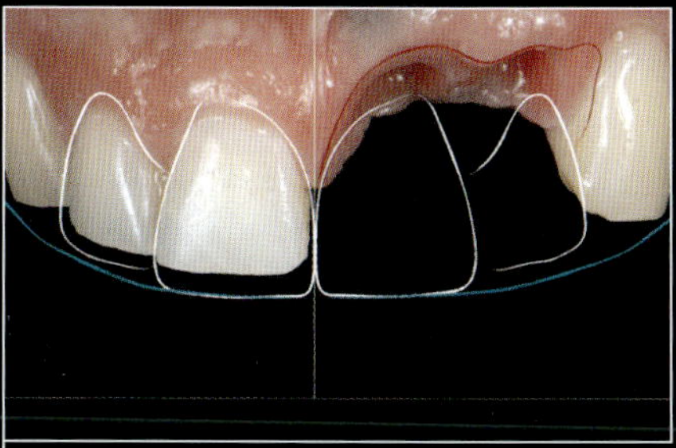
2

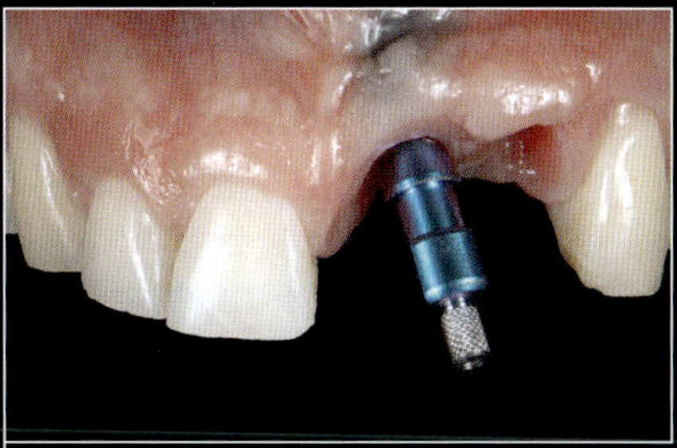
3a

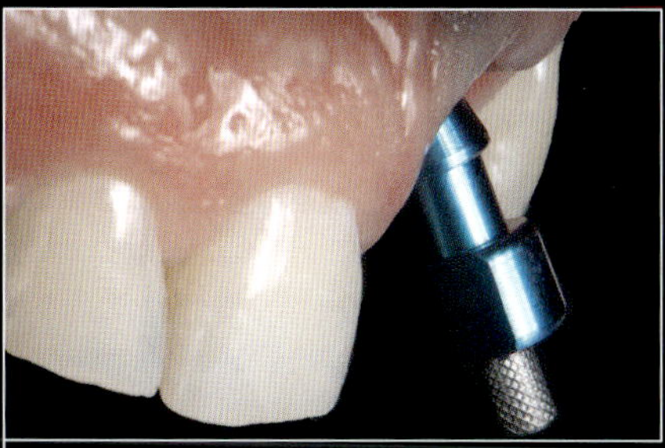
3b

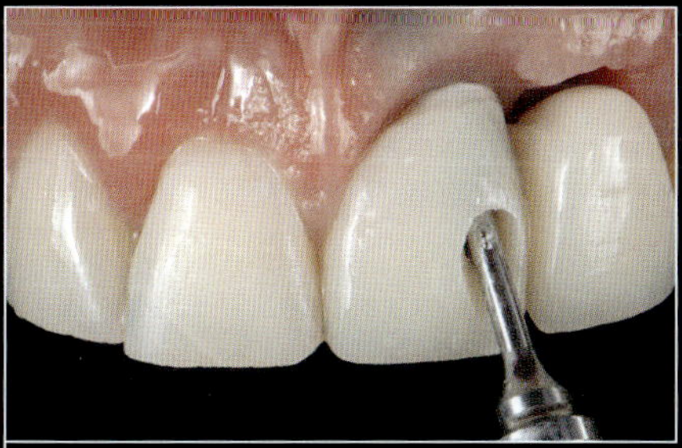
4a

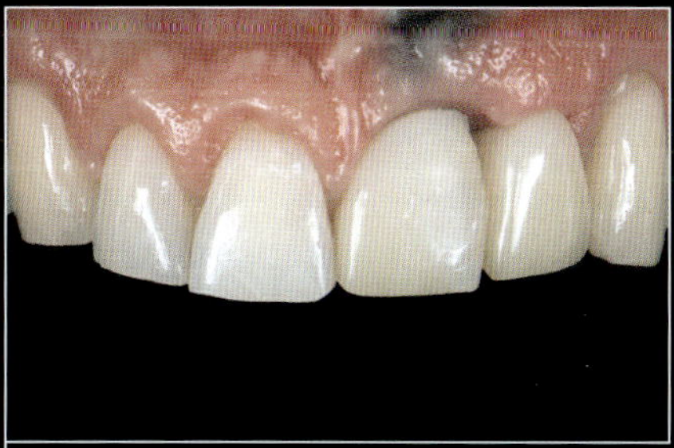
4b

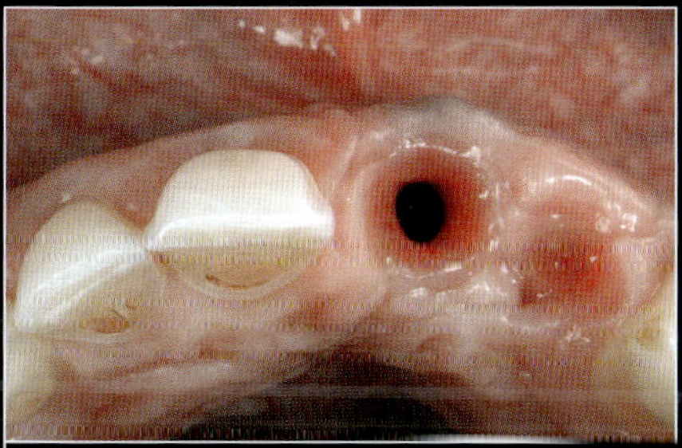
5a

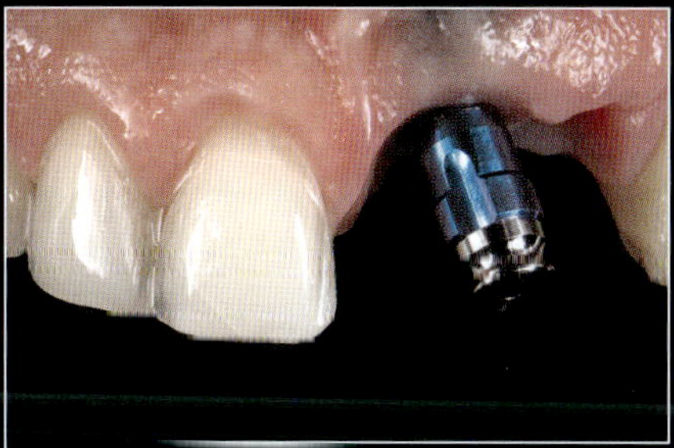
5b

Fig 1a Pretreatment intraoral situation.

Fig 1b Metal abutment and screw poorly positioned.

Fig 1c Gingival discrepancy and poor anatomical tooth shape.

Fig 2 Treatment plan (Digital Smile Design, C. Coachman and M. Voigt).

Figs 3a and 3b Transfer coping for poorly positioned implant.

Fig 4a Provisional placement with lateral incisor implant buried.

Fig 4b Remarkable esthetic improvement after healing of the crown, adaptation of the provisional, and gingival grafting.

Fig 5a Minimally invasive preparation of the right central and lateral incisors and gingival conditioning at the site of the left central and lateral.

Fig 5b Transfer coping.

Laboratory Phases

In the laboratory, the dental technician faced the multiple challenges of gingival discrepancy, poor implant positioning, and difference between the implant and prepared tooth substrates. To solve these issues, the work was divided into several laboratory phases.

Phase I: Fabricating the Infrastructure

This first phase consisted of finding a solution for the implant restoration. In terms of the poor implant position, one might consider cementing the final restoration. However, cementation of prostheses on malpositioned implants may not guarantee long-term success. Thus, a customized screw-retained implant restoration was advocated, since it has many clinical advantages as far as long-term maintenance. For that, a customized abutment was created to correct the positioning for the implant restoration. A UCLA abutment was used in association with a prefabricated extension device for lingual access (micro-UCLA, SignoVinces). After casting, two screw points, a main thread following the long axis of the implant and a secondary palatal thread for correct positioning of the final restoration, were determined (Figs 6a and 6b). Next, the dentogingival framework was fabricated (Figs 6c to 6e).

Phase II: Matching the Substrates

After completion of the metal framework, application of ceramic was initiated. It was decided to create a balance in the gingival area—which was incorrect in the previous dentogingival prosthesis—thus creating a suitable architecture to construct the ideal tooth anatomy.

To ensure better esthetic integration among the implant restorations and ceramic veneers, the left central and lateral incisor teeth were customized on the dentogingival prosthesis to provide similar characteristics to the right central and lateral incisors. Thus, artificial ceramic veneer preparations were fabricated in the dentogingival prosthesis following a similar veneer preparation design and abutment shade of the natural contralateral teeth. The fabrication of customized artificial ceramic veneer preparations into a prosthesis decreases the necessary number of bake corrections, thus avoiding modifications in optical and mechanical properties of the final prosthesis. In addition, the opportunity to fabricate all porcelain veneers at the same time improves the predictability of color and shape. However, an additional step is added to the restorative phase: bonding the porcelain veneers to the dentogingival prosthesis. One may consider the adhesive interface between ceramics a concern; however, bonding ceramic to ceramic is more predictable than bonding to dental structure and, should any adjustments be necessary in the future, repairs can be easily performed.

By using digital photographs with color scales, it was possible to reproduce the details of tooth substrate shape and color, as well as the gingival area, to match the remaining teeth (Fig 7), thereby facilitating the manufacture of ultra-thin restorations without concern for the differences in tooth substrate (Fig 8). Also, an intraoral proof was used to check adaptation and the correct implant placement, and new photographs were taken to verify color and shape of the created substrates.

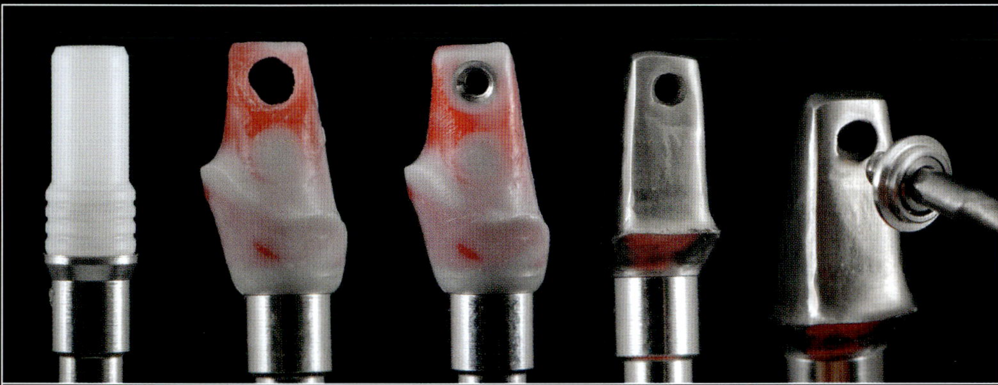
6a

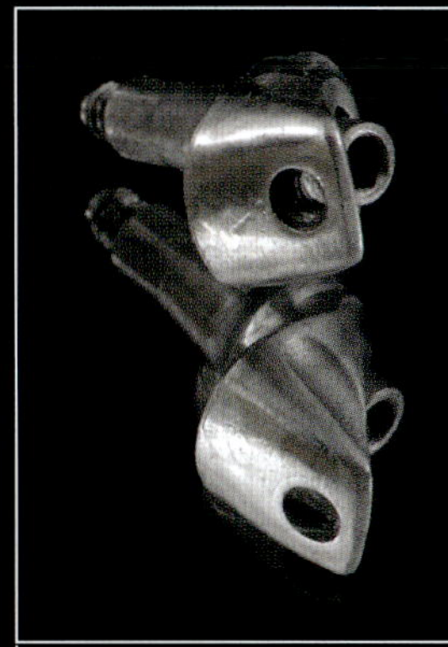
6b

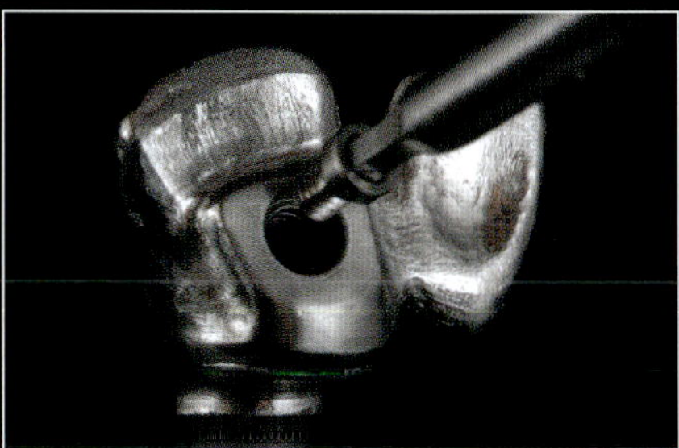
6c

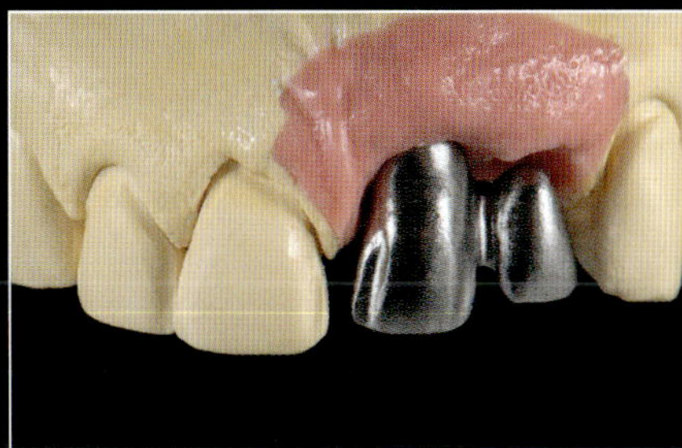
6d

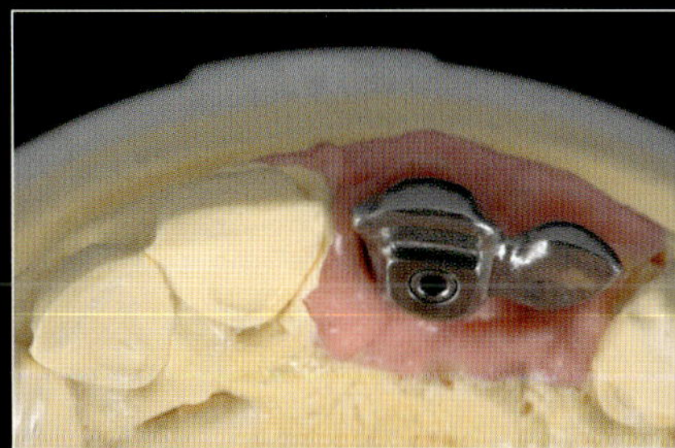
6e

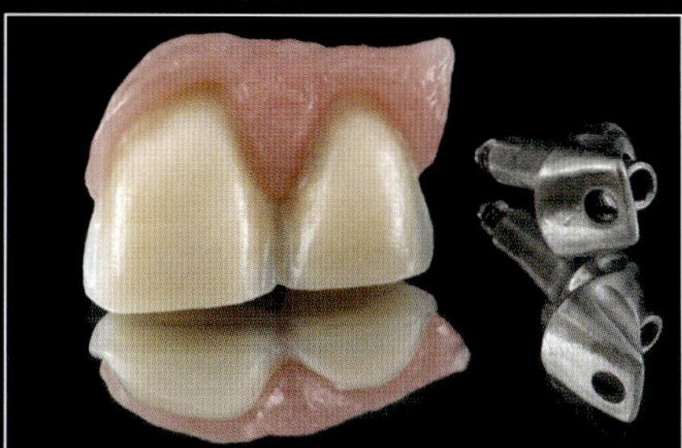
7a

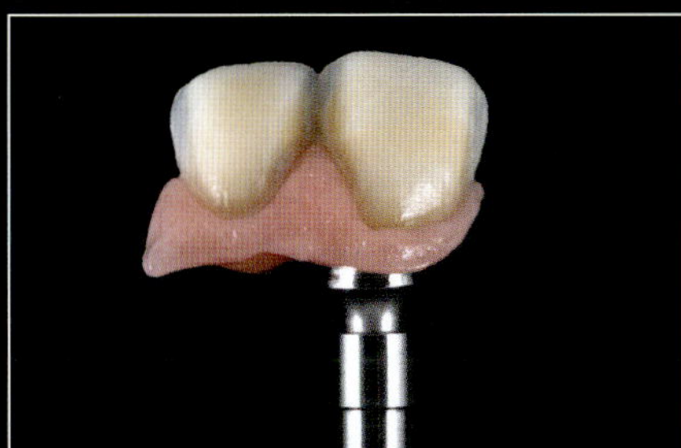
7b

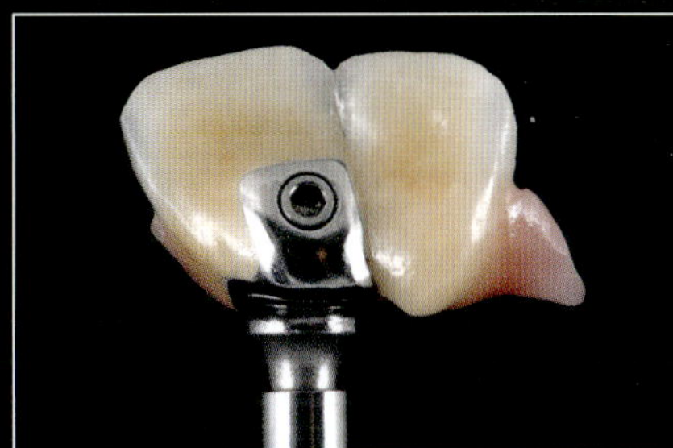
7c

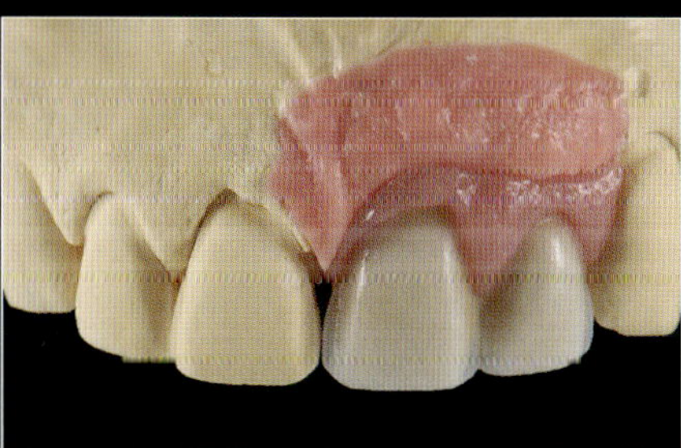
8a

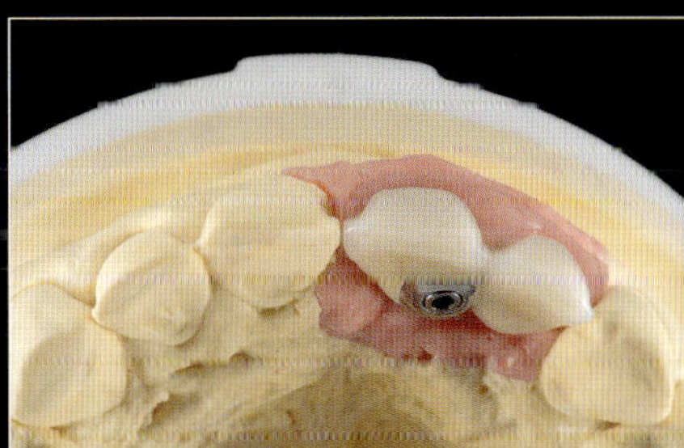
8b

Fig 6a Metal abutment with main and secondary palatal screw access holes.
Fig 6b Metal framework on the abutment after casting.
Figs 6c to 6e Metal framework and abutment.
Figs 7a to 7c Dentogingival prosthesis after ceramic application.
Figs 8a to 8c Die cast reproducing the color and shape of dental substrates.

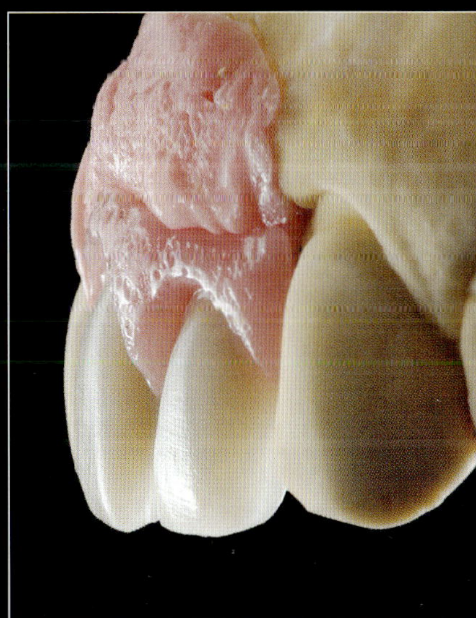
8c

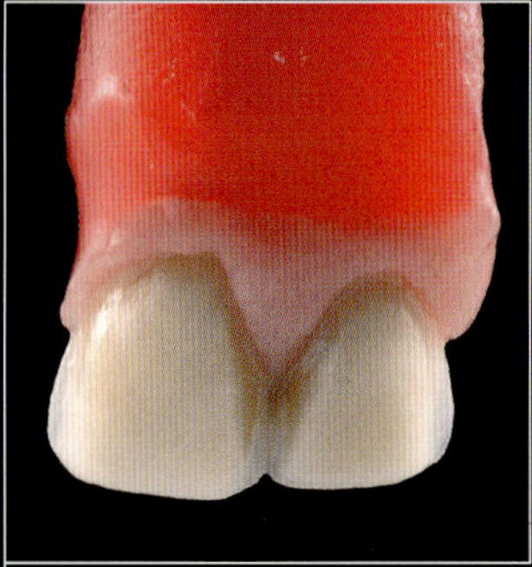
9a

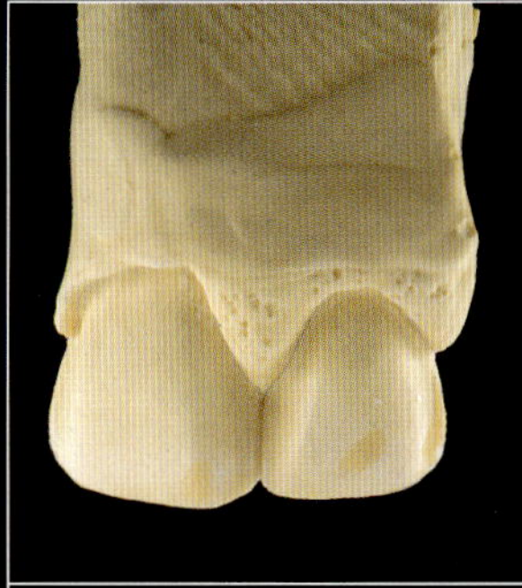
9b

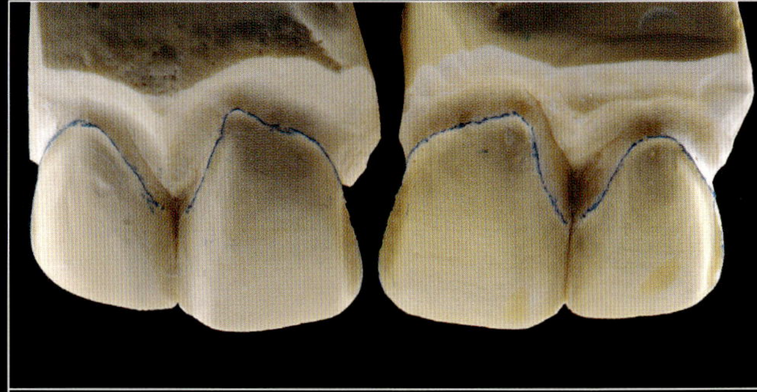
9c

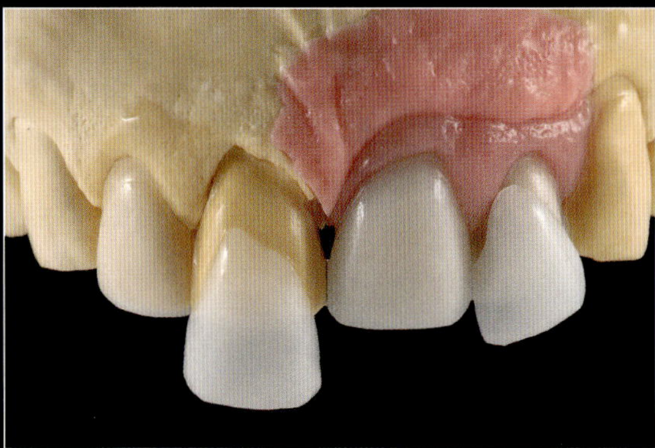
10a

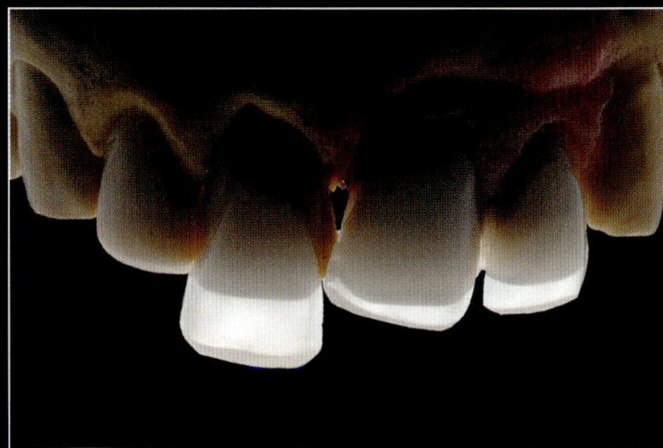
10b

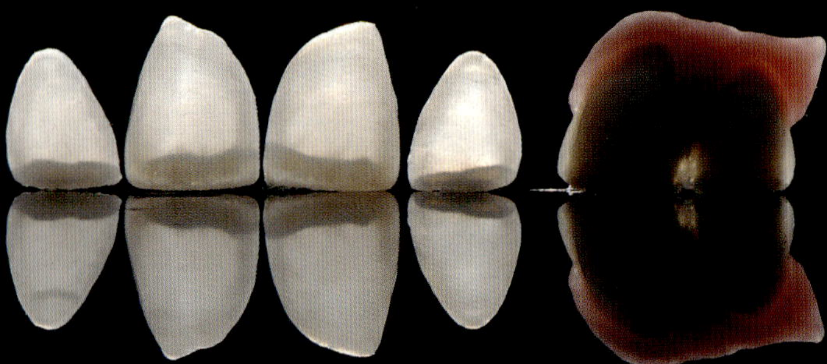
10c

Fig 9a Wax application for reproducing the ceramic structure.

Fig 9b Die cast.

Fig 9c Die cast of the four teeth. Note the shape similarity of the dies, which will facilitate a more uniform and predictable ceramic application.

Figs 10a to 10c Translucent, thin veneers placed. Remaining teeth matching.

Phase III: Duplicating the Infrastructure

A wax-up of the ceramic structure was fabricated, removing retentions and creating dies. This duplication was made with polyvinyl siloxane (same used in refractory die duplication), and a replica was made in plaster, obtaining a working die cast for waxing the veneers (Fig 9).

Phase IV: Manufacture of Ceramic Veneer Restorations

Lithium disilicate–based ceramic veneers were chosen instead of feldspathic veneers to avoid a new impression as well as to allow try-in after the bisque bake phase plus possible corrections that could present a problem for feldspathic veneers.

The LT A1 (IPS e.max Press, Ivoclar Vivadent) ingot was selected. It would provide the acceptable final color and translucency for the restorations (Fig 10). Opalescent enamel effect was then applied. After try-in to check the final color and shape, the final glazing and texturing were performed (Fig 11). The restorations were tried-in again (Figs 12 and 13), and cementation for implant placement was performed in the same laboratory.

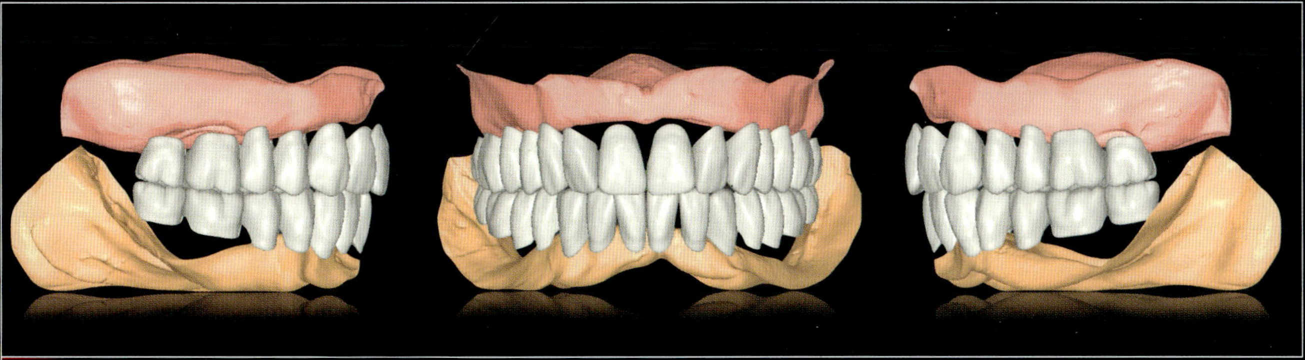

10

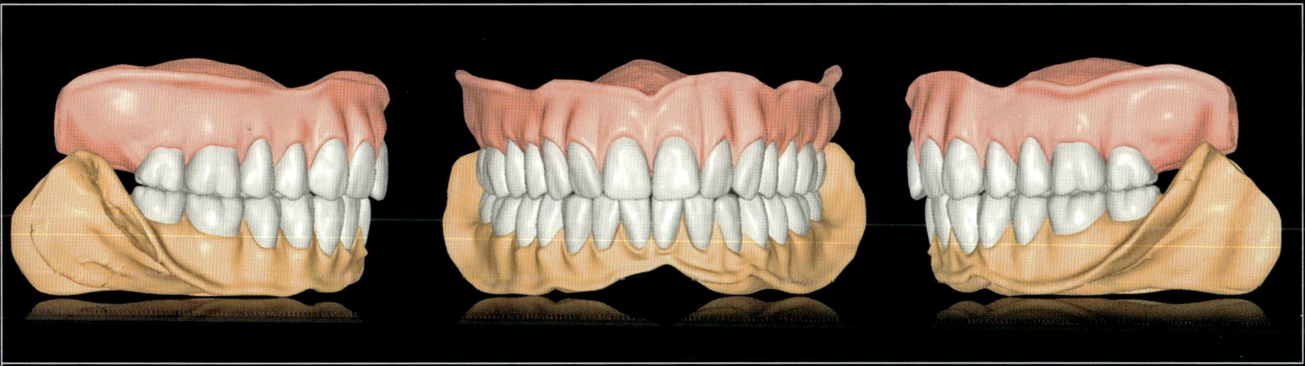

11

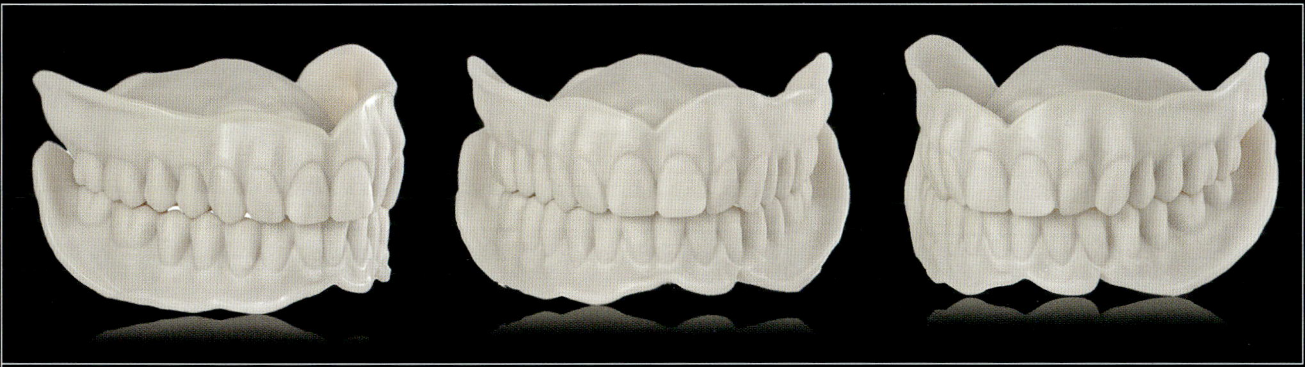

12

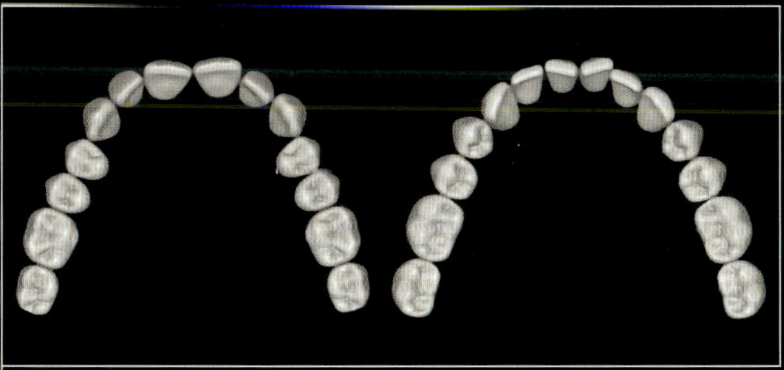

13

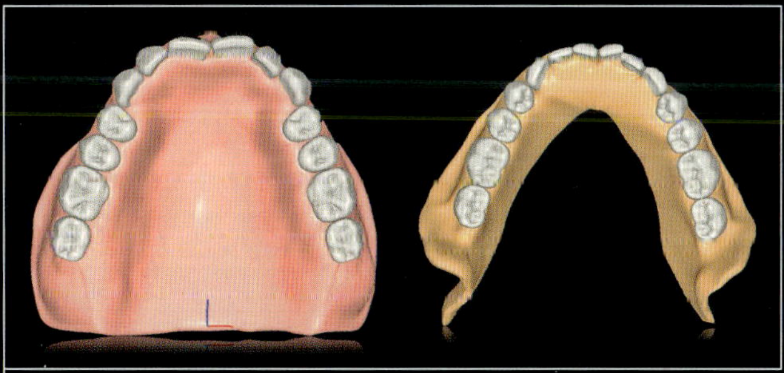

14

Fig 10 Digital image of first teeth setup: bold maxillary lateral incisors and minor mandibular incisor crowding.
Fig 11 Digital image of completed denture after festooning (first setup).
Fig 12 Try-in denture (first setup).
Fig 13 Teeth alignment (first setup). 3D printed dentures ready for try-in.
Fig 14 Teeth alignment in denture (first setup).

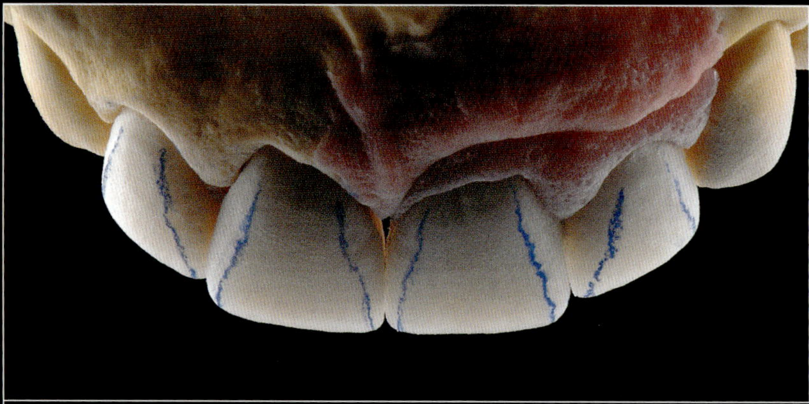

11

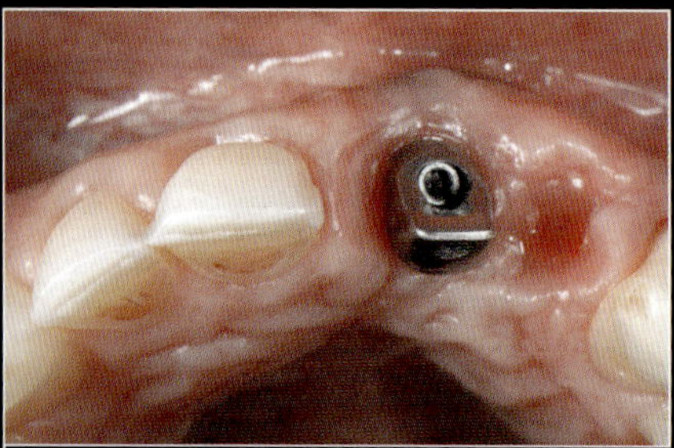

12a

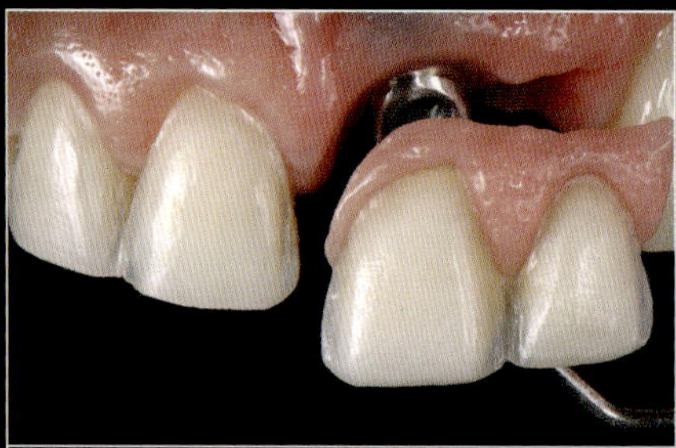

12b

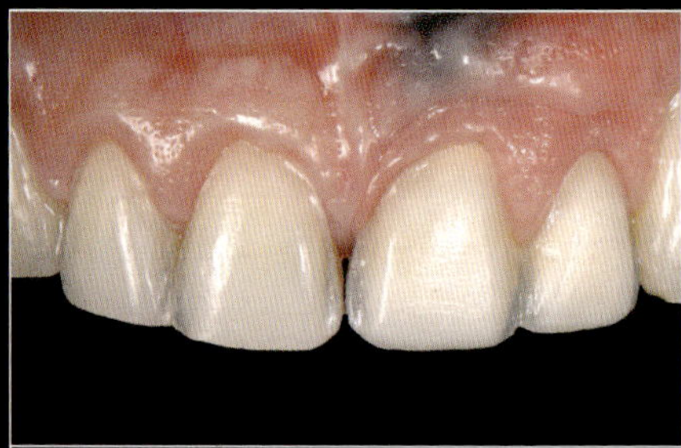

12c

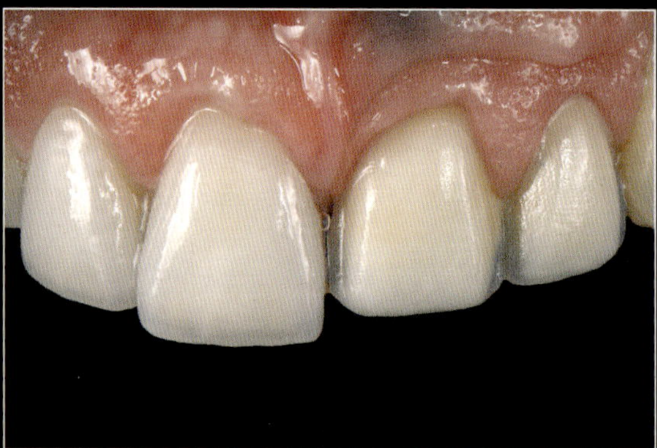

13a

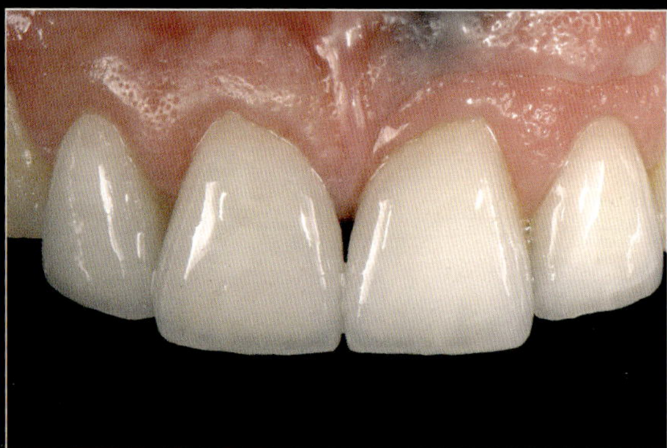

13b

Fig 11 Brightness definition areas.

Fig 12a Abutment placement.

Figs 12b and 12c Dentogingival ceramic structure insertion.

Figs 13a and 13b Final try-in for shape and color assessment.

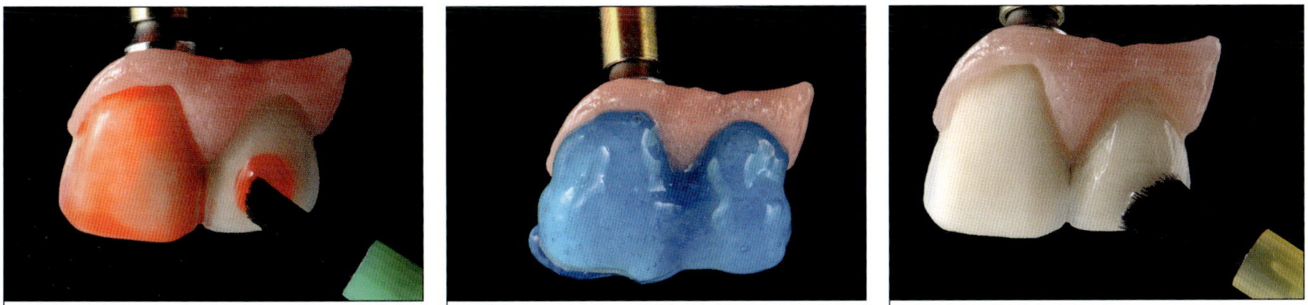

14a 14b 14c

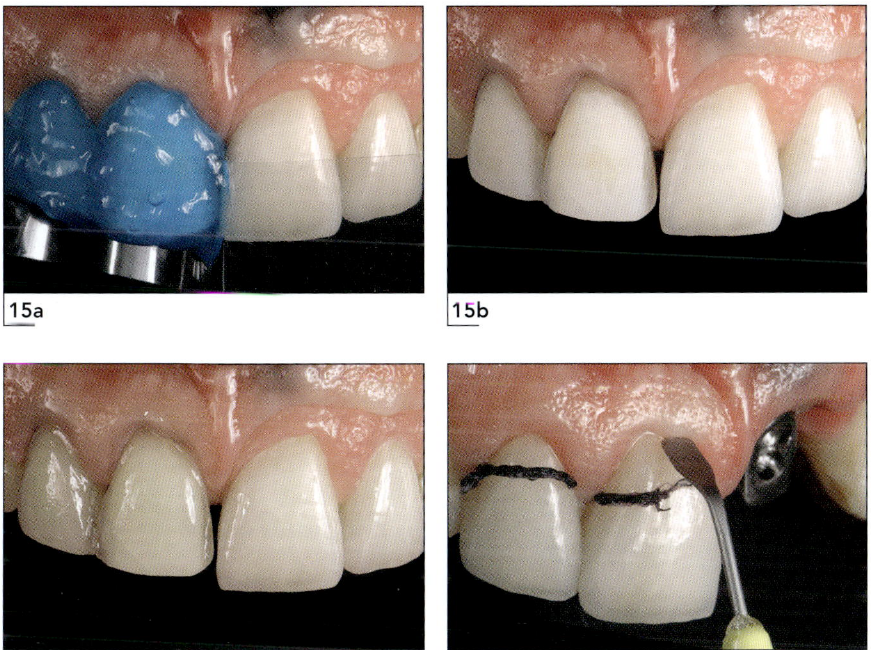

15a 15b 15c 15d

Fig 14a Hydrofluoric acid application.

Fig 14b Phosphoric acid application for residual removal.

Fig 14c Silane application for 60 seconds.

Fig 15a Phosphoric acid application for 30 seconds.

Fig 15b After air jets were used for drying, enamel preparation was completed.

Fig 15c Thin adhesive layer application.

Fig 15d Excess resin cement removed with a scalpel.

Phase V: Final Delivery

The artificial ceramic teeth on the dentogingival prosthesis were etched with 10% hydrofluoric acid for 90 seconds (Fig 14a), followed by rinsing and drying. To remove glass particle debris, 35% phosphoric acid was applied (Fig 14b), followed by rinsing and drying. Silane was subsequently applied for 60 seconds (Fig 14c) and air dried, after which a thin layer of adhesive was placed, air-thinned, and left uncured. Ceramic veneer restorations in lithium disilicate were treated similarly as described above with the exception that the lithium disilicate glass-ceramic was etched for 20 seconds. The veneers were bonded to the dentogingival prosthesis and light polymerized for 60 seconds on each restoration. Polishing was performed using silicone carbide points (Exa-Cerapol, Edenta AG Dental Produkte).

The implant abutment was retained by 35 N torque at the main abutment followed by sealing with Teflon tape. Next the dentogingival prosthesis was placed and the secondary palatal access hole was screw retained at 10 N.

The porcelain veneers were then carefully bonded (Variolink Veneer, Ivoclar Vivadent) to the right central and lateral incisors (Figs 15a to 15c). Retraction cords were removed by using a clinical probe, and the excess resin cement was removed with a scalpel (Fig 15d). After the veneers were bonded to the natural teeth, the dentogingival prosthesis was removed and interproximal space verified for any debris before the final placement of the implant restoration. Occlusal adjustments were made, and maintenance appointments were scheduled (Figs 16 and 17).

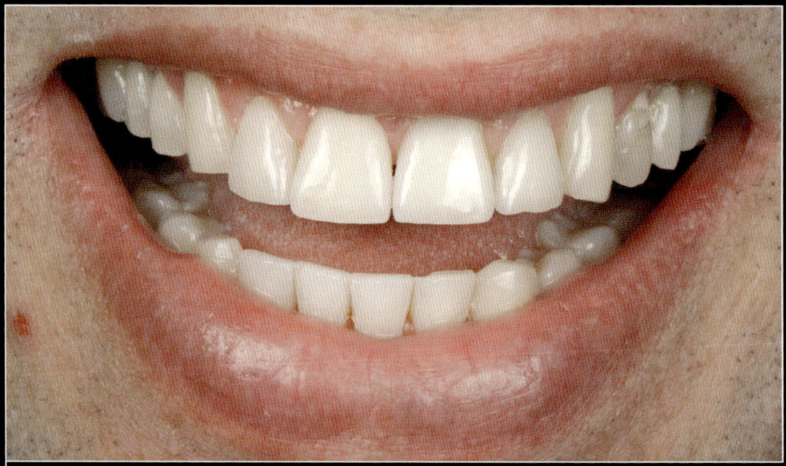

16a

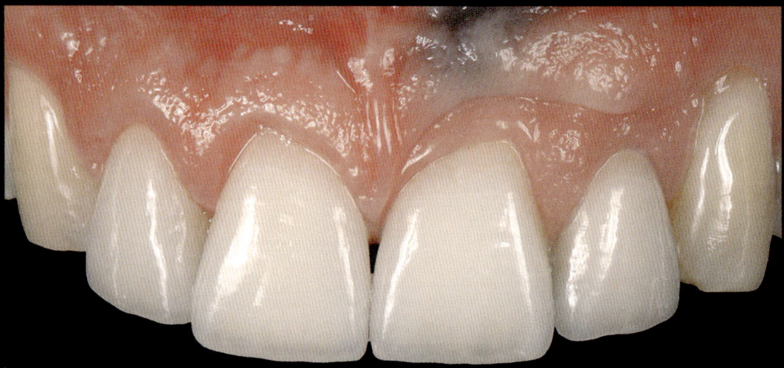

16b

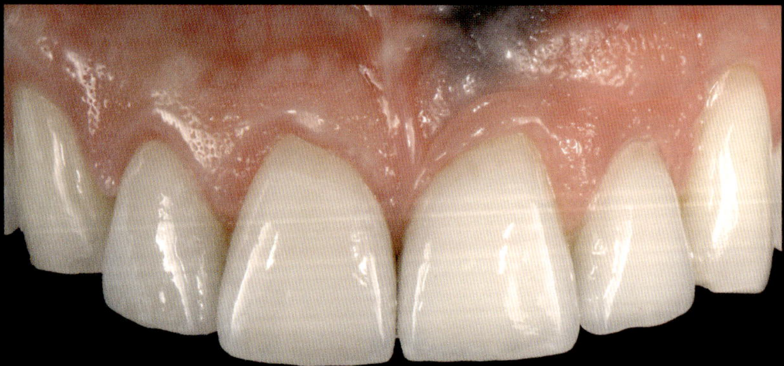

17

Figs 16a and 16b Final aspect after cementing.
Fig 17 Two-year follow-up.

CONCLUSIONS

The procedures described in this article represent a plausible solution for malpositioned implants that can provide patients with satisfactory esthetic, biologic, and functional outcomes with favorable predictability. The dental technician must have the training to be able to observe and report possible eventual side effects of such complex restorations.

REFERENCES

1. Henry PJ, Laney WR, Jemt T, et al. Osseointegrated implants for single-tooth replacement: A prospective 5-year multicenter study. Int J Oral Maxillofac Implants 1996;11:450–455.
2. Dominguez E, Vazquez M, González-Martín O, Alandez J. Mucogingival therapy to treat implant fenestration in the esthetic zone: A case report after 2 year follow up. Int J Esthet Dent 2014;9:40–53.
3. Su H, Gonzalez-Martin O, Weisgold A, Lee E. Considerations of implant abutment and crown contour: Critical contour and subcritical contour. Int J Periodontics Restorative Dent 2010;30: 335–343.
4. Joly JC, Mesquita CPF, Carvalho SR. Flapless aesthetic crown lengthening: A new therapeutic approach. Rev Mex Periodontol 2011;2(3):103–108.
5. Magne P, Belser UC. Novel porcelain laminate preparation approach driven by a diagnostic mock-up. J Esthet Restorative Dent 2004;16:7–16.
6. Gürel G. Predictable, precise, and repeatable tooth preparation for porcelain laminate veneers. Pract Proced Aesthet Dent 2003;15:17–24.

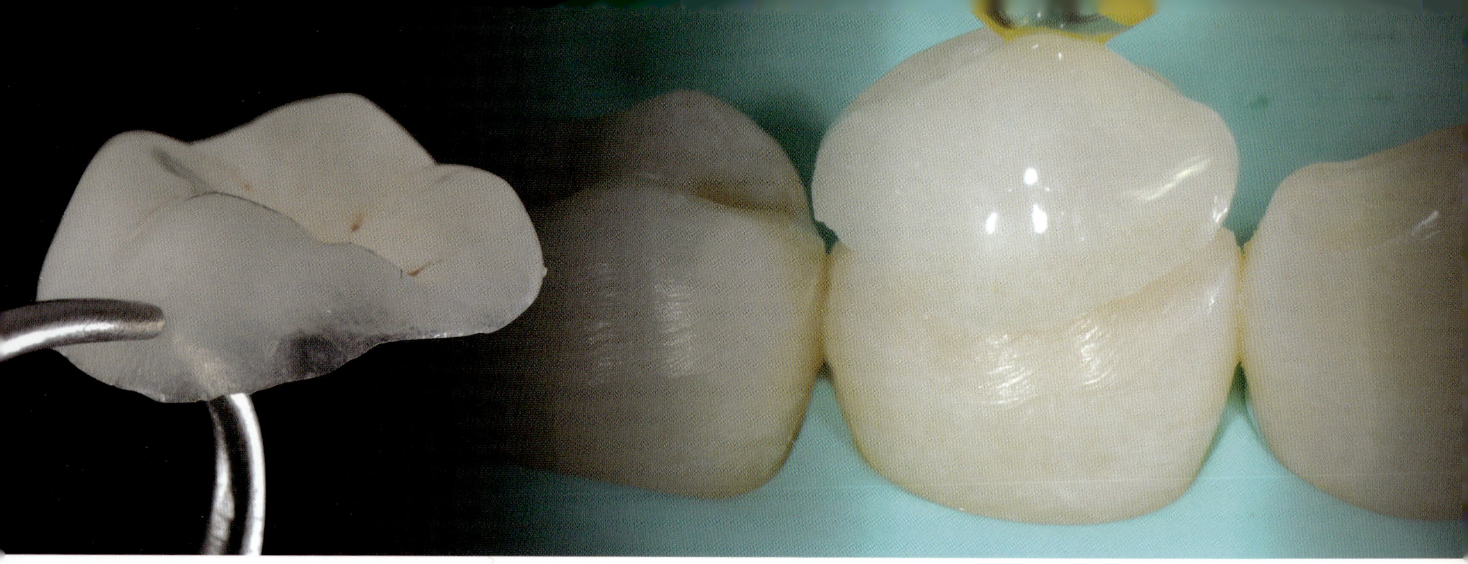

Minimally Invasive Prosthetic Procedures (MIPP): Classification and Clinical Cases

Leonardo Bacherini, DDS[1]
Mauro Fradeani, MD, DDS[2]

The treatment of patients with a worn dentition has become more and more common nowadays due to an increase of this type of pathology, which also affects the younger population.[1] For this reason, the clinician must adopt a precautionary and conservative treatment approach to preserve as much tooth structure as possible while also reestablishing the proper relationship between function, esthetics, and longevity of the restorations.

An understanding of different types of wear, well described in the literature by several authors, is very important for the clinician, because the longevity of the restorations will be greatly influenced by the type of wear.[2] Most authors now agree on the multifactorial nature of dental wear.[3] Often different types of wear are present in a patient with a worn dentition, and diagnosis can be challenging for the clinician who must formulate a proper treatment plan.[4] Among different types of wear, attrition is the most important, because it increases the risk of failure of restorations due to abnormal occlusal loads they will be subjected to. Thus, when treating patients suffering from wear by attrition, the clinician should consider the possibility of eliminating or reducing occlusion as a causative factor.

It is still not yet clear whether occlusion plays a role in the onset and persistence of the parafunction that causes wear. However, the clinician must not ignore which functional parameters to evaluate, so to eventually correct them in order to solve the problem of wear by attrition.[5] A more comprehensive approach to treatment should comply with two of the cornerstones of modern dentistry: minimally invasive treatment and the combination of function and esthetics.[6]

The purpose of a comprehensive treatment plan should be not only to restore the initial volume that was lost as a result of wear but also to determine whether

[1]Private Practice, Sieci-Pontassieve-Firenze, Italy.
[2]Private Practice, Pesaro, Italy.

Correspondence to: Dr Leonardo Bacherini, Studio Odontoiatrico, Piazza Aldo Moro, 7, Sieci-Pontassieve (FI), 50065, Italy.
Email: leonardo@dentsign.it

the stomatognathic system is in a state of equilibrium, knowing that any possible alteration could damage one of its components, such as the temporomandibular joint (TMJ), muscles, or teeth.[5] Most of the time, TMJ disorders, occlusal instability, and tooth wear are due to abnormal muscle activity.

Sometimes, however, in the absence of parafunction, an inadequate dental occlusal relationship can cause excessive wear, especially in the anterior teeth.[5,7] For example, a restricted envelope of function often leads to localized wear only on the anterior teeth, resulting in a loss of anterior guidance, which is a factor considered to be very important for maintaining equilibrium in the stomatognathic system.

The loss of anterior guidance will determine both working and balancing contacts in the posterior area during excursive movements. Balancing contacts are considered responsible for abnormal muscle activity.[8]

Whenever evaluating a patient with a worn dentition limited to the anterior, both esthetic and functional parameters should be considered during the treatment plan formulation. The main goal is the achievement of the correct relationship between the maxillary and mandibular anterior teeth during function so to minimize the possible tooth wear over time. The ratio between overbite and overjet that determines the anterior guidance can be used as a predictor of attrition-type tooth wear of the maxillary and mandibular incisors.[9]

The reestablishment of the equilibrium of the stomatognathic system is the key to slowing the rate of wear by attrition and to subsequently increasing the longevity of the restoration. To accomplish this, functional parameters must be evaluated, managed, and corrected. The centric relation (CR), the vertical dimension of occlusion (VDO), and the relationship between the anterior teeth are to be considered as the most important factors. The proper management of these three parameters will allow the clinician not only to restore esthetics and function, but also to respect the modern concepts of minimal invasiveness while achieving maximum longevity of the final restoration.[10]

FUNCTIONAL PARAMETERS

Centric Relation

CR is the position usually used in more extensive prosthetic cases. When a limited number of restorations are required and no specific occlusal scheme has to be followed, a confirmatory approach can be adopted. In that case, maximal intercuspation (MI), or acquired occlusion, must be used.

Centric relation is considered the most physiological position for articulation and musculature, as well as the most stable position from an orthopedic standpoint.[5] It is the only one considered repeatable during occlusal recording techniques, such as the bilateral manipulation, Lucia jig, leaf gauge, and anterior deprogrammer techniques.[11]

It is advisable to put the mandible in CR (reorganization approach) in the following situations:

- Prosthetic rehabilitation of one or both arches
- Rehabilitation two or more quadrants
- Rehabilitation of the anterior area where dental attrition is evident

In the presence of dental attrition, the clinician can often identify a forward slide of the mandible from CR position to MI position. In this case it is mandatory to follow the reorganization approach so to guide the mandible in CR, thus sometimes resulting in the creation of a space between the maxillary and mandibular anterior teeth. In these cases, the lack of anterior guidance will be compensated by the design of the restoration, which from the buccal side will be extended to the palatal surface (full veneers). This new crown design does not require any tooth preparation on the palatal side, and at the same time it allows the creation of contact with the mandibular incisors. In this full-veneer restoration design, the complete maintenance of the enamel on all tooth surfaces allows very predictable bonding and consequently ensures an exceptional resistance to fracture.[12]

Vertical Dimension of Occlusion

If the prosthetic rehabilitation involves at least one complete arch, the possibility of increasing the distance between the two arches should be carefully considered to minimize the invasiveness of the prosthetic procedure. When new space is created between the two arches, the need for tooth structure removal will be tremendously reduced.[6]

Whenever indicated, permanent increase of the VDO up to 5 mm represents a safe and predictable procedure without detrimental consequences. The associated signs and symptoms that sometimes can occur are self-limiting, with a tendency to resolve within 2 weeks.[13] Therefore, even when there has been no loss of VDO, the strategy of increasing the distance between the two arches has to be evaluated in order to minimize or even eliminate the need to remove dental tissue in a traditional way. Tooth preparation can be minimized, especially on the anterior teeth, where a remarkable space between the two arches can be achieved.

Although many clinicians, not sufficiently trained, persist in thinking that in these extensive rehabilitation cases it is sufficient to use the acquired position (MI), it must be emphasized, as widely suggested by many experts in the field, that increasing the VDO necessarily involves positioning the mandible in CR (reorganization approach).[14–16] This is especially true considering that once the dentist starts to grind the teeth of an entire arch, the MI position (which is a dental-related position) will be automatically lost.[17]

Reduced Ceramic Thickness

Another important consideration of the minimally invasive prosthetic procedure (MIPP)[6] is the possibility of reducing the thickness of the ceramic material. When supported by enamel, minimally invasive lithium disilicate occlusal restorations have a high load-bearing capacity with a very high resistance to fracture.[18] Adhesive bonding of the restorations, mainly in enamel and fabricated with an etchable ceramic material, is likely the key element for the success of the restoration.

MIPP CLASSIFICATIONS

Confirmatory Approach—Maximal Intercuspation

- **MIPP 0:** Additional restorations (anterior, posterior) with no preparation, mainly on enamel
- **MIPP 1:** Partial restorations (anterior veneers, posterior restorations) with minimal tooth preparation, mainly on enamel

Reorganization Approach—Centric Relation and Modified Vertical Dimension

- **MIPP 2A:** Partial restorations (veneers, posterior restorations) with minimal tooth preparation, mainly on enamel in CR
- **MIPP 2B:** Full-coverage veneers (patient with open bite in CR) with minimal tooth preparation, mainly on enamel
- **MIPP 3A:** One arch in CR with VDO alteration and tooth structure preservation, mainly on enamel
- **MIPP 3B:** Two arches in CR with VDO alteration and tooth structure preservation, mainly on enamel

The following two clinical cases demonstrate the advantages of the approach described above.

CASE 1

MIPP 2B

A 30-year-old woman presented to the second author's clinic expressing esthetic concerns about her teeth based on the shortening of her anterior teeth over time (Fig 1). Her request was to restore the appearance of her smile so as to find a new harmony with her face; however, she did not want to be submitted to any invasive treatment.

This case shows that an esthetic issue may also include different functional aspects to be evaluated and corrected.

CASE 1

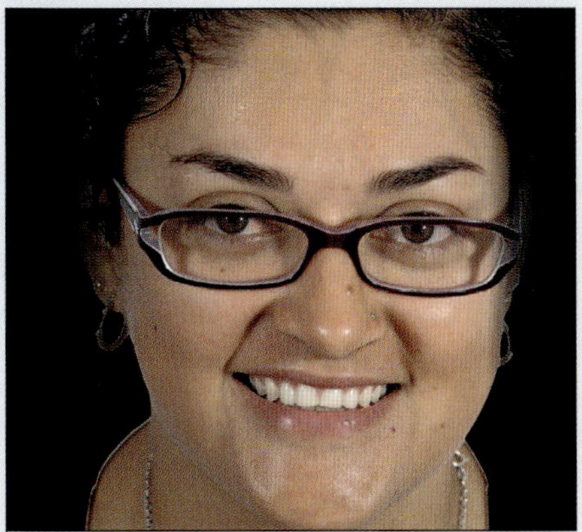

1

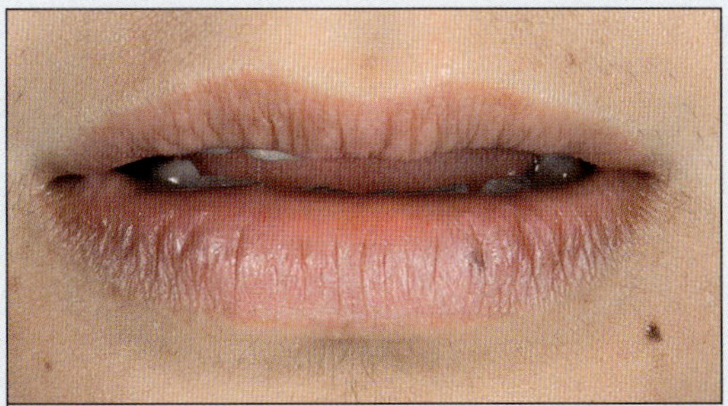

2

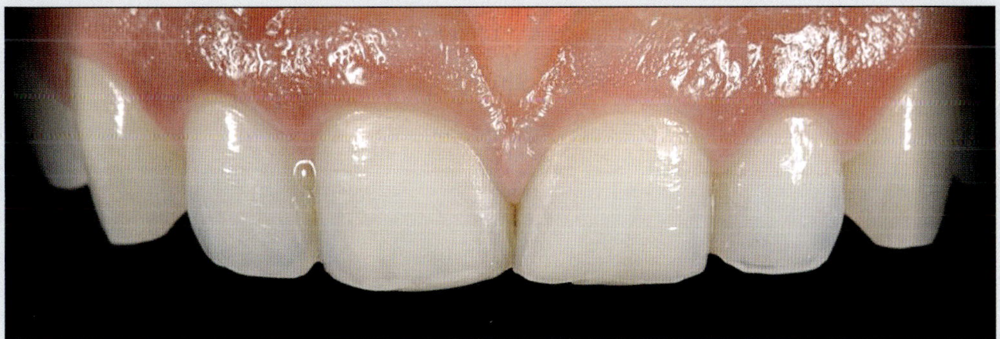

3

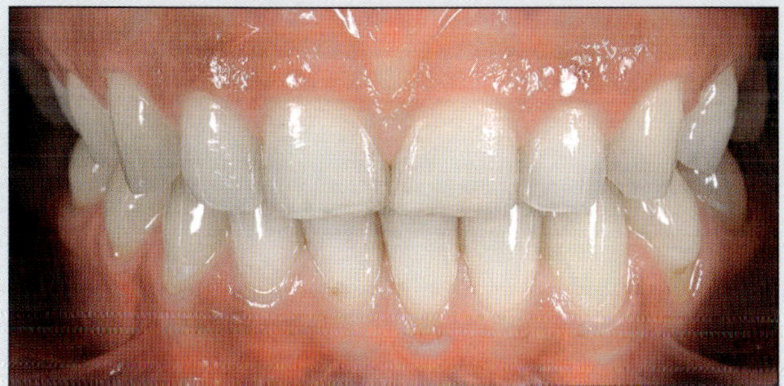

4a

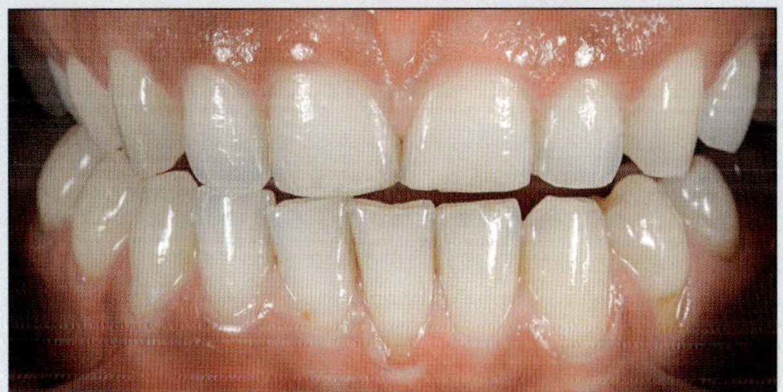

4b

Fig 1 Initial presentation of the patient, who was uncomfortable with the appearance of her smile.
Fig 2 No display of teeth in the resting position.
Fig 3 Frontal view of the maxillary anterior teeth affected by dental attrition.
Figs 4a and 4b Static and dynamic evaluation of the occlusion. Note the lack of anterior guidance due to wear of the anterior teeth.

Esthetic analysis: Main issues

- Lack of proper tooth exposure at rest (Fig 2)
- Flattened incisal edges
- Reduced length of the maxillary incisors (Fig 3)

Functional analysis: Main issues

- Attrition of the anterior teeth
- Reduced overjet and minimal overbite (Fig 4a)
- Lack of anterior guidance (Fig 4b)

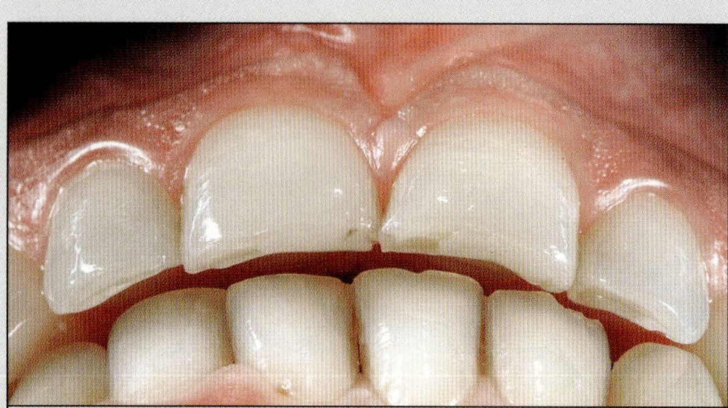

5

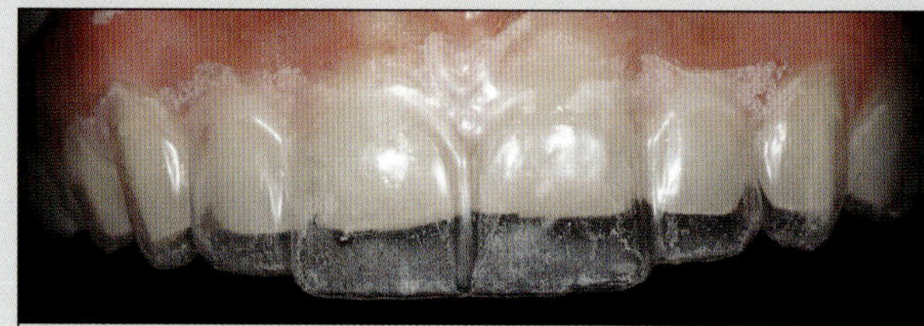

6

Fig 5 After selective grinding to position the mandible in CR, an open bite remained between the maxillary and mandibular anterior teeth.

Fig 6 Direct mock-up performed with a transparent matrix and flowable composite resin.

- Posterior interferences during excursive movements
- Discrepancy between CR and MI

Step 1

- Compilation of the esthetic checklist.[19] The purpose is to analyze the esthetic and functional needs of the patient to highlight the most important parameters to be altered, so as to obtain a complete integration of the restoration.
- Functional evaluation. The aim is to reestablish an ideal incisal length and to recreate an adequate ratio between overbite and overjet with an appropriate anterior guidance.

Step 2

- Alginate impressions of both arches, facebow record, and CR occlusal registration were taken to mount the study casts in a semiadjustable articulator. The purpose was to previsualize the amount of tooth structure to be removed to place the mandible in CR through a selective grinding procedure.
- A simulated selective grinding on the stone casts was performed. The proposed clinical procedure was considered noninvasive. Therefore, together with the patient, it was decided to follow the same procedure in the mouth.

Step 3

- Selective grinding procedure in the patient's mouth. An open space was formed on the anterior area of the mouth after the completion of the procedure, with the mandible in CR position (Fig 5).

Step 4

- New alginate impressions and a new facebow registration were taken. The laboratory chart[20] was transmitted to the dental technician for fabrication of the wax-up.

Step 5

- A diagnostic wax-up of the anterior maxillary and mandibular teeth was completed, and a silicone index was fabricated. An intraoral mock-up of the proposed anterior restorations was made with a transparent matrix and flowable composite resin (Fig 6), and modifications were made to improve the esthetics of the teeth.
- An impression of the mock-up was taken to guide the technician in fabricating the definitive restorations.

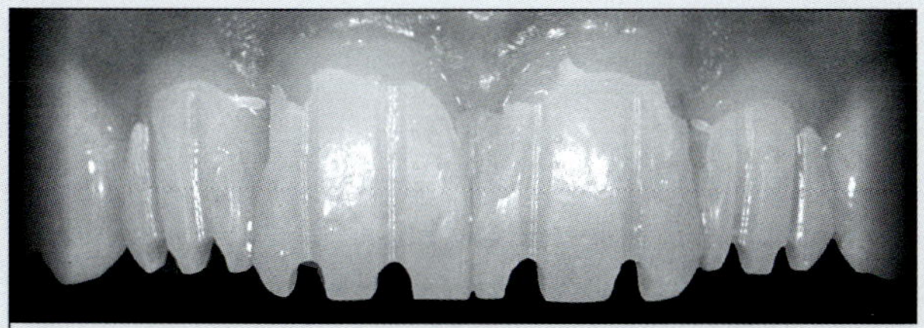
7

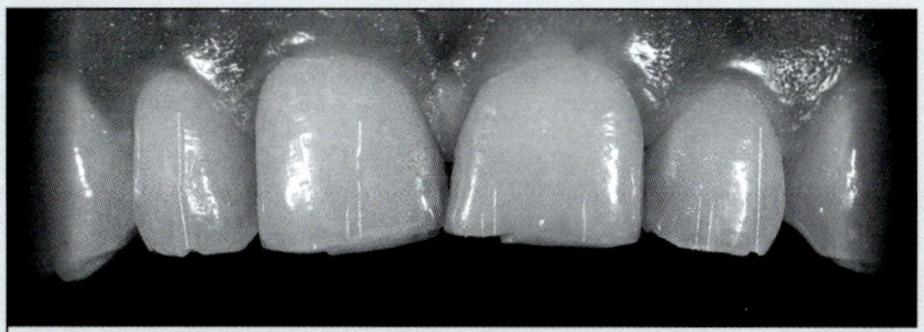
8

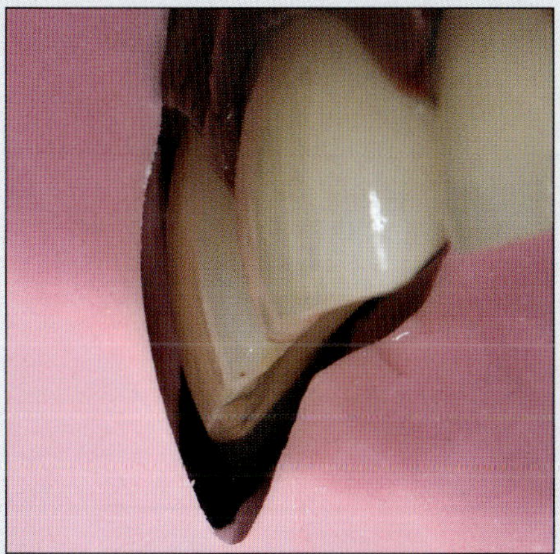
9

Fig 7 The mock-up represents the preview of the final volume of the restorations. Tooth preparation was performed through the mock-up to precisely calibrate the tooth reduction.

Fig 8 After removing the mock-up, it is possible to notice that the calibrated reduction performed to create enough space for the restorative material is only slightly visible on the teeth.

Fig 9 A silicone index made from the wax-up was used to check the amount of space available for the full-veneer restorations.

Figs 10a and 10b Definitive tooth preparations of the four maxillary anterior teeth. Note the amount of enamel still present on the entire surface. Dentin was present only on the incisal margins due to tooth wear. The palatal surface remained completely untouched.

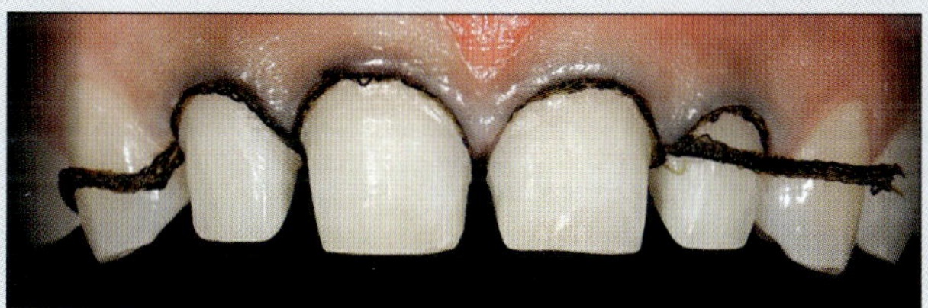
10a

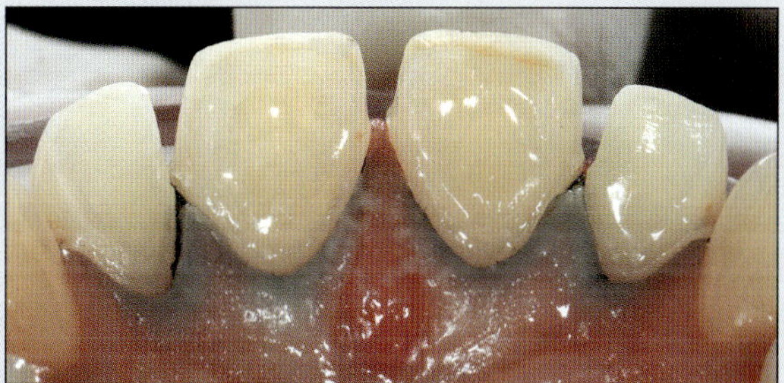
10b

Step 6

- Tooth preparation, final impressions, and provisional restorations. A calibrated tooth preparation was performed through the composite resin mock-up (Figs 7 and 8). Because of the planned volume increase in the labial and incisal areas (Fig 9), a sufficient amount of space was gained for the restorative material. On the palatal tooth surfaces, because of the amount of space gained by placing the mandible in CR, no grinding procedure was necessary to create full-coverage restorations (full veneers). With this minimally invasive technique, the surfaces of the final preparations were completely covered by enamel, except for a small portion of dentin already present in the incisal area due to the original wear. To obtain a better integration with the surrounding tissue, a very light chamfer was chosen for the finish line configuration (Fig 10).
- A final impression was taken with polyvinyl siloxane material using a one-step double-mix technique. The shell of the provisional restorations was fabricated at the new VDO with the modified indirect technique (MIT),[20] then relined and cemented temporarily with dual-curing resin-based cement (Telio CS Link, Ivoclar Vivadent).

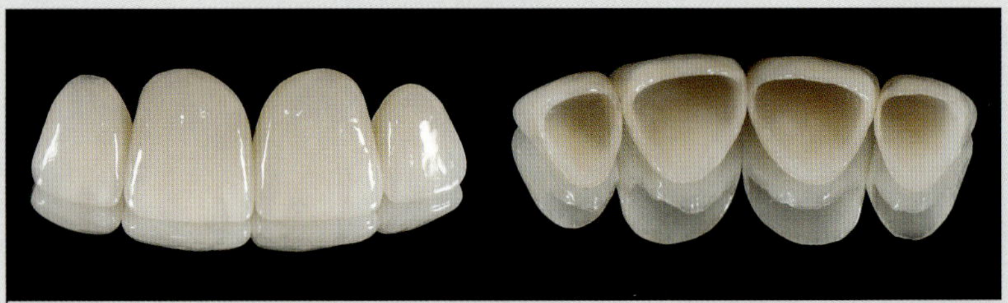
11a

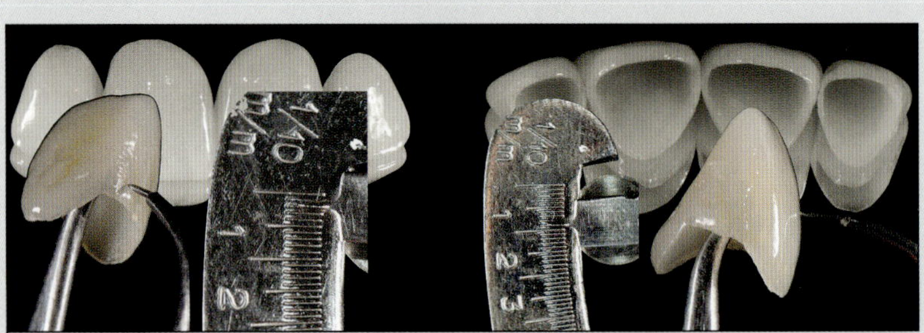

11b

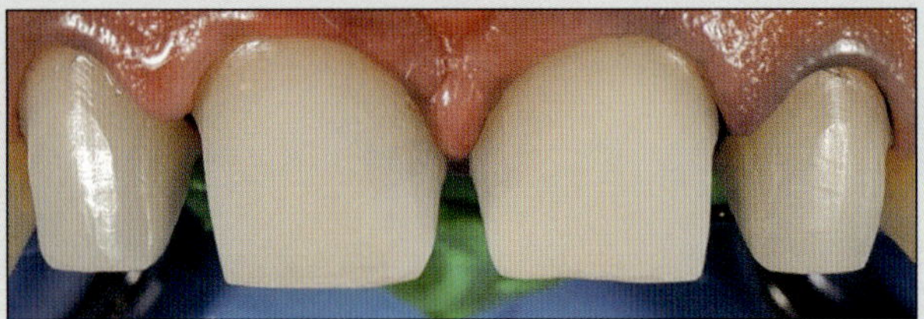
12a

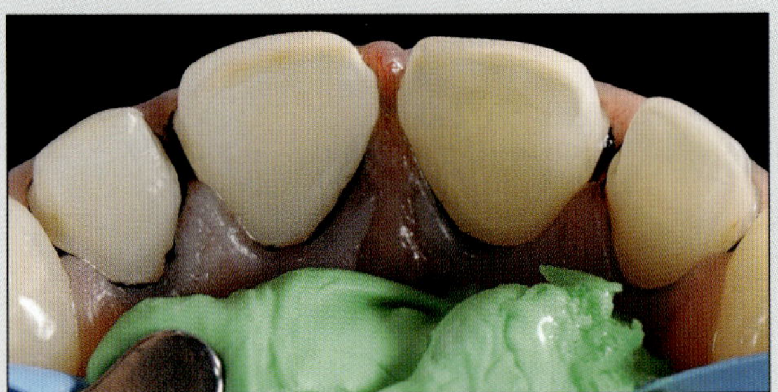
12b

Figs 11a and 11b Full veneers ready for cementation.
Figs 12a and 12b After the etching procedure, it is possible to better appreciate the amount of enamel present.

Step 7

- Try-in and cementation. Four maxillary bilayered lithium disilicate full veneers were fabricated in the laboratory with a reduced thickness (0.2 to 0.8 mm) (Fig 11).
- Cementation followed a precise protocol. Retraction cords were placed in the sulcus of every prepared tooth to minimize the humidity from the crevicular fluid and to act as a barrier for the penetration of the resin cement to the base of the sulcus. In addition, rubber dam was used to isolate the anterior area from saliva and humidity. The inner surfaces of the restorations were etched with 4.5% hydrofluoric acid (Ivoclar Vivadent) for 20 seconds, thoroughly rinsed with water, and placed in an ultrasonic bath with distilled water for 3 minutes. After thorough air drying, the intaglio surface was silanized (Monobond-S, Ivoclar Vivadent) and dried for 60 seconds.
- Tooth preparations were cleaned with pumice and rubber burs (Opticlean, Kerr), etched for 30 seconds on enamel and 15 seconds on dentin with 37.5% phosphoric acid (Ultra-Etch, Ultradent Products), rinsed, and dried (Fig 12). Both fitting surfaces, restorations and teeth, were coated with the adhesive system (OptiBond FL, Kerr), and because of the reduced thickness of the ceramic restorations, a light-curing composite resin cement (Variolink Veneer, Ivoclar Vivadent) was selected to lute the restorations.

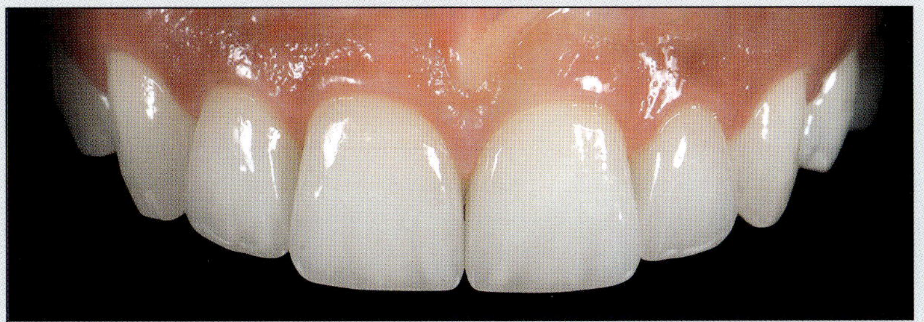

13

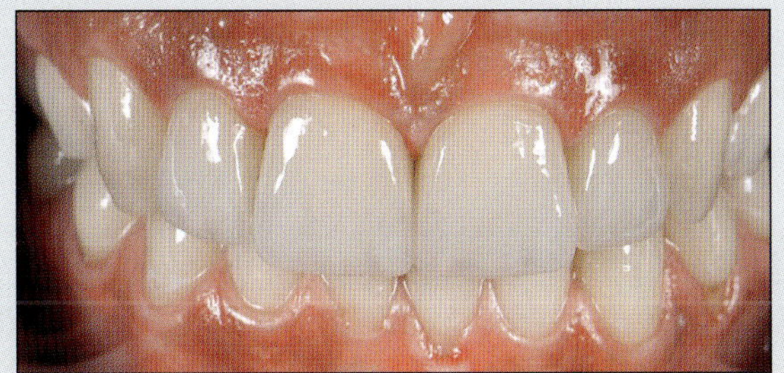

14a

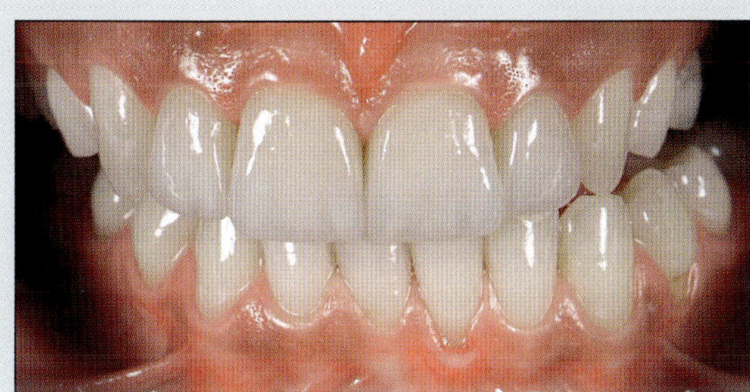

14b

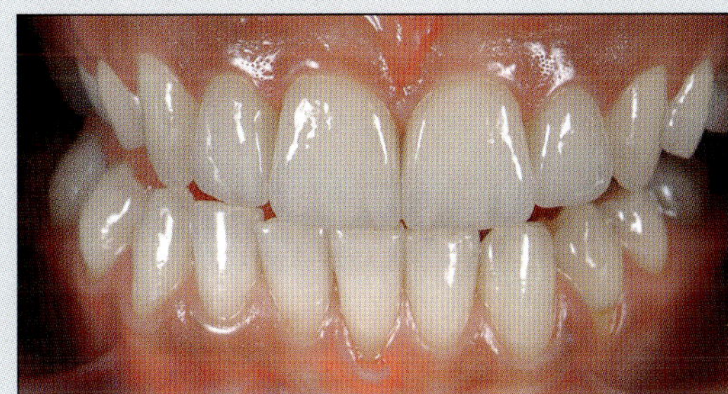

14c

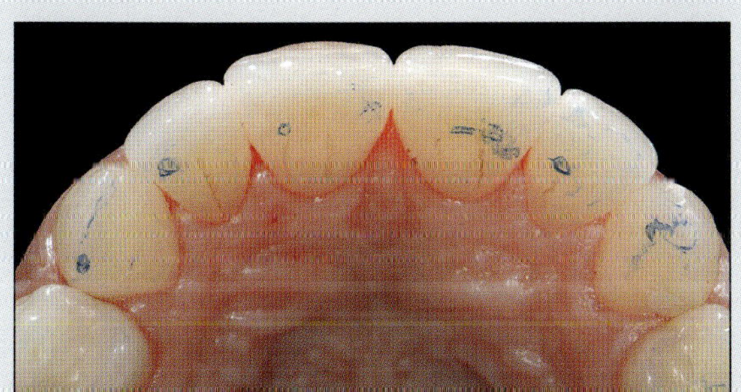

15

Fig 13 Definitive maxillary anterior restorations after cementation.

Figs 14a to 14c Static and dynamic final evaluation of the treatment. Note the new anterior guidance (*b and c*).

Fig 15 Occlusal view of the full veneers, where it is possible to appreciate the occlusal contacts obtained with full veneers.

Step 8

- Fine-tuning of the occlusal adjustment and final polishing were completed. Posttreatment photographs were taken immediately (Figs 13 to 19) and after 6 years (Figs 20 and 21).

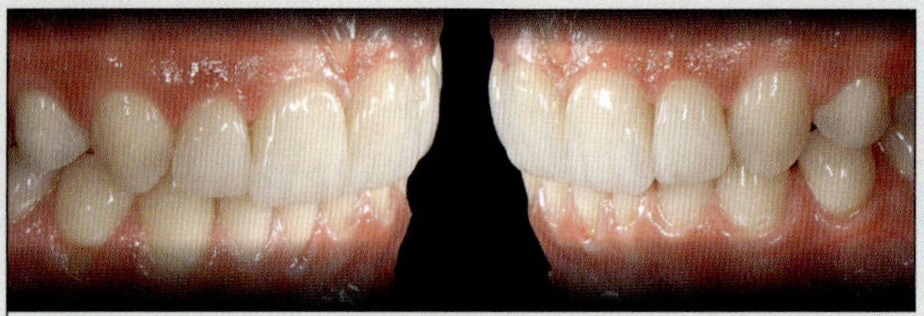

16

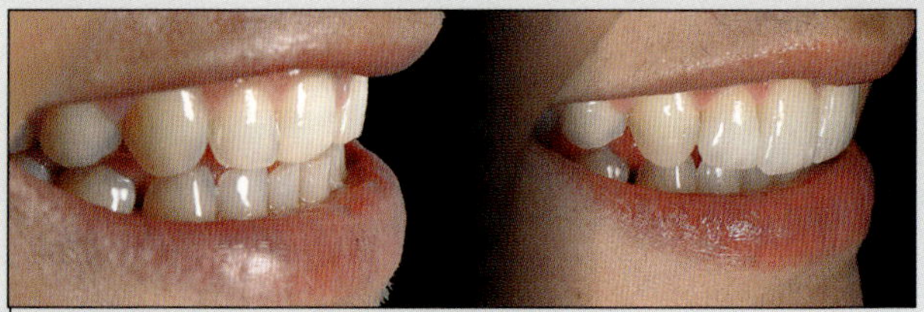

17

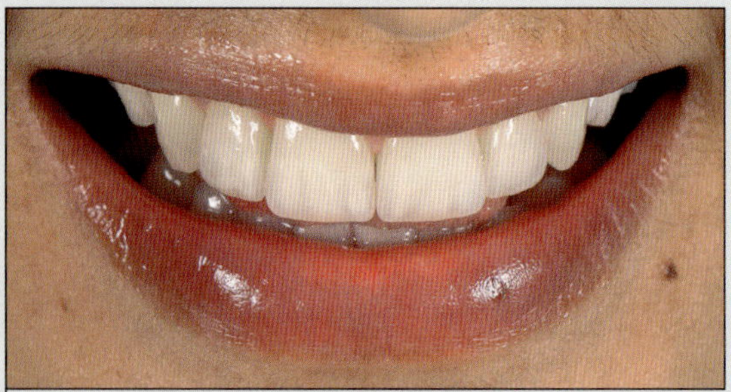

18

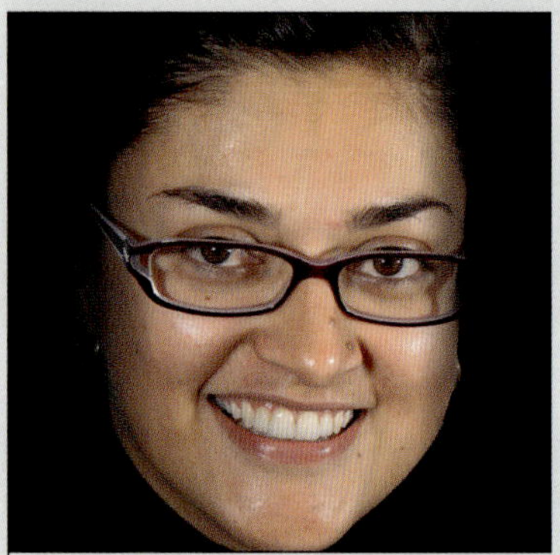

19

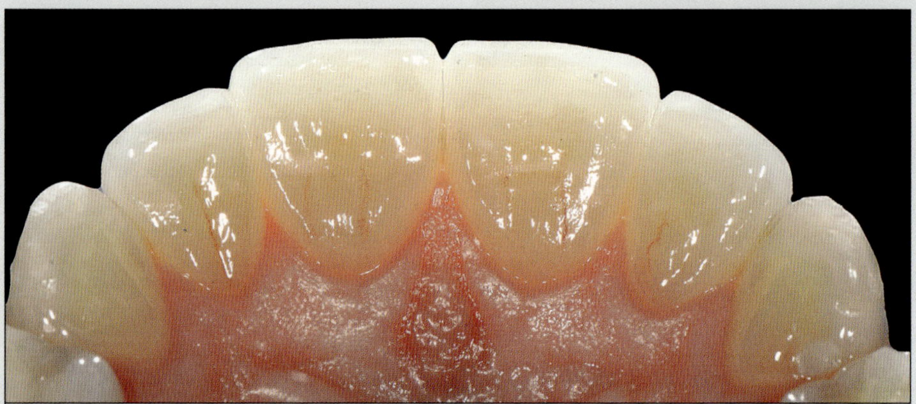

20

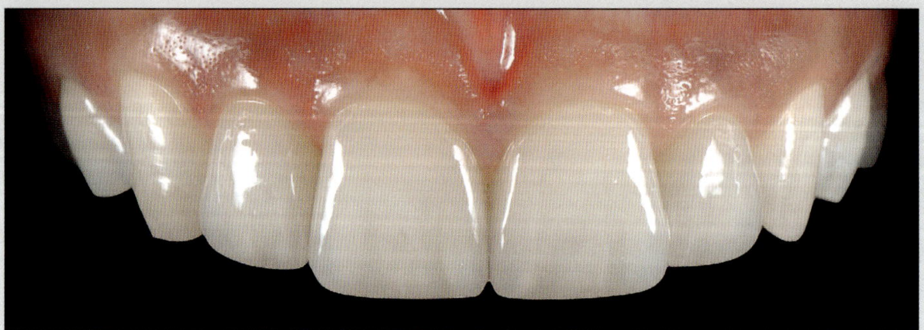

21

Fig 16 Lateral view of the esthetic and functional rehabilitation.
Fig 17 Lateral view of the change in the dentolabial relationship: *(left)* before and *(right)* after.
Fig 18 The new smile of the patient.
Fig 19 Final appearance of the patient with her new smile in harmony with the face.
Fig 20 Occlusal view of the restorations after 6 years in service. No signs of wear present.
Fig 21 Frontal view after 6 years.

CASE 2

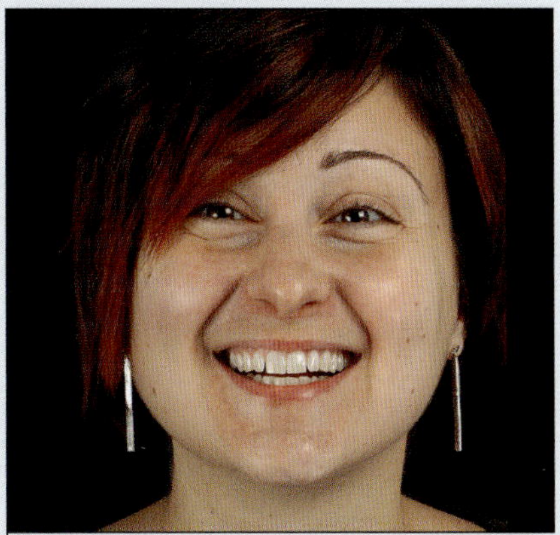

Fig 22 Initial presentation: Patient is uncomfortable with the appearance of her teeth.

Fig 23 Photographic progression of the smile for the facial analysis.

Fig 24 Photographic progression of the smile is useful for completing the dentolabial analysis.

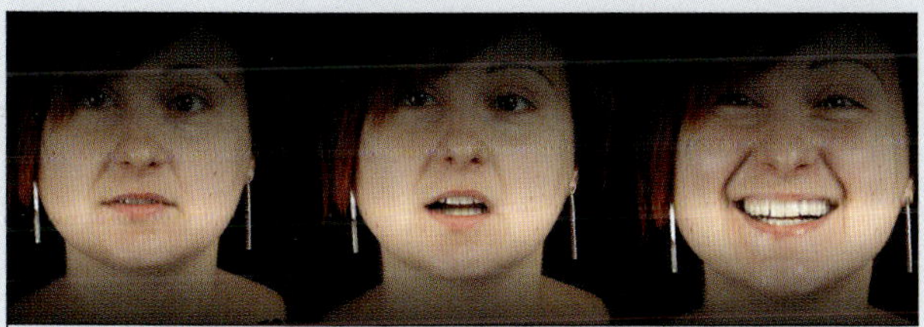

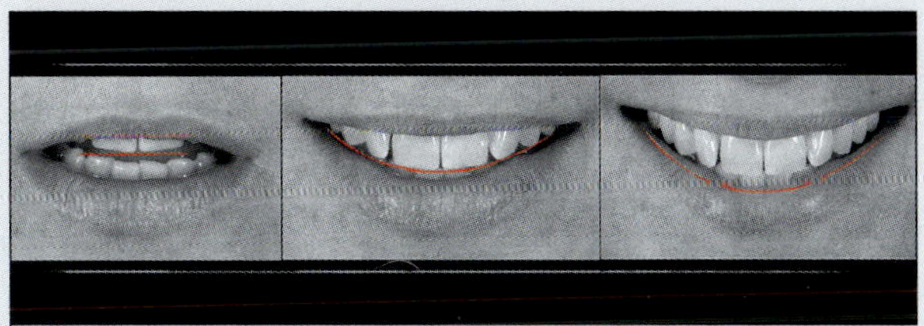

CASE 2

MIPP 3B

A 38-year-old woman presented to the first author's clinic, stating that she was unhappy with the appearance of her teeth (Fig 22). She requested a prosthetic treatment to improve her smile, and she emphasized her desire to have highly esthetic restorations without any invasive treatment. Particularly, she was complaining about the diastemata between her maxillary anterior teeth, and she had noticed a progressive wear of some of the incisors over time.

Esthetic analysis: Main issues

- Presence of diastemata between some maxillary anterior teeth
- Imperfect dental arrangement with rotation of some teeth
- Unsatisfactory tooth shape in the maxillary anterior area

Functional analysis: Main issues

- Attrition of the anterior teeth
- Nonphysiologic wear for the patient's young age
- Reduced overjet and minimal overbite (restricted envelope of function)
- Lack of anterior guidance
- Posterior interferences during excursive movements
- Discrepancy between CR and MI
- Muscle tenderness

Step 1

- Compilation of the esthetic checklist.[19] The purpose is to analyze the esthetic and functional parameters of the patient to highlight the most important ones to be altered, so as to obtain a complete integration of the restoration (Figs 23 to 28).
- Functional evaluation. The aim is to reestablish an ideal incisal length and to recreate an adequate ratio between overbite and overjet with an appropriate anterior guidance (Figs 29 to 32).

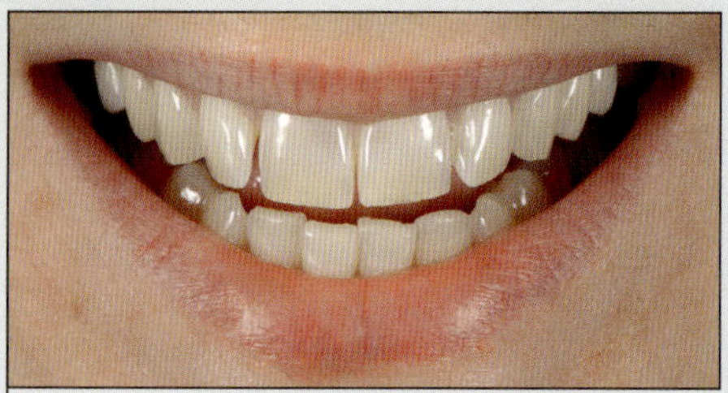
25a

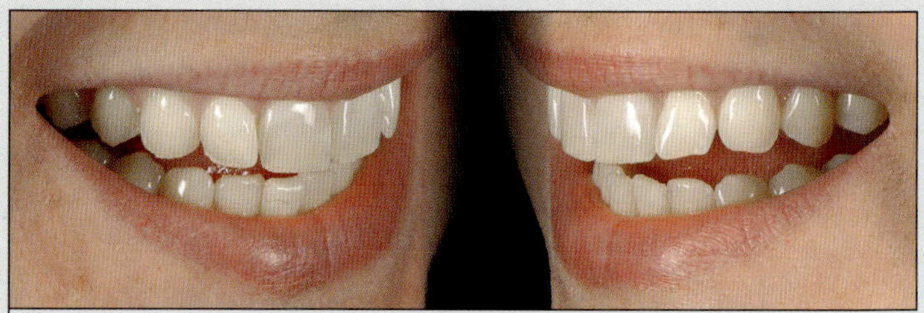
25b

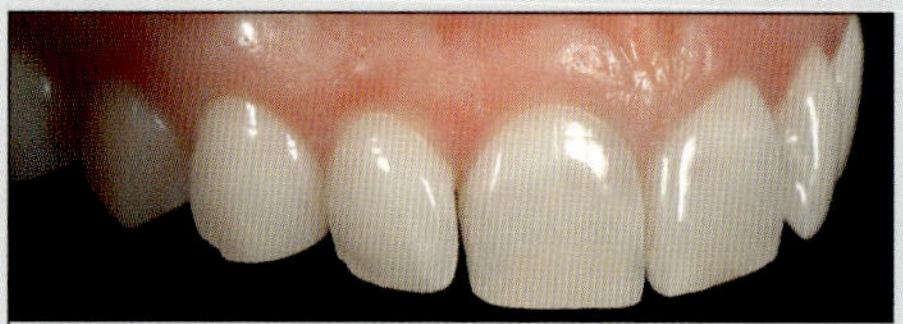
26a

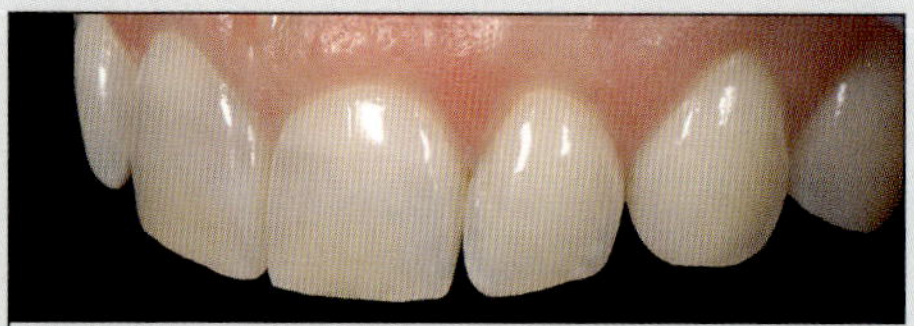
26b

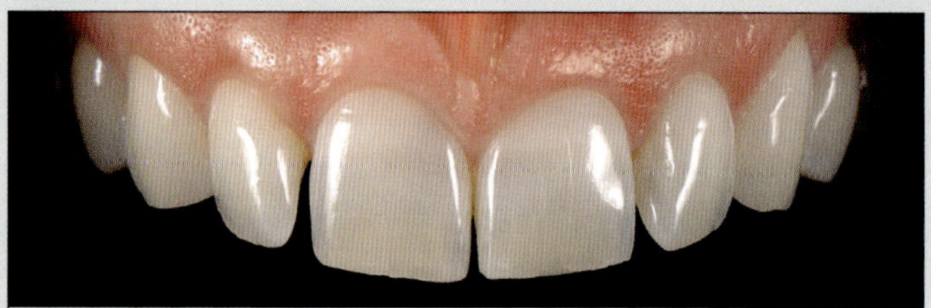
26c

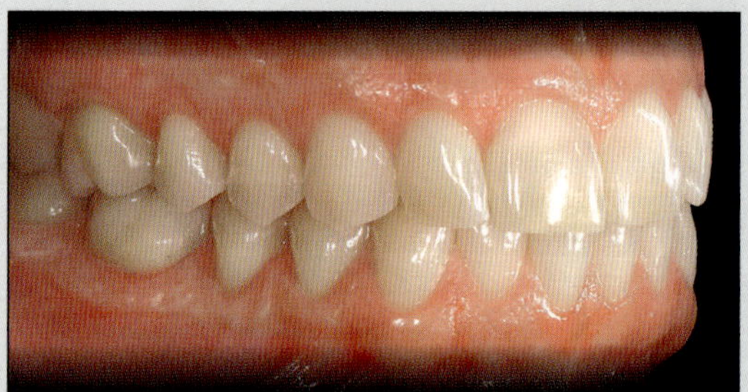
27a

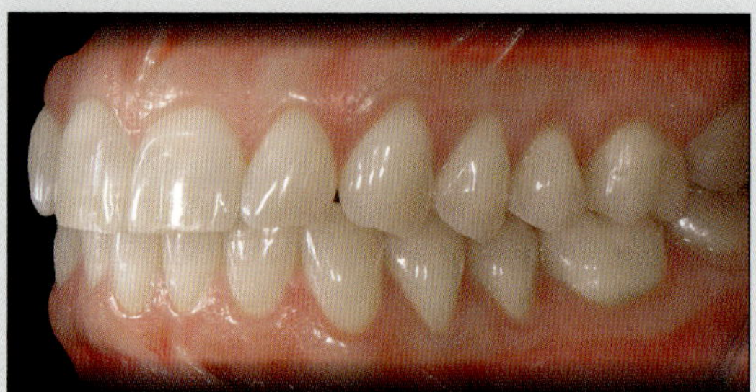
27b

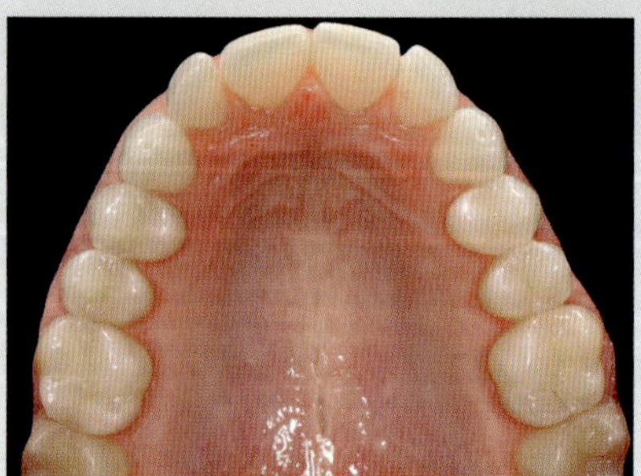
28a

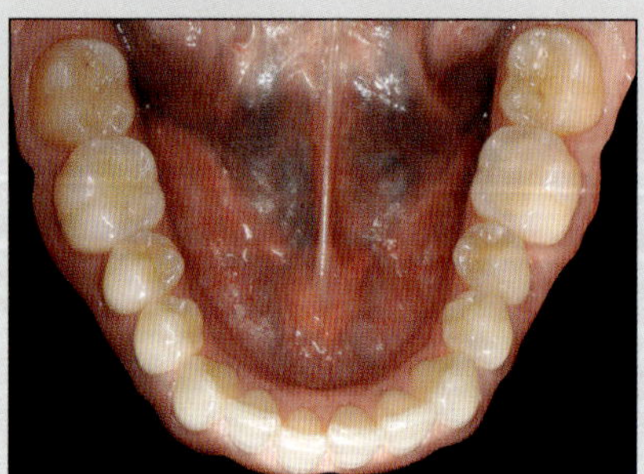
28b

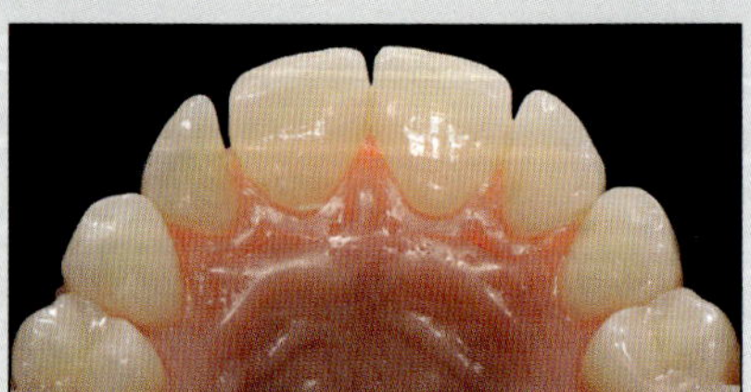
28c

Figs 25a and 25b Details of the dentolabial analysis.

Figs 26a to 26c View of the maxillary anterior teeth, where it is possible to appreciate an unpleasant tooth arrangement with some diastemata and wear.

Figs 27a and 27b Lateral views of the occlusion.

Figs 28a to 28c Occlusal view of maxillary and mandibular arches. Note the wear of the incisal margin considered nonphysiologic for the age of the patient.

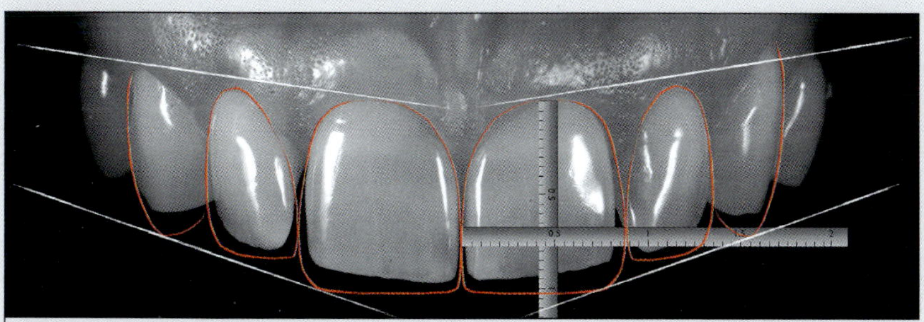

29

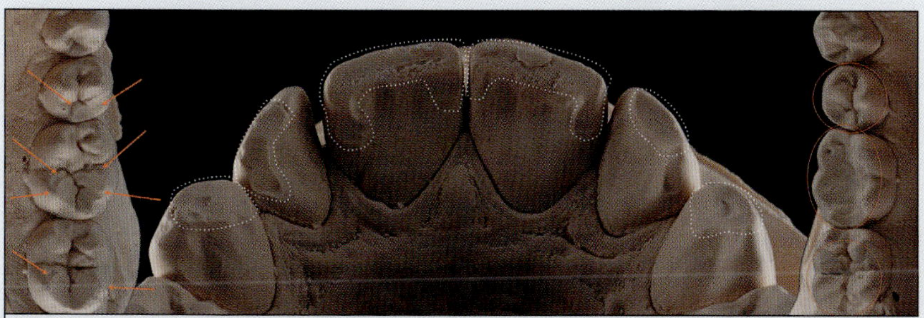

30

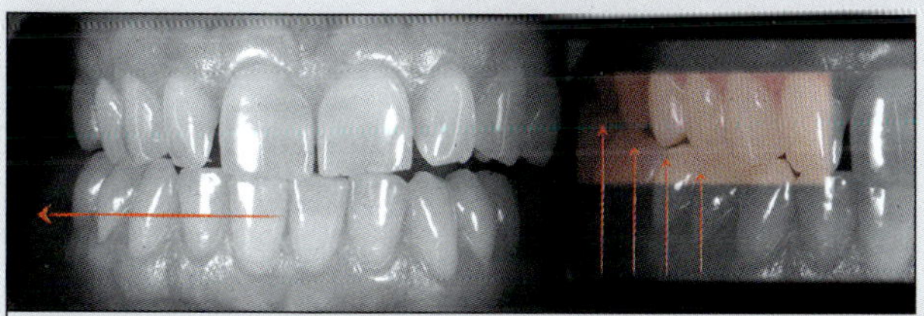

31a

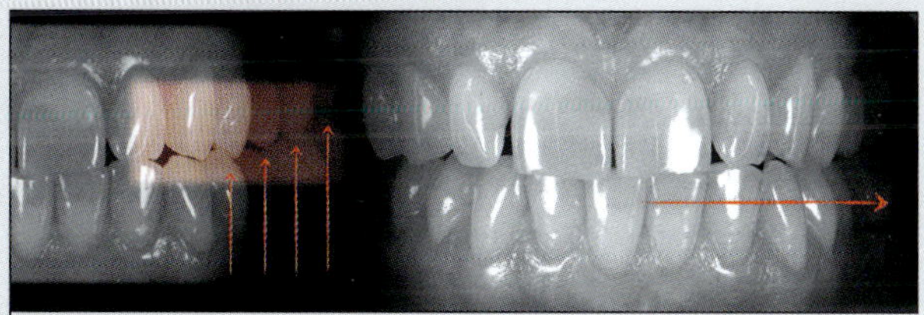

31b

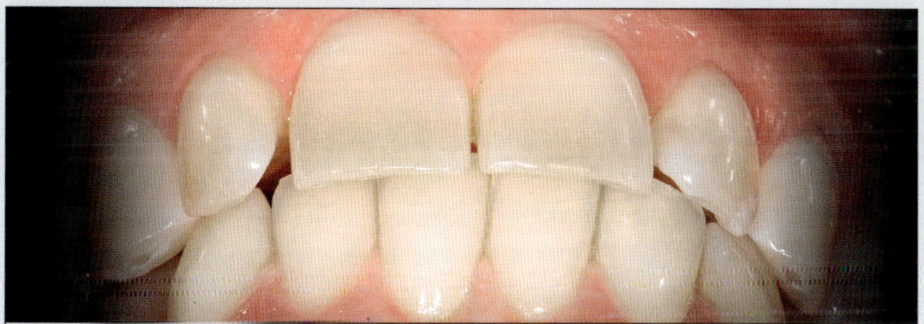

32

Fig 29 Complete dental analysis with the proposed new ideal dental composition.

Fig 30 Analysis of wear facets was important to analyze the type of wear and to formulate a proper treatment plan. Note the large amount of working and balancing contacts.

Figs 31a and 31b Functional analysis demonstrates the absence of canine guidance with many posterior contacts during excursive movement.

Fig 32 Relationship between anterior teeth. Note the reduced amount of overbite and overjet.

Step 2

- Alginate impression, facebow record, and CR record (Fig 33). The aim of this step, as in Case 1, was to evaluate if, with a selective grinding procedure, it would be possible to reestablish a new anterior relationship and consequently to perform a restorative treatment that respected the esthetic and functional parameters.
- The specific aim was to achieve an adequate anterior dental composition, an ideal overbite-overjet relationship, and a shallower anterior guidance.

Step 3

- Selective grinding on the stone casts. As this procedure was considered very invasive and not useful in

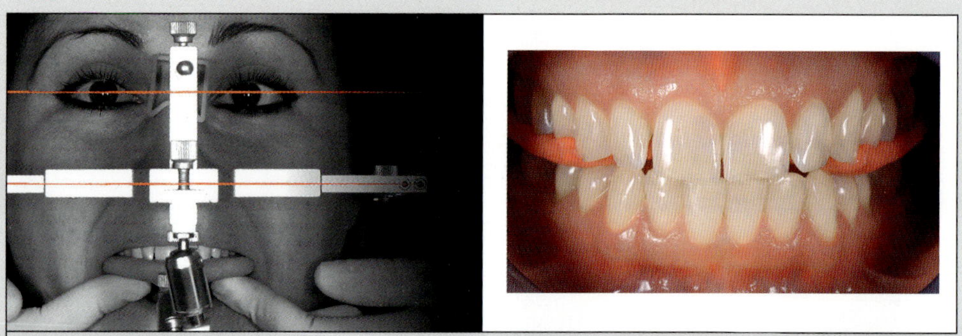

33

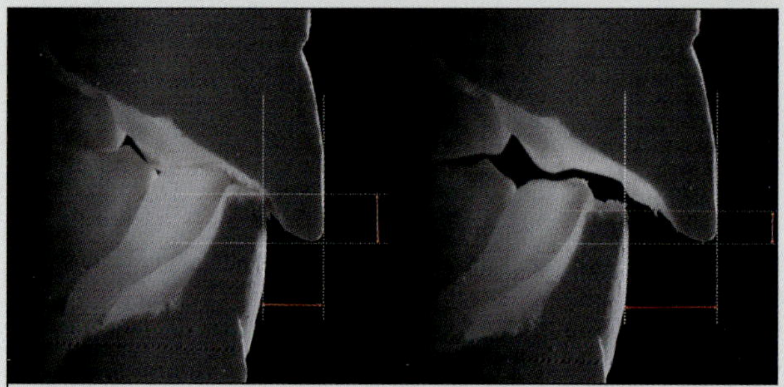

34

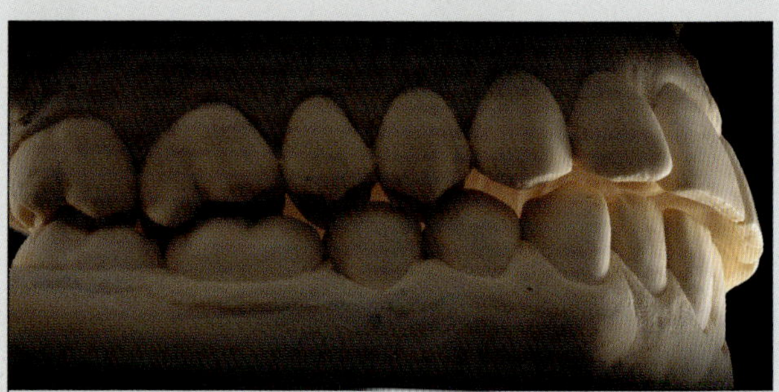

35

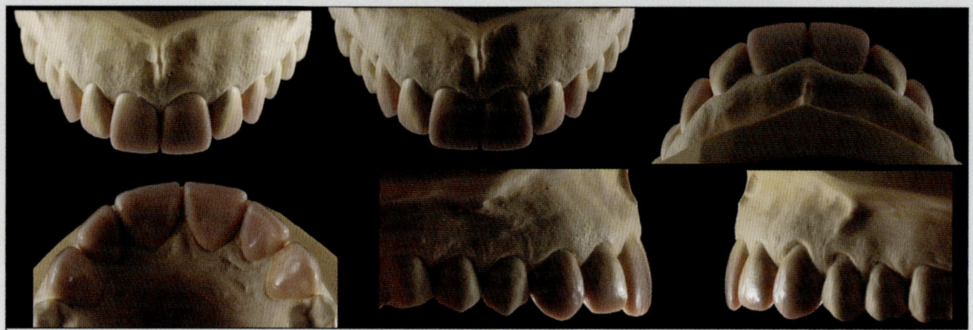

36

Fig 33 Initial facebow and CR registration were taken to make the wax-up of the maxillary anterior teeth. After a complete esthetic and functional analysis, all data were sent to the lab to fabricate the diagnostic wax-up.

Fig 34 A new relationship is created between the anterior teeth after increasing the VDO in CR.

Fig 35 The space between the two arches available for the restorative material is shown. The new relationship between the anterior teeth will allow the development of a new anterior guidance.

Fig 36 Wax-up of the maxillary anterior teeth to optimize both esthetic and functional parameters.

reestablishing a proper anterior relationship, it was decided, in accordance with the patient, not to replicate it in the mouth.

Step 4

- Formulation of an alternative treatment plan. Orthodontic treatment was proposed but not accepted by the patient.
- After placing the stone casts in the articulator, it was decided to increase the VDO in CR position in order to reestablish more adequate functional and esthetic parameters with a minimally invasive procedure (Figs 34 and 35).
- The diagnostic wax-up clearly confirmed the possibility of recreating a new anterior relationship with an ideal overbite-overjet ratio, a pleasant dental composition, and a shallow anterior guidance (Fig 36).

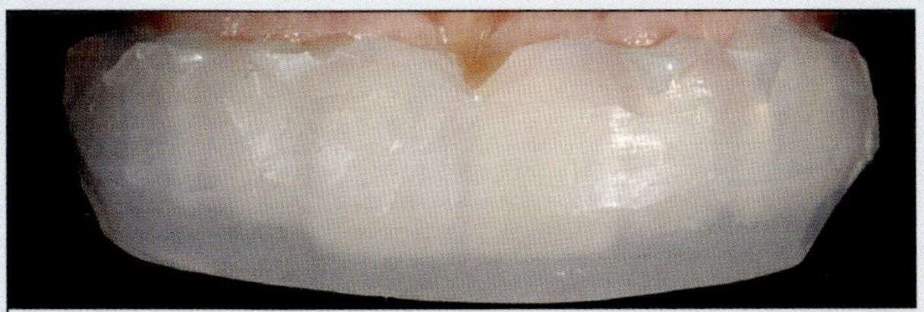

37a

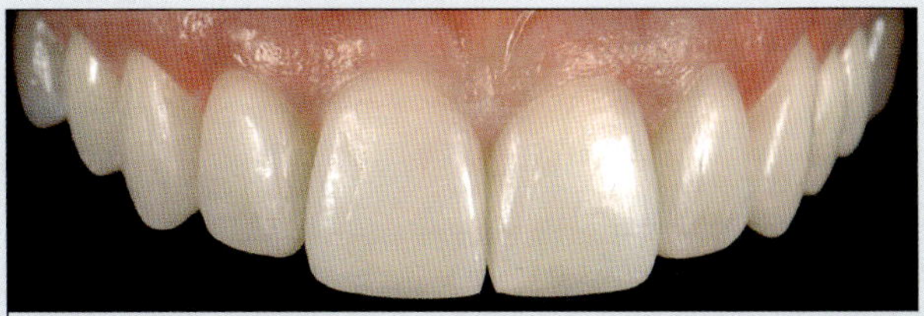

37b

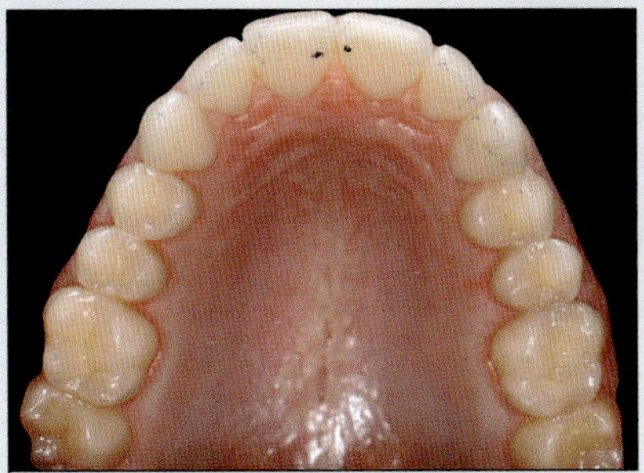

38a

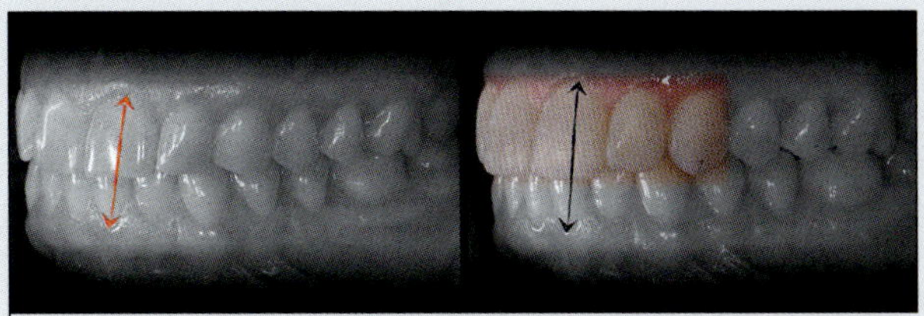

38b

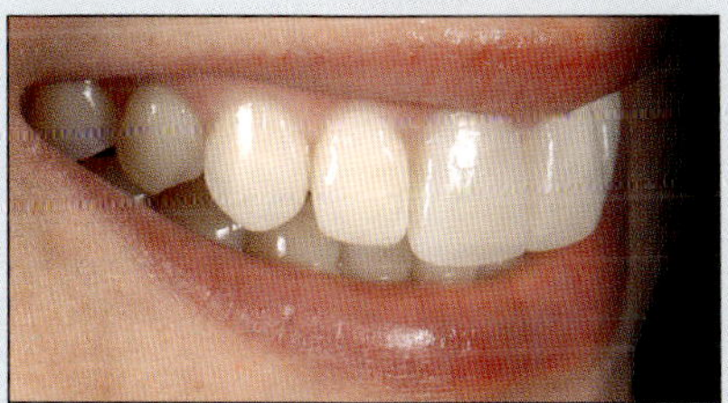

39a

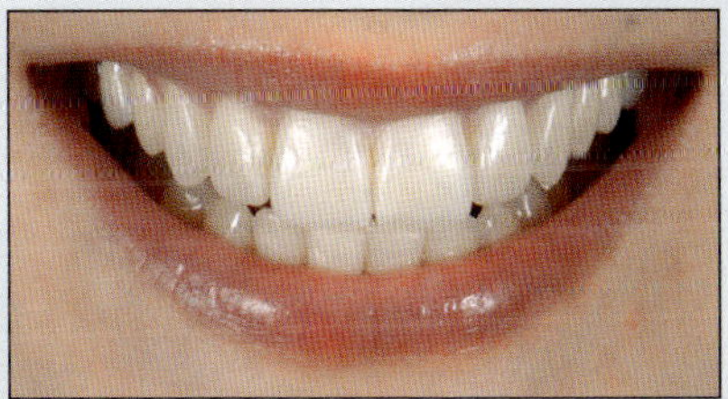

39b

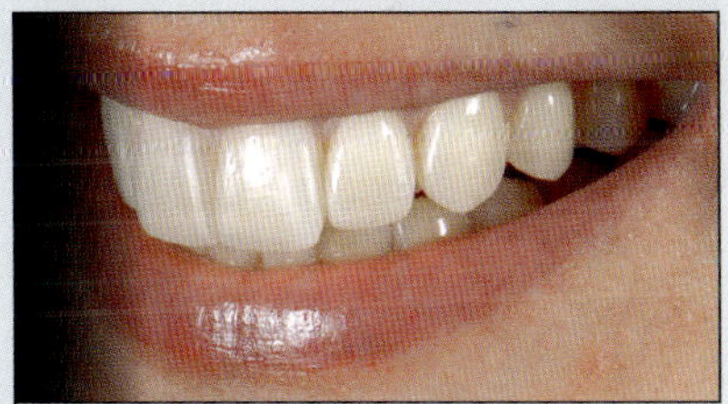

39c

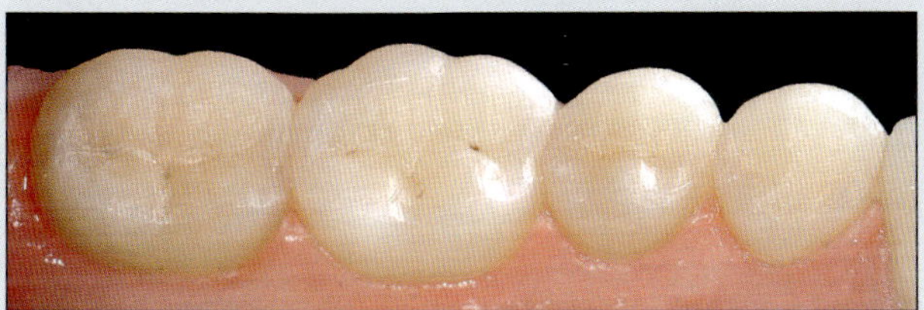

40a

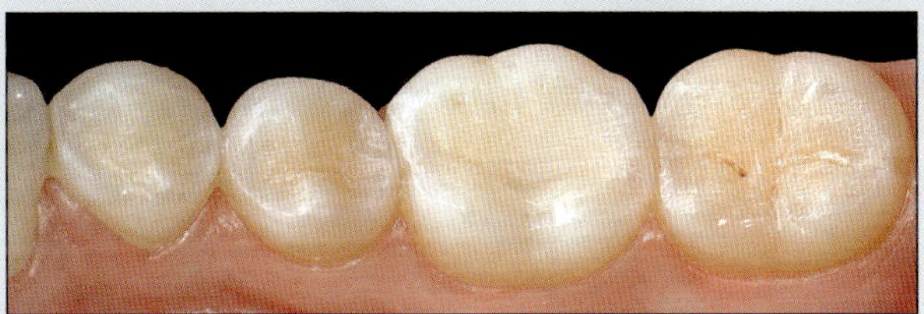

40b

Figs 37a and 37b Indirect mock-up fabricated with a transparent matrix and flowable composite resin.

Figs 38a and 38b The mock-up is adjusted in the patient's mouth to allow the clinician to precisely define the new VDO and the new relationship between the two arches.

Figs 39a to 39c A new dentolabial relationship with the mock-up on the maxillary anterior teeth was tested.

Figs 40a and 40b Preparation design in the occlusal surfaces of the mandibular posterior teeth was performed, avoiding interproximal area involvement with the aim of maintaining as much enamel as possible.

Step 5

- Mock-up of the anterior teeth (Figs 37 and 38). The aim of this step was to determine—and to adjust directly in the patient's mouth—the anterior component of the occlusion (anterior guidance). Moreover, an esthetic evaluation of the new anterior dental composition was done, checking the relationship between anterior teeth, face, and lips (Fig 39). With the mock-up in situ to serve as a jig, a new facebow record and CR registration were taken, thus maintaining the proposed VDO.

Step 6

- With the anterior mock-up in situ, a minimal preparation of the posterior mandibular teeth was performed (Fig 40). As the VDO increase provided 0.5 mm of additional space at the level of the second

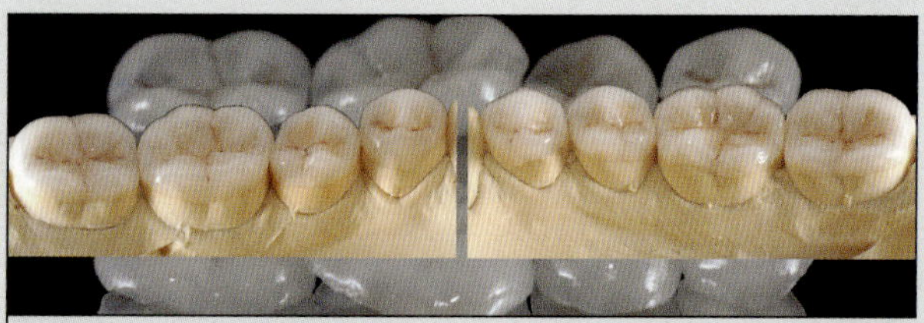

41a

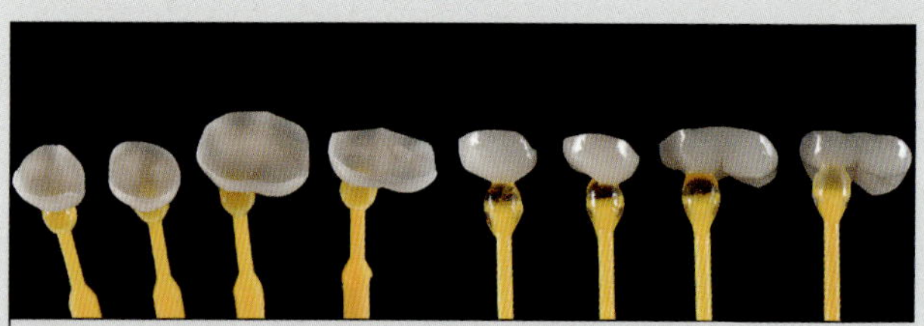

41b

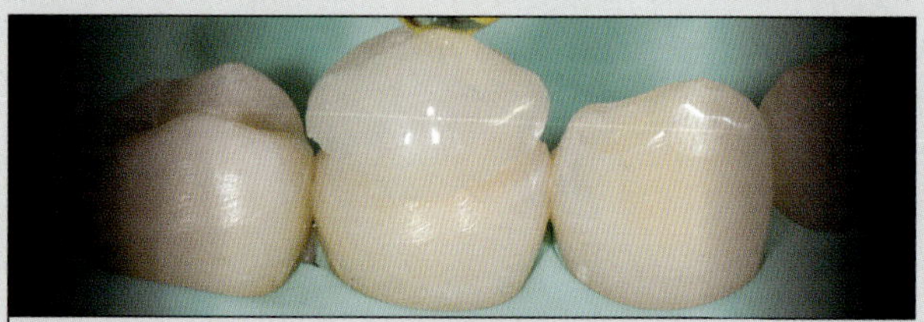

41c

Figs 41a to 41c Definitive mandibular posterior restorations fabricated using monolithic lithium disilicate. Note the minimal thickness of the partial-coverage restorations, which were luted with a three-step adhesive bonding protocol.

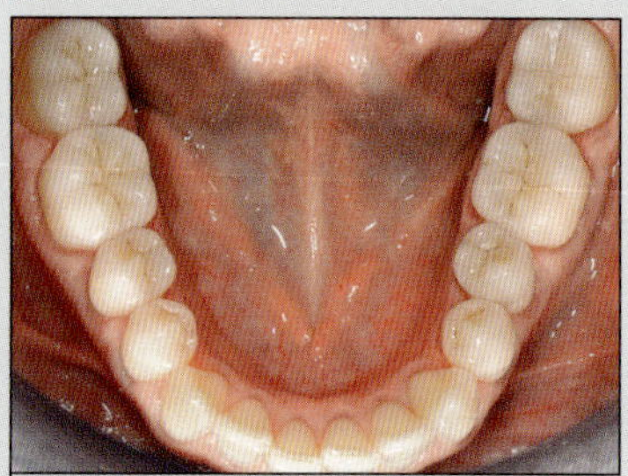

42

Fig 42 Occlusal view of the mandibular arch with partial-coverage restorations in place.

molar, tooth preparation on the mandibular posterior teeth was performed just to round some line angles and to facilitate the esthetic integration of the definitive restorations. A very light chamfer finish line was chosen for the buccal areas for esthetic optimization. The interdental contact points were maintained, as the interdental area of every tooth was found to be free of caries.

Step 7

- A final impression of the mandibular arch with polyvinyl siloxane material was taken with the one-step double-mix technique.

Step 8

- Posterior provisional restorations were not necessary. As the VDO increase provided sufficient space for the restorative material, the centric cusps of the prepared teeth in the mandibular posterior areas were not reduced.
- After removing the mock-up on the anterior area, the mandible went back to its original position thanks to the maintenance of the untouched cusps. As a result of this procedure, it was not necessary to fabricate and position a provisional restoration in the posterior area.

Step 9

- Definitive posterior restorations (Fig 41) and maxillary anterior provisionals. The mandibular posterior monolithic partial-coverage ceramic restorations were fabricated together with a shell for the provisional restorations for the maxillary anterior teeth.

Step 10

- Bonding of the mandibular posterior partial-coverage restorations followed a precise protocol (Fig 42). The inner surfaces of the restorations were etched with 4.5% hydrofluoric acid for 20 seconds, thoroughly rinsed with water, and placed in an ultrasonic bath with distilled water for 3 minutes. After thorough air drying, the intaglio surfaces were silanized with Monobond-S and dried for 60 seconds. Tooth preparations were cleaned with pumice and rubber burs (Opticlean), etched for 30 seconds on enamel and 15 seconds on dentin with 37.5% phosphoric acid (Ultra-Etch), rinsed, and dried. Both fitting surfaces, restorations and teeth, were coated with the adhesive

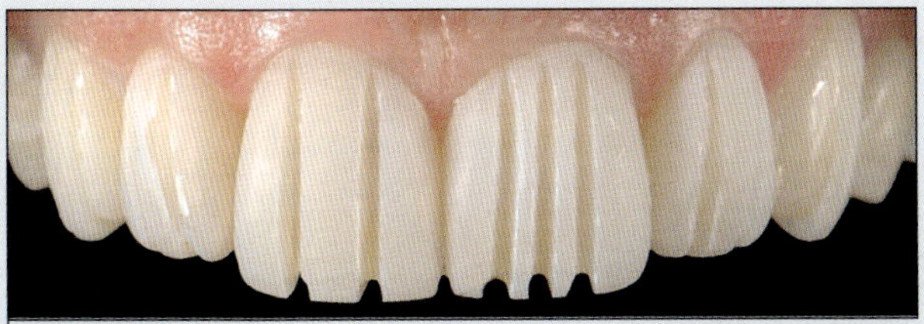

43a

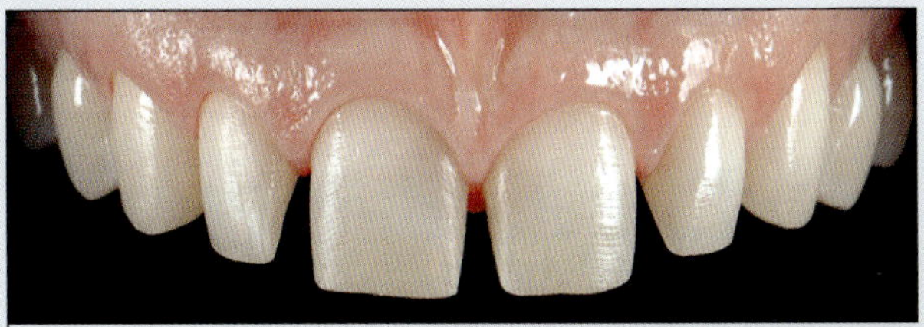

43b

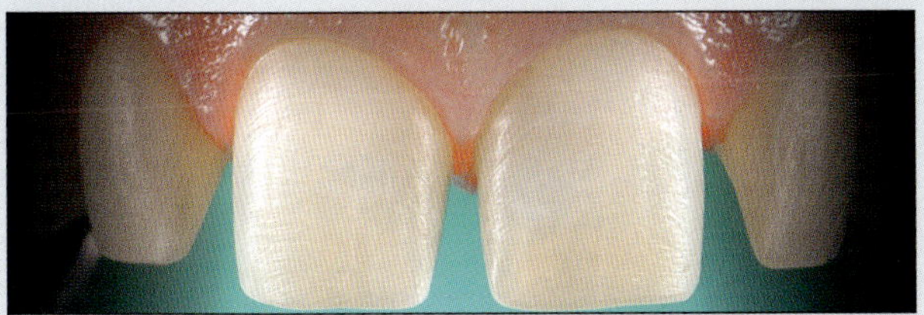

43c

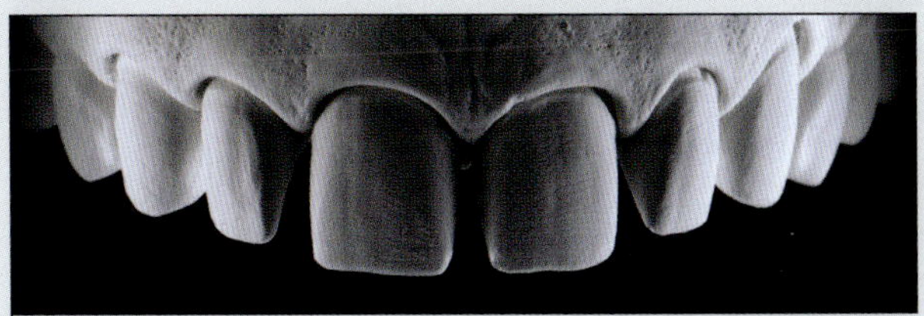

44a

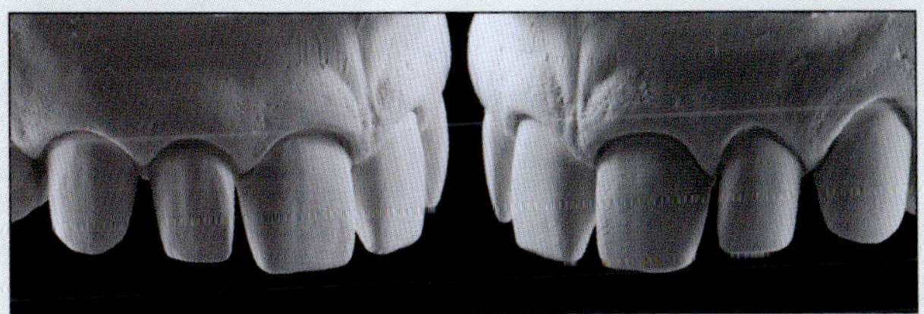

44b

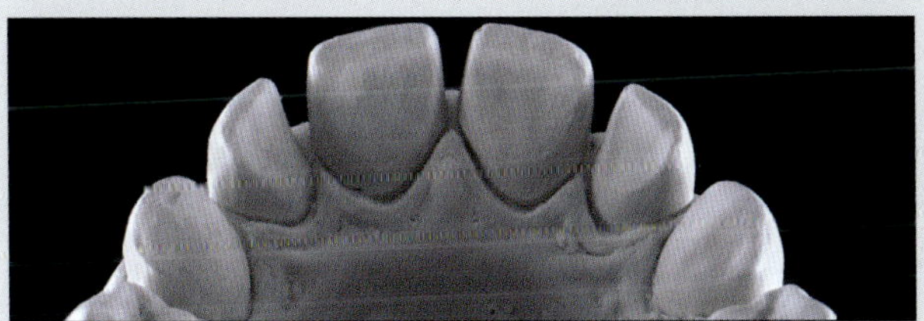

44c

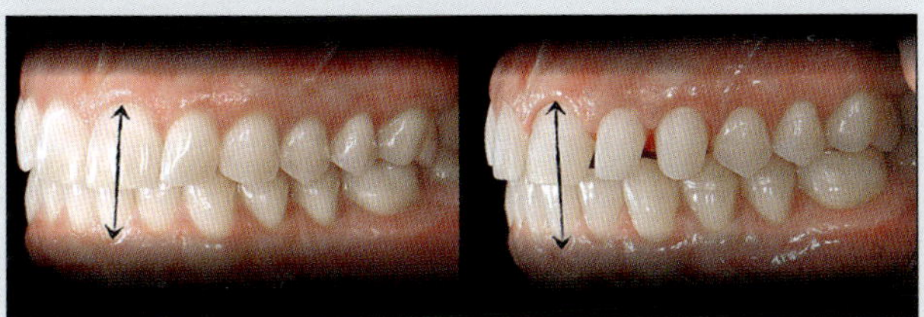

45a

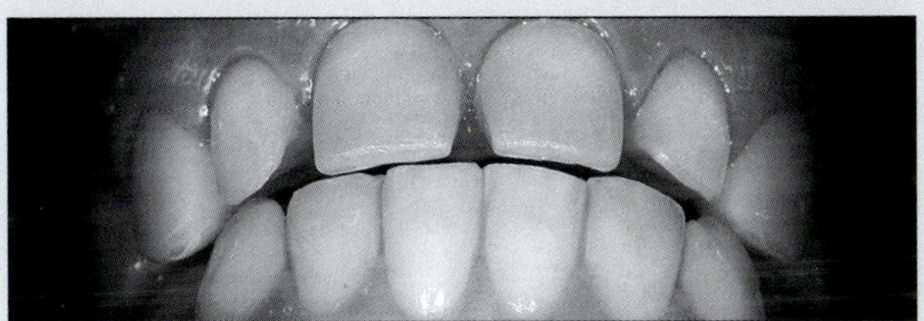

45b

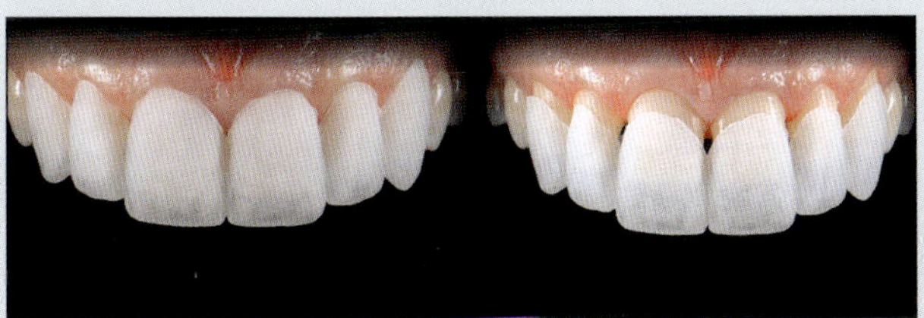

46a

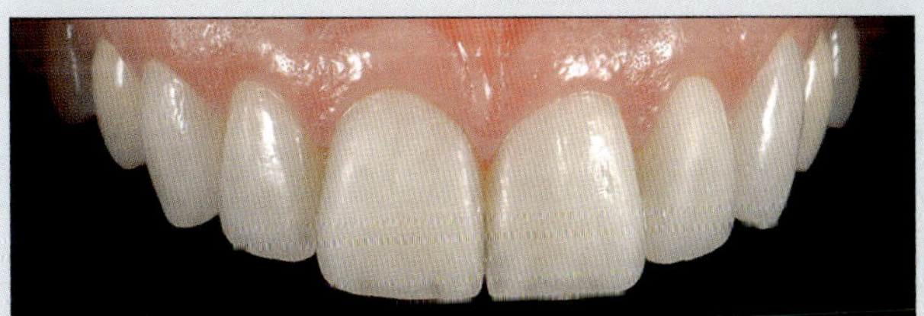

46b

Figs 43a to 43c Definitive preparation of the anterior teeth using a minimally invasive procedure. Note that a very light tooth preparation was completed on the enamel.

Figs 44a to 44c On the stone casts, it is possible to see the design of the preparations, with a delicate chamfer finish line that extends to the palatal area to better define the limit of the preparation and to obtain a more natural integration of the restoration with the surrounding tissue.

Figs 45a and 45b After the VDO increase and establishment of the CR position, a large amount of space was present between the anterior teeth. The full-veneer design of the restorations allowed re-creation of contact with the mandibular teeth and a new and more physiologic function.

Figs 46a and 46b Using the modified indirect technique (MIT[20]) and a very minimal tooth preparation, it is possible to reline and refine the shell of the provisional restoration.

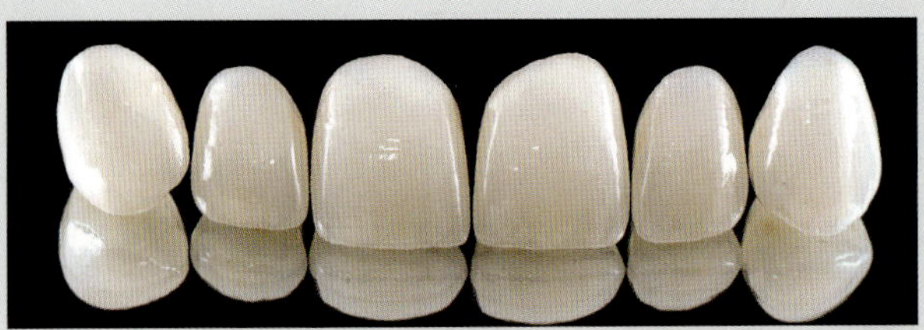

47a

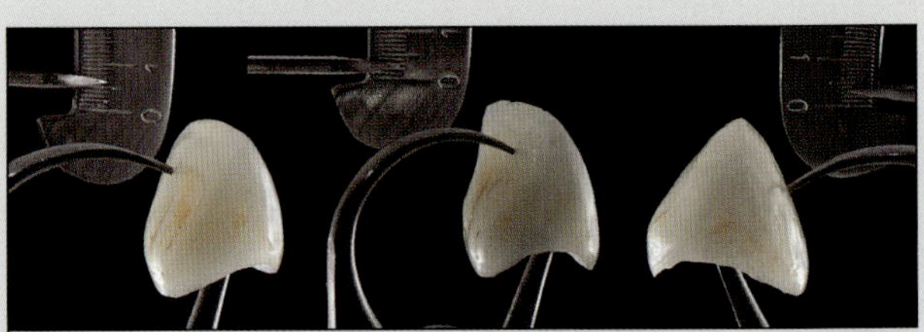

47b

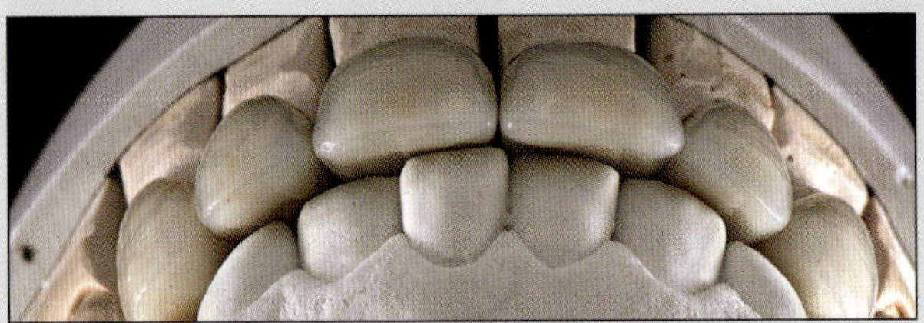

47c

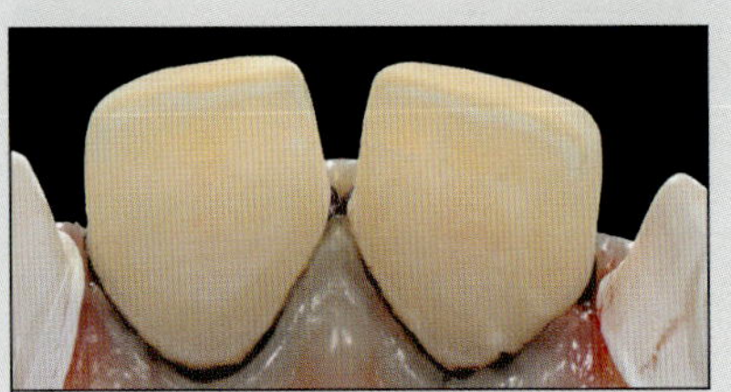

48

Figs 47a to 47c Maxillary bilayered full veneers fabricated with lithium disilicate. Note the thickness of the restoration and the new relationship between maxillary and mandibular teeth.

Fig 48 Maxillary central incisors ready for the bonding procedure after etching with phosphoric acid. Note the amount of enamel remaining on the palatal surfaces because of the space gained by increasing the VDO.

system (OptiBond FL); because of the reduced thickness of the ceramic restorations, a light-curing composite resin cement (Variolink Veneer) was selected to lute the restorations.

Step 11

- Tooth preparation of the maxillary anterior teeth (Figs 43 and 44). Once the posterior mandibular partial restorations were cemented, a new mock-up of the maxillary anterior teeth was made with the aim of guiding the preparations using a minimally invasive procedure.
- Moreover, because of the space gained in the palatal area by the increase of the VDO (already achieved after having positioned the eight posterior restorations), a full-veneer design was chosen for the final preparations. The prepared teeth were covered completely by enamel, even though a delicate chamfer finish line configuration was performed on the margins to obtain a better esthetic integration of the restoration (Figs 45 and 46).

Step 12

- Bilayered lithium disilicate maxillary anterior restorations were fabricated. The final impression of the anterior tooth preparations was taken with the definitive posterior partial restorations in situ. Maxillary bilayered full veneers were fabricated and cemented following a three-step adhesive bonding protocol (Figs 47 and 48).

Step 13

- Occlusal adjustment and final polishing. By guiding the mandible in CR with the bimanual manipulation (Dawson maneuver), a precise final occlusal adjustment was performed. The goal was to obtain well-distributed and synchronized posterior contacts, delicate contacts on the anterior teeth, and no posterior contacts during excursive movements (Figs 49 to 56).

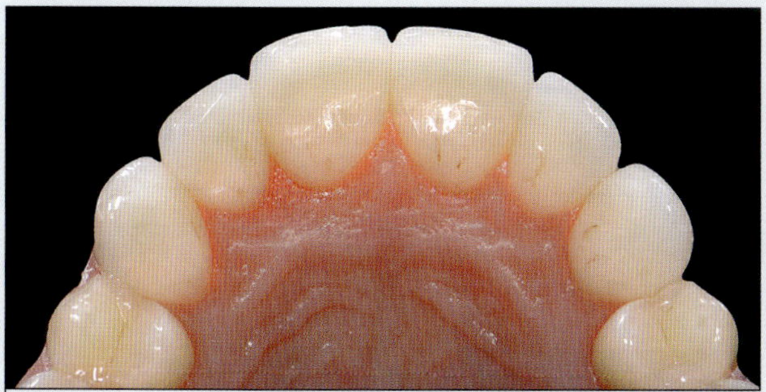

49

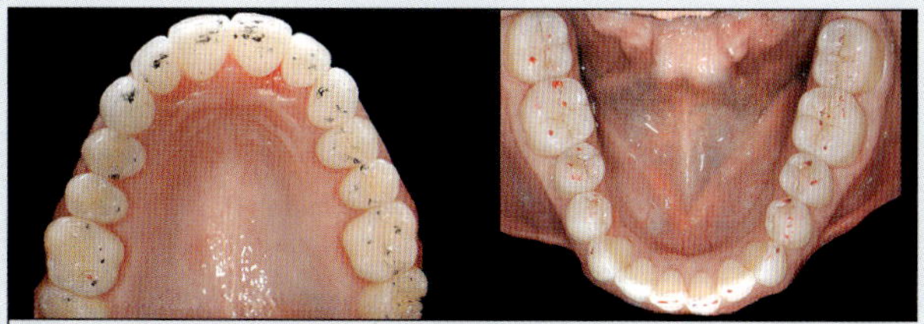

50

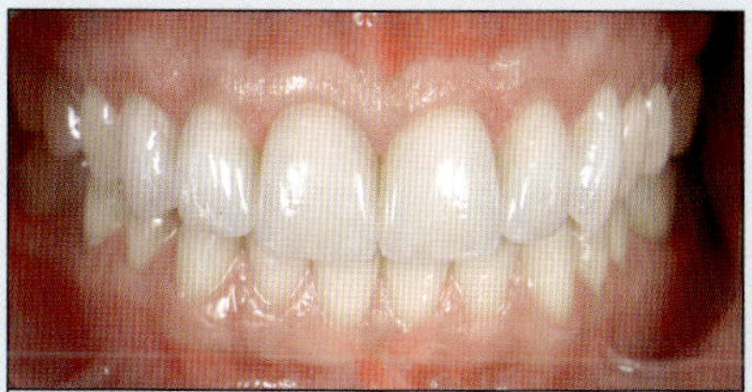

51a

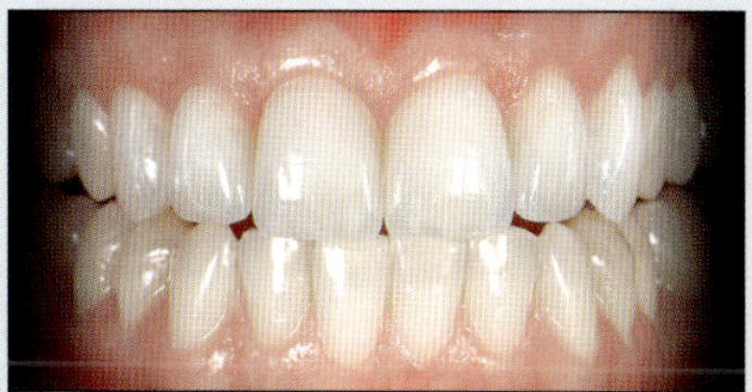

51b

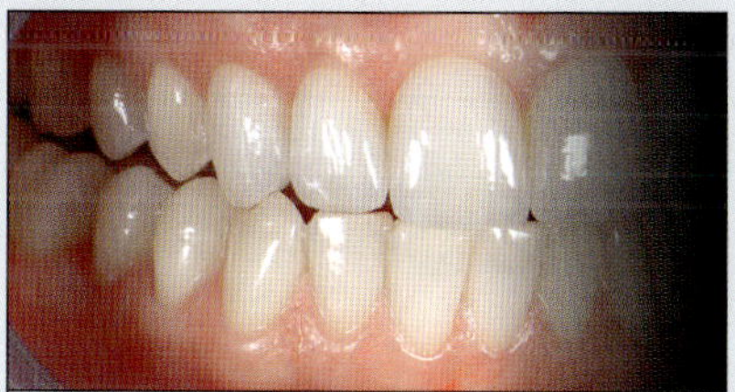

51c

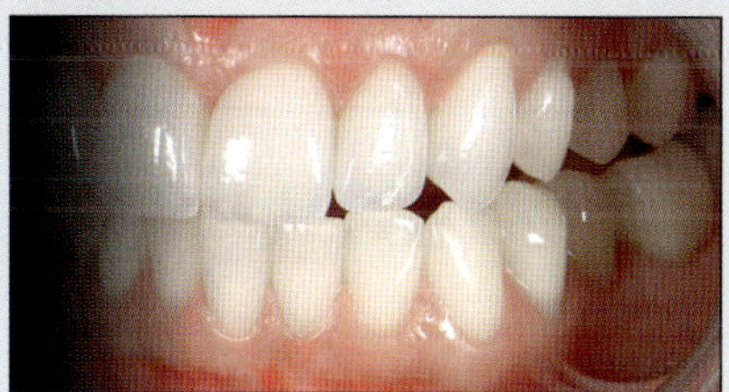

51d

Fig 49 Occlusal view of the definitive maxillary anterior full veneers after cementation.

Fig 50 New occlusion of the patient with well-distributed and synchronized posterior contacts, delicate contacts on the anterior teeth, and no posterior contacts during excursive movements.

Figs 51a to 51d Final dynamic evaluation of the new occlusion. Note the disocclusion of posterior teeth during excursive movements.

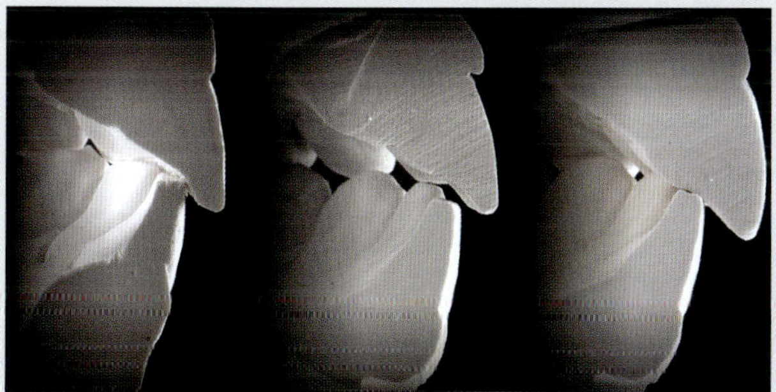

52a

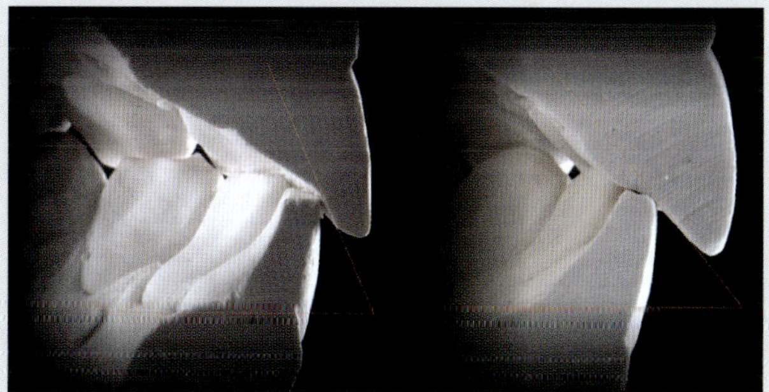

52b

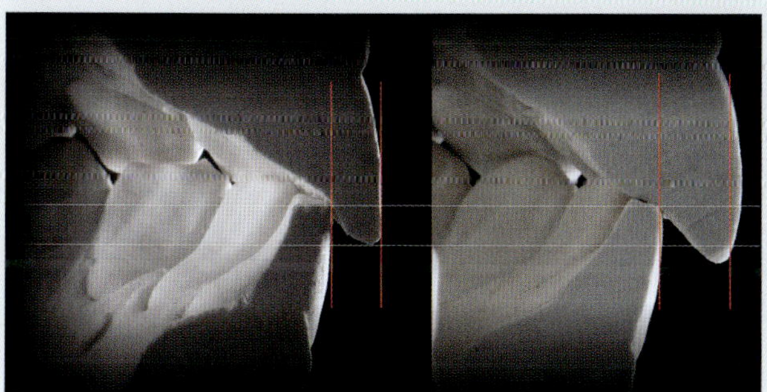

52c

Figs 52a to 52c Diagram of the evolution of the treatment from the initial presentation to the definitive restorations. Note the new overjet and overbite and the new anterior guidance with a flatter angle. Reducing the angle of guidance may reduce the muscle activity. An initial restricted envelope of function was reduced with the treatment.

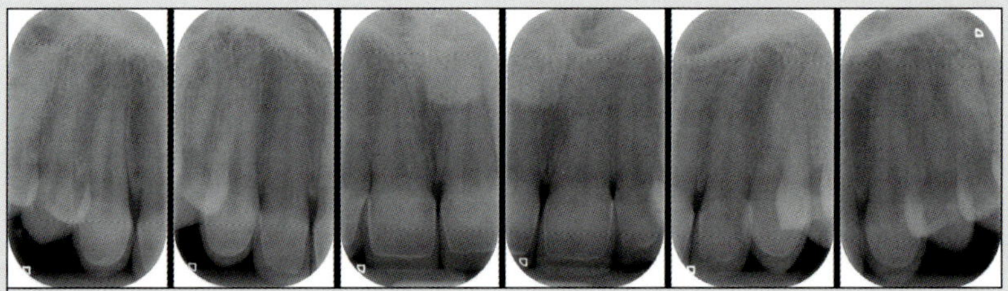

53

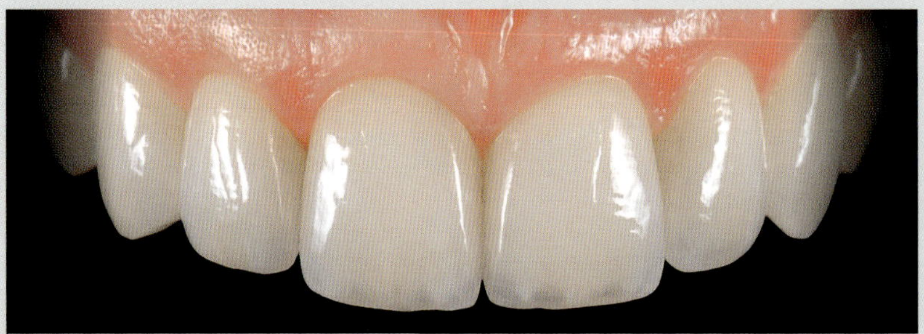

54

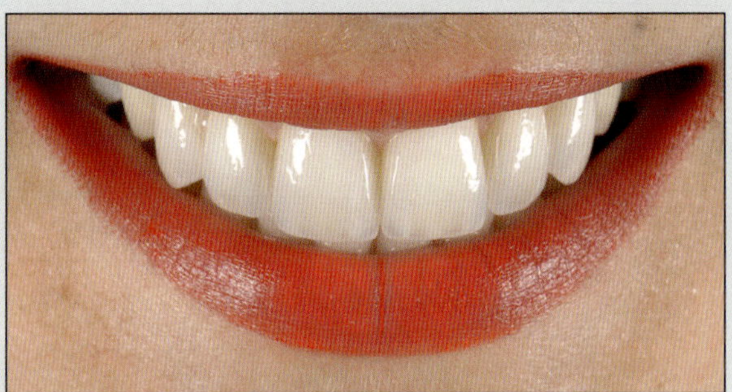

55a

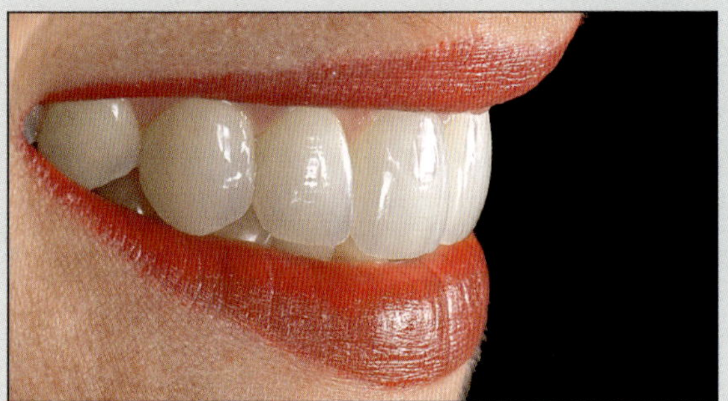

55b

Fig 53 Final radiographs of the maxillary anterior teeth show the minimal invasiveness of the treatment.

Fig 54 New anterior dental composition.

Figs 55a and 55b Final integration of the treatment with the lips of the patient.

Fig 56 Satisfactory integration of the rehabilitation in relation to the lips and the face of the patient.

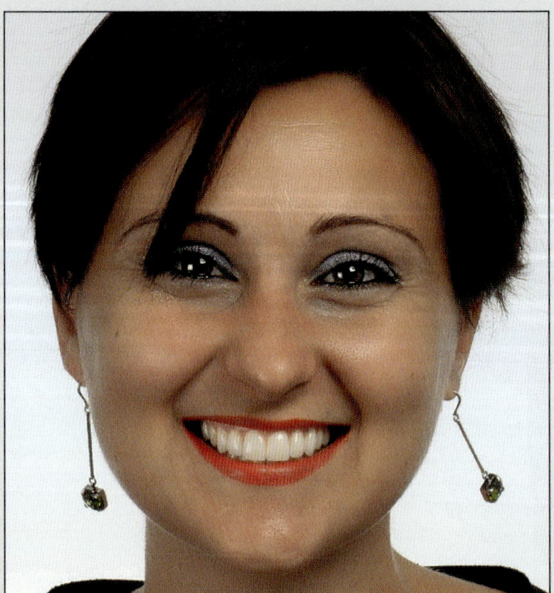

56

CONCLUSIONS

Because of the proper management of CR, with or without a VDO increase, a new relationship between the two arches was obtained, and all the functional and esthetic parameters were optimized.

When facing these types of clinical cases, the prosthodontist needs to consider that by limiting his or her intervention to a cosmetic treatment, there may be a risk of failure of the restorations due to an improper relationship between the maxillary and mandibular anterior teeth during function.

From an esthetic point of view, a good integration of the restoration with the face, the lips, and the surrounding tissue was obtained, and the patients were truly happy with their new smiles. From a functional point of view, a new relationship between the anterior teeth was obtained with an improved overbite-overjet relationship and a new flatter anterior guidance, thus improving the envelope of function. This ensures a better distribution of load and a more physiologic occlusion. Once again, the goal of the prosthetic treatment in these patients is to reestablish a new equilibrium in the stomatognathic system and to guarantee the longevity of the restorations.

ACKNOWLEDGMENTS

The authors would like to thank Mr Giancarlo Barducci, CDT, for his precious work in fabricating all the restorations in this article.

REFERENCES

1. Bardsley PF. The evolution of tooth wear indices. Clin Oral Investig 2008;12(suppl 1):S15–S19.
2. Paesani DA (ed). Bruxism: Theory and Practice. Chicago: Quintessence, 2010.
3. Grippo JO, Simring M, Schreinder S. Attrition, abrasion, corrosion and abfraction revisited: A new perspective on tooth surface lesions. J Am Dent Assoc 2004;135:1109–1118.
4. Lee A, He LH, Lyons K, Swain MV. Tooth wear and wear investigations in dentistry. J Oral Rehabil 2012;39:217–225.
5. Dawson PE. Functional Occlusion: From TMJ to Smile Design. St Louis: Mosby Elsevier, 2006.
6. Fradeani M, Barducci G, Bacherini L, Brennan M. Esthetic rehabilitation of a severely worn dentition with minimally invasive prosthetic procedures (MIPP). Int J Periodontics Restorative Dent 2012;32:135–147.
7. Silness J, Johnannessen G, Røynstrand T. Longitudinal relationship between incisal occlusion and incisal tooth wear. Acta Odontol Scand 1993;51:15–21.
8. Spear F. Fundamental occlusal therapy considerations. In: McNeill C (ed). Science and Practice of Occlusion. Chicago: Quintessence, 1997:421–436.
9. Yaffe A, Hochman N, Ehrlich J. A functional aspect of anterior attrition or flaring and mode of treatment. Int J Prosthodont 1992;5:284–289.
10. Bacherini L, Brennan M, Bocabella L, Vigiani P. Esthetic rehabilitation of a severely discolored dentition with a minimally invasive prosthetic procedure (MIPP). Quintessence Dent Technol 2013;36:59–76.
11. McKee JR. Comparing condylar position repeatability for standardized versus nonstandardized methods of achieving centric relation. J Prosthet Dent 1997;77:280–284.
12. Silva NR, Bonfante EA, Martins LM, et al. Reliability of reduced-thickness and thinly veneered lithium disilicate crowns. J Dent Res 2012;91:305–310.
13. Abduo J. Safety of increasing vertical dimension of occlusion: A systematic review. Quintessence Int 2012;43:369–380.
14. Spear F, Kinzer F. Approaches to vertical dimension. In: Cohen M (ed). Interdisciplinary Treatment Planning: Principles, Design, Implementation. Chicago: Quintessence, 2008:249–281.
15. Becker CM, Kaiser DA. Evolution of occlusion and occlusal instruments. J Prosthodont 1993;2:33–43.
16. Keshvad A, Winstanley RB. An appraisal of the literature on centric relation. Part III. J Oral Rehabil 2001;28:55–63.
17. Okeson JP. Management of Temporomandibular Disorders and Occlusion. St Louis: Mosby Elsevier, 2012.
18. Ma L, Guess PC, Zhang Y. Load-bearing properties of minimal-invasive monolithic lithium disilicate and zirconia occlusal onlays. Finite element and theoretical analyses. Dent Mater 2013;29:742–751.
19. Fradeani M. Esthetic Rehabilitation in Fixed Prosthodontics, Vol 1. Esthetic Analysis: A Systematic Approach to Prosthetic Treatment. Chicago: Quintessence, 2004.
20. Fradeani M, Barducci G (eds). Esthetic Rehabilitation in Fixed Prosthodontics. Vol 2: Prosthetic Treatment: A Systematic Approach to Esthetic, Biologic, and Functional Integration. Chicago: Quintessence, 2004.

BIOMATERIALS UPDATE

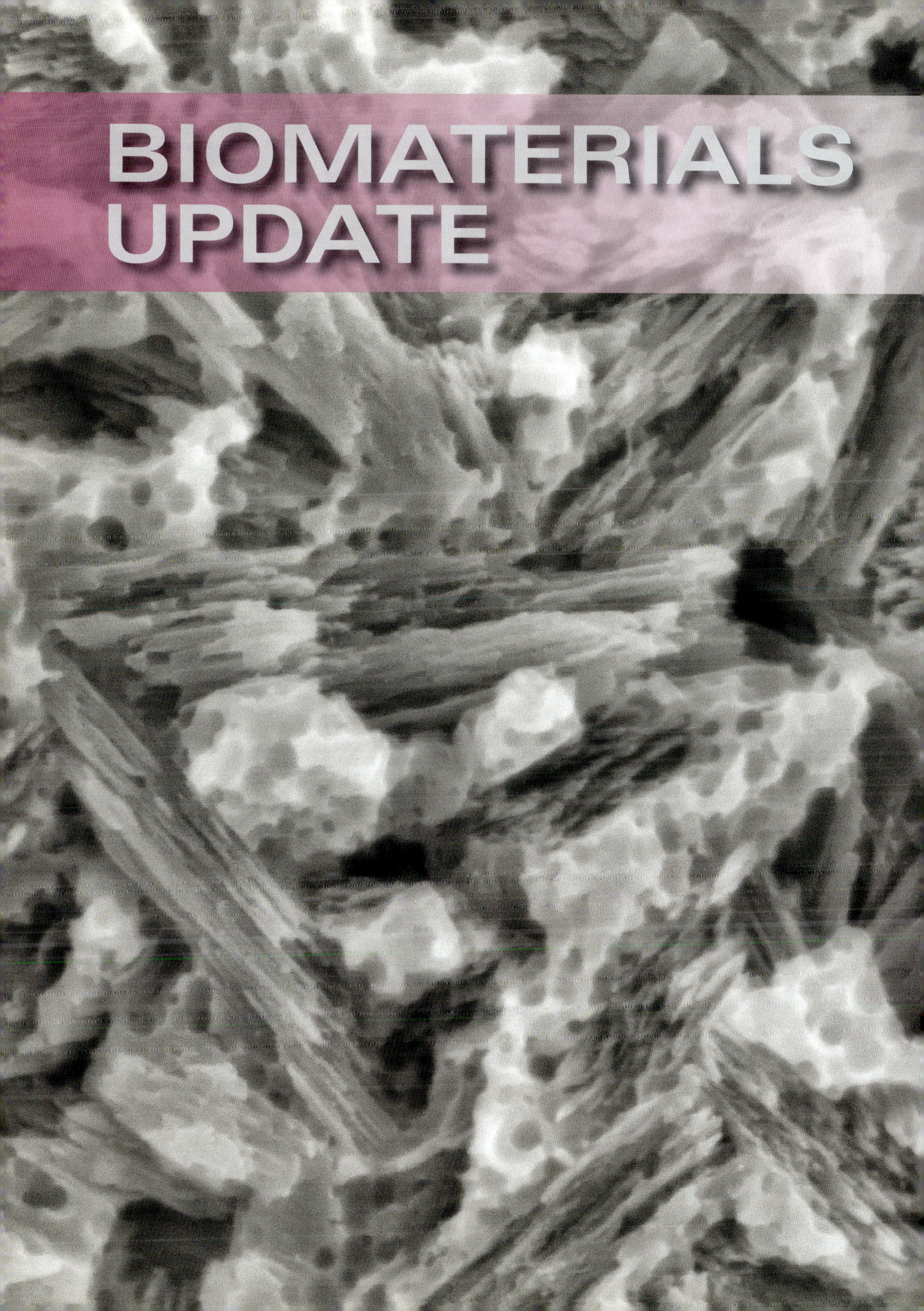

CAD/CAM High-Strength Glass-Ceramics

Neimar Sartori, DDS, MS, PhD[1]
Gilberto Tostado, DDS[2]
Jin-Ho Phark, DMD, Dr Med Dent[3]
Kazunari Takanashi, RDT[4]
Richard Lin, DDS[5]
Sillas Duarte, Jr, DDS, MS, PhD[6]

[1]Assistant Professor, Division of Restorative Sciences; Assistant Director, Advanced Program in Operative Dentistry, Ostrow School of Dentistry, University of Southern California, Los Angeles, California, USA.

[2]Resident, Advanced Program in Prosthodontics, Division of Restorative Sciences, Ostrow School of Dentistry, University of Southern California, Los Angeles, California, USA.

[3]Assistant Professor, Division of Restorative Sciences; Director of Biomaterials Laboratory, Ostrow School of Dentistry, University of Southern California, Los Angeles, California, USA.

[4]Director, Oral Design Center of Los Angeles, Los Angeles, California, USA.

[5]Assistant Professor, Director, CAD/CAM Technologies, Division of Restorative Sciences, Ostrow School of Dentistry, University of Southern California, Los Angeles, California, USA.

[6]Associate Professor and Chair, Division of Restorative Sciences; Director, Advanced Program in Operative Dentistry, Ostrow School of Dentistry, University of Southern California, Los Angeles, California, USA.

Correspondence to: Dr Neimar Sartori, Division of Restorative Sciences, Ostrow School of Dentistry, University of Southern California, 925 W 34th Street, DEN 4365, Los Angeles, CA 90089-0641. Email: sartori@usc.edu

The increased demand for high-quality, natural-looking restorations fabricated in a single appointment has fueled the development of newer restorative materials and technologies.[1] Highly esthetic ceramic restorations can be fabricated in less than an hour using computer-aided design/computer-assisted manufacture (CAD/CAM) technology.[2,3]

The main disadvantage of esthetic all-ceramic restorations made of feldspathic porcelain or leucite-reinforced glass-ceramic has been related to their relatively low flexural strength (130 to 160 MPa). However, the development of high-strength glass-ceramic with higher flexural strength (210 to 540 MPa) offers an alternative to conventional feldspathic or leucite-reinforced ceramics.[4] Lithium disilicate and zirconia-reinforced lithium silicate high-strength glass-ceramics provide an adequately esthetic appearance without requiring the addition of veneering ceramic, resulting in superior structural integrity.[5] Furthermore, high-

strength glass-ceramics can be used to fabricate ultrathin restorations (less than 0.5 mm thickness) with adequate optical and mechanical properties, as well as improved marginal integrity.

In 1998, lithium disilicate glass-ceramic (IPS Empress II, Ivoclar Vivadent) using the lost-wax press technique was introduced. Lithium disilicate glass-ceramic was designed for single-tooth and anterior three-unit fixed partial denture (FPD) restorations.[6,7] The survival rate of a lithium disilicate all-ceramic system (IPS Empress II) has been shown to be within acceptable limits for anterior (97.5%) and posterior (98%) full-coverage crowns after 10 years.[8] However, the survival rates reported for FPD restorations made of the same material ranged from 50% after 2 years[9] to 70% after 5 years.[10]

A second generation of lithium disilicate glass-ceramic (IPS e.max Press, Ivoclar Vivadent) was released to the market in 2001.[7] This newer formulation includes a microstructure with a higher amount of smaller lithium disilicate crystals (approximately 70%). By increasing the percentage of lithium disilicate crystals on the glass-ceramic material, the optical and mechanical properties are improved.[11] A long-term prospective study of monolithic posterior three-unit FPD restorations fabricated of IPS e.max Press revealed a survival rate of 87.9 % after 10 years.[12]

With the popularization of CAD/CAM technologies, lithium disilicate glass-ceramic (IPS e.max CAD, Ivoclar Vivadent) for CAD/CAM milling was introduced in 2005.[13] Recently, two zirconia-reinforced lithium silicate glass-ceramics for fabrication of monolithic restorations using CAD/CAM technology also became available (Suprinity, VITA; Celtra Duo, Dentsply).[3] Due to strength and versatility, CAD/CAM lithium disilicate and zirconia-reinforced lithium silicate glass-ceramic blocks can be used for fabrication of numerous types of restorations (partial-coverage and full-coverage crowns, implant abutments, and three-unit FPDs). The aim of this article is to review the biomaterial properties of CAD/CAM high-strength glass-ceramics.

HIGH-STRENGTH GLASS-CERAMICS

Glass-ceramics are polycrystalline materials produced through controlled crystallization of base glass. The process of controlled crystallization of glasses is essential to produce a ceramic with acceptable optical and mechanical properties.[14] Controlled nucleation and crystallization of glasses can be obtained by employing catalysts or nucleation agents.[15] The crystallization process occurs in two different stages: *(1)* nucleation (formation of the crystals) followed by *(2)* crystal growth.

Controlling nucleation is of paramount importance to produce a suitable glass-ceramic material. Nucleation is the beginning of chemical or physical transformation in glass composition (phase separation), in which a small number of ions become arranged in a pattern characteristic of a solid crystal.[16] The addition of nucleating agents, ie, phosphorus pentoxide (P_2O_5), to lithium disilicate compounds provides controlled nucleation and crystal growth.[14,17–19] The microstructure of a given glass-ceramic material can be adjusted depending on the type and amount of nucleation agent incorporated into the compound.

In addition to the nucleation agents, raw powders should be incorporated into a binary quartz and lithium dioxide ($Li_2O–SiO_2$) system composition to enhance the chemical durability[20] and mechanical properties of glass-ceramics.[3,11,21,22] Examples of raw powders are aluminum oxide (Al_2O_3), potassium oxide (K_2O), aluminum metaphosphate ($Al[PO_3]_3$), zirconium oxide (ZrO_2), zinc oxide (ZnO), and calcium oxide (CaO). These raw powders are mixed and heated to form a new glass.[23] After cooling down, this new glass is then thermically treated to allow the crystallization of the glass-ceramic components.[11]

The process of crystallization of a lithium disilicate glass-ceramic, nucleation, and crystal growth is complex, intriguing, and temperature dependent.[11] The rise of the temperature between 500°C and 560°C forms nanophases of lithium phosphate (Li_3PO_4) and nucleation of lithium metasilicate (Li_2SiO_3) and lithium disilicate ($Li_2Si_2O_5$).[14] From 560°C to 750°C, growth of lithium metasilicate crystals and agglomeration of lithium disilicate nanophases (crystal size smaller than 100 nm) occur.[24] When the temperature reaches 820°C, lithium metasilicate is completely decomposed and lithium disilicate crystals grow quickly, reaching maximum growth rate at a temperature of 850°C.[14,17,24]

As a result of this crystallization process, lithium disilicate represents the main crystal phase (approximately 70%) of the glass-ceramic microstructure (Fig 1).[6] The needlelike lithium disilicate crystals (3 to 6 μm

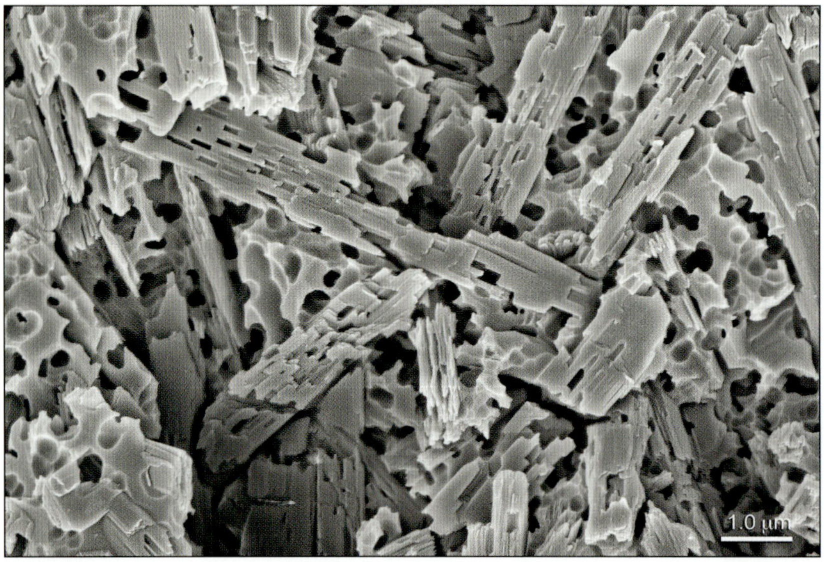

Fig 1 Microstructure of pressed lithium disilicate glass-ceramic (IPS e.max Press) after crystallization followed by etching with 5% hydrofluoric acid for 20 seconds (magnification × 10,000).

in length)[11] are embedded in a glassy matrix of lithium orthophosphate (Li_3PO_4).[6] The surface on the lithium disilicate crystals presents multiple holes (0.1 to 0.3 µm in length), indicating the location of the previous crystal precipitation (small holes on the surface of the crystals; see Fig 1).[6]

CLASSIFICATION OF CAD/CAM HIGH-STRENGTH GLASS-CERAMICS

CAD/CAM high-strength glass-ceramics can be classified as lithium disilicate–reinforced or zirconia-reinforced lithium silicate glass-ceramics.

CAD/CAM Lithium Disilicate–Reinforced Glass-Ceramic

IPS e.max CAD is an example of a CAD/CAM lithium disilicate–reinforced glass-ceramic. Because crystallized lithium disilicate CAD blocks would be difficult to mill using chairside milling units, an intermediate product, lithium metasilicate glass-ceramic, was developed using the two-stage crystallization process.[25,26] In the first stage of crystallization, lithium metasilicate is precipitated by controlled double nucleation and then pressure-casted in the block shape. These partially crystallized IPS e.max CAD blocks have a bluish appearance with approximately 40% by volume of lithium metasilicate platelet-shaped crystals embedded in a glassy phase, with crystal size ranging from 0.2 to 1.0 µm and a nanocrystalline disilicate matrix[11] (Fig 2). This partially crystallized CAD/CAM block exhibits a flexural strength of 130 to 150 MPa, which can withstand the stresses during the milling process without chipping of margins while allowing intraoral occlusal adjustment.[11,26]

After milling and try-in of the restoration in its blue stage, it is then heat treated at 850°C.[13] During this process, lithium metasilicate glass-ceramic is transformed into lithium disilicate glass-ceramic. After crystallization, the restoration presents a toothlike color, with excellent chemical durability of less than 100 µg/cm^2, strength of 360 ± 60 MPa, and toughness of 2 MPa·m$^{1/2}$.[25]

The chemical composition of crystalized IPS e.max CAD is identical to that of IPS e.max Press. However, due to the difference in size of the lithium disilicate crystals, the microstructure of IPS e.max CAD is slightly different. CAD/CAM lithium disilicate glass-ceramic consists of 70% by volume fine-grain needlelike lithium disilicate crystals with length of approximately 1.5 µm embedded into a glassy matrix (Fig 3), whereas for the pressed version (IPS e.max Press) the lithium disilicate crystals can grow up to 7 µm.[25] CAD/CAM lithium disilicate glass-ceramic appears to have a more

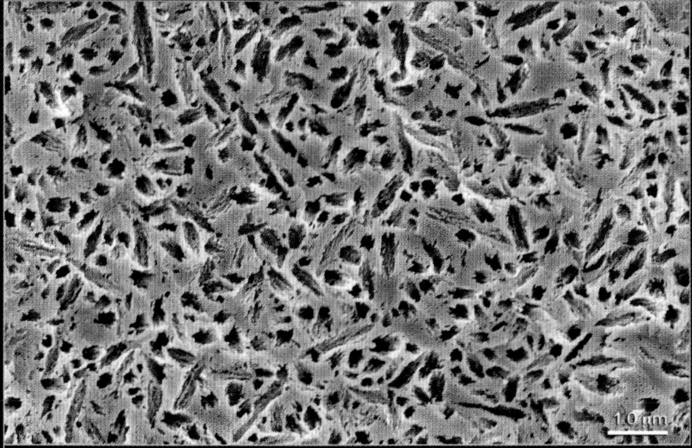

2

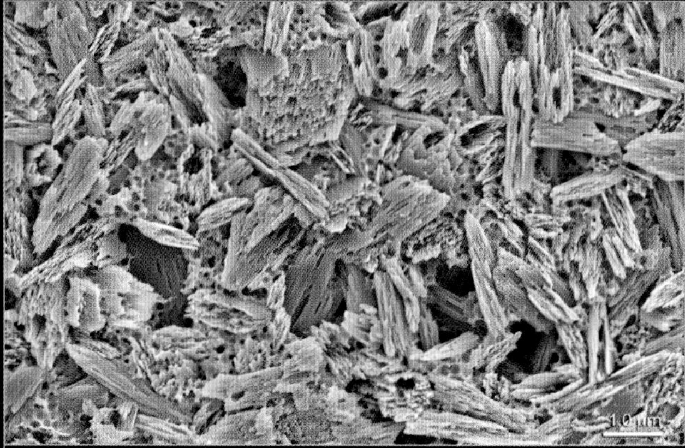

3

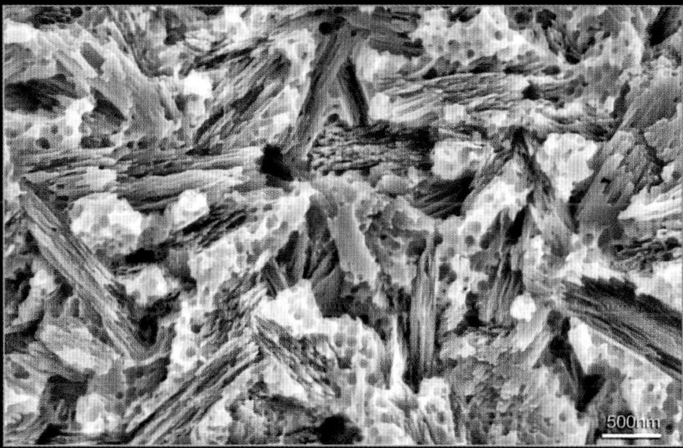

4

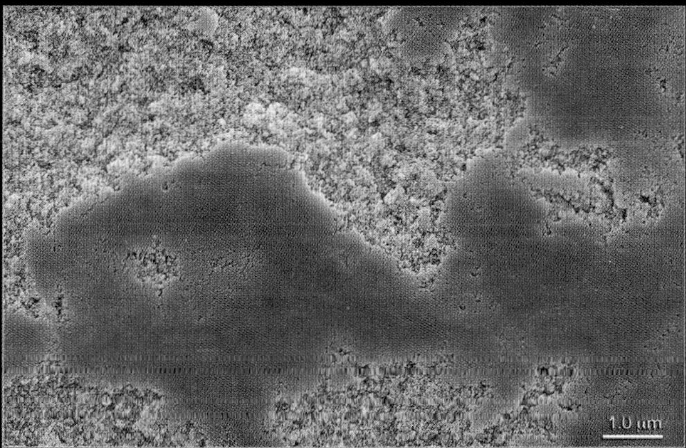

5

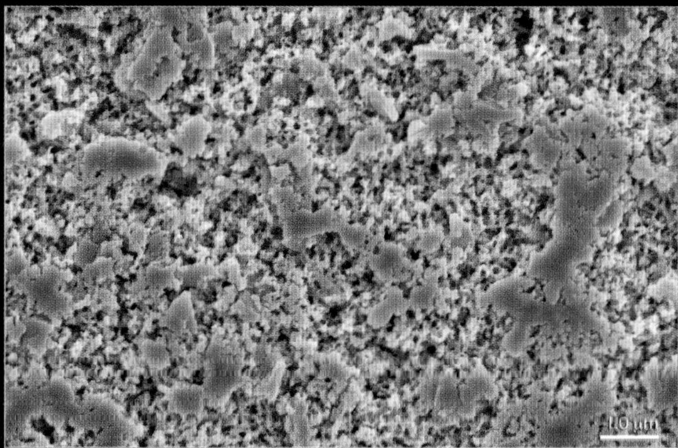

6

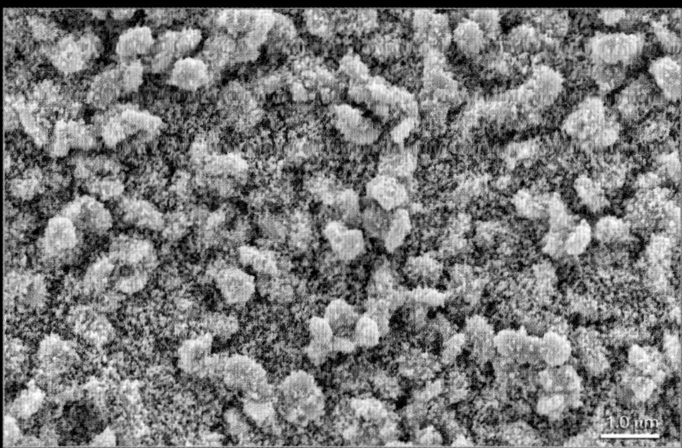

7

homogenous microstructure, in which the lithium disilicate crystals are more densely adhered to the glass-ceramic matrix (Fig 4).

Because of its favorable translucency and shade assortment, CAD/CAM lithium disilicate glass-ceramic can be used as monolithic restorations or as a core material for subsequent layering with veneering ceramics. Clinical results revealed a 97% survival rate after 7 years for partial-coverage restorations fabricated using CAD/CAM technology.[5]

CAD/CAM Zirconia-Reinforced Lithium Silicate Glass-Ceramic

Two zirconia-reinforced lithium silicate ceramics are available for CAD/CAM restorations: VITA Suprinity (VITA Zahnfabrik) and Celtra Duo (Dentsply). Both materials rely on the addition of 10% by weight zirconium oxide to lithium silicate glass compositions to improve their mechanical and optical properties. Zirconia-reinforced lithium silicate glass-ceramics have mechanical properties comparable with those of lithium disilicate glass-ceramics.[27] After crystallization, a dual microstructure is obtained of lithium metasilicate and lithium disilicate crystals embedded in glassy matrix containing zirconium oxide.[28]

VITA Suprinity

VITA Suprinity CAD/CAM blocks are composed of silicon dioxide (SiO_2), lithium oxide (Li_2O), potassium oxide (K_2O), phosphorus pentoxide (P_2O_5), aluminium oxide (Al_2O_3), zirconium dioxide (ZnO_2), cerium (IV) oxide (CeO_2), and pigments. These CAD/CAM blocks are produced in three distinct stages.[29,30] Initially, zirconium dioxide, silicon dioxide, lithium oxide, and other ceramic components are heated at a temperature of 1,500°C to melt all components. After creating a homogenous solution, the melted glass is poured into molds to form blocks.[30] The resulting glass block is brittle and not suited for the CAD/CAM milling process; thus, a second heating treatment is necessary. In the second heating stage (from 500°C to 600°C), the crystals within the glass matrix form lithium metasilicate[30] and the glass block achieves adequate mechanical properties to withstand the stresses of the milling process. The resulting translucent glass-ceramic block is then made commercially available (Fig 5).

After milling, the translucent glass-ceramic restoration must be recrystallized at a temperature of 840°C for 8 minutes. The crystallization forms a homogeneous structure of lithium disilicate with a subsidiary crystal phase containing zirconium oxide[30] (Fig 6).

Celtra Duo

Celtra Duo can be classified as zirconia-reinforced lithium silicate CAD/CAM blocks containing 10% zirconia.[31] The microstructure consists of a large amount of ultrafine lithium silicate crystals with an approximate size of 0.5 to 0.7 μm embedded in the glass matrix[31] (Fig 7). According to the manufacturer, zirconia is completely dissolved into the glass matrix.

Celtra Duo blocks as supplied are already sintered, and, theoretically, no additional sintering steps are needed. However, if additional heat treatment is performed (ie, for external staining and glazing), the flexural strength is increased by 76%.[31]

Fig 2 Microstructure of CAD/CAM lithium disilicate–reinforced glass-ceramic (IPS e.max CAD) before crystallization (blue stage), showing the glassy matrix impregnated with metasilicate crystals (magnification × 10,000).

Fig 3 Microstructure of CAD/CAM lithium disilicate–reinforced glass-ceramic (IPS e.max CAD) after crystallization followed by etching with 5% hydrofluoric acid for 20 seconds (magnification × 10,000).

Fig 4 Higher magnification of CAD/CAM lithium disilicate–reinforced glass-ceramic (IPS e.max CAD) after crystallization followed by etching with 5% hydrofluoric acid for 20 seconds (magnification × 20,000).

Fig 5 Microstructure of CAD/CAM zirconia-reinforced lithium silicate glass-ceramic (VITA Suprinity) before crystallization (magnification × 10,000).

Fig 6 Microstructure of CAD/CAM zirconia-reinforced lithium silicate glass-ceramic (VITA Suprinity) after crystallization followed by etching with 5% hydrofluoric acid for 20 seconds (magnification × 10,000).

Fig 7 Microstructure of CAD/CAM zirconia-reinforced lithium silicate glass-ceramic (Celtra Duo) after etching with 5% hydrofluoric acid for 30 seconds (magnification × 10,000).

Table 1 Mechanical Properties of CAD/CAM Glass-Ceramics

Material	Elastic modulus (GPa)	Fracture toughness (MPa√m)	Flexural strength (MPa)
Enamel	87–100[32]	0.6–1.5[33]	470 (intrarod)–978 (multiple rods)[34]
Dentin	17–40[35]	2.3[36]	212[37]
IPS e.max Press (Ivoclar Vivadent)	95[26]	2.75[26]	400[26]
IPS e.max CAD (Ivoclar Vivadent)	95[26]	2.25[26]	360[26]
VITA Suprinity (VITA Zahnfabrik)	70[29]	2.0[29]	420[29]
Celtra Duo (Dentsply) after milling	70[31]	2.0[31]	210[31]
Celtra Duo (Dentsply) after crystallization	—	—	370[31]

MATERIAL PROPERTIES

Mechanical Properties

Although most clinical situations involve complex three-dimensional loading, three of the most important mechanical properties of a material are modulus of elasticity, fracture toughness, and flexural strength. The basic mechanical properties for the high-strength glass-ceramics are displayed in Table 1.

The interlocking arrangement of the lithium disilicate crystal microstructure increases the flexural strength and toughness of the glass-ceramic, reducing crack propagation within the glass matrix.[13] The improved homogeneity of CAD/CAM high-strength glass-ceramics allows fabrication of ultrathin monolithic restorations.[5]

Optical Properties

High strength glass-ceramics are available in different shades and translucencies. The shade of high-strength glass-ceramics is controlled by pigments (usually metal oxides) dissolved into the glass matrix.

IPS e.max CAD blocks are available in 16 different Vita shades and 4 bleach (BL) shades. Different translucencies, such as low translucency (LT), high translucency (HT), and medium opacity (MO), are available for different types of processing techniques. VITA Suprinity blocks are available in 8 different Vita shades (0M1, A1, A2, A3, A3.5, B2, C2, and D2) and 2 different translucencies (translucent: T, and high translucent: HT). Celtra Duo blocks are available in low translucency (LT) and high translucency (HT). LT blocks are available in 5 shades (A1, A2, A3, A3.5, and B2), while HT blocks are limited to 3 shades (A1, A2, A3).

There is a significant change in the translucency and opacity of milled CAD/CAM glass-ceramic restorations after the crystallization process (Fig 8). None of the tested highly translucent CAD/CAM glass-ceramics exhibited opalescence when used with the thickness recommended by the manufacturer (after crystallization) (Fig 9). When highly translucent CAD/CAM glass-ceramics were compared, zirconia-reinforced lithium silicate glass-ceramics presented as more opaque than lithium disilicate–reinforced glass-ceramics.

The fluorescence of CAD/CAM reinforced glass-ceramics was also evaluated in our laboratories (Fig 10). All of the tested restorative ceramics displayed significantly lower fluorescence than that of the natural tooth. Lithium disilicate glass-ceramic (IPS e.max CAD) exhibited low fluorescence, within the bluish wavelength range. Zirconia-reinforced lithium silicate glass-ceramics emitted low and incorrect fluorescence, with a greenish fluorescent hue discrepant from that of the natural tooth.[38]

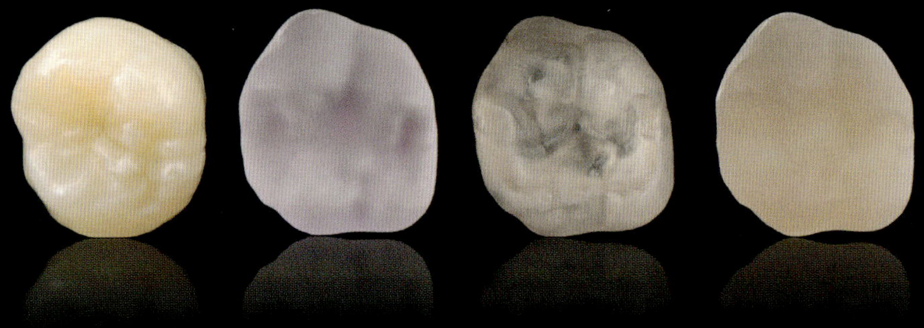

8a

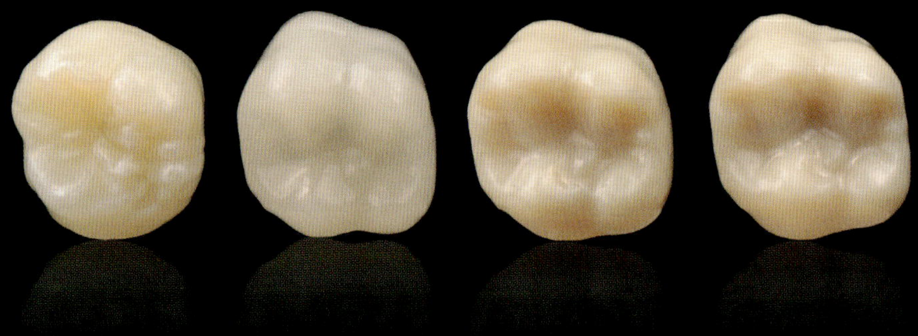

8b

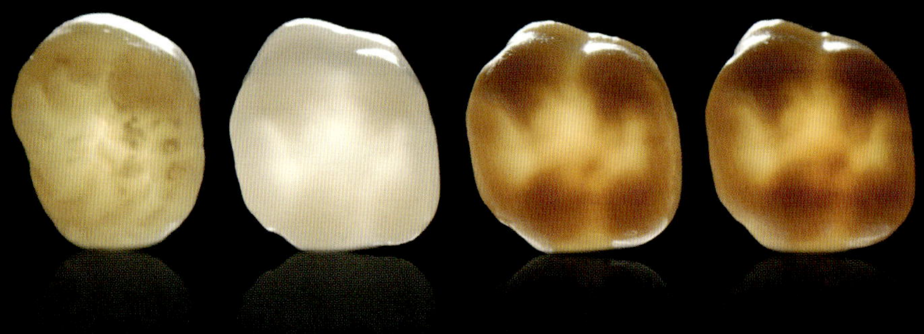

9

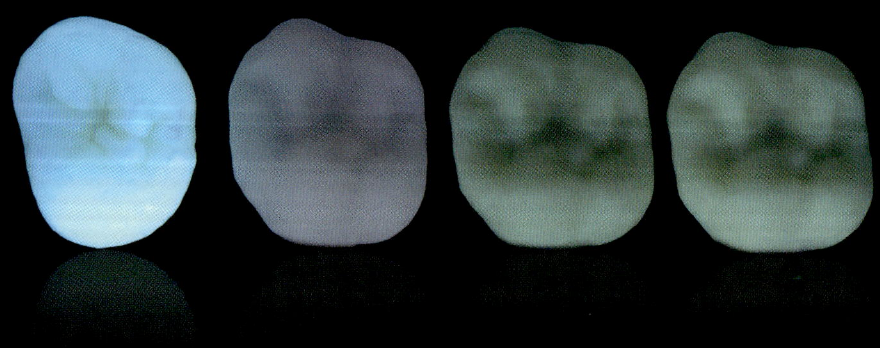

10

Figs 8a and 8b Milled CAD/CAM restorations *(a)* before and *(b)* after crystallization: *(left to right)* natural tooth, IPS e.max CAD, VITA Suprinity, and Celtra Duo.

Fig 9 Translucency of different CAD/CAM high-strength glass-ceramics compared to natural tooth: *(left to right)* natural tooth, IPS e.max CAD, VITA Suprinity, and Celtra Duo.

Fig 10 Fluorescence of different CAD/CAM high-strength glass-ceramics compared to natural tooth: *(left to right)* natural tooth, IPS e.max CAD, VITA Suprinity, and Celtra Duo.

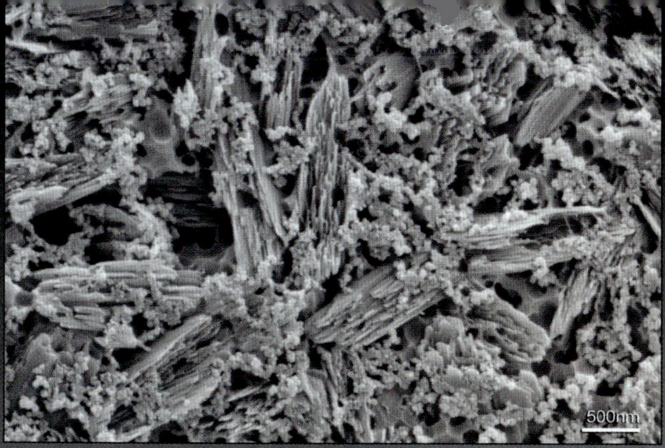

Fig 11 Microstructure of IPS e.max CAD etched with hydrofluoric acid showing crystalline precipitates (magnification × 20,000).

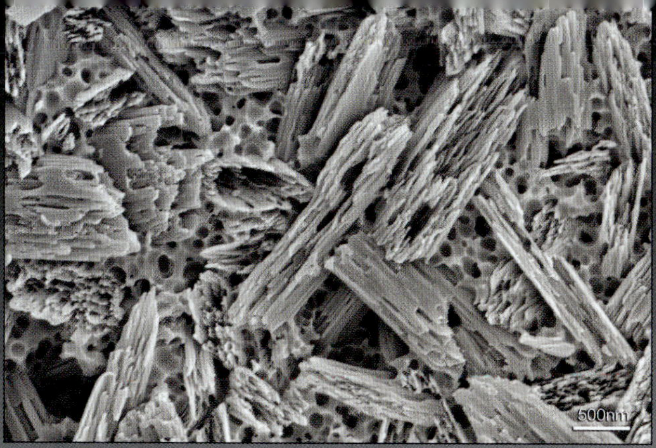

Fig 12 Microstructure of IPS e.max CAD after etching with hydrofluoric acid followed by cleaning with 35% phosphoric acid (magnification × 20,000). Note that the crystalline precipitates were completely removed.

ADHESIVE LUTING

An important advantage of CAD/CAM high-strength glass-ceramics is their ability to be adhesively luted. Acidic treatment of the restoration modifies the surface by creating microporosites that allow micromechanical interlocking of resin cements to the restorative material. Adhesive luting is fundamental for minimally invasive and conservative restorations.

To develop a microretentive surface, the intaglio surface must be etched using 5% hydrofluoric acid for different times for different materials according to manufacturers' recommendations (20 seconds for e.max CAD and e.max Press, 20 seconds for Suprinity, and 30 seconds for Celtra Duo).[11,29,31] The hydrofluoric acid must be rinsed off with forceful water spray. The surface must then be cleaned from crystalline precipitates that accumulate within the microporosities after etching[32] (Fig 11). Crystalline precipitates may compete with the adhesive cement, decreasing the bond strength. Thus, after etching, the intaglio surface must be cleaned with 35% phosphoric acid under scrubbing motion for 60 seconds or by immersion in an ultrasonic bath for 1 to 3 minutes in 98% alcohol (Fig 12). The intaglio surface must be dried and silane coupling agent applied. The silane should be allowed to react for 1 minute. The silanol group will bond to the glass network while the organofunctional group will copolymerize with the methacrylate of the resin cement. Recent data from our laboratories suggested that methacryloyloxydecyl dihydrogen phosphate (MDP)-containing silane yielded higher bond strengths to zirconia-reinforced lithium silicate glass-ceramics than that of conventional silanes.

CONCLUSIONS

CAD/CAM high-strength glass-ceramics present adequate optical and mechanical properties. Monolithic CAD/CAM lithium disilicate–reinforced glass ceramic has shown adequate clinical longevity, whereas CAD/CAM zirconia-reinforced lithium silicate glass-ceramic needs further independent clinical investigation. Monolithic restorations fabricated using CAD/CAM technology are reliable restorative options for dental rehabilitation. Figures 13 to 27 demonstrate their use in the restoration of a patient with amelogenesis imperfecta.

Fig 13 Preoperative view of a patient with amelogenesis imperfecta removing her dentures.

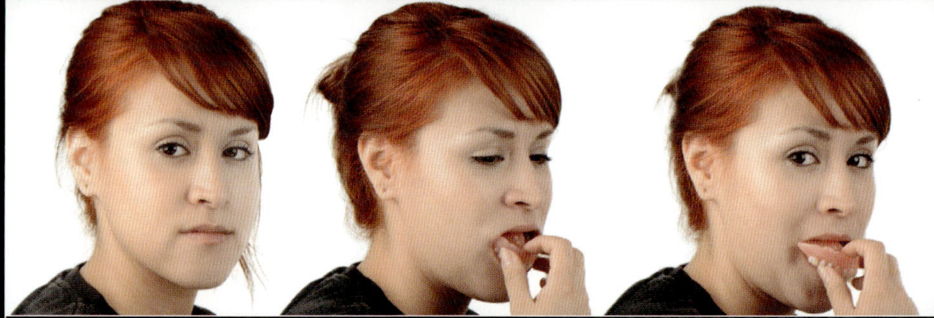

13

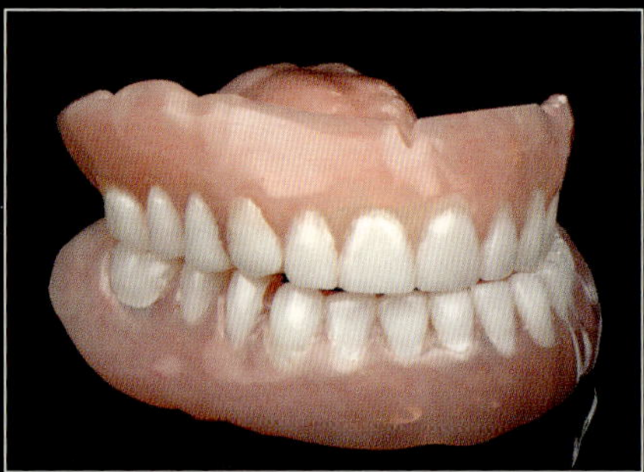

14a

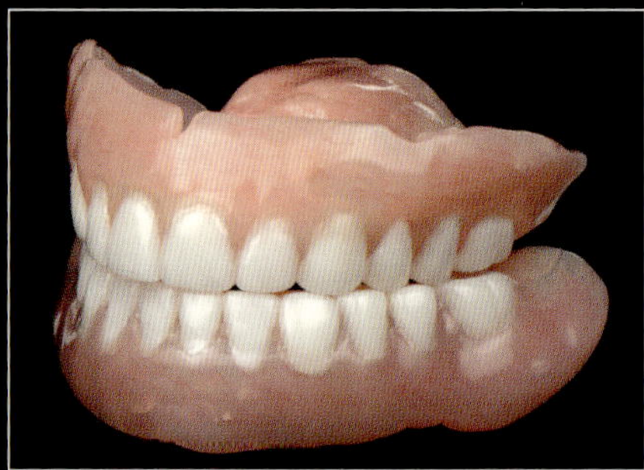

14b

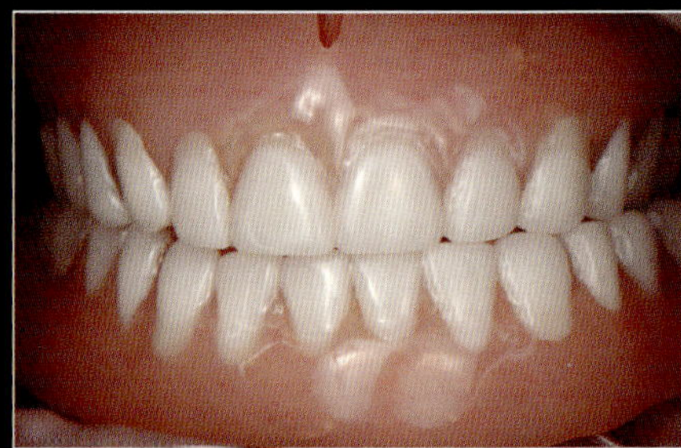

15

Figs 14a and 14b The patient wore maxillary and mandibular complete dentures for over 10 years.

Fig 15 Preoperative intraoral view with the complete dentures.

Fig 16 Preoperative computed tomography scan revealed that the patient had had orthognathic surgery to correct a skeletal Class III malocclusion. At that time the complete dentures were used as reference to establish the position of her maxilla. Presence of impacted teeth can also be seen.

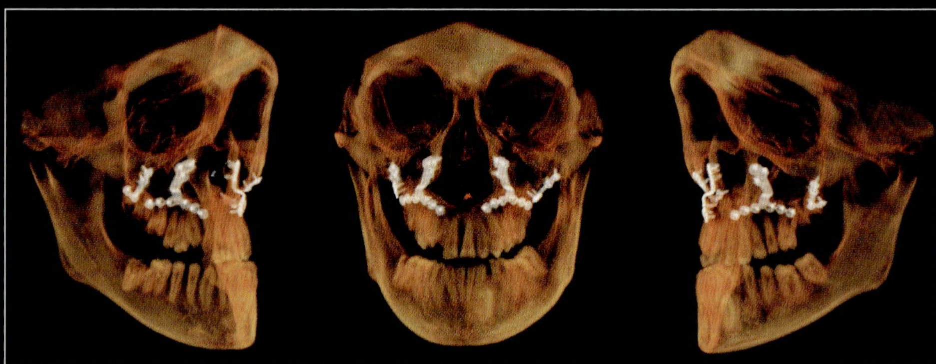

16

Fig 17 Preoperative view of the patient's smile without the complete dentures.

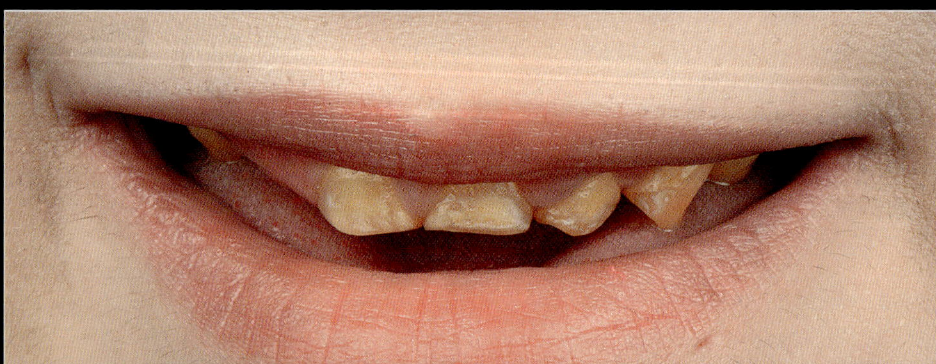

17

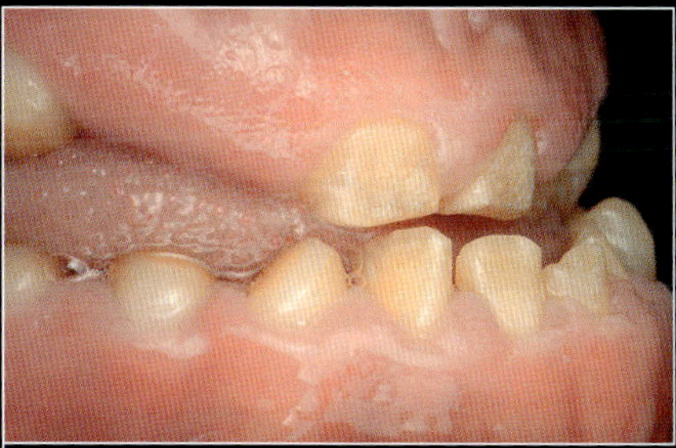
18a

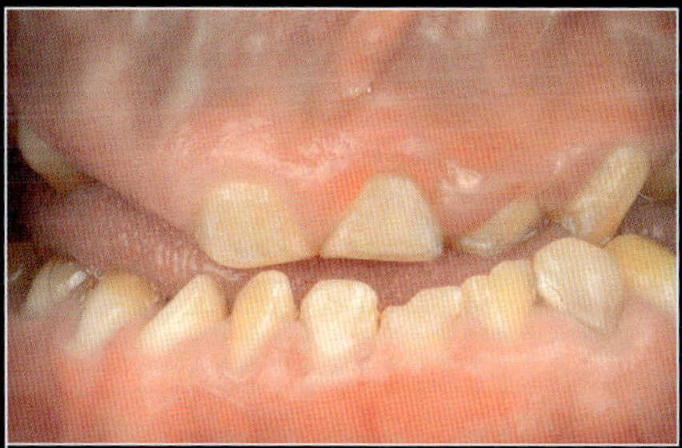
18b

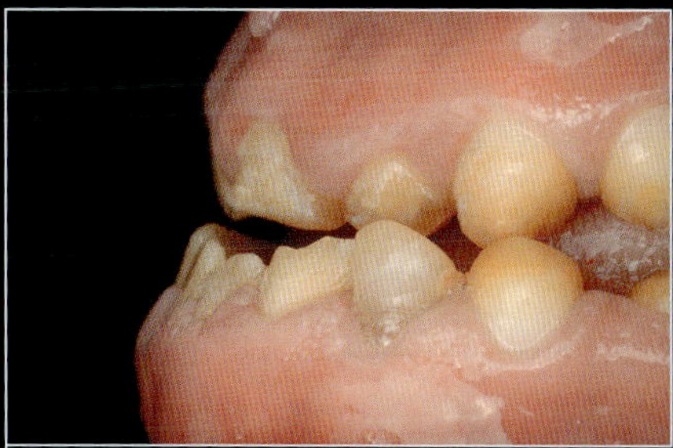
18c

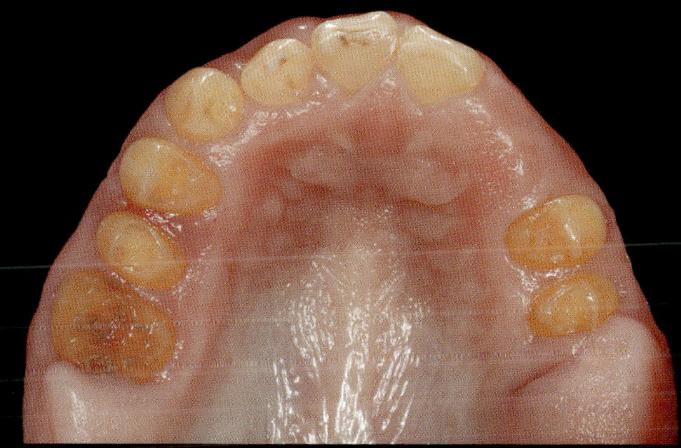
19a

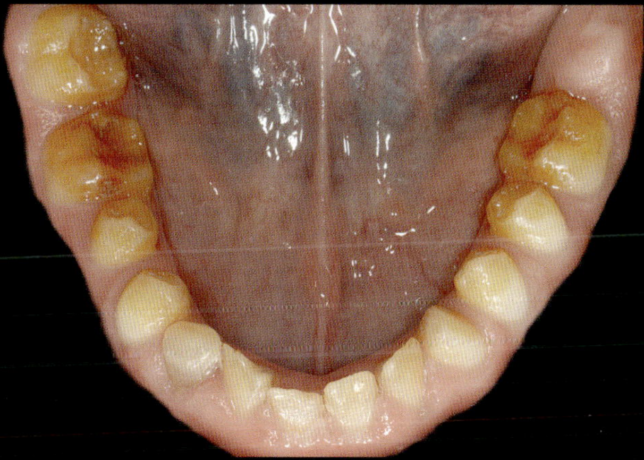
19b

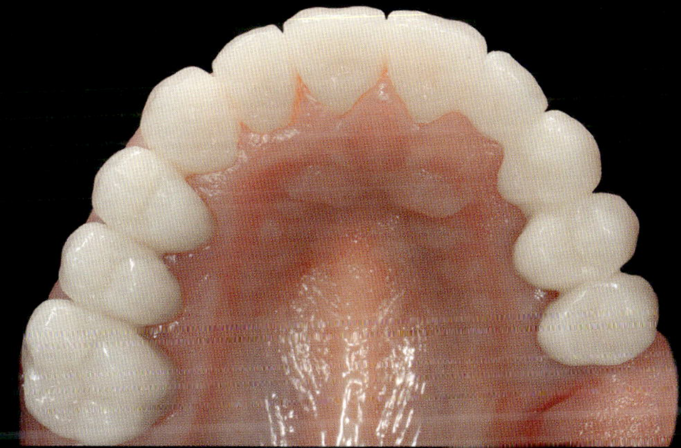
20a

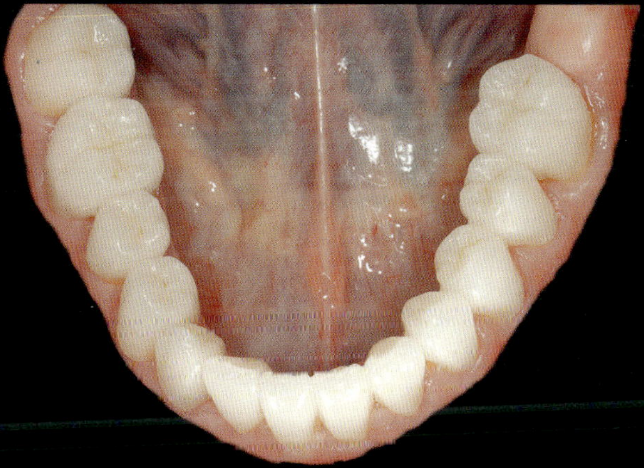
20b

Figs 18a to 18c Preoperative intraoral views of the patient displaying amelogenesis imperfecta, prognathism, and negative overjet (malocclusion Class III according to Angle's classification).

Figs 19a and 19b Preoperative view of maxillary and mandibular arches. After careful analysis of the treatment plan options, it was determined that a nonpreparation full-mouth adhesive rehabilitation would the ideal treatment option.

Figs 20a and 20b Maxillary and mandibular polymethyl methacrylate (PMMA) provisional restorations at the correct vertical dimension of occlusion (VDO) were fabricated based on the wax-up. No tooth preparation was performed.

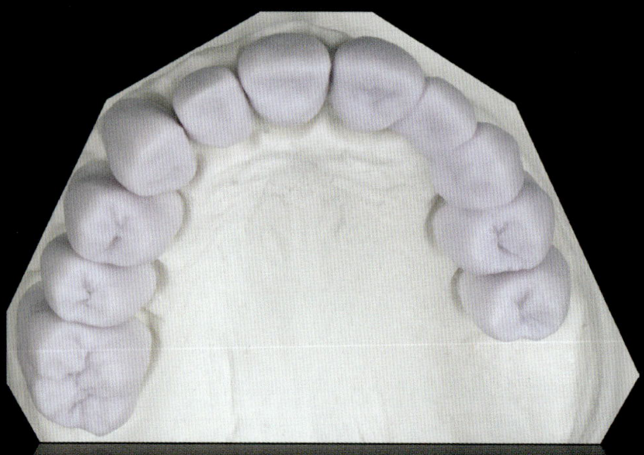

21a

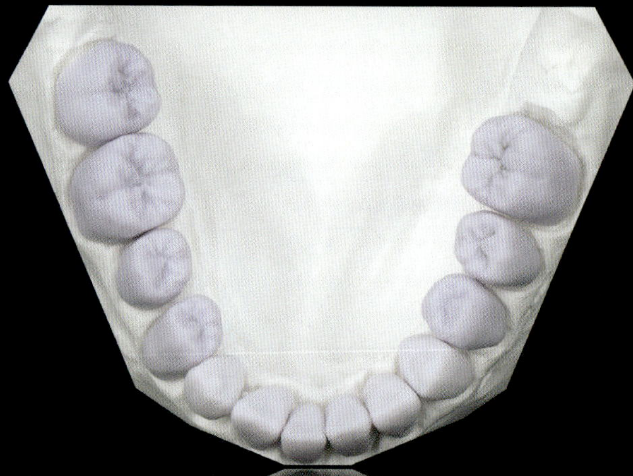

21b

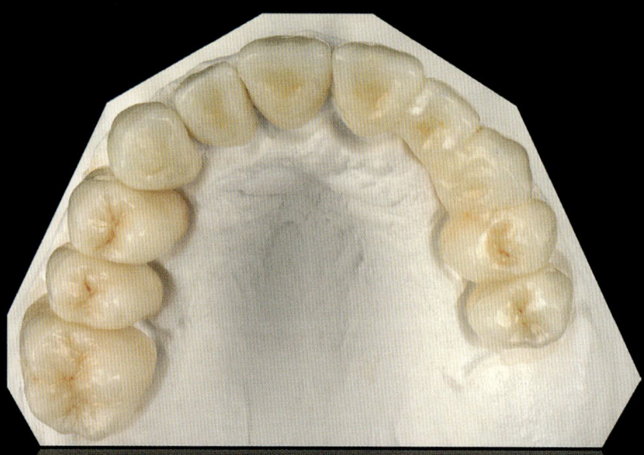

22a

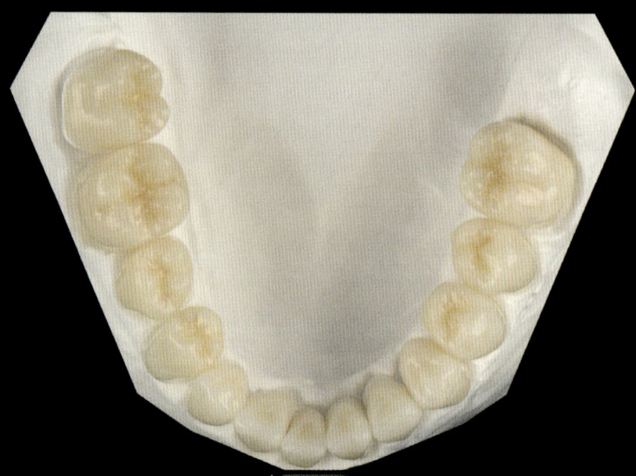

22b

Figs 21a and 21b CAD/CAM monolithic restorations in the blue stage. CAD/CAM monolithic restorations (up to 0.3-mm thickness) were milled with lithium disilicate–reinforced glass-ceramic (IPS e.max CAD) based the wax-up (CAD/CAM biocopy).

Figs 22a and 22b CAD/CAM lithium disilicate–reinforced glass-ceramic monolithic restorations after external characterization, glazing, and crystallization.

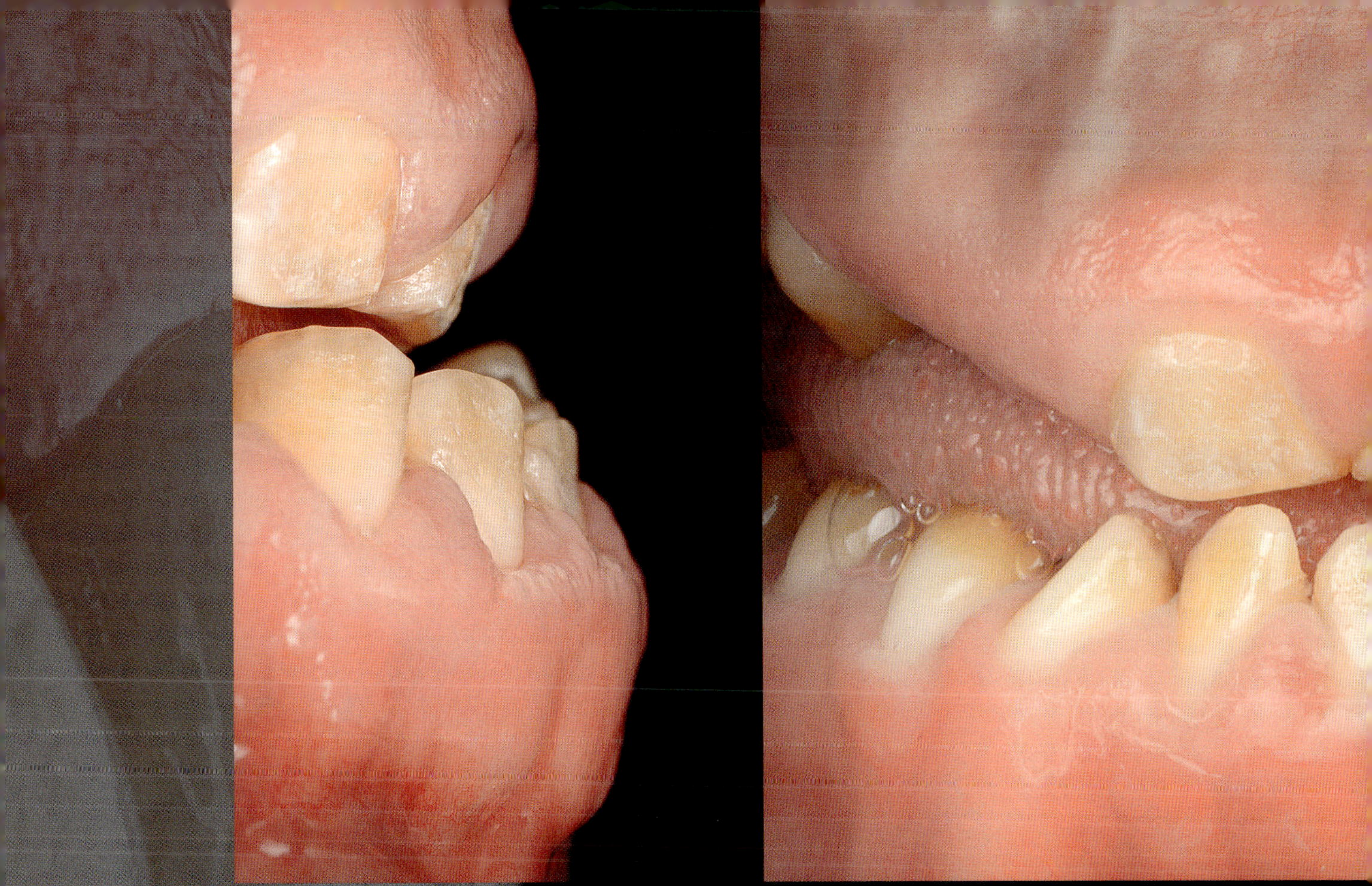

Preoperative intraoral views show prognathism and negative overjet, and postoperative views show positive overjet and overbite after correction of VDO.

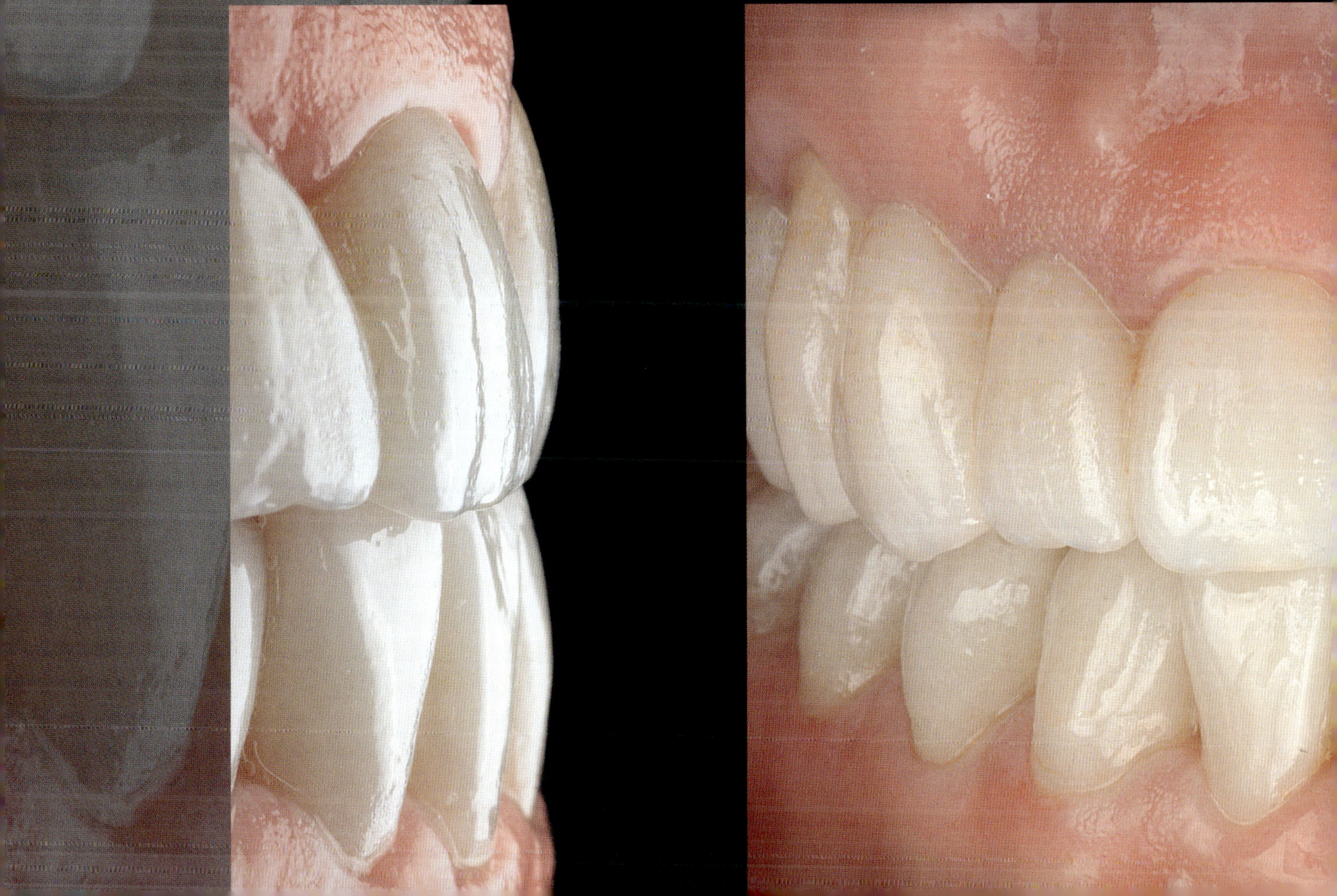

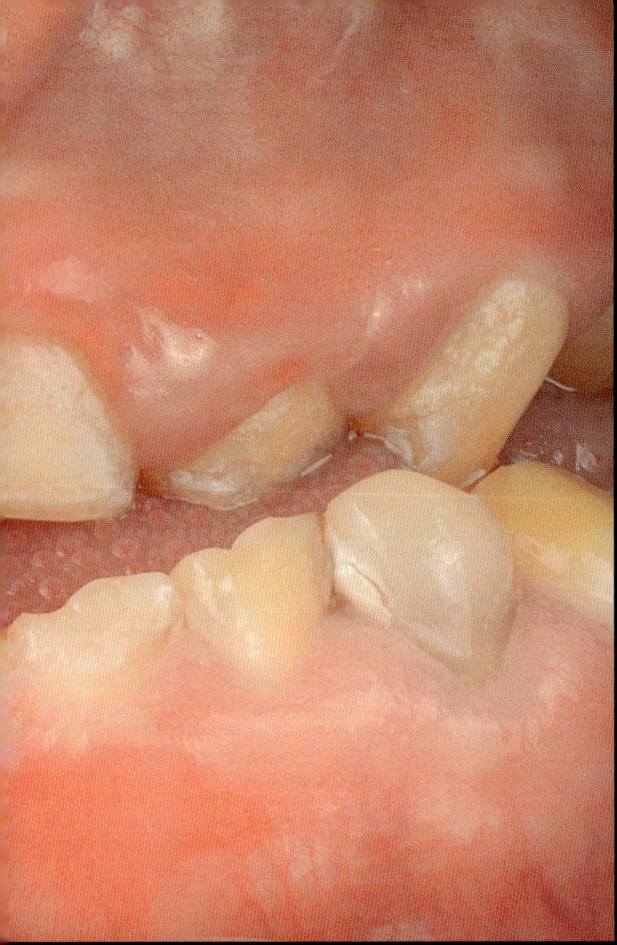
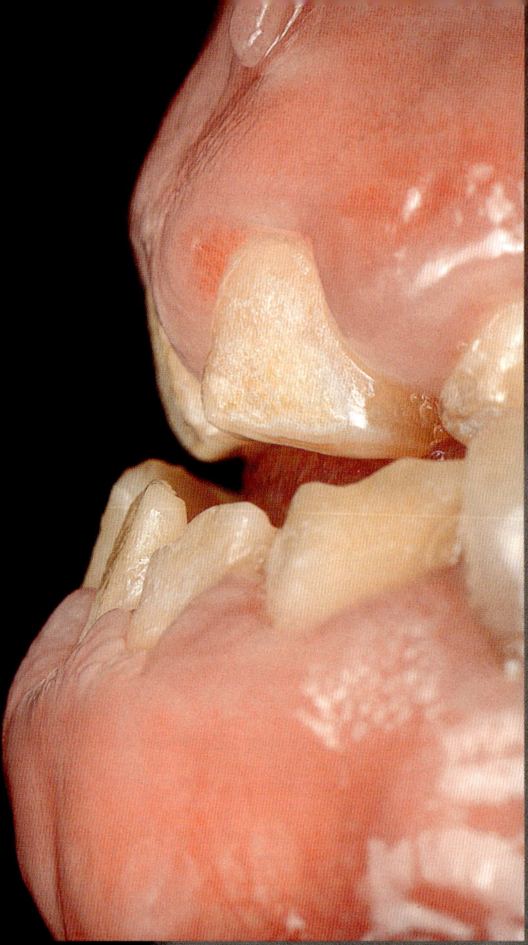
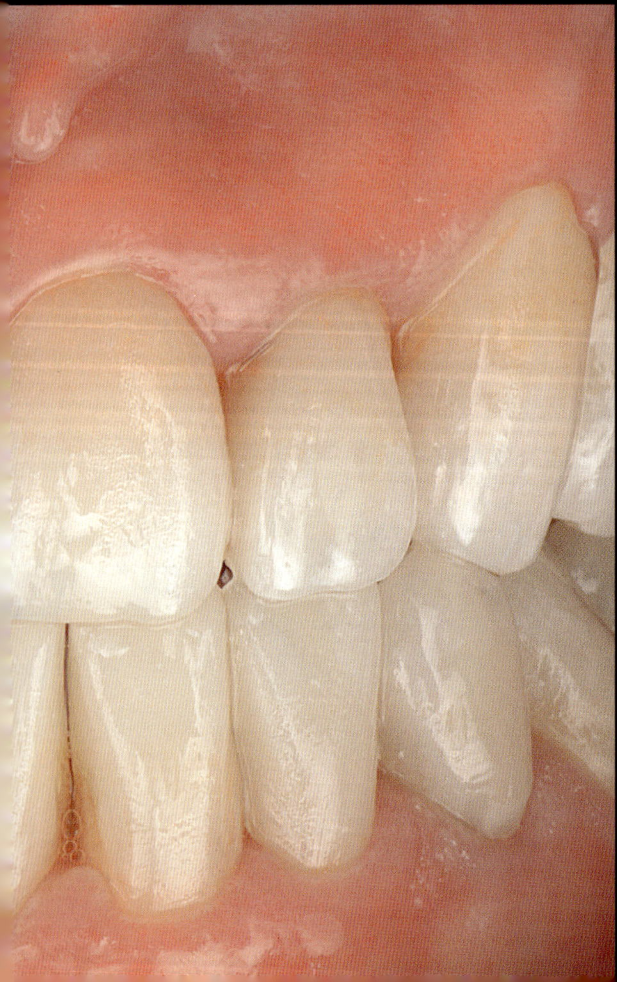
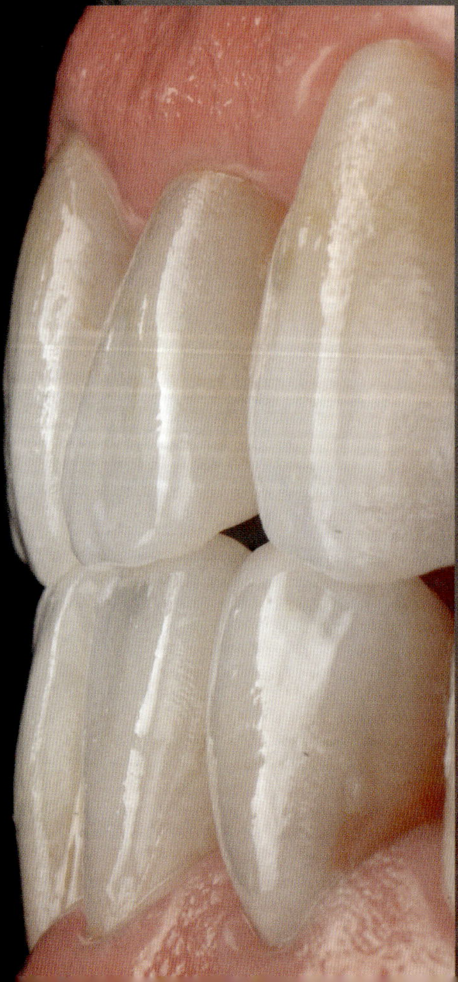

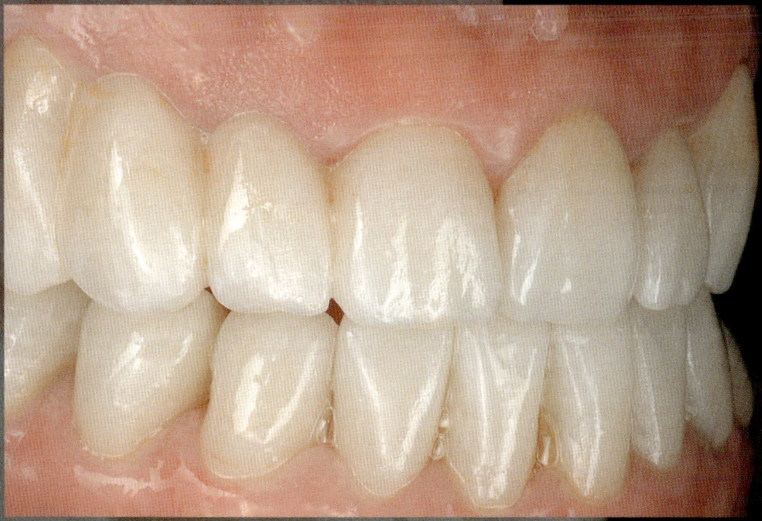
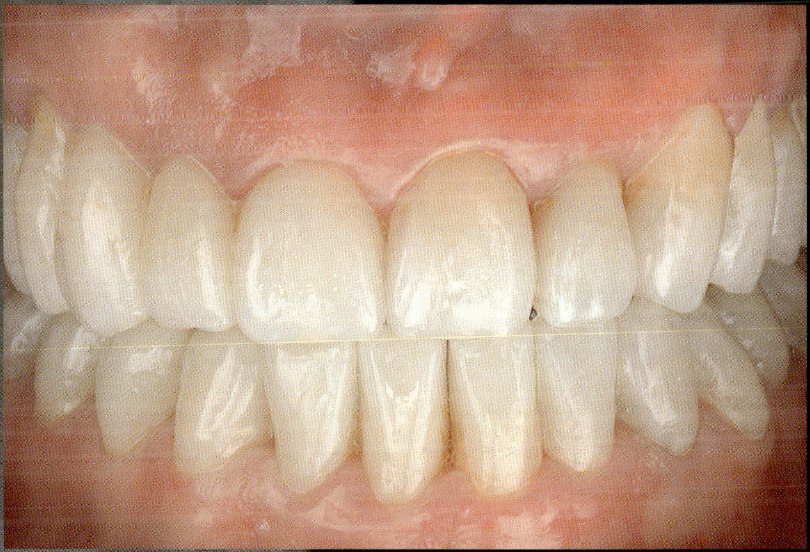
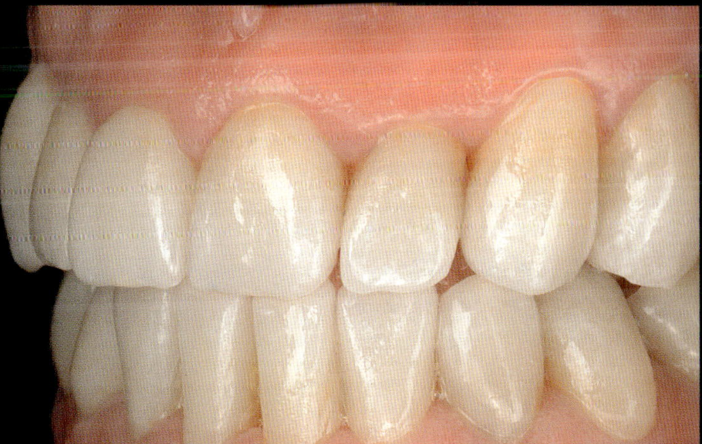

Right, frontal, and left views of the amelogenesis imperfecta teeth restored using nonpreparation monolithic CAD/CAM restorations.

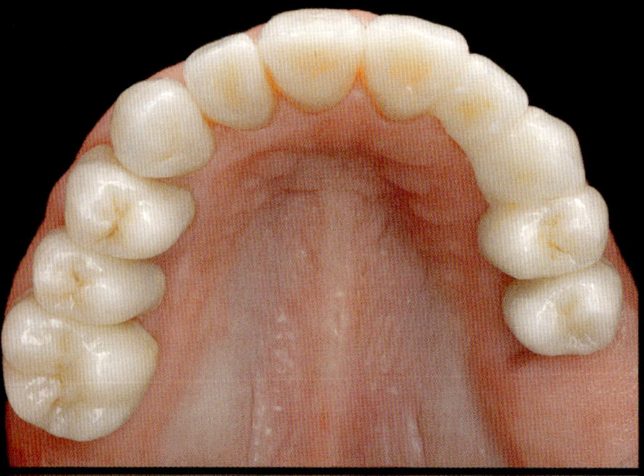

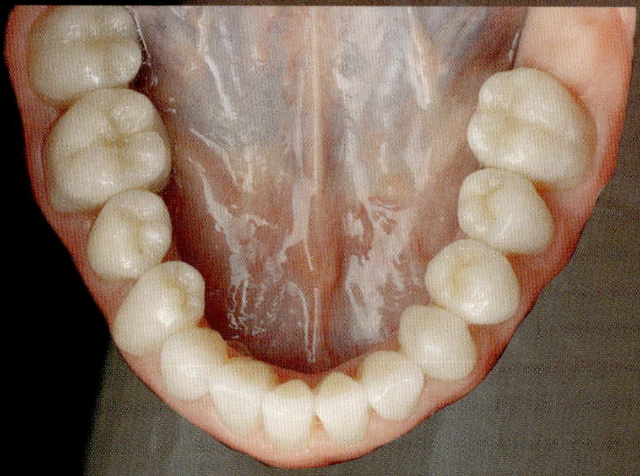

Postoperative view of maxillary and mandibular arches after adhesively luting the CAD/CAM restorations.

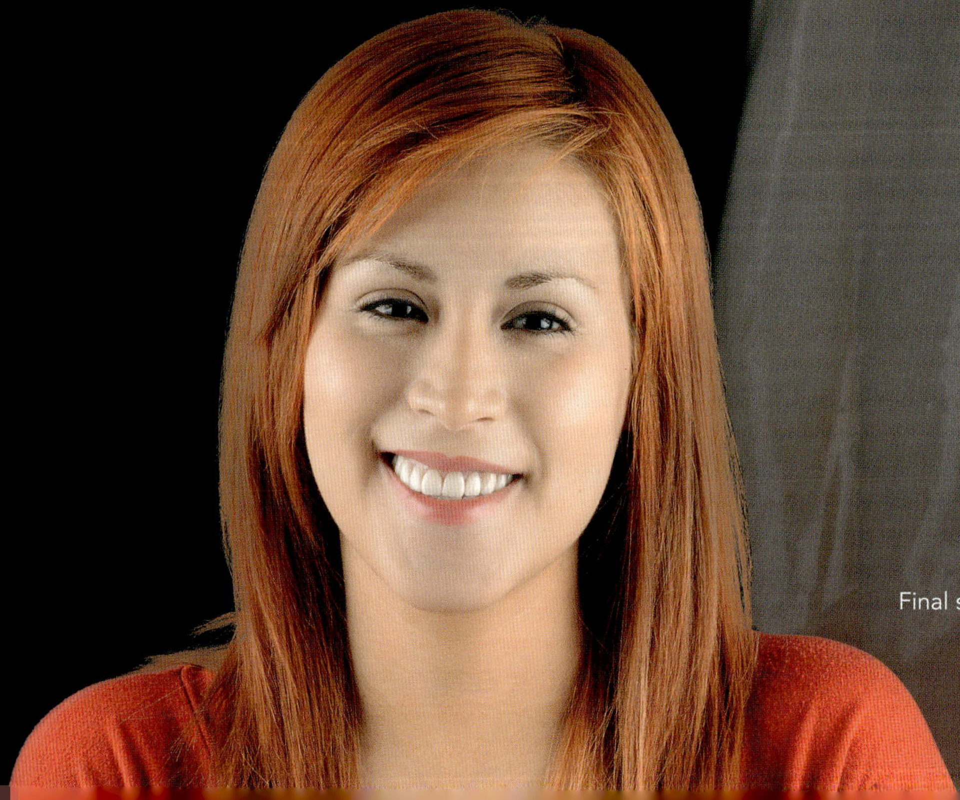

Final smile of the patient.

REFERENCES

1. Haselton DR, Diaz-Arnold AM, Hillis SL. Clinical assessment of high-strength all-ceramic crowns. J Prosthet Dent 2000;83:396–401.
2. El-Meliegy E, van Noort R. Glasses and Glass Ceramics for Medical Applications. New York: Springer, 2012.
3. Denry I, Kelly JR. Emerging ceramic-based materials for dentistry. J Dent Res 2014;93:1235–1242.
4. Anusavice KJ. Phillips' Science of Dental Materials. St. Louis: Elsevier, 2013.
5. Guess PC, Selz CF, Steinhart YN, Stampf S, Strub JR. Prospective clinical split-mouth study of pressed and CAD/CAM all-ceramic partial-coverage restorations: 7-year results. Int J Prosthodont 2013;26:21–25.
6. Höland W, Schweiger M, Frank M, Rheinberger V. A comparison of the microstructure and properties of the IPS Empress 2 and the IPS Empress glass-ceramics. J Biomed Mater Res 2000;53:297–303.
7. Schultheis S, Strub JR, Gerds TA, Guess PC. Monolithic and bilayer CAD/CAM lithium-disilicate versus metal-ceramic fixed dental prostheses: Comparison of fracture loads and failure modes after fatigue. Clin Oral Investig 2013;17:1407–1413.
8. Valenti M, Valenti A. Retrospective survival analysis of 261 lithium disilicate crowns in a private general practice. Quintessence Int 2009;40:573–579.
9. Taskonak B, Sertgoz A. Two-year clinical evaluation of lithia-disilicate-based all-ceramic crowns and fixed partial dentures. Dent Mater 2006;22:1008–1013.
10. Marquardt P, Strub JR. Survival rates of IPS empress 2 all-ceramic crowns and fixed partial dentures: Results of a 5-year prospective clinical study. Quintessence Int 2006;37:253–259.
11. IPS e.max Scientific Documentation. Ivoclar-Vivadent, 2009.
12. Kern M, Sasse M, Wolfart S. Ten-year outcome of three-unit fixed dental prostheses made from monolithic lithium disilicate ceramic. J Am Dent Assoc 2012;143:234–240.
13. Hench LL, Day DE, Holand W, Rheinberger VM. Glass and medicine. Int J Appl Glass Sci 2010;1:104–117.
14. Höland W, Apel E, vant't Hoen C. Studies of crystal phase formations in high-strength lithium disilicate glass-ceramics. J Non-Cryst Solids 2006;352:4041–4050.
15. Stookey SD. Catalyzed crystallization of glass in theory and practice. Ind Eng Chem 1959;51:805–808.
16. Höland W, Beall GH; American Ceramic Society. Glass-Ceramic Technology, ed 2. Hoboken: Wiley, 2012.
17. Monmaturapoj N, Lawita P, Thepsuwan W. Characterisation and properties of lithium disilicate glass ceramics in the SiO_2-Li_2O-K_2O-Al_2O_3 system for dental applications. Adv Mater Science Eng 2013;2013:1–11.
18. Goharian P, Nemati A, Shabanian M, Afshar A. Properties, crystallization mechanism and microstructure of lithium disilicate glass-ceramic. J Non-Cryst Solids 2010;356:208–214.
19. Höland W, Beall GH; American Ceramic Society. Composition systems for glass-ceramics. In: Glass-Ceramic Technology, ed 2. Hoboken: Wiley, 2012:75–206.
20. Tulyaganov DU, Agathopoulos S, Kansal I, Valério P, Ribeiro MJ, Ferreira JMF. Synthesis and properties of lithium disilicate glass-ceramics in the system SiO_2-Al_2O_3-K_2O-Li_2O. Ceram Int 2009;35:3013–3019.
21. Beall GH. Glass-ceramics: Recent development and application. Ceram Trans 1993;30:241–266.
22. Beall GN. Design of glass-ceramics. Solid State Sci 1989;3:333–354.
23. Headley TJ, Loehman RE. Crystallization of a glass-ceramic by epitaxial growth. J Am Ceram Soc 1984;67:620–625.
24. Apel E, Hoen C, Rheinberger V, Höland W. Influence of ZrO_2 on the crystallization and properties of lithium disilicate glass-ceramics derived from a multi-component system. J Eur Ceram Soc 2007;27:1571–1577.
25. Höland W, Schweiger M, Watzke R, Peschke A, Kappert H. Ceramics as biomaterials for dental restoration. Expert Rev Med Devices 2008;5:729–745.
26. Guess PC, Schultheis S, Bonfante EA, Coelho PG, Ferencz JL, Silva NRFA. All-ceramic systems: Laboratory and clinical performance. Dent Clin of North Am 2011;55:333.
27. Denry I, Kelly JR. Emerging ceramic-based materials for dentistry. J Dent Res 2014;93:1235–1242.
28. Krüger S, Deubener J, Ritzberger C, Höland W. Nucleation kinetics of lithium metasilicate in ZrO_2-bearing lithium disilicate glasses for dental application. Int J Adv Glass Sci 2013;4:9–19.
29. VITA Suprinity: Technical and Scientific Documentation. VITA Zahnfabrik, 2013.
30. Durschang B, Probst J, Thiel N, Bibus J, Vollmann M, Schusser U [inventors]. Fraunhofer-Gesellschaft, Degudent, Vita Zahnfabrik, assignees. Lithium disilicate glass-ceramic, method for production thereof and use thereof. US patent application 20120309607 A1, 6 December 2012.
31. Celtra Duo. Dentsply, 2013.
32. Park S, Quinn JB, Romberg E, Arola D. On the brittleness of enamel and selected dental materials. Dent Mater 2008;24: 1477–1485.
33. Bechtle S, Habelitz S, Klocke A, Fett T, Schneider GA. The fracture behaviour of dental enamel. Biomaterials 2010;31:375–384.
34. Bechtle S, Ozcoban H, Lilleodden ET, et al. Hierarchical flexural strength of enamel: Transition from brittle to damage-tolerant behaviour. J R Soc Interface 2012;9:1265–1274.
35. Ziskind D, Hasday M, Cohen SR, Wagner HD. Young's modulus of peritubular and intertubular human dentin by nano-indentation tests. J Struct Biol 2011;174:23–30.
36. Yan J, Taskonak B, Mecholsky JJ Jr. Fractography and fracture toughness of human dentin. J Mech Behav Biomed Mater 2009, 2:478–484.
37. Plotino G, Grande NM, Bedini R, Pameijer CH, Somma F. Flexural properties of endodontic posts and human root dentin. Dent Mater 2007;23:1129–1135.
38. Rey Duro F, Souza Andrade J, Duarte Jr S. Fluorescence. Clinical evaluation of new composite resins. Quintessence Dent Technol 2012;35:145–156.
39. Duarte Jr S, Phark J-H, Blatz M, Sadan A. Ceramic systems: An ultrastructural study. Quintessence Dent Technol 2010;33:42–60.

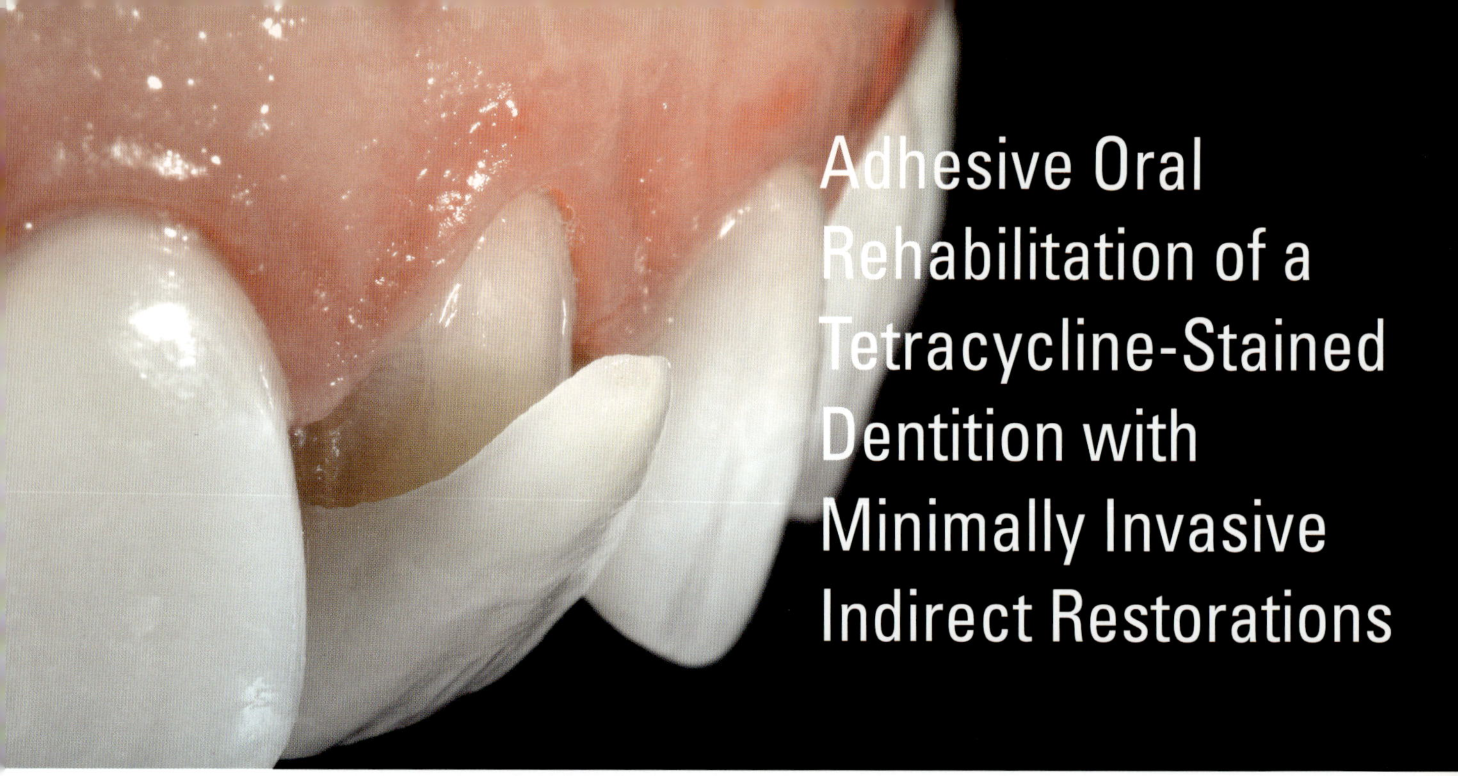

Adhesive Oral Rehabilitation of a Tetracycline-Stained Dentition with Minimally Invasive Indirect Restorations

Oswaldo Scopin de Andrade, DDS, MS, PhD[1]
Messias Rodrigues, DDS, MS[2]
Ronaldo Hirata, DDS, MS, PhD[3]
Luiz Alves Ferreira, CDT[4]

The evolution of materials science has allowed the use of adhesive procedures even in patients requiring complex oral rehabilitation.[1–5] Currently, invasive tooth preparations that remove excessive enamel and dentinal structure are being gradually replaced by adhesive dentistry concepts, even in fixed prosthodontics.[5,6] However, in patients exhibiting a severely discolored dentition, clinicians and technicians face problems in applying these concepts, established and documented in the scientific literature, because most of those conservative techniques are designed for teeth with minor color alterations.

For the severely discolored dentition, traditional restorative dentistry has had limitations—such as those seen in earlier concepts of ceramic build-up in which many layers of material were necessary to mask the discoloration, requiring the removal of more tooth structure. This invasive preparation may expose more dentin, increasing the chance of postoperative sensitivity and jeopardizing clinical longevity. Moreover, depending on the approach and ceramic selection, the esthetic result sometimes may not satisfy the patient or dentist. With the evolution of ceramic materials, it is now possible to fabricate thin restorations that mask tooth discoloration and have bonded characteristics.[7,8] Lithium disilicate glass ceramic (LDGC) can be used in monolithic form, or it can be reduced followed by a veneering build-up with a fluorapatite-based ceramic.[9,10] This type of ceramic can be etched and silanized for

[1]Director, Advanced Program in Implant and Esthetic Dentistry, Senac University, São Paulo, Brazil.

[2]Assistant Professor, Orthodontics, School of Dentistry, UNITAU, Taubaté, São Paulo, Brazil.

[3]Assistant Professor, Biomaterials and Biomimetics, New York University College of Dentistry, New York, New York, USA.

[4]Dental Technician and Ceramist, Specialized Dental Laboratory, São Paulo, Brazil.

Correspondence to: Dr.Oswaldo Scopin de Andrade, Rua Barão de Piracicamirim 889 #61, Piracicaba-SP-Brazil, CEP 13.416-005. Email: osda@terra.com.br

bonding to tooth structure.[11] The use of a ceramic with adhesive characteristics and a range of options for fabricating the restoration allows the dentist and ceramist to preserve sound tooth structure.[12]

The purpose of this article is to present a clinical case highlighting specific topics in applying the adhesive oral rehabilitation (AOR) concept in a severely discolored dentition.

CASE REPORT

A 46-year-old female patient presented to a private office with a complaint about esthetic aspects of her smile. The patient stated that she had been trying to solve her problem for years. She was aware that the color change of her teeth was caused by excessive intake of tetracycline during childhood. Another issue pointed out by the patient was that she never pursued any restorative treatment for fear that the excessive enamel preparation required for a ceramic material could reduce the lifespan of her natural dentition. So, for years she had been trying every type of bleaching technique available to improve her esthetics. At the time of her initial consultation, she realized that bleaching was no longer an option and she requested a prosthetic treatment, emphasizing that the damage to her natural dentition should be minimal.

Diagnostic and Initial Approach

The initial clinical examination included intraoral analysis of occlusion, periodontal health, and preexisting restorations, plus digital radiography and photography. Clinical examination showed that the patient had a gummy smile; however, the patient's major concern was only the color of her teeth. She reported previous orthodontic treatment to improve tooth alignment. The photographs showed important details necessary to select the best treatment option for the patient. Several initial photographs were taken to analyze various aspects of the dentition:

- Lips in resting position—the anterior tooth display (Fig 1a)
- Discrete smile—initial tooth display (Fig 1b)
- Frontal forced smile—total tooth display in frontal view (Fig 1c)
- Lateral forced smile—total tooth display in both lateral views (Figs 1d and 1e)
- Photographs with lip retractor—details about periodontal architecture and general anatomy
- Facial photograph—teeth in relation to face

A polyvinyl siloxane (PVS) impression material was selected to produce the initial study cast. This material was selected because it is a very precise material that allows the technician to obtain more than one cast from the same impression. The dental technician performed an initial additive wax-up[7,12] with no preparation of the teeth (Fig 2). By building an overcontoured anatomy, it was easy to analyze the initial requirements for the case; also, it allowed the clinician, ceramist, and patient to understand if, in this specific case, a conservative approach could be performed.

Because the patient had a high lip line and a gummy smile, no incisal lengthening or changing of the vertical dimension of occlusion (VDO) was planned. In planning an AOR, the ceramist should be made aware of such details by the clinician before the wax-up procedure. Because most of the initial planning is performed by additive procedures only, and no stone was prepared on the cast, no facebow record was taken or used in any phase of this case. The casts were mounted in a semiadjustable articulator based on initial patient photography. In cases of full-mouth rehabilitation, it is advisable to split the rehabilitation into steps, preserving references that facilitate recording the occlusion and mounting the articulator. For patients with no planned changes in VDO, the following clinical sequence is preferred:

1. Maxillary restorations, second premolar to second premolar
2. Mandibular restorations, second premolar to second premolar
3. First molar restorations, right side
4. First molar restorations, left side

Each area selected to be restored is completed before starting the contralateral side to allow total control and maintenance of the original VDO and occlusal pattern of the patient.

CASE REPORT

Figs 1a to 1e Initial photography sequence for treatment planning, showing adequate tooth display at resting position and the anatomy of the patient's smile.

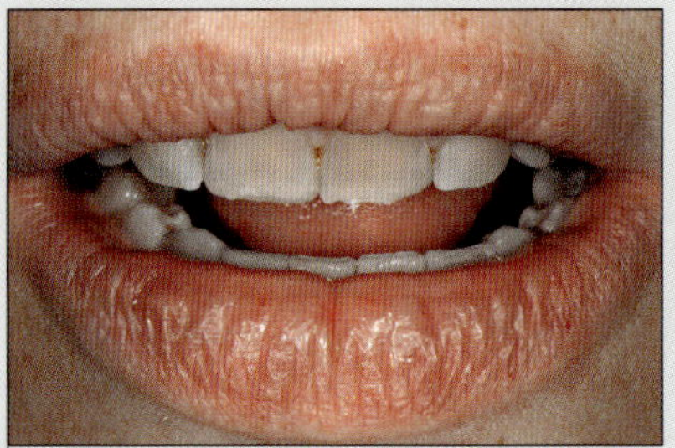
1a

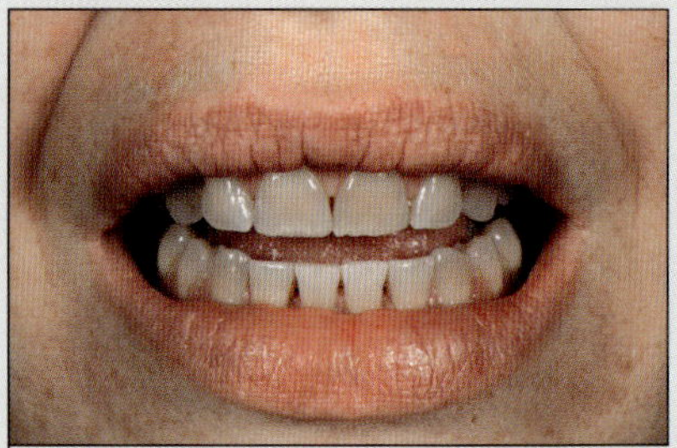
1b

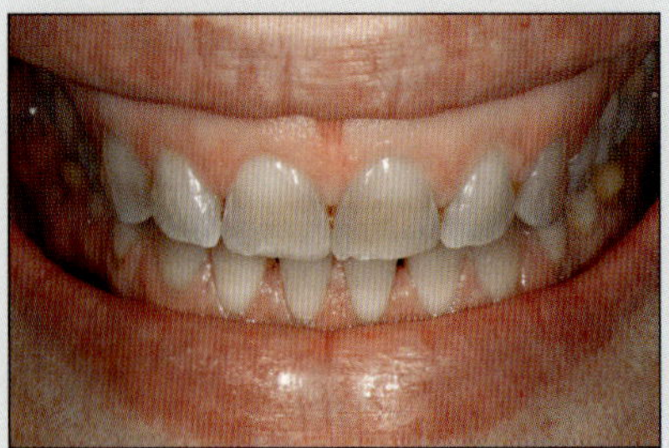
1c

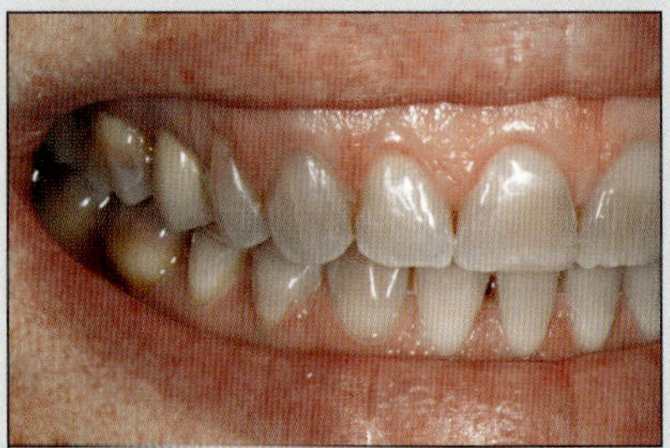
1d

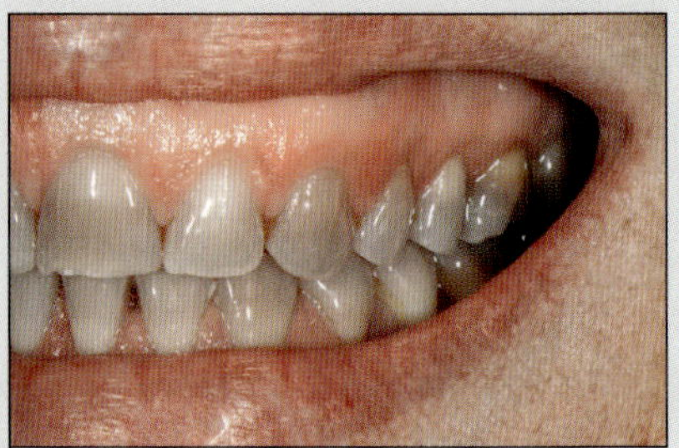
1e

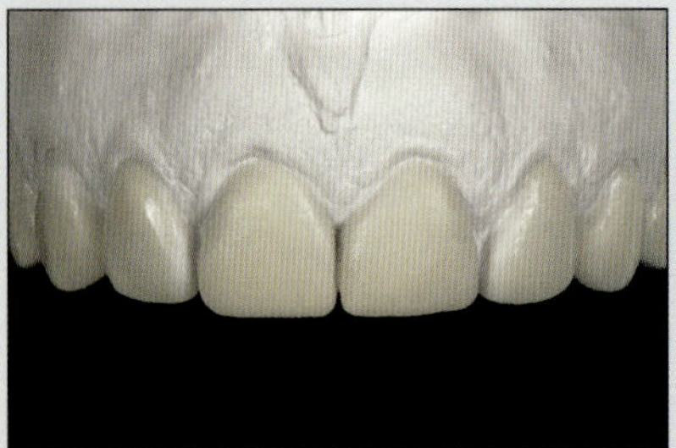
2a

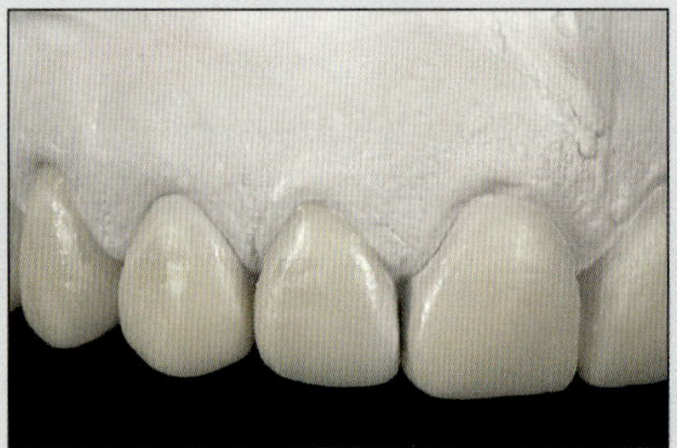
2b

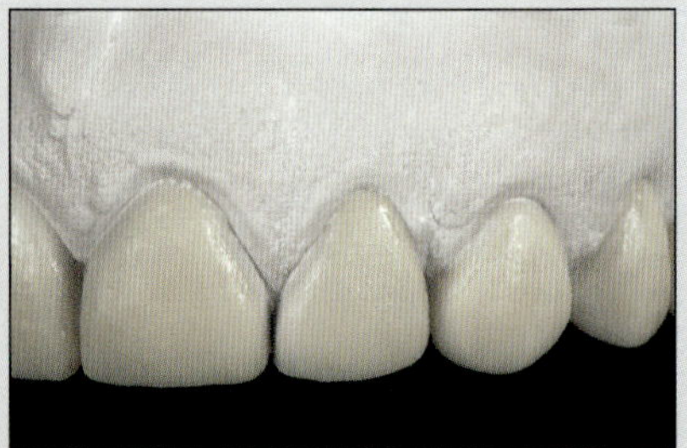
2c

Figs 2a to 2e Additive wax-up for the mock-up of the proposed treatment and evaluation of clinical and laboratory options.

Figs 2f and 2g Close-up views of the maxillary left canine: *(f)* after additive wax-up and *(g)* intact.

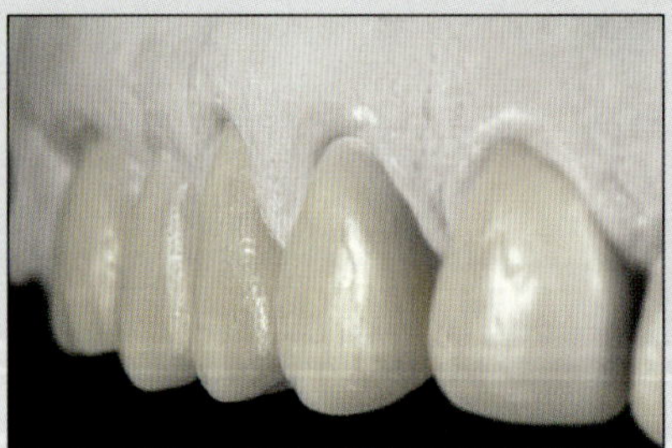
2d

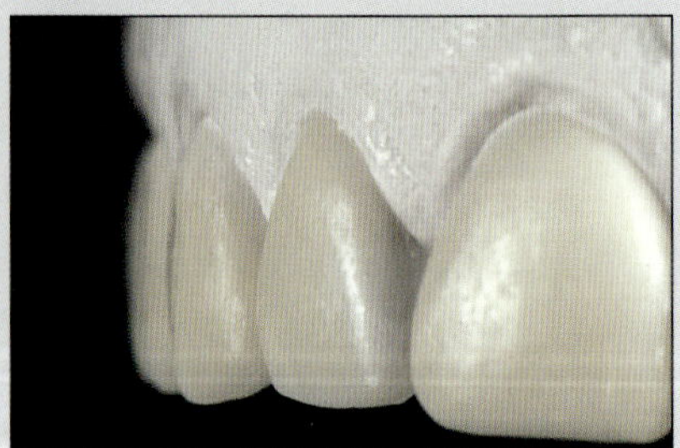
2e

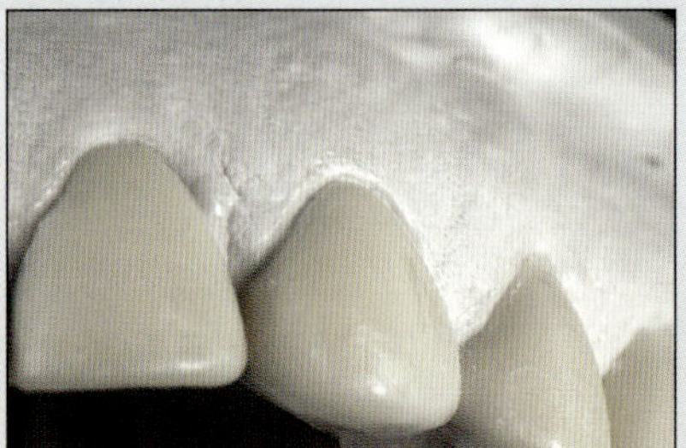
2f

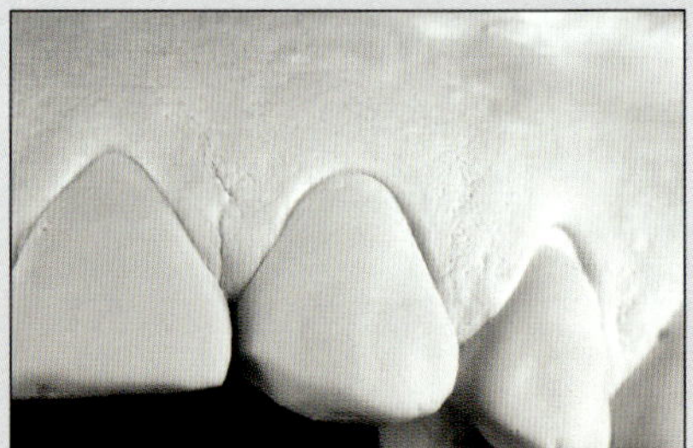
2g

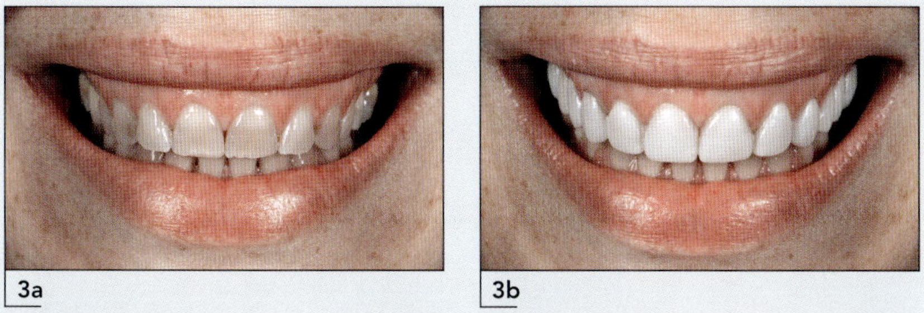

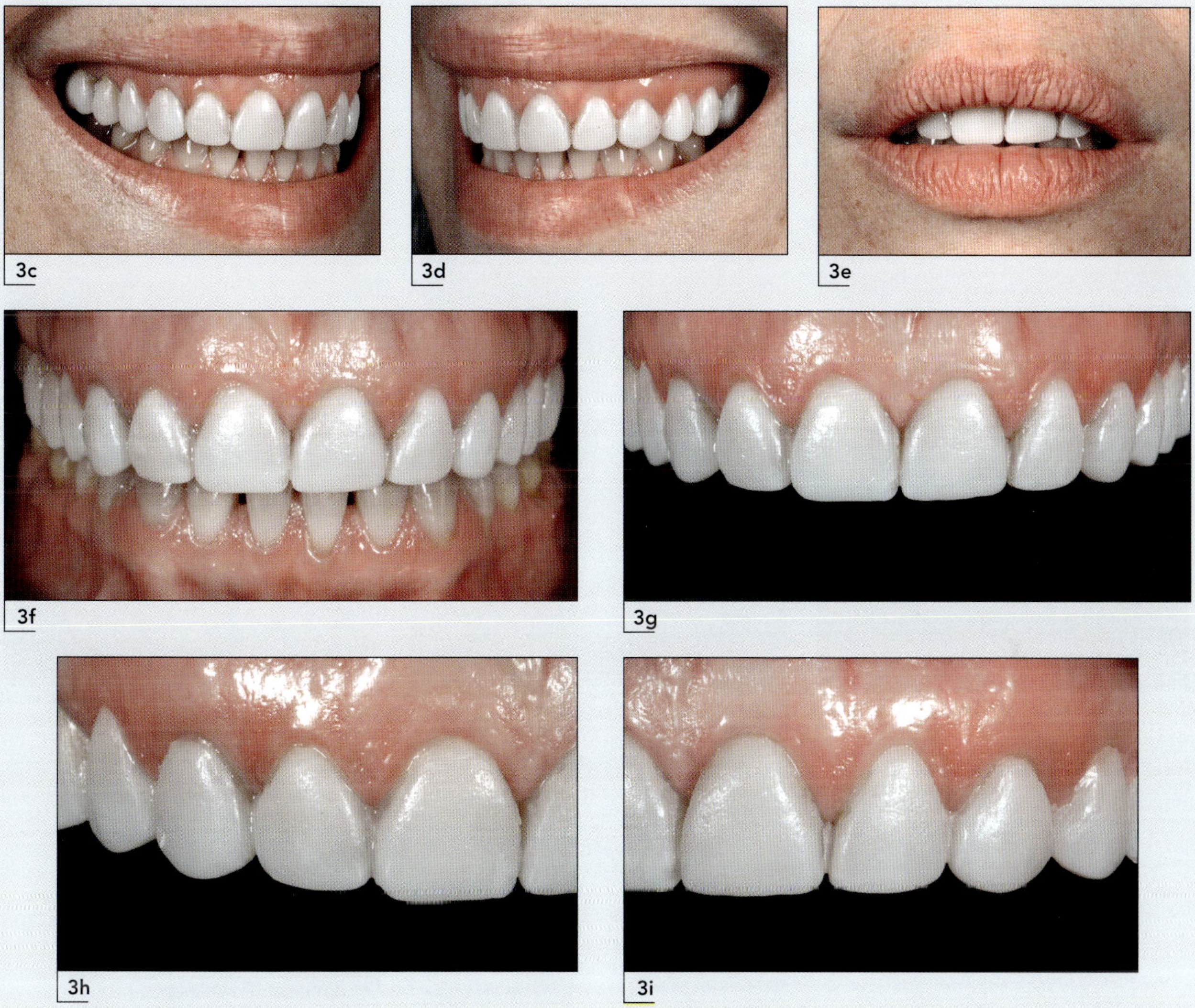

Figs 3a and 3b Frontal views of the patient's smile before and after the mock-up.

Figs 3c and 3d Lateral views of the smile with the mock-up in position.

Fig 3e Resting position with the mock-up in place.

Figs 3f to 3i Intraoral views of the mock-up.

Bis-acrylic Resin Direct Maxillary Mock-up

The initial wax-up was completed only for the maxillary arch, to analyze if it would be possible to perform a minimally invasive adhesive oral rehabilitation, as requested by the patient. A silicone index was fabricated on a duplicated cast of the wax-up. The reason was to preserve the initial wax-up. An intraoral mock-up of the initially proposed treatment was made with a bis-acrylic resin (Systemp II C&B, Ivoclar Vivadent). New photographs were taken, and the simulation was analyzed by the patient and clinician (Fig 3). In this initial phase of the treatment, it was important to discuss all possibilities and their clinical sequencing with the patient.

The patient approved the smile anatomy. Next, the bis-acrylic resin shells were carefully removed from the patient's mouth, trying to preserve each shell that sim-

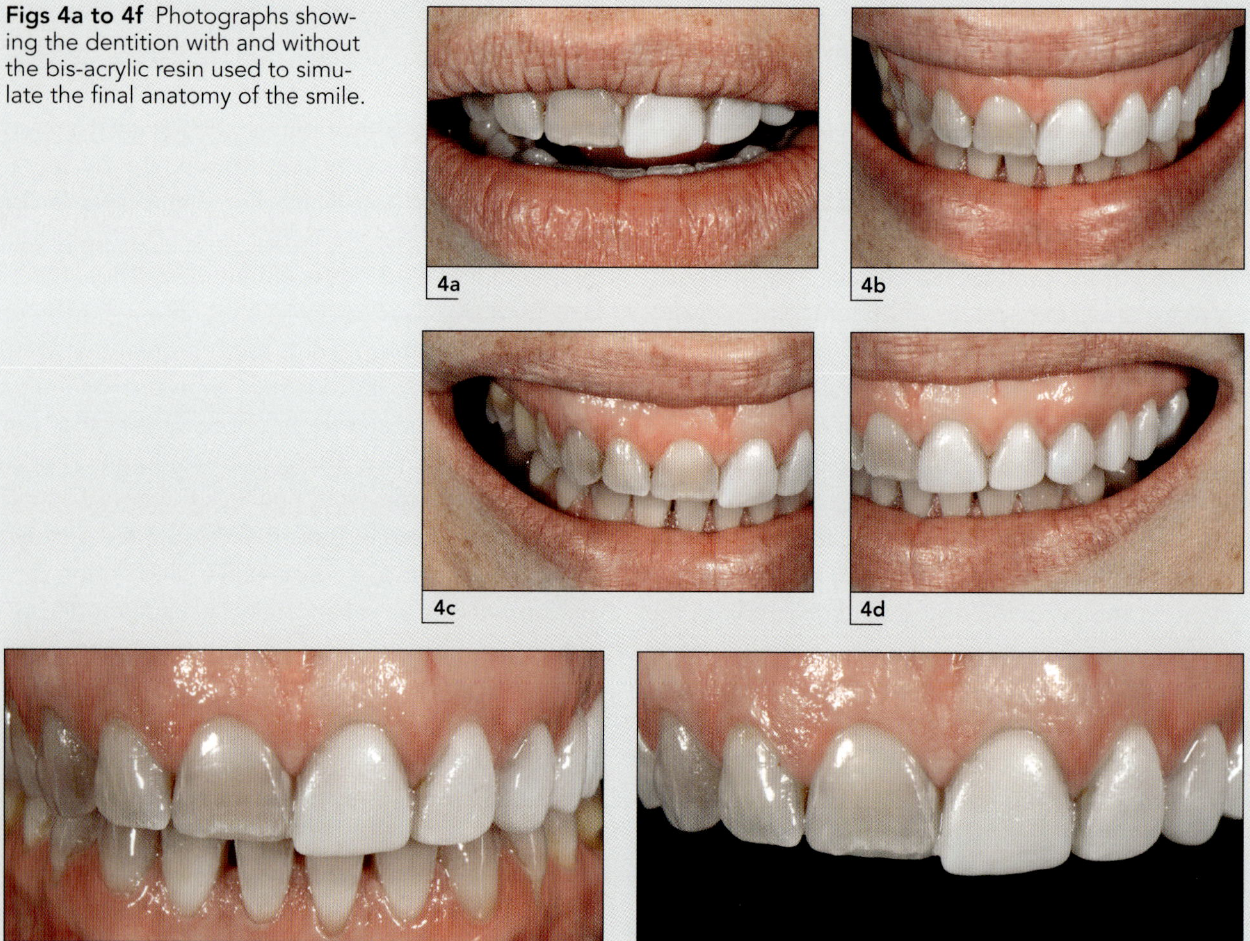

4a 4b 4c 4d 4e 4f

Figs 4a to 4f Photographs showing the dentition with and without the bis-acrylic resin used to simulate the final anatomy of the smile.

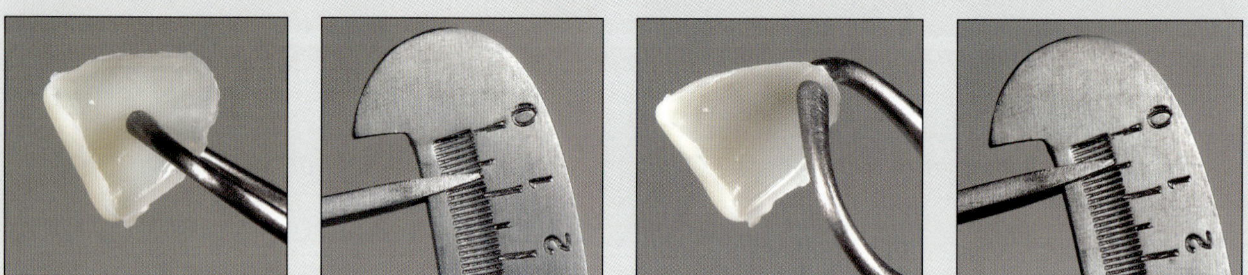

5a 5b 5c 5d

Figs 5a to 5d Measurement of the resin shell with a caliper. This information is utilized to predict the final thickness of the laminate veneer.

ulated the wax-up. An important set of photographs for explaining the treatment to the patient is the "half mock-up," in which the simulation is removed from one hemiarch so that the patient can easily see the difference (Fig 4). Each resin shell was measured in three different areas: cervical, middle, and close to the incisal edge. This information was used to analyze and predict the ceramic thickness required to block the discolored dentition (Fig 5). In this patient there was adequate space for ceramic material to make laminate veneers; however, as this was a case with severe discoloration, additional analysis had to be carried out before tooth preparation.

Prepreparation Ceramic Test

When space is available for the ceramic material, prior to tooth preparation a prepreparation evaluative test can be done. This test helps the ceramist to determine which ingot of LDGC should be pressed and also orients the clinician to which areas may require tooth preparation.

The laboratory sent to the clinician, in this case, two laminate veneers made in lithium disilicate (IPS e.max Press, Ivoclar Vivadent) in two different shades (Fig 6). For the maxillary right central incisor, a low-translucency bleach (LT B1) ingot was used, and for the left central incisor, a high-translucency bleach (HT BL3) ingot was used. This "ceramic mock-up" is an important tool for conservative tooth preparation. The role of this test was to allow the clinician to analyze prior to preparation the potential of the material to block the dark shade of the tooth substrate. The communication between clinician and ceramist is extremely important; therefore, before tooth preparation, the ceramist performed a digital photography analysis and suggested that interproximal preparation would be necessary for a better esthetic result and more natural optical characteristics.

Maxillary Tooth Preparations

Even in a severely discolored dentition, a conservative approach is indicated to preserve enamel as much as possible. Three important factors should be analyzed prior to tooth reduction to determine the need for and amount of reduction.[13]

1. *Space and thickness of the final restoration.* This was confirmed during the mock-up session by measuring the thickness of the bis-acrylic resin shell of each tooth. LDGC was the material selected for this patient because it allows the fabrication of pressed laminate veneers with thicknesses between 0.3 and 0.5 mm, providing durability and lifelike esthetics.
2. *Shade and color modification.* This was inspected and evaluated during the prepreparation ceramic test. The ceramic mock-ups were made from two different ceramic ingots.
3. *Path of insertion.* This is determined so that tooth reduction will be limited to that which permits the insertion of the restoration onto the tooth preparation.

During the mock-up session it was possible to analyze and check the thickness of the final anatomy. Note that there was no need to prepare the teeth on the basis of the first factor. For the second factor, it was confirmed that, for better esthetics, interproximal preparation would be recommended. Thus, the final and third step was to define and determine the path of insertion. In this patient, tooth preparation was restricted to controlled enamel removal of identifiable areas with ridges and surface irregularities that would restrict the insertion of the final restoration, because the first two factors were previously checked and analyzed before tooth reduction. If these three factors are carefully evaluated, a conservative preparation can be performed even in cases of severe shade modification. Another important issue is that there was no need to place the preparation inside the gingival sulcus; in healthy periodontal tissue it is always preferable to preserve the original and natural gingival architecture.

The final tooth preparations from canine to canine are shown in Fig 7. The maxillary right second premolar had a previously placed porcelain-fused-to-metal crown that was removed; a zirconia-based crown was planned because of the presence of a metal post and core that could not be removed. Following tooth preparation, impression procedures were carried out with a PVS material (Virtual, Ivoclar Vivadent).

Final Shade Selection for the Maxillary Teeth

Even when the prepreparation ceramic test has been performed, it is important to reposition the selected ceramic mock-up, which is a try-in restoration, onto the prepared tooth and to retake digital photographs (Fig 8a). For this patient, the ceramist recommended taking photographs of the tooth substrate shade (Fig 8b) and the final desired shade (Fig 8c).

Provisional Restorations

For cases involving laminate veneers, delivery of an adequate provisional restoration is always a challenge.[9]

Fig 6 Two laminate veneers made prior to tooth preparation for the prepreparation ceramic test.

Figs 7a to 7c Final preparations for ceramic laminate veneers, canine to canine.

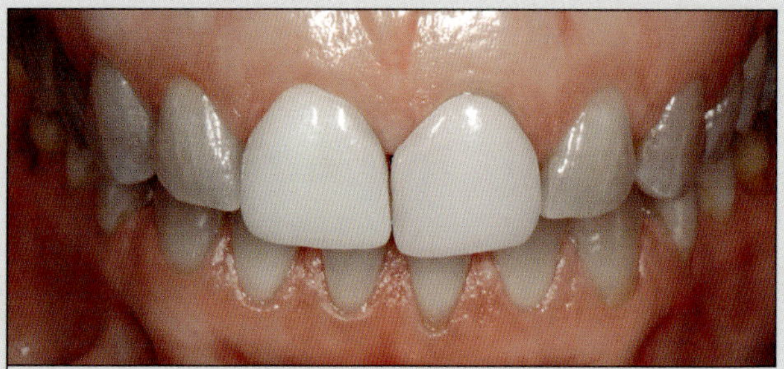

6

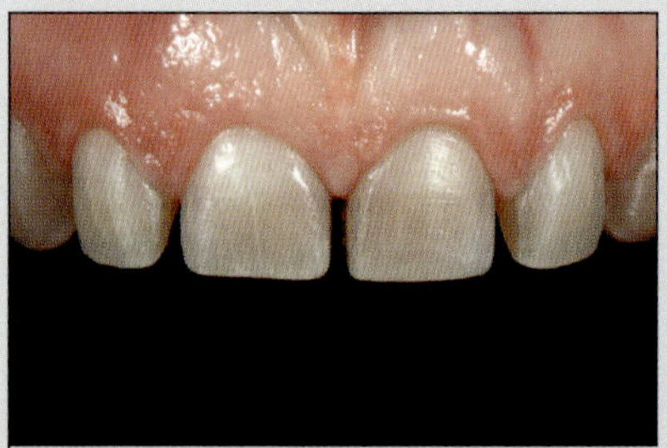

7a

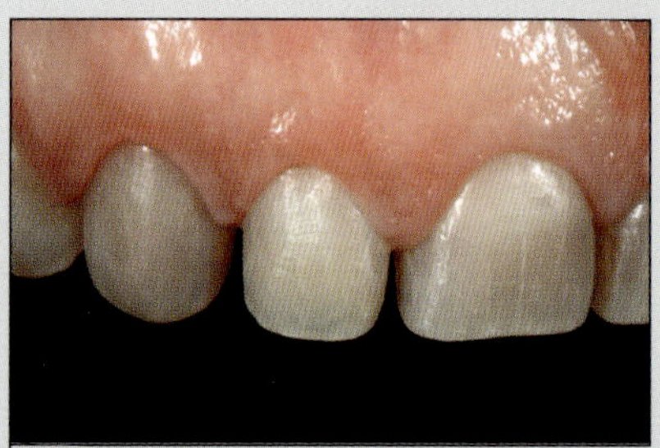

7b

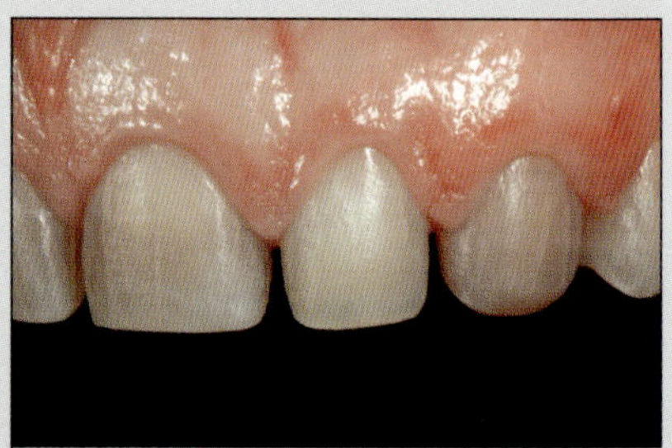

7c

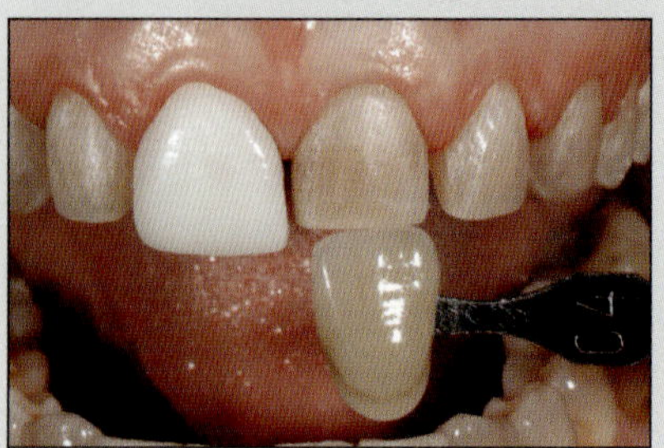

8a

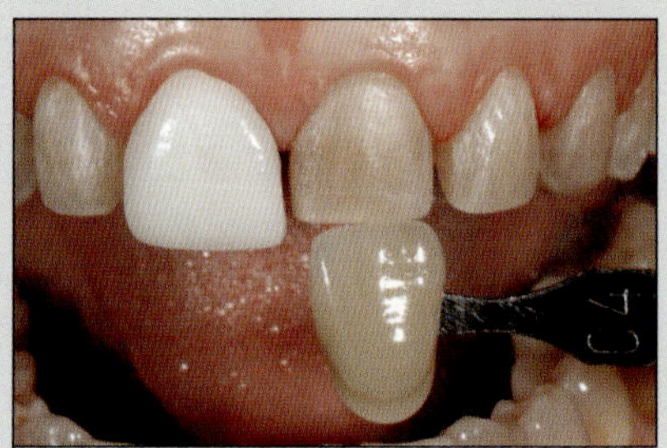

8b

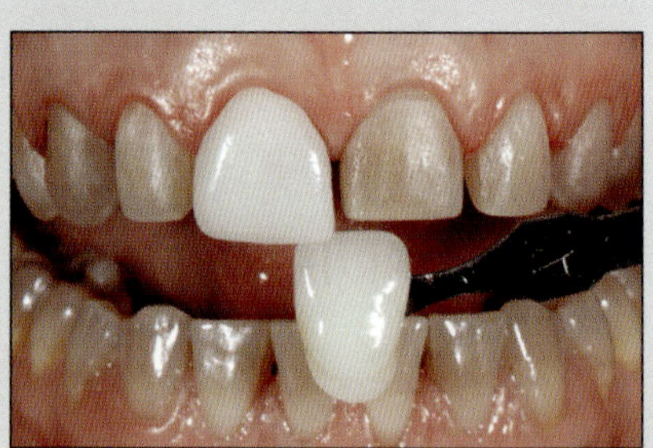

8c

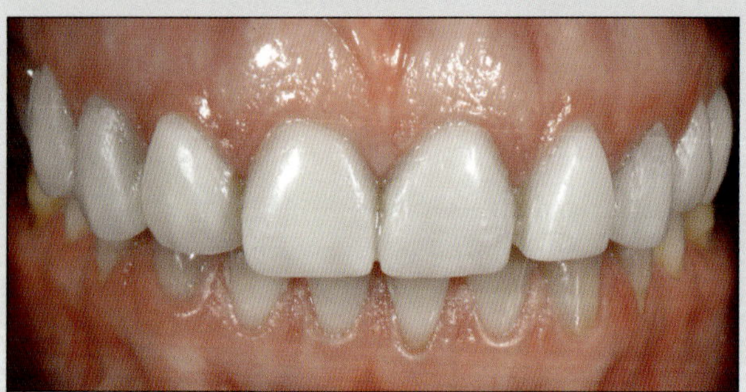

9a

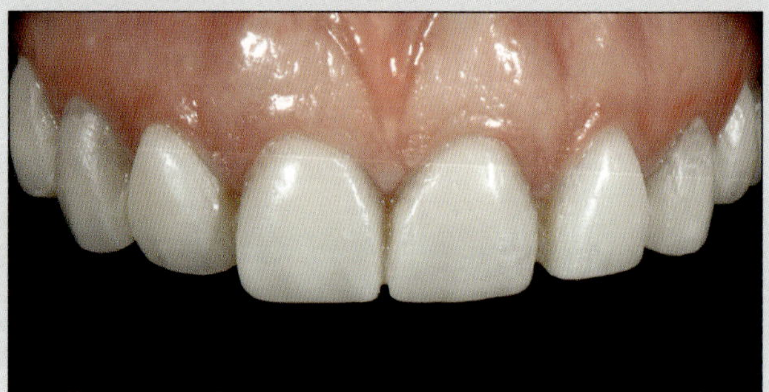

9b

Fig 8a Selected IPS e.max Press ingot (LT B1) in position after tooth preparation.

Figs 8b and 8c Photographs with the Vita Shade guide of the tooth substrate and the desired shade.

Figs 9a and 9b Intraoral view of the acrylic resin provisionals after being luted and polished.

In a discolored dentition, highly esthetic provisional restorations become a more difficult task. When adequate space is present, the authors prefer to utilize conventional acrylic resin provisionals made at the laboratory. The restorations were made as sets of two splinted provisionals: first and second premolar, canine and lateral incisor, and two central incisors. After being relined, finished, and polished, the provisionals were luted with light-curing resin cement (Variolink Veneer, Ivoclar Vivadent) (Fig 9). Tooth preparations were restricted to enamel, and, to facilitate removal of the provisional, no etching or adhesive was applied to the teeth. Retention was achieved by mechanical retention of the relined acrylic resin and the resin cement.

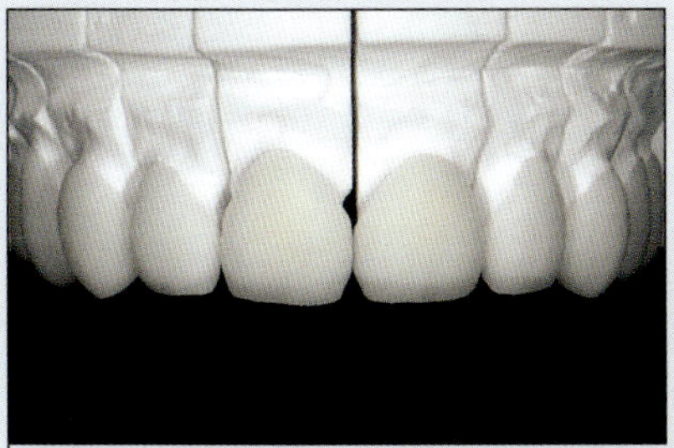

10a

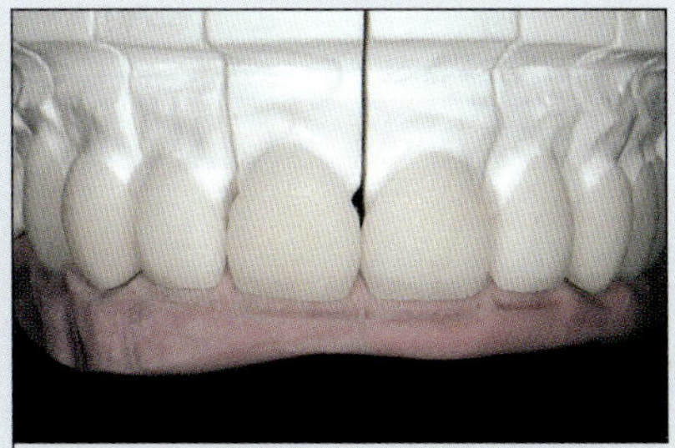

10b

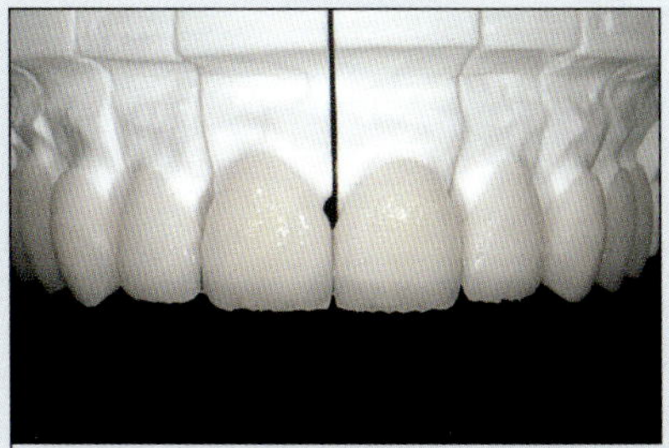

10c

Fig 10a IPS e.max Press core made in shade LT B1 ready to be veneered.

Figs 10b and 10c Initial ceramic stratification with IPS e.max Ceram.

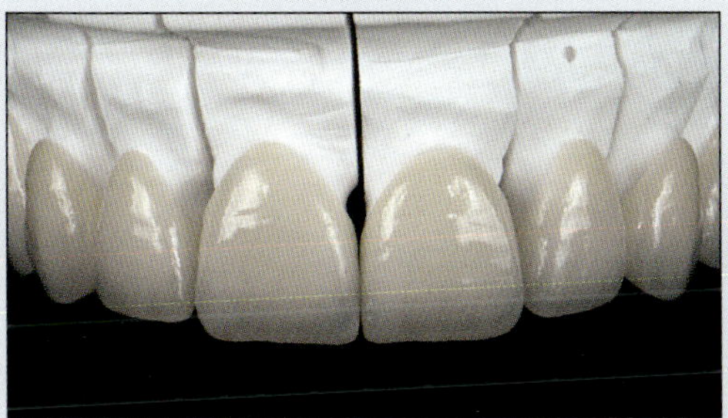

11a

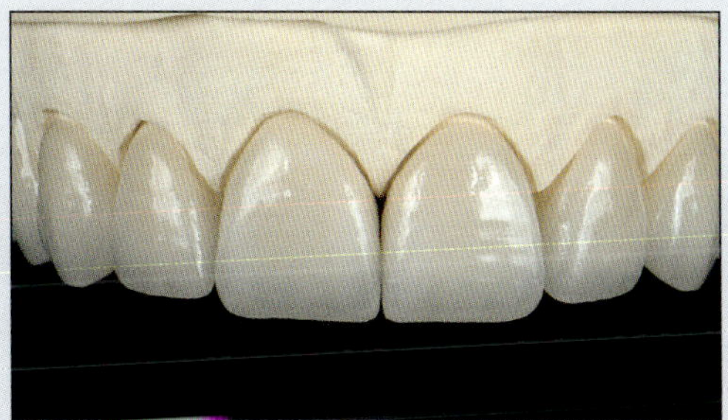

11b

Figs 11a and 11b Definitive restorations fitted and adjusted on both casts.

Laboratory Procedures

The impressions were sent to the ceramist. At the laboratory, two casts were made to develop the definitive restorations. IPS e.max Press LT B1 ingots had been selected previously during the planning phase. The ingots were pressed to produce the cores (Fig 10a), which were reduced and layered with a fluorapatite-based ceramic (Figs 10b and 10c) that is compatible with LDGC. The current trend is to work only with monolithic LDGC, which is then stained. However, the fluorescence of this material in the monolithic approach is only obtained with a special glaze (FLUO Glaze Paste, Ivoclar Vivadent), which may be removed during intraoral polishing, changing its optical and esthetic characteristics. Therefore, if there is space available, as detected in the planning phase, the authors always prefer to layer the lithium disilicate core with a compatible ceramic (IPS e.max Ceram, Ivoclar Vivadent), which improves esthetics and optical long-term results. The definitive ceramic laminate veneers were checked on both casts for gingival contour, marginal adaptation, and interproximal contacts (Fig 11).

Try-in and Bonding Procedures for Definitive Maxillary Restorations

The soft tissue was healthy enough after 2 weeks for definitive bonding. The well-adapted provisionals were easy to clean as a result of the careful and precise tooth preparation, which preserved enamel and positioned the finish lines at the level of the gingival crevice (Fig 12). After removal of the provisional restorations, the tooth surfaces were cleaned with pumice and water (Fig 13). Next, each individual laminate veneer was checked for marginal adaptation and interproximal contacts (Fig 14). A try-in paste was used to select the best shade of resin cement. A high-value light-curing resin cement shade (Variolink Veneer +1, Ivoclar Vivadent) was selected for final bonding. After esthetic approval by the patient, the laminate veneers were prepared for bonding. The intaglio surface was etched with 9% hydrofluoric acid for 20 seconds. The etched surfaces were rinsed and cleaned with 35% phosphoric acid for 10 seconds. The veneers were once more rinsed and air dried. A silane coupling agent was applied for 2 minutes and dried. The intaglio surfaces

Figs 12a and 12b Maxillary right central and lateral incisors immediately after provisional removal.

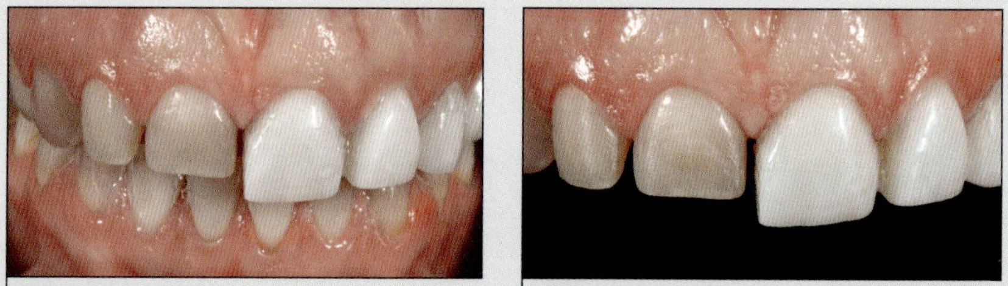

12a 12b

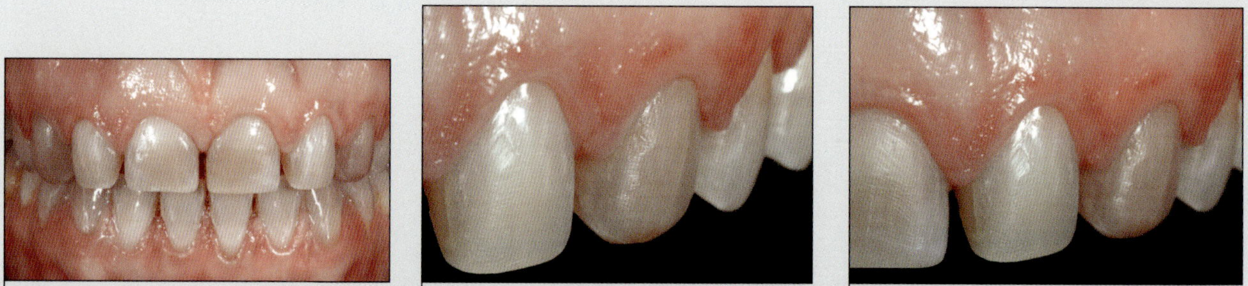

13a 13b 13c

Figs 13a to 13c Frontal and close-up views after provisional removal. Note the quality and health of the gingival tissue.

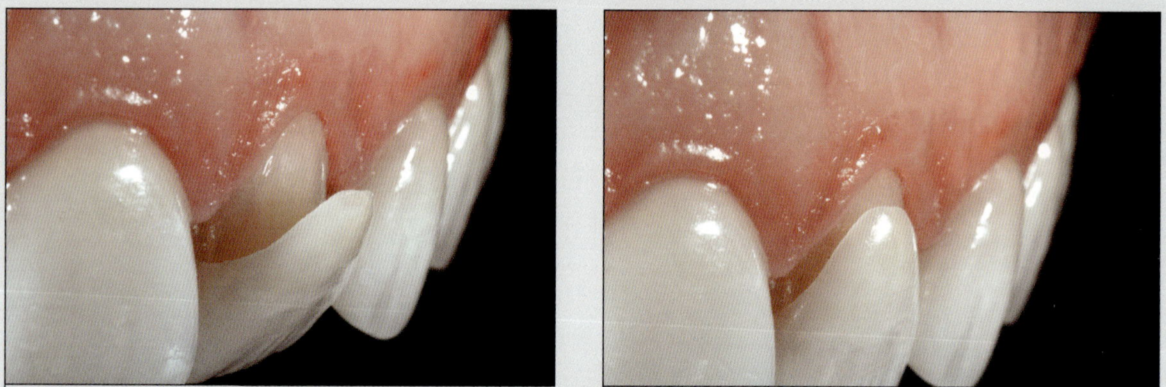

14a 14b

Figs 14a to 14c Close-up views of the insertion of the laminate veneer on the left lateral incisor.

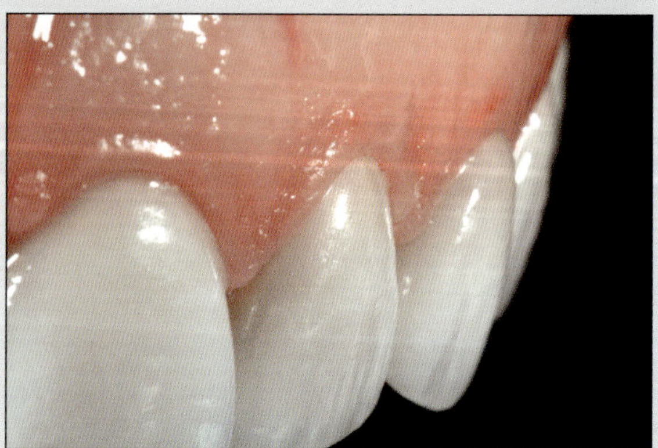

14c

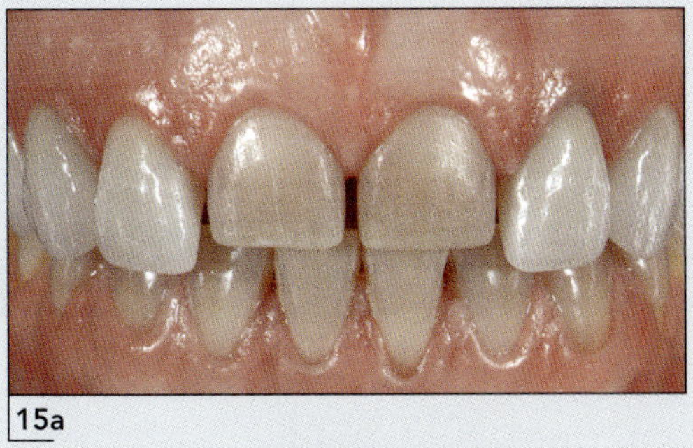

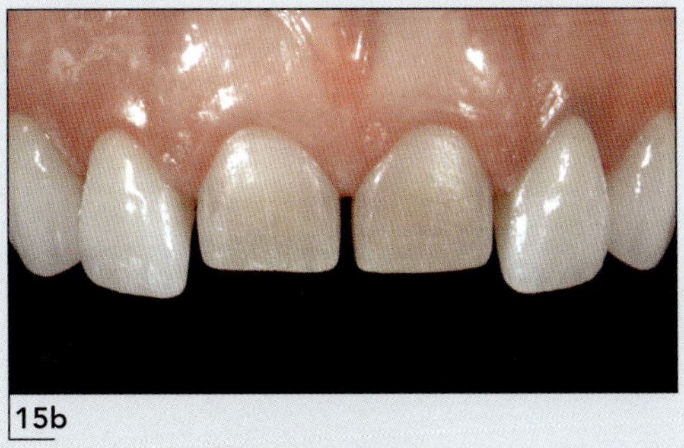

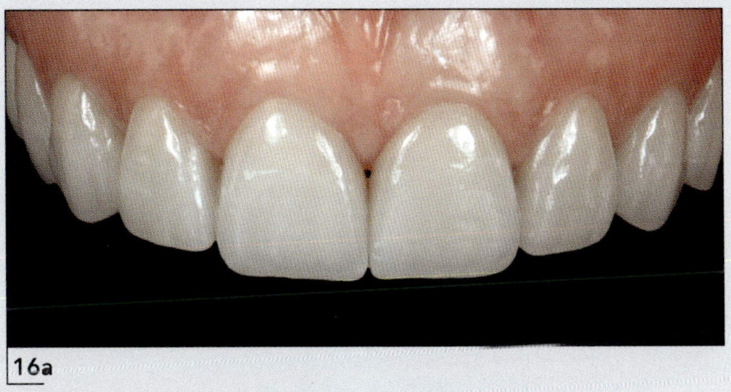

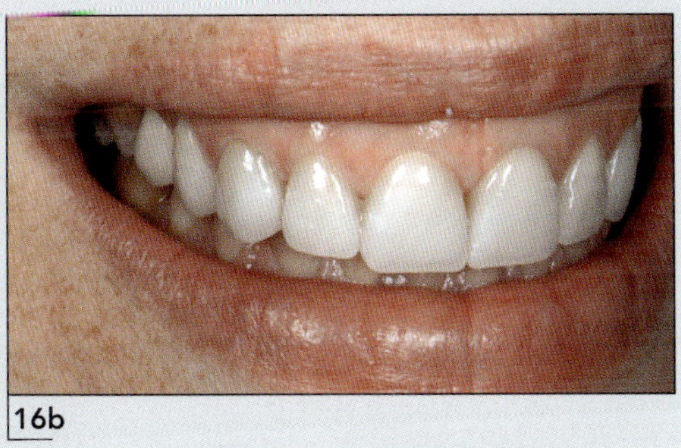

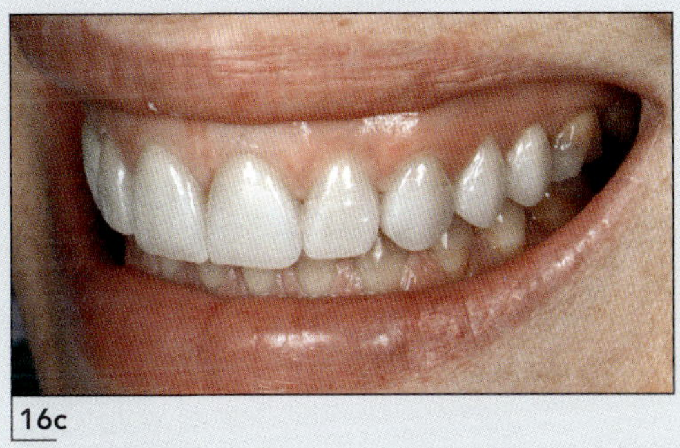

Figs 15a and 15b Frontal view immediately before the bonding process of the maxillary central incisors.

Figs 16a to 16c Final result of the ceramic laminate veneer restorations from the right first premolar to the left second premolar. The right second premolar was restored with a zirconia-based crown.

were coated with a hydrophilic adhesive resin (Excite F, Ivoclar Vivadent), air thinned for evaporation of the solvent, and left uncured.

The tooth preparations were etched with 35% phosphoric acid for 30 to 60 seconds, washed, and air dried. The same adhesive that was used for the veneers was applied to the tooth structure in the same manner. The ceramic restorations were loaded with the selected light-curing resin cement and positioned on the teeth. All excess resin cement was carefully removed before light curing. An LED light-curing unit (Bluephase, Ivoclar Vivadent) in low-power mode was used to cure each surface for 40 seconds. A water-soluble glycerin gel was used to air block, and the margin of the restoration was polymerized again for 40 seconds per surface. The excess resin cement was removed with a scalpel and composite resin strips. Only one laminate veneer was bonded at a time for better control of the bonding and cleaning process. The last two veneers to be bonded were the central incisors (Fig 15). The zirconia crown on the maxillary right second premolar was the only exception and was luted with a resin cement with monomer acid (Panavia F 2.0, Kuraray). The final maxillary restorations are shown in Fig 16.

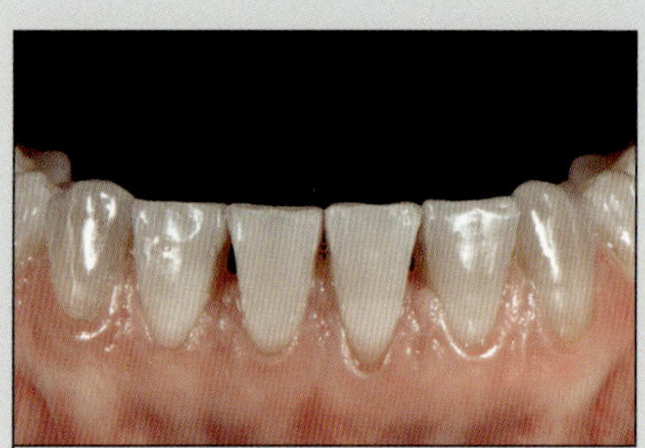

17a

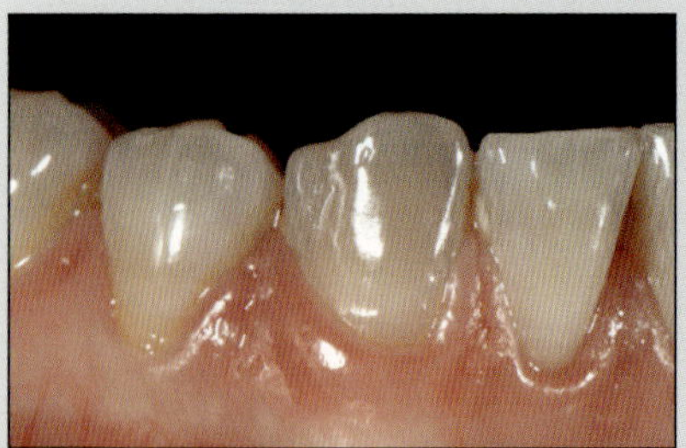

17b

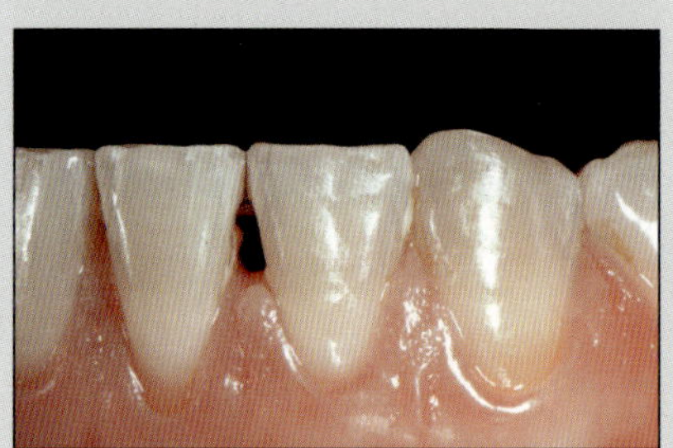

17c

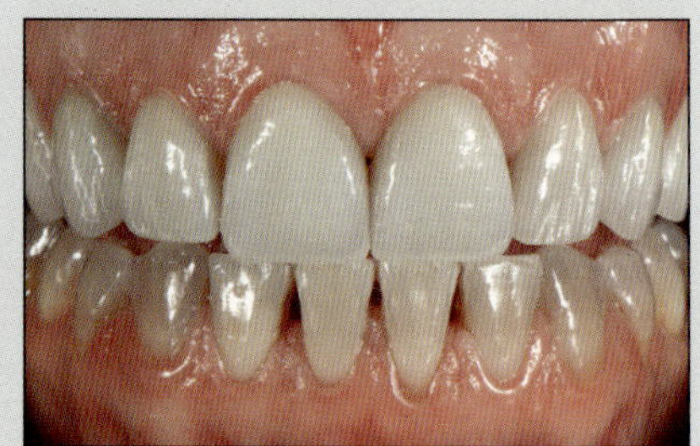

17d

Figs 17a to 17d Anterior mandibular dentition before tooth preparation. The patient at this time wore a bonded lingual orthodontic retainer from canine to canine.

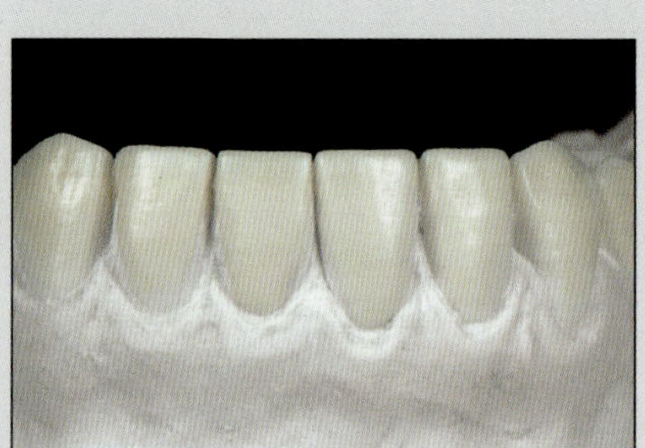

18a

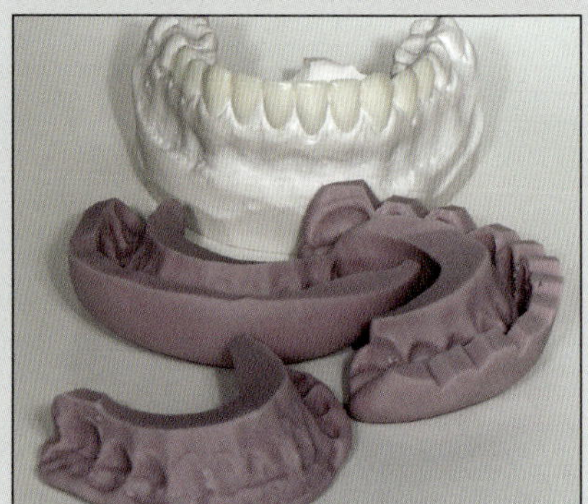

18b

Fig 18a Close-up view of the wax-up of the mandibular anterior dentition.

Fig 18b Silicone indices made to guide the tooth preparations for the laminate ceramic veneers.

Mandibular Tooth Preparations

After final bonding, polishing, and finishing procedures for the maxillary teeth from premolar to premolar, the next step was to rehabilitate the mandibular arch. The initial situation prior to preparing the mandibular arch is shown in Fig 17. As previously noted, for better occlusal records and mounting on the articulator, one arch was prepared and finished at a time. A new PVS impression was taken of the maxillary restored arch to articulate with the wax-up of the anterior mandibular teeth (Fig 18a). For this area, a 0.5-mm incisal reduction was done before the wax-up of the final anatomy. This was necessary because changing the VDO was not indicated in this patient. Silicone indices were made to control tooth reduction (Fig 18b).

The patient wore an orthodontic retainer from mandibular canine to canine that was removed prior to tooth preparation. For the mandibular arch, the same conservative approach was used. In this way, an accurate and precise tooth preparation concept had to be applied because the amount of enamel was limited. In Fig 19, a prepared tooth can be compared with an intact one. Definitive preparations are shown in Fig 20. In the premolar area, special attention had to be given to avoid excessive removal of tooth structure at the cervical margin. The impression was taken and sent to the laboratory for fabrication of the ceramic veneers from

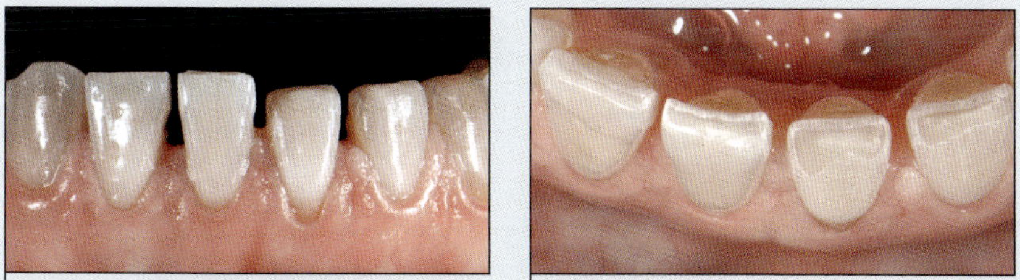

19a 19b

Figs 19a and 19b Comparison of the prepared teeth at the left side of patient's mouth with the intact teeth at the right side. Note that the removal of the orthodontic retainer opened small diastemata between the incisors.

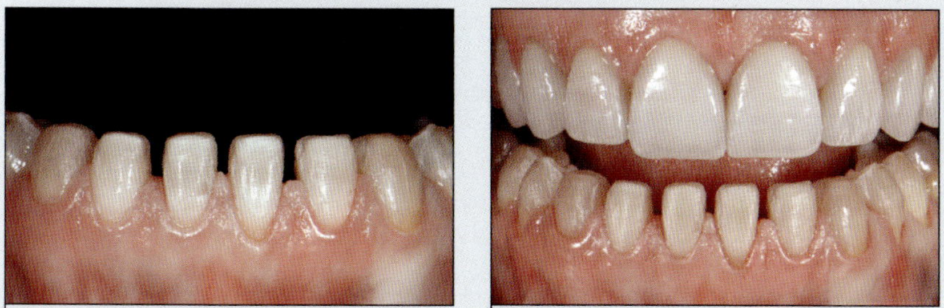

20a 20b

Figs 20a and 20b Final tooth preparations for the mandibular anterior and premolar teeth.

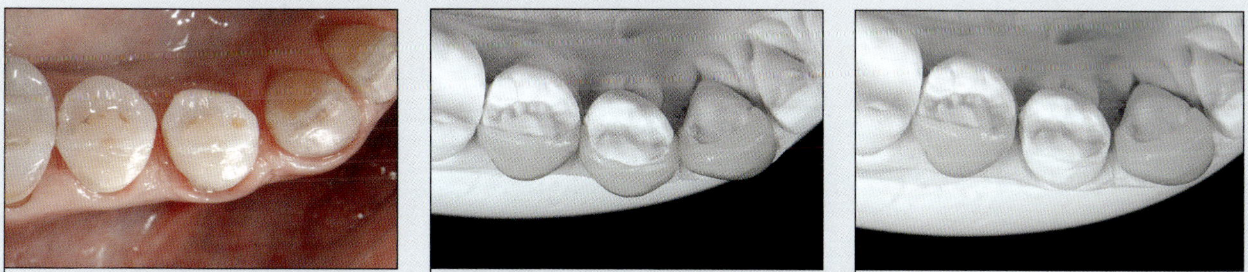

21a 21b 21c

Fig 21a Occlusal view of the final preparations for ceramic laminate veneers on the right canine and premolars.
Figs 21b and 21c Occlusal view of the veneers on the master cast. The path-of-insertion test before bonding showed that the restoration of the first premolar should be done after the canine and second premolar.

second premolar to second premolar. It is important to emphasize that the path of insertion of a laminate veneer in this specific case is from buccal to lingual at the premolar area, so it was not necessary to remove a large amount of sound tooth structure at the gingival margin. Figure 21a shows the conservative preparations on the right canine and premolars. The definitive laminate ceramic veneers on those teeth are shown in Figs 21b and 21c. Regarding the path of insertion of those elements, the sequence for bonding was determined on the cast; in this case, the canine and second premolar veneers were bonded before the veneer on the first premolar. If a different sequence had been selected, it is likely that an insertion problem would have resulted in excessive adjustments, compromising the final result and marginal adaptation.

Figure 22a shows the tooth preparations on the left canine and premolars; an important highlight of this photograph is that the left lateral incisor had yet to be prepared. As mentioned before, the molars were the last to be prepared. Note that in this area it was not necessary to prepare the interproximal surfaces between the first and second premolars. Definitive restorations of this area are shown in Figs 22b and 22c.

All the steps until the final bonding were carried out exactly as for the maxilla. As the provisionals were well adapted, the gingival tissue was stable and healthy for final bonding. Figure 23 shows the situation immediately after cementation of the veneers on the right side of the mandible.

Fig 22a Intraoral view of the ceramic laminate veneer preparations of the left canine and premolars.

Fig 22b Occlusal view of the veneers for the left canine and premolars positioned on the cast.

Fig 22c Close-up lateral view of veneer for the left second premolar.

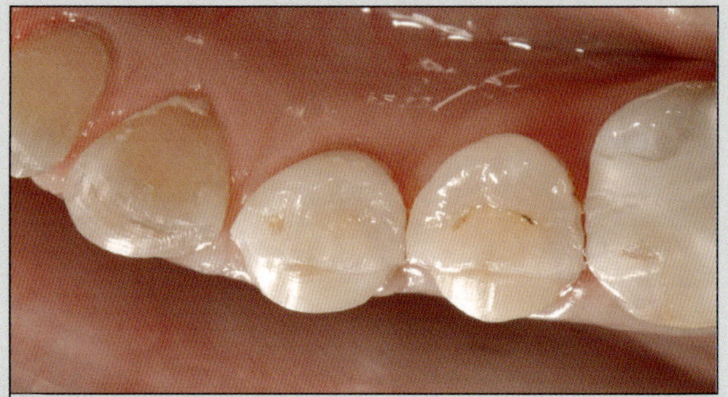

22a

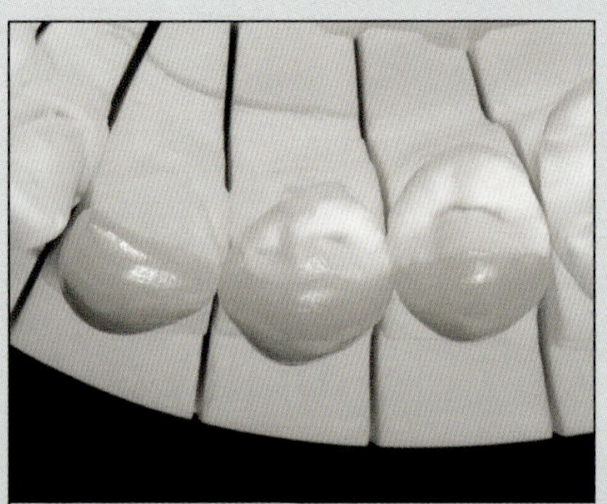

22b

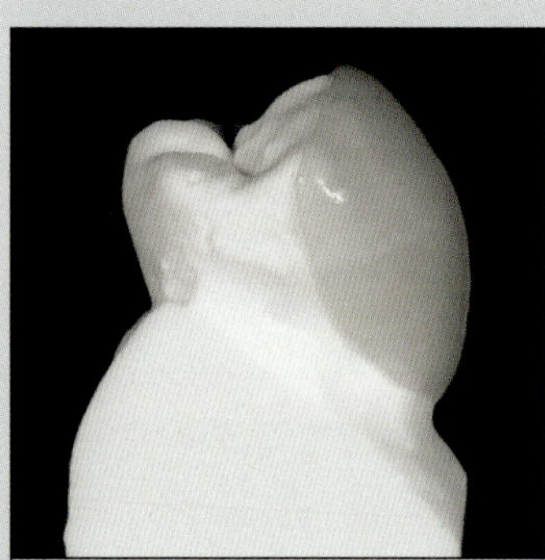

22c

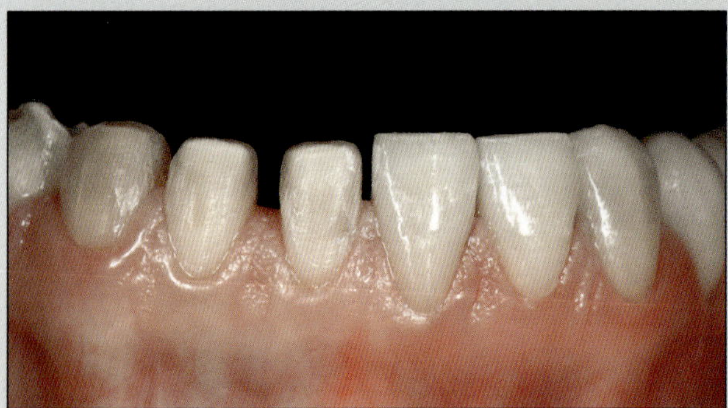

23a

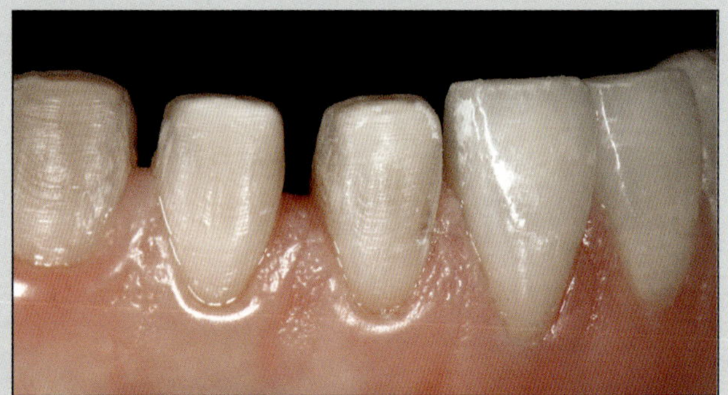

23b

Figs 23a and 23b Immediately after the bonding procedure on the left second premolar to left central incisor. Observe the immediate result of the adhesive cementation on the gingival tissue when properly executed.

Restoration of the Molar Teeth

With the approach of restoring first the maxillary anterior dentition and premolars followed by the same regions in mandibular arch, it was possible to have better occlusal control of the case. When there is no need to change the VDO, it is always important to maintain a reference to record and articulate the original occlusion so that the VDO will be maintained. In this case, the molars, which were the final teeth to be restored, helped in this important role. Overlays and onlays were fabricated for the maxillary and mandibular molars. The final result can be seen in Fig 24. At the end of the treatment, the patient was provided with an occlusal nightguard.

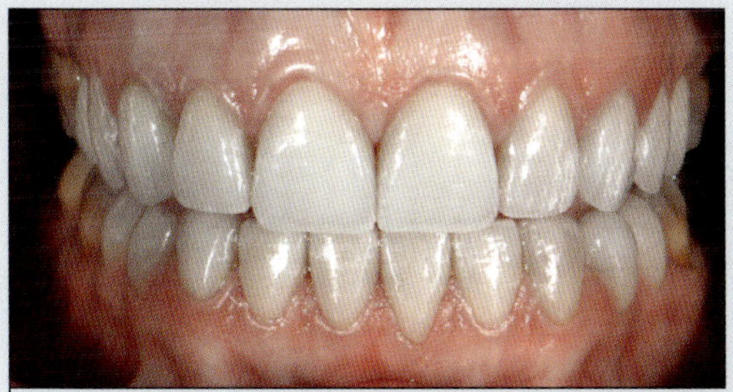
24a

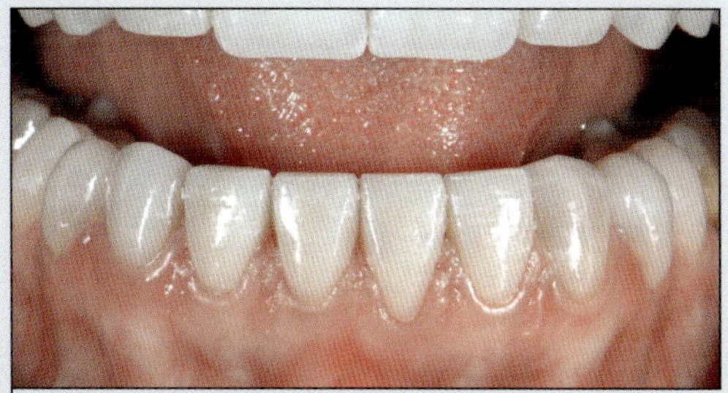
24b

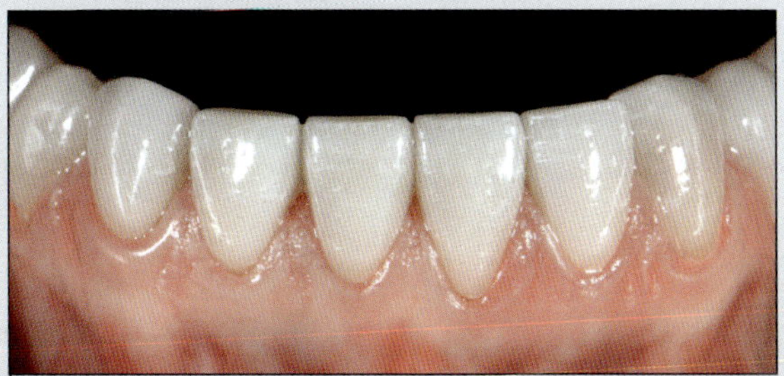
24c

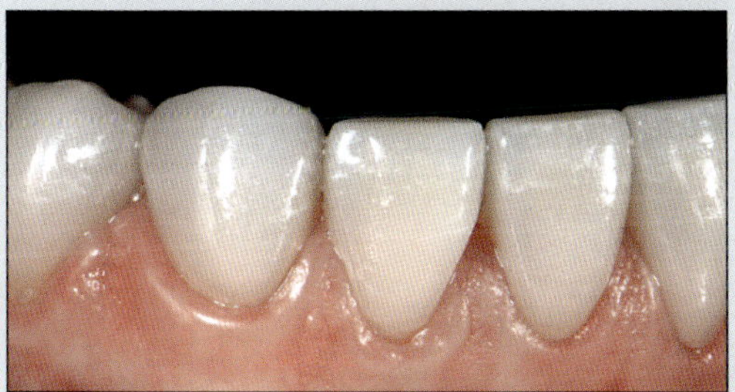
24d

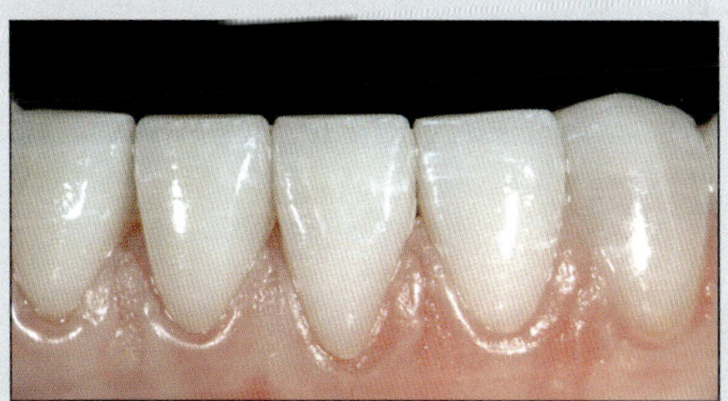
24e

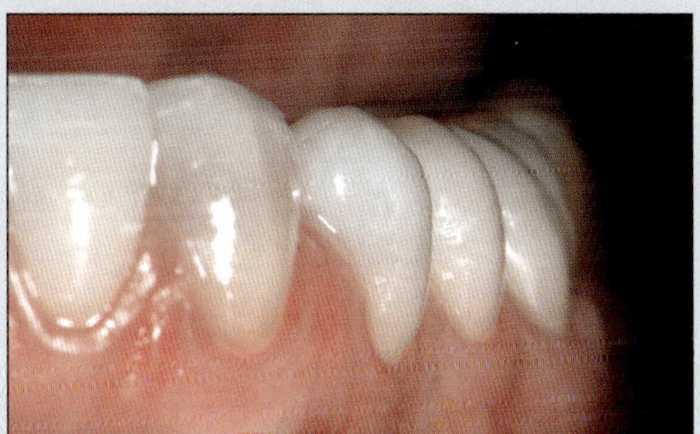
24f

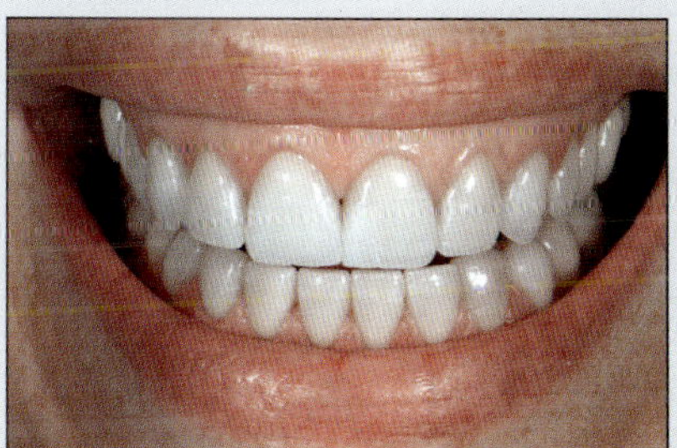
24g

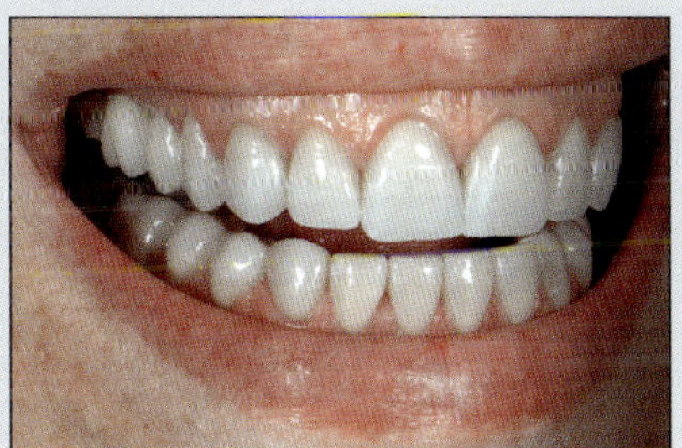
24h

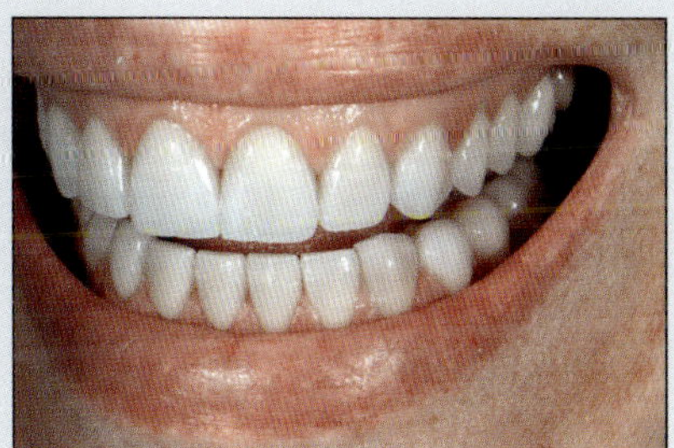
24i

Figs 24a to 24o Final result 5 months after the adhesive oral rehabilitation customized for the patient's discolored dentition.

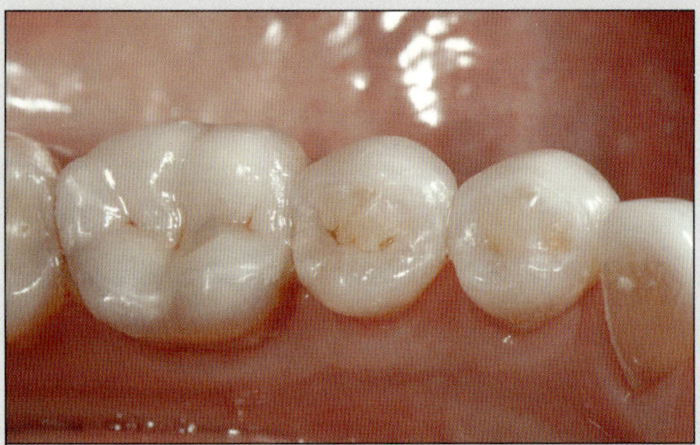

24j

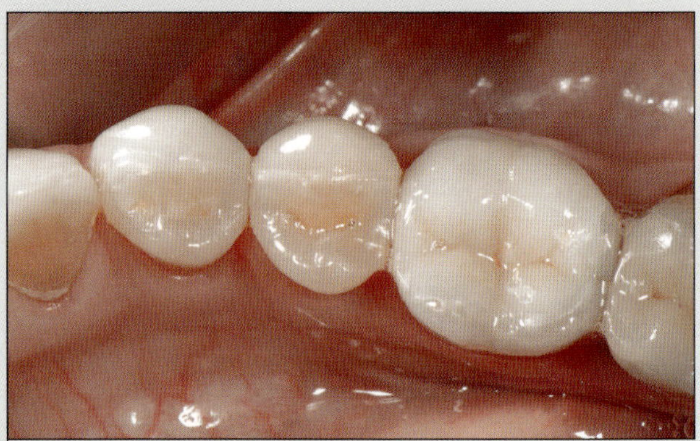

24k

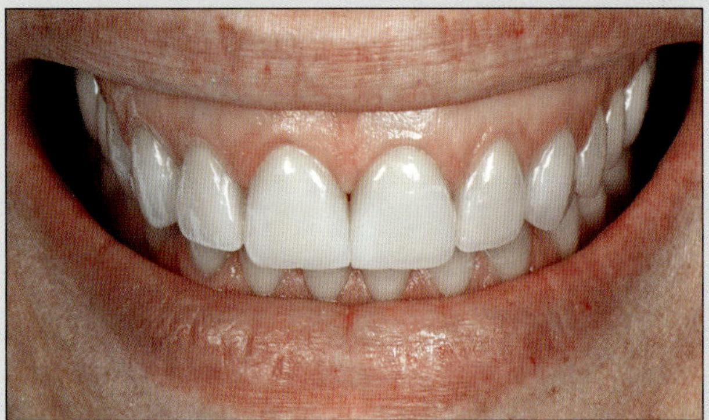

24l

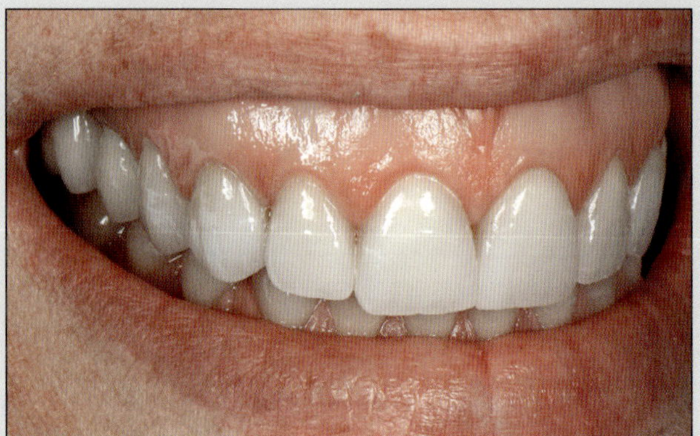

24m

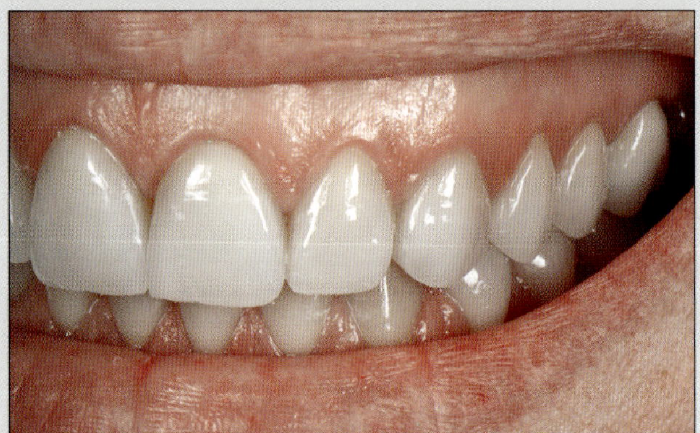

24n

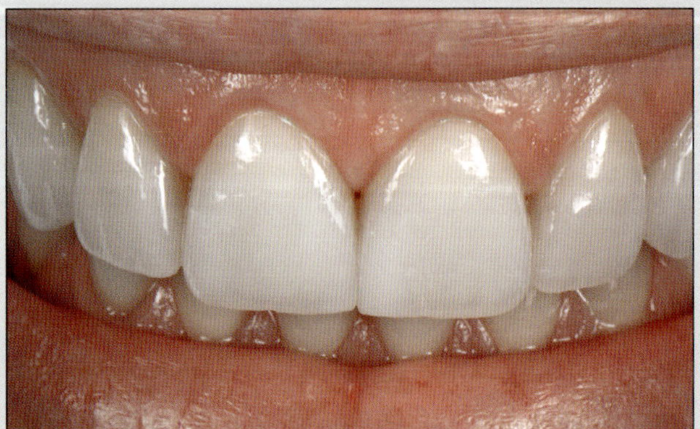

24o

CONCLUSIONS

The adhesive oral rehabilitation concept implies the use of minimally invasive procedures even in cases of severely discolored dentitions with tetracycline staining. Utilizing controlled diagnostic procedures, it is possible to predict the final anatomy of the oral rehabilitation to provide the patient esthetic and functional conservative restorations. Combining ceramic materials with adhesive characteristics, it is possible to fabricate conservative laminate veneers that preserve dental hard tissue while achieving long-term results.

REFERENCES

1. Vailati F, Belser UC. Full-mouth adhesive rehabilitation of a severely eroded dentition: The three-step technique. Part 1. Eur J Esthet Dent 2008;3:30–44.
2. Vailati F, Belser UC. Full-mouth adhesive rehabilitation of a severely eroded dentition: The three-step technique. Part 2. Eur J Esthet Dent 2008;3:128–146.
3. Vailati F, Belser UC. Full-mouth adhesive rehabilitation of a severely eroded dentition: The three-step technique. Part 3. Eur J Esthet Dent 2008;3:236–257.
4. Vailati F, Bruguera A, Belser UC. Minimallly invasive treatment of initial dental erosion using pressed lithium disilicate glass-ceramic restorations: A case report. Quintessence Dent Technol 2012;35:65–78.
5. Scopin de Andrade O, Rodrigues M, Hirata R, Ferreira LA. Adhesive oral rehabilitation: Maximizing treatment options with minimally invasive indirect restorations. Quintessence Dent Technol 2014;37:71–93.
6. Fradeani M, Barducci G, Bacherini L, Brennan M. Esthetic rehabilitation of a severely worn dentition with minimally invasive prosthetic procedures (MIPP). Int J Periodontics Restorative Dent 2012;32:135–147.
7. Gurel G. The Science and Art of Porcelain Laminate Veneers. Berlin: Quintessence, 2003.
8. Bacherini L, Brennan M, Bocabella L, Vigiani P. Esthetic rehabilitation of a severely discolored dentition with minimally invasive prosthetic procedures (MIPP). Quintessence Dent Technol 2013;36:59–76.
9. Scopin de Andrade O, Borges G, Stefani A, Fujiy F, Battistella P. A step-by-step ultraconservative esthetic rehabilitation using lithium disilicate ceramic. Quintessence Dent Technol 2010;33:114–131.
10. Scopin de Andrade O, Romanini JC, Hirata R. Ultimate ceramic veneers: A laboratory-guided ultraconservative preparation concept for maximum enamel preservation. Quintessence Dental Technol 2012;34:29–43.
11. Duarte S Jr, Phark JH, Blatz M, Sadan A. Ceramic systems: An ultrastructural study. Quintessence Dent Technol 2010;33:42–60.
12. Magne P, Belser U. Bonded Porcelain Restorations in the Anterior Dentition: A Biomimetic Approach. Chicago: Quintessence, 2002.
13. Scopin de Andrade O, Kina S, Hirata R. Concepts for an ultraconservative approach to indirect anterior restorations. Quintessence Dent Technol 2011;34:103–119.

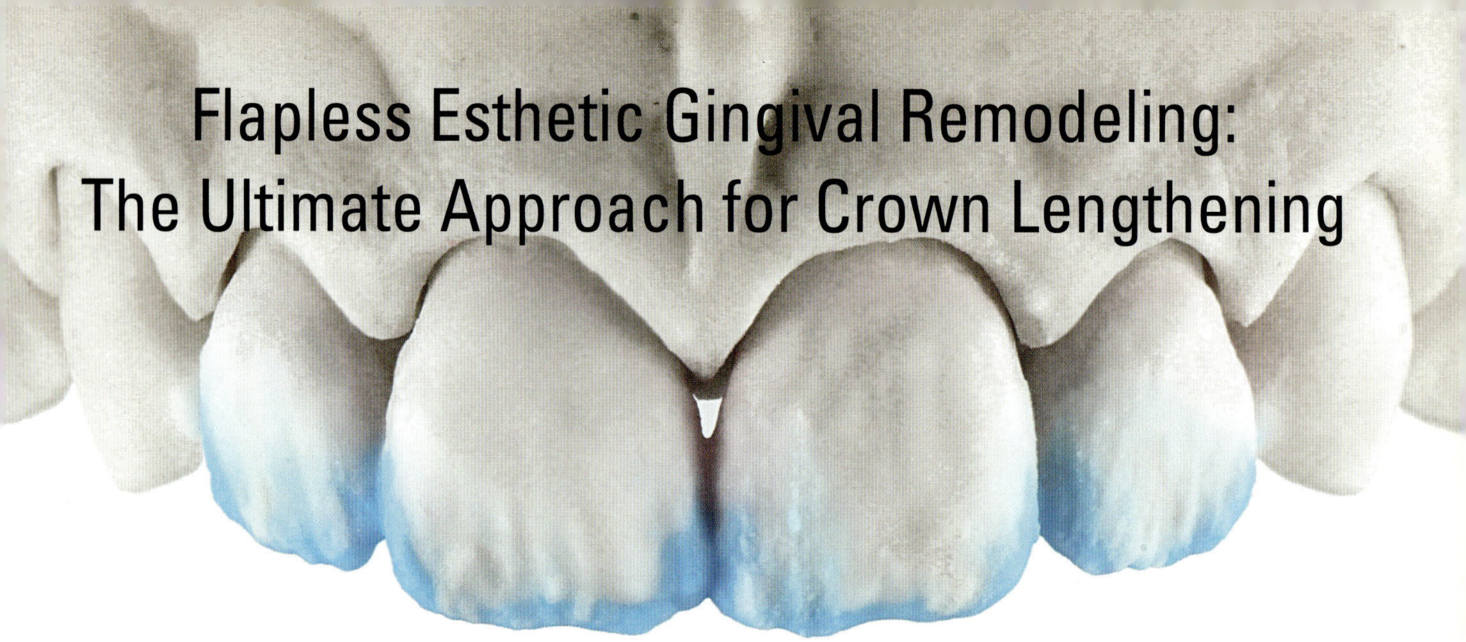

Flapless Esthetic Gingival Remodeling: The Ultimate Approach for Crown Lengthening

Ivan Contreras Molina, DDS, MSc, PhD[1]
Gildardo Contreras Molina, DDS[2]
Isis Carvalho Encarnação, DDS, MSc, PhD[1]
Cristiano Soares, CDT[3]
Luiz Narciso Baratieri, DDS, MSc, PhD[4]

The integration of knowledge from various specialties of dentistry has become essential for comprehensive diagnosis, planning, and implementation of simple restorative treatments to extensive rehabilitations. The evolution and scientific development of the materials available as well as the improvement of surgical techniques have contributed to the achievement of dramatic results in the dental practice.

This case report demonstrates the relationship between periodontics and restorative dentistry, ultimately aimed at obtaining a harmonious, balanced smile. Without such multidisciplinary interaction, a minimally invasive approach would not be possible for both surgical and restorative procedures.[1]

The case involves one of the most widely used minimally invasive procedures for correcting excessive gingival exposure while smiling: periodontal plastic surgery without flaps, also known as "the flapless procedure."[2–4] This technique requires osteotomy, when indicated, via the gingival sulcus through the use of micro-chisels. This article proposes a new approach to correct excessive gingival exposure, one of the problems that most negatively affects the smile, with reduced surgical time, without sutures, and with minimal surgical trauma, ultimately leading to an excellent postoperative phase.

CASE REPORT

A 23-year-old male patient came to the Dental Clinic at Federal University of Santa Catarina, Florianópolis, Brazil, requesting a solution to improve his smile, specifically the color and shape of his teeth (Fig 1).

[1]Graduate, PhD in Dentistry, Federal University of Santa Catarina, Florianópolis, Brazil.
[2]Professor, Department of Surgery, University Michoacana de San Nicolas de Hidalgo, Morelia, Mexico.
[3]Dental Technician, Campinas, Brazil.
[4]Professor, Department of Dentistry, Federal University of Santa Catarina, Florianópolis, Brazil.

Correspondence to: Dr Ivan Contreras Molina, Privada Plan de Ayutla #39, Col. Chapultepec sur, Morelia, Mexico.
Email: dr.ivancontreras@gmail.com

CASE REPORT

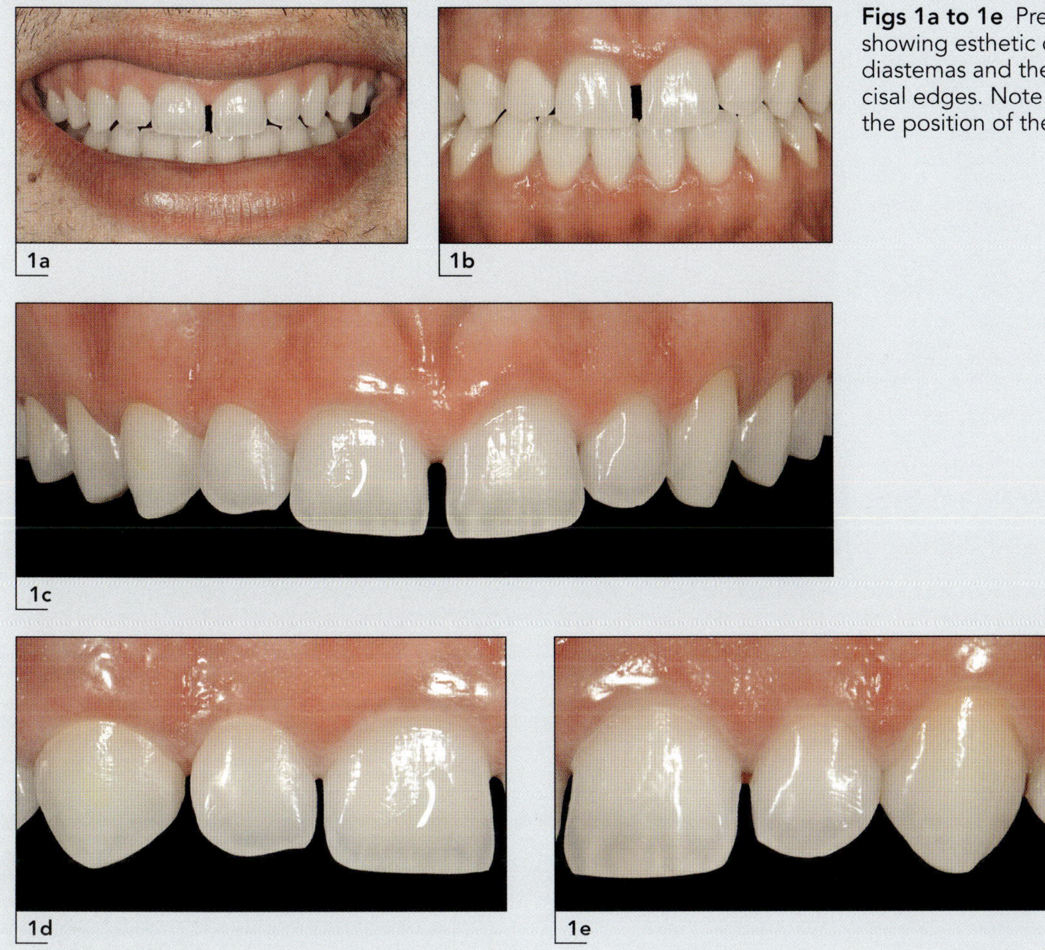

Figs 1a to 1e Preoperative situation showing esthetic deficiencies due to diastemas and the location of the incisal edges. Note the discrepancy of the position of the gingival margin.

Phase 1: Treatment Planning and Surgical Phases (Figs 2 to 4)

The first aim was to precisely obtain the dimensions of the biologic width for each of the teeth involved in order to determine whether osteotomy would be required. The periodontal probe is gently positioned into the gingival sulcus with light pressure to determine the probing depth; some pressure is then applied on the probe until it is inserted to the bone crest (bone probing depth). The biologic width of the given tooth is determined by the subtraction of the values of its bone probing depth and the gingival probing depth. A 15-mm periodontal probe is used to obtain the measurements to the nearest 0.5 mm (Fig 2). The incision is positioned on the CEJ level when sound teeth are treated, or along the desired position of the future gingival margin when restorative procedures are indicated as in this case (Fig 3a). The tissue collar band is then removed using periodontal curettes (Fig 3b).

The next step is to determine whether bone contouring is required. Once again, bone probing depth is determined (Fig 3c), and if the obtained value is less than the individual tooth's biologic width, osteotomy is performed (Fig 3d). The osteotomy, when indicated, is performed through the gingival sulcus using the appropriate delicate micro-chisels with small movements (Figs 3e and 3f). After the osteotomy, probing is performed once again to check the newly established biologic space (Figs 3g and 3h).[5,6] Because of the thin to moderate tissue biotype observed in this case, osteoplasty or reduction of bone thickness was not performed. Figures 4a and 4b shows the result obtained after 8 days and 90 days, respectively.

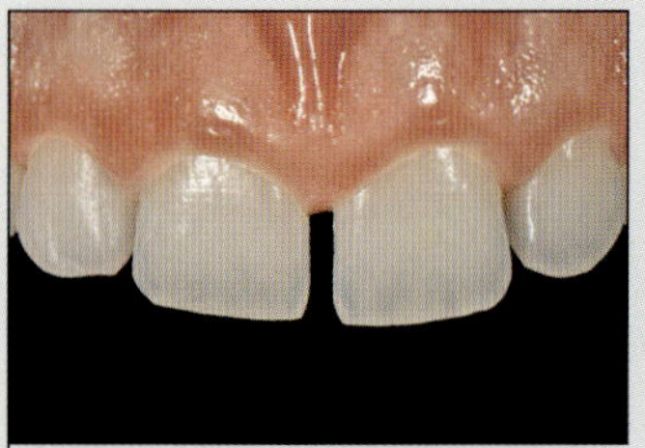
2a

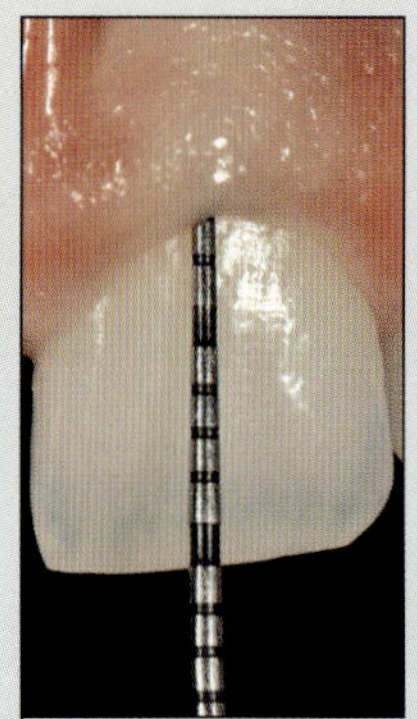
2b

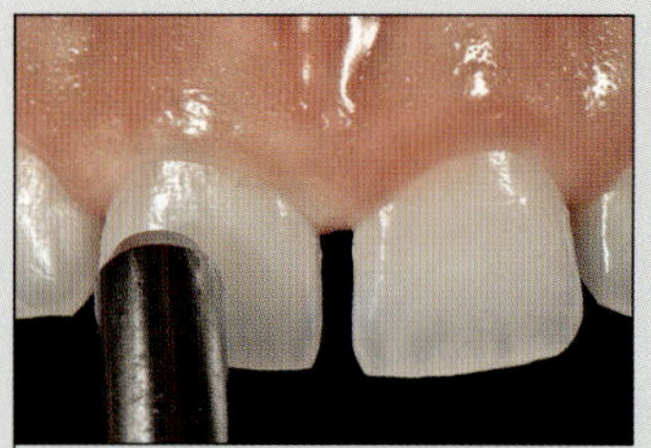
2c

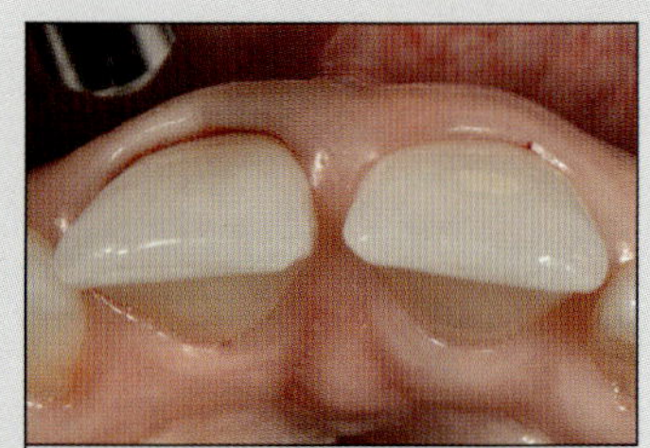
2d

Fig 2a Intraoral view of the maxillary anterior teeth.

Fig 2b Probing to determine the sulcus depth, cementoenamel junction, and bone crest.

Figs 2c and 2d Use of an air jet inside the sulcus, showing a visual reference of the cementoenamel junction.

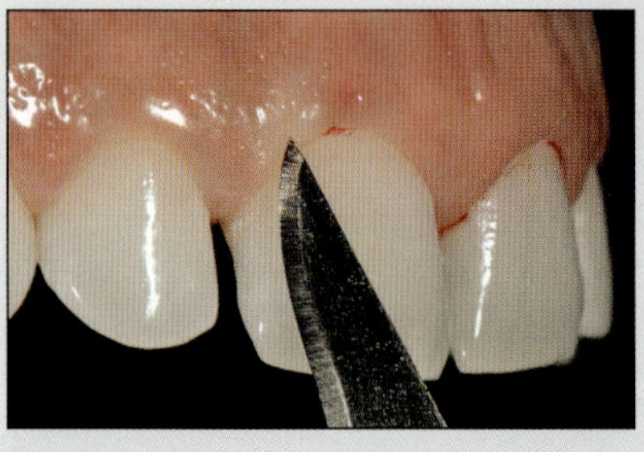

Fig 3a Gingival recontouring with an internal bevel surgical technique.

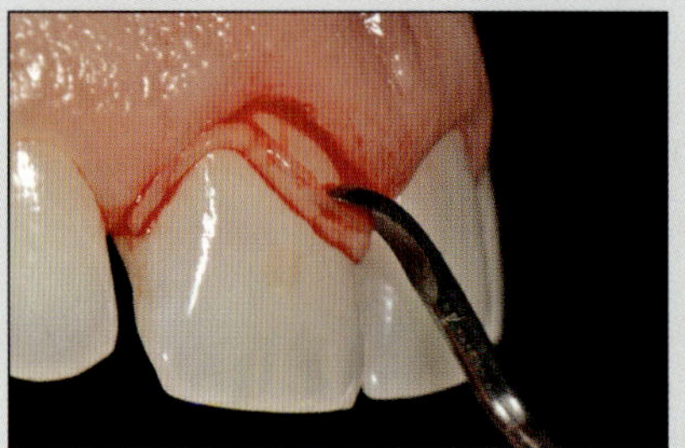

Fig 3b Sharp curette is used to remove excess tissue.

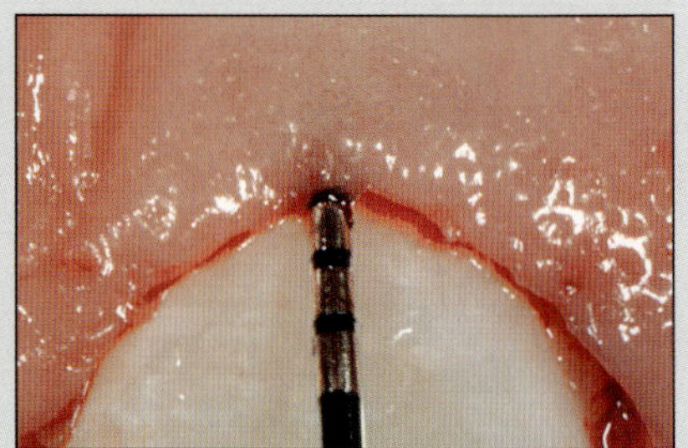

Fig 3c Bone probing, defining the need to perform osteotomy.

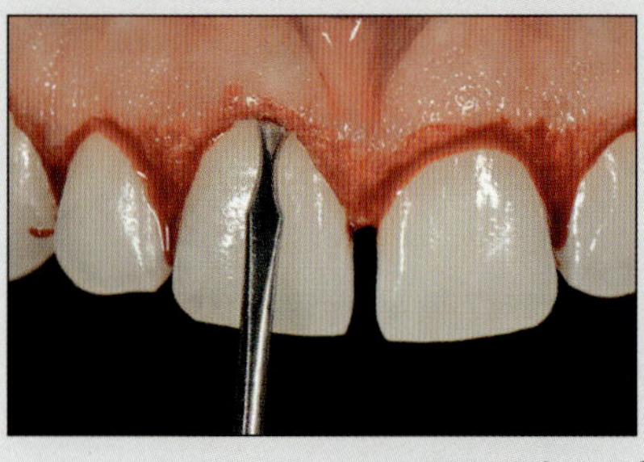

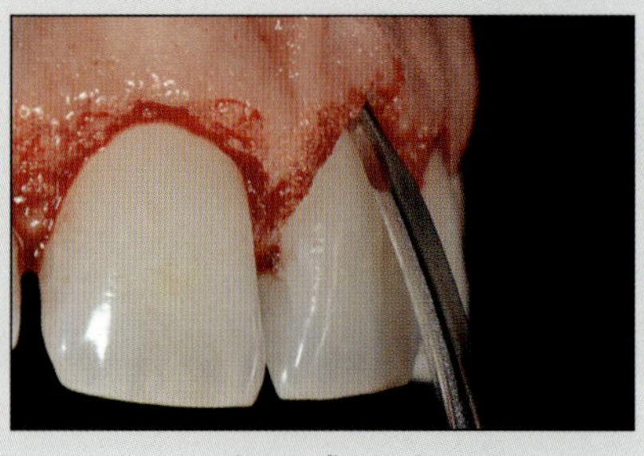

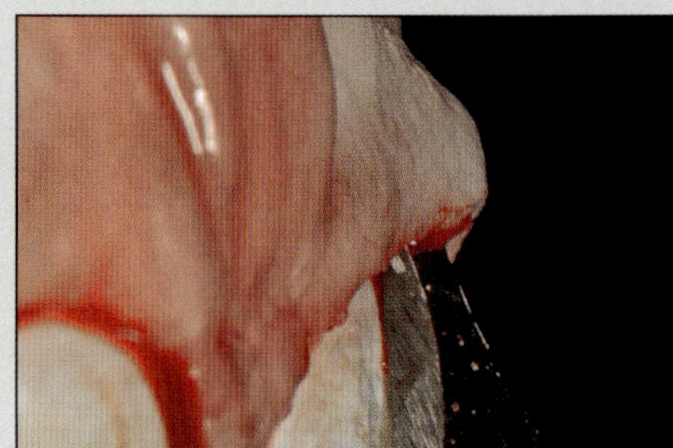

Figs 3d to 3f Osteotomy without flap elevation using a micro-chisel.

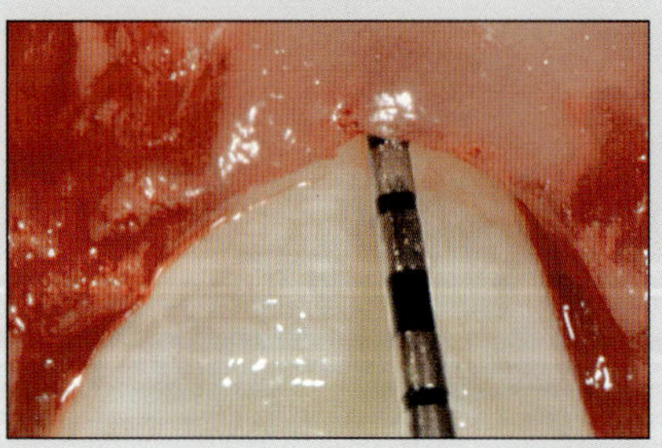

Fig 3g After osteotomy, a second probing is carried out to check the new biologic space.

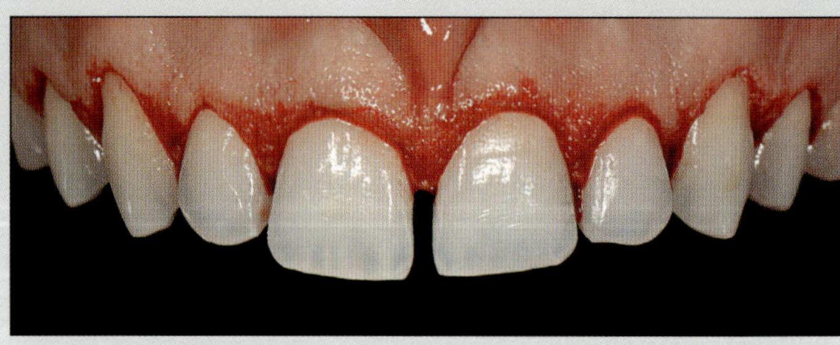

Fig 3h Immediate postoperative view.

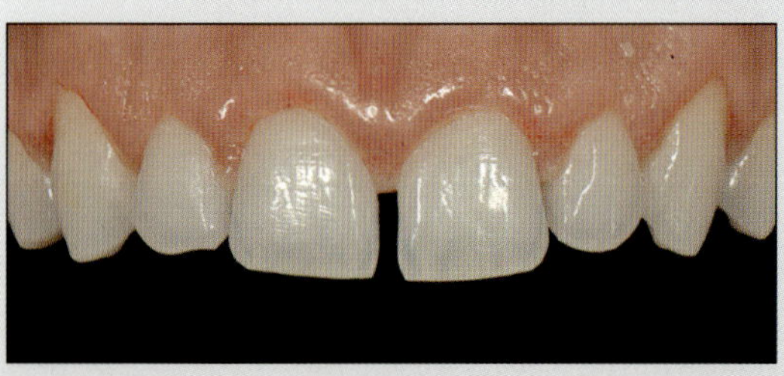

Fig 4a Clinical appearance 8 days after surgery.

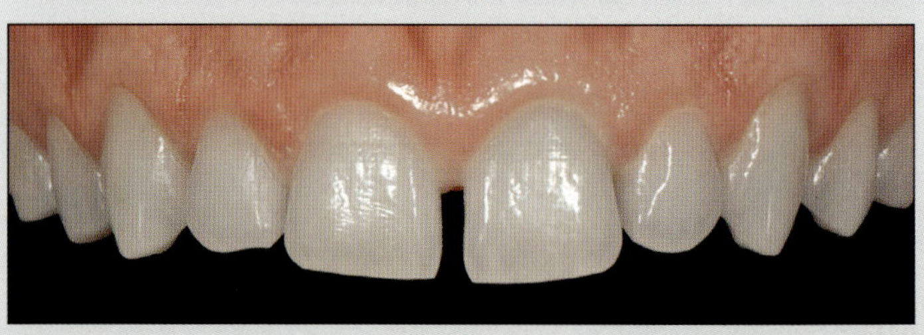

Fig 4b Clinical appearance 90 days after surgery.

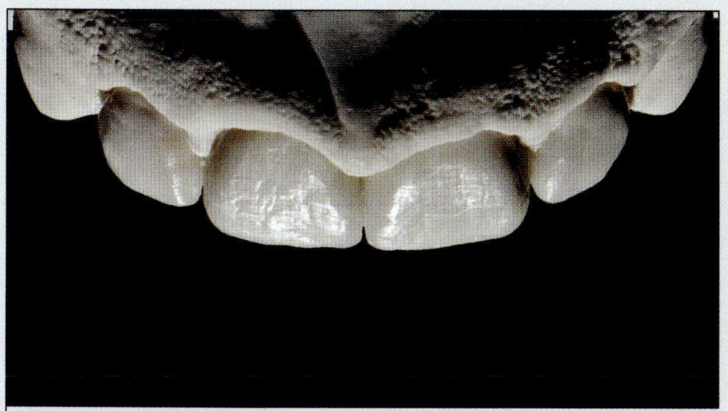

5a

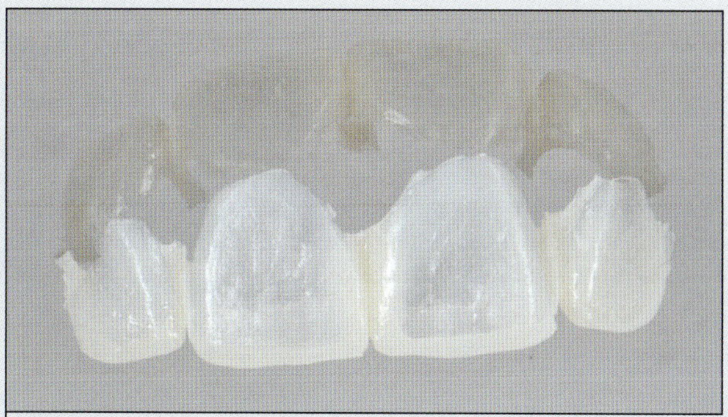

5b

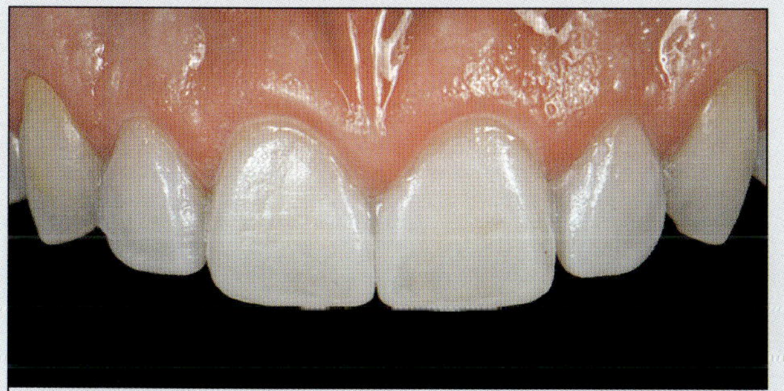

5c

Fig 5a Initial additive wax-up for the mock-up procedure.

Fig 5b Mock-up fabricated with bis-acrylic resin loaded into a vinyl polysiloxane template.

Fig 5c Anticipated view of the final restorations with the mock-up.

Fig 5d Patient's smile with mock-up in place. The patient and the clinician are able to check the esthetic potential of the restorations.

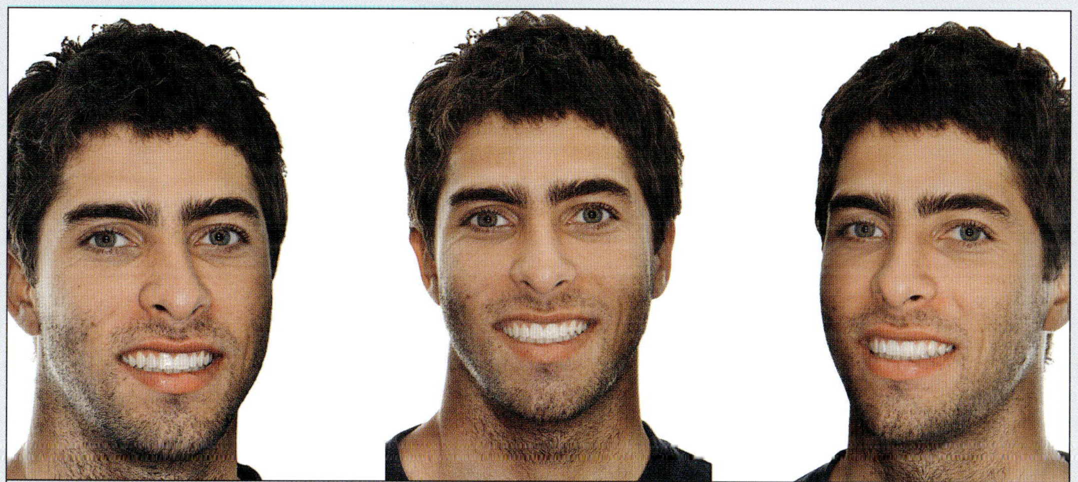

5d

Phase 2: Mock-up and Preparation (Figs 5 to 8)

A conservative approach requires accurate tooth preparation to restore the original volume. A few basic principles can be followed to save a significant amount of sound tooth tissue. The mock-up (Telio, Ivoclar Vivadent) shown in Fig 5 was used on the teeth as a guide during the preparation step.[7] In this case, the distal areas showed the greatest retention (Fig 6a). The retentive areas were marked in the incisal region with a pencil (Figs 6b to 6d). An EVA handpiece and diamond disks (Sof-Lex, 3M ESPE) were used to smooth the angles.

The final ultraconservative preparations are shown in Fig 7. A single retraction cord was used for gingival displacement for the double-mix single impression technique with polyvinyl siloxane (Fig 8).[8]

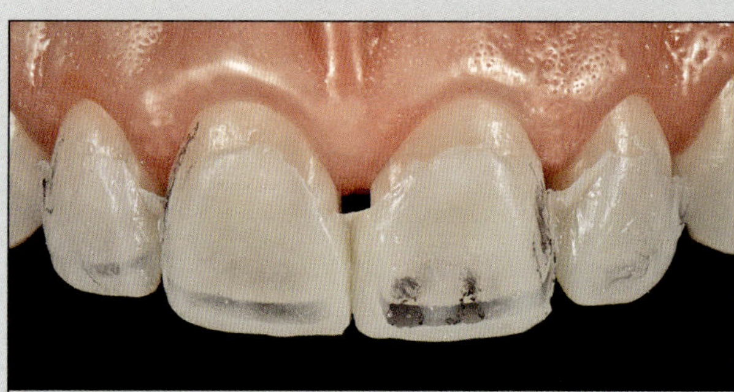

6a

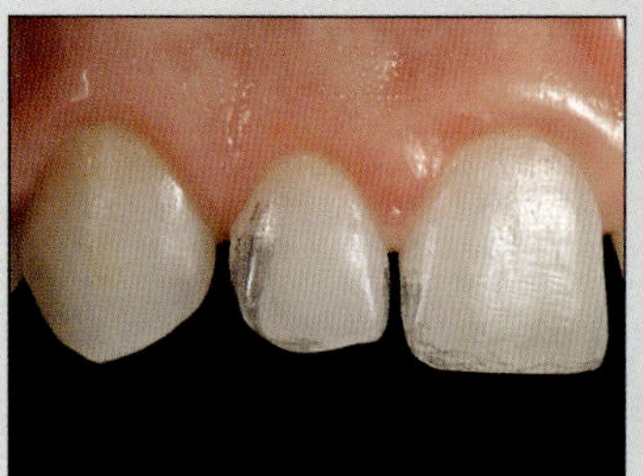

6b

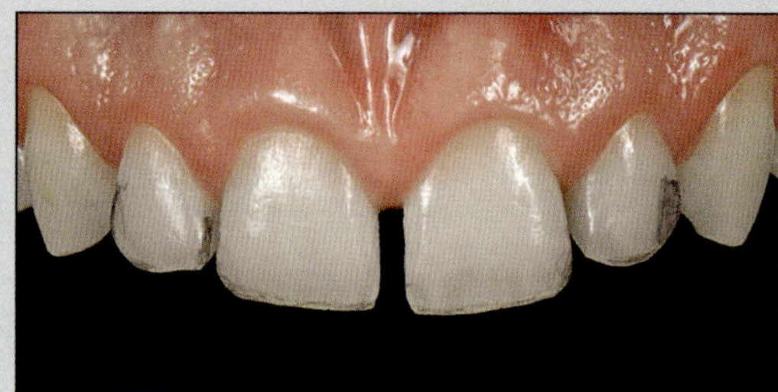

6c

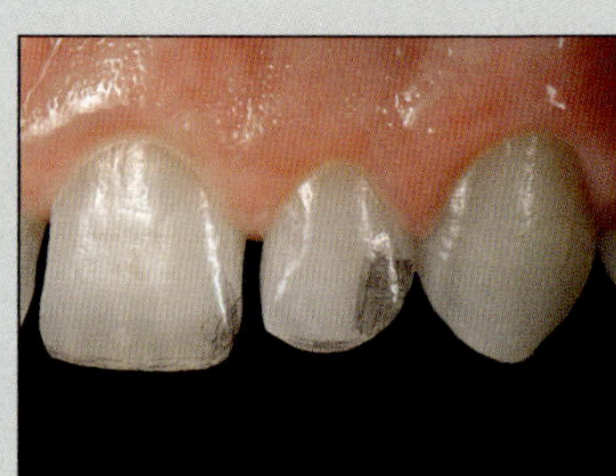

6d

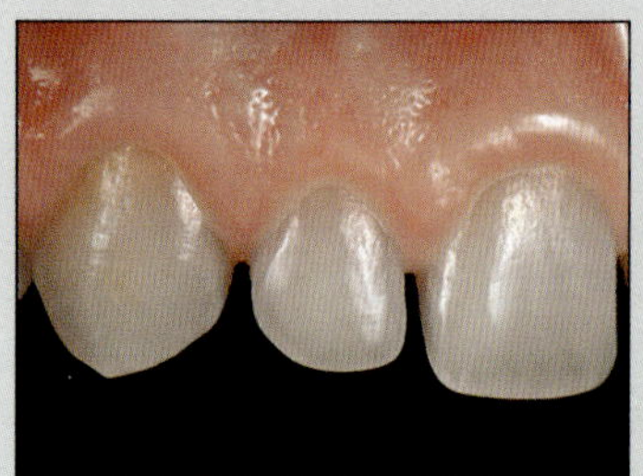

7a

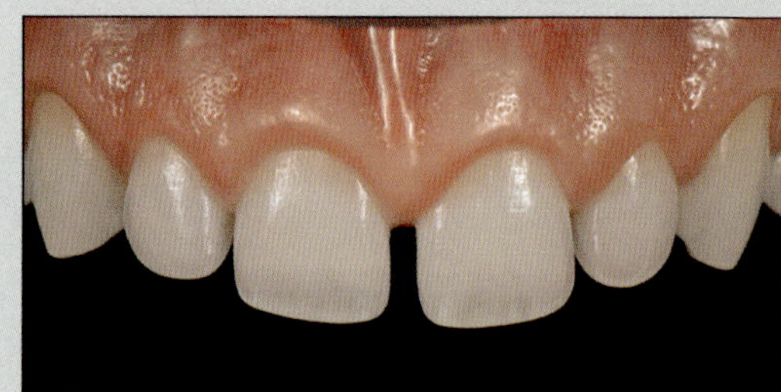

7b

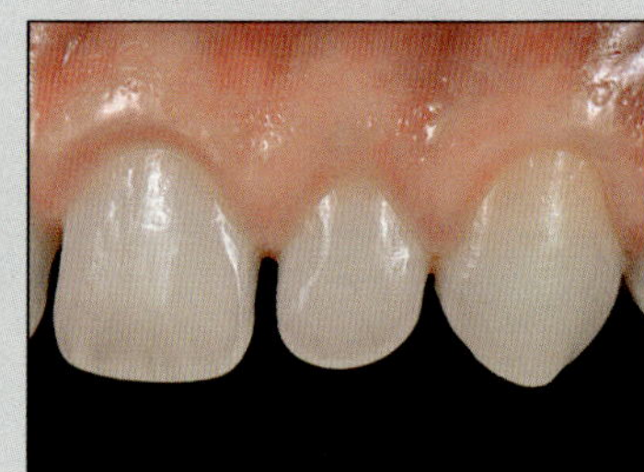

7c

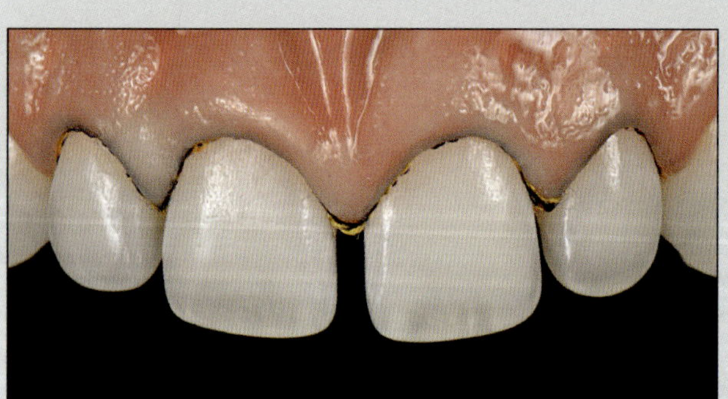

8a

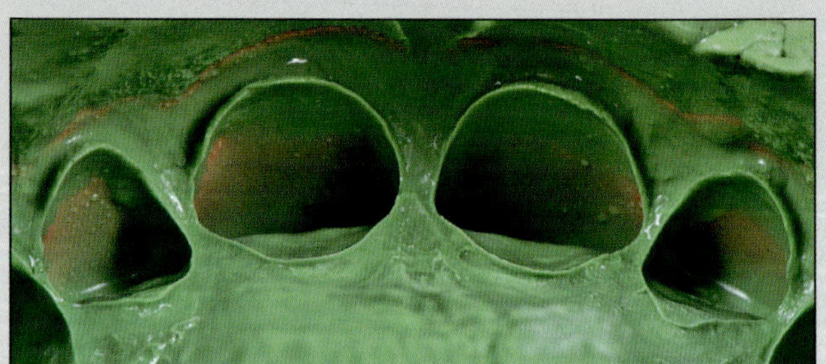

8b

Fig 6a Mock-up in place to view the space for the restorations.

Figs 6b to 6d The retentive areas of the teeth were marked with pencil and carefully corrected to facilitate insertion of the future restorations.

Figs 7a to 7c Close-up views of the ultraconservative veneer preparations.

Figs 8a and 8b Final impression using polyvinyl siloxane and a single-cord technique.

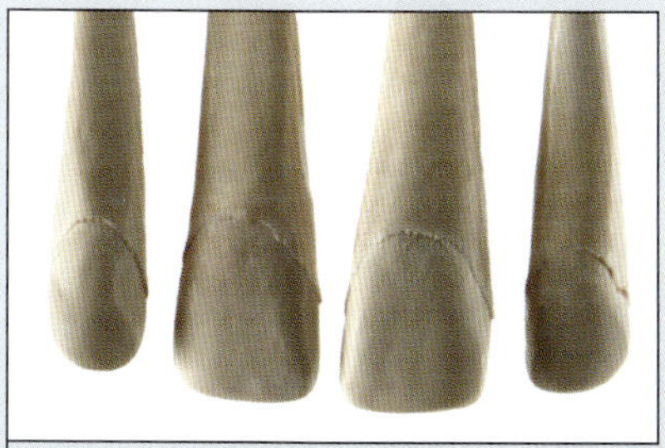
9a

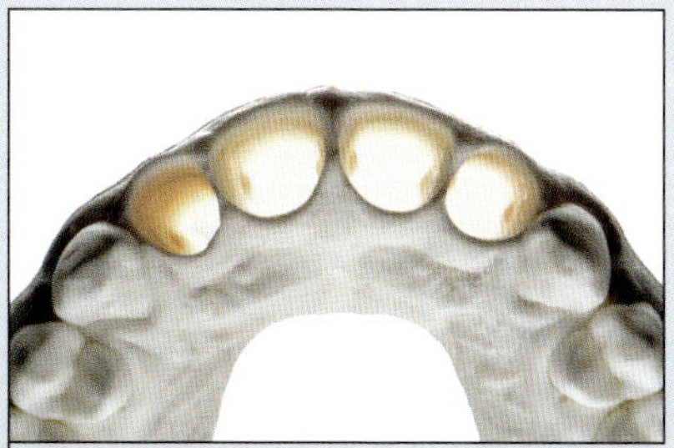
9b

Fig 9a Alveolar dies.

Fig 9b Alveolar cast.

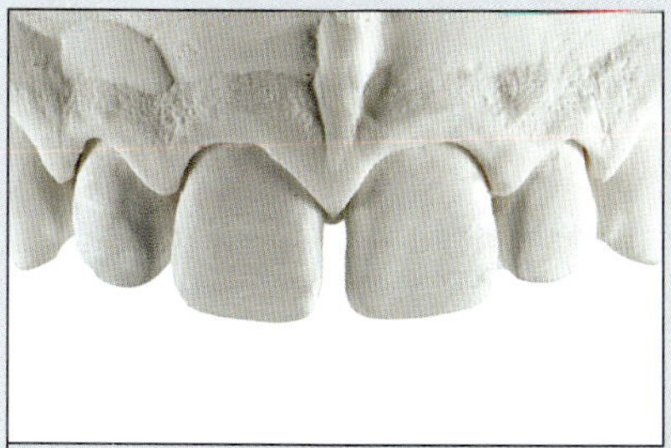
9c

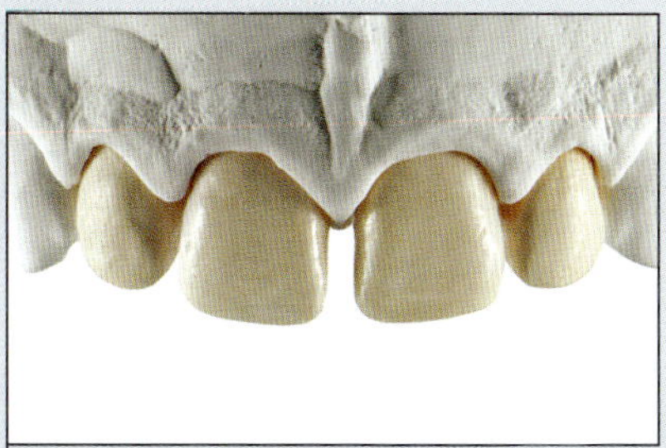
9d

Figs 9c and 9d Alveolar cast with the correct emergence profile and dies in position.

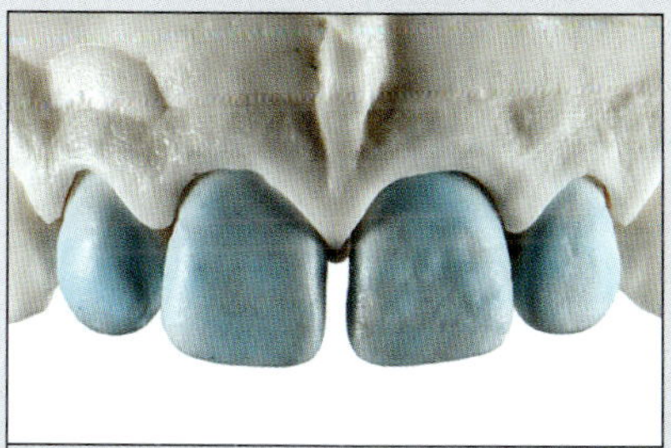
9e

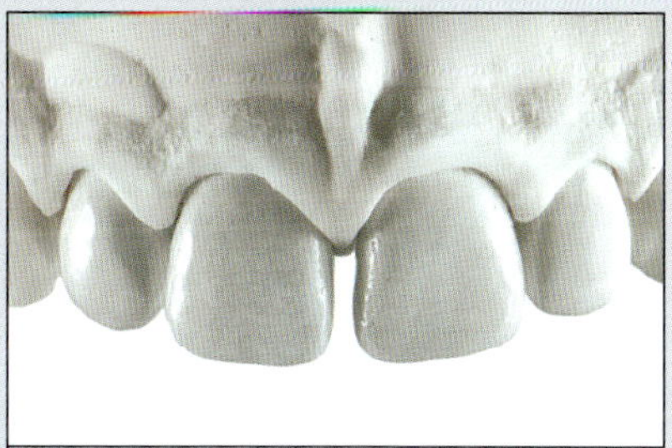
9f

Fig 9e Wash and biscuit firings with opalescent E1, fluorapatite-rich, leucite-reinforced glass ceramics (IPS d.Sign, Ivoclar Vivadent).

Fig 9f Note the smoothness of the ceramic after the first firing. In this step, a temperature 60°C above normal was used.

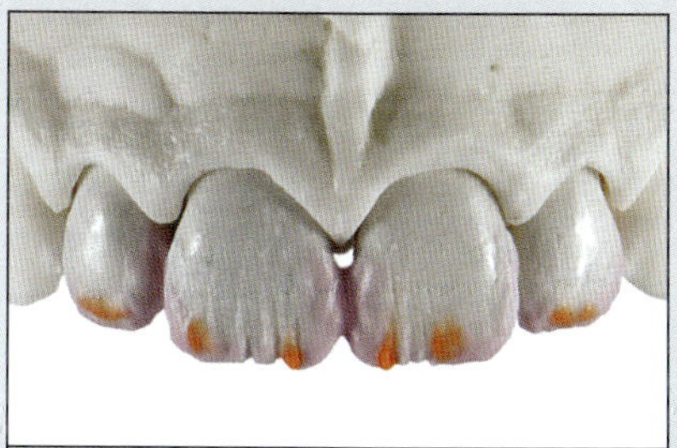
9g

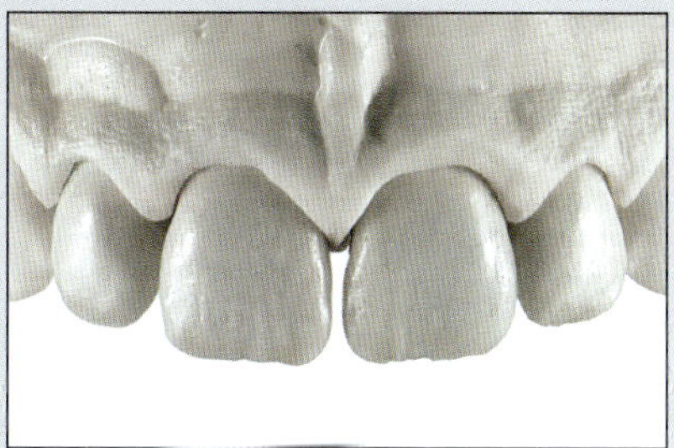
9h

Fig 9g Opaque dentin (DDA1 + 20% Bleach 2) and mamelon masses (MM Salmon) were used.

Fig 9h Final firing of the core completed.

Phase 3: Restorative Phase (Figs 9 to 14)

Four feldspathic ceramic veneers (IPS d.Sign, Ivoclar Vivadent) were fabricated using the refractory die technique for closing the diastema between the maxillary central and lateral incisors (Fig 9). All restorations were checked for marginal fit and proximal contacts.[9] The final shade was evaluated using a glycerin-based try-in paste (Variolink Try-in, Ivoclar Vivadent), resulting in the selection of a clear translucent resin cement (Fig 10).

Figs 9i and 9j View of the application of the proximal (DA1 + 20% Bleach 2), enamel (E1 + E2 1:1, in the incisal angles) and the incisal edge (E1 + 10% Tblue) masses.

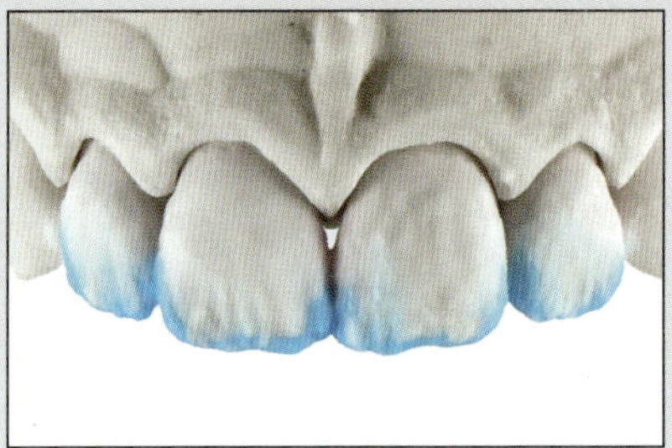

9i

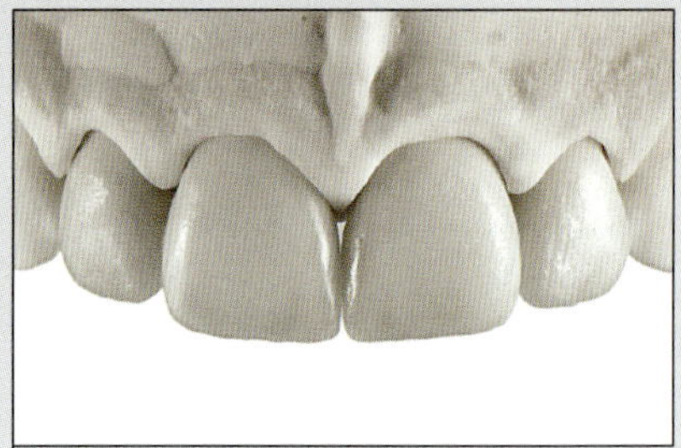

9j

Fig 9k Demarcation of the labial surfaces and angles of transition.

Fig 9l Smoothing of the angles of transition to establish a correct width-to-shape ratio.

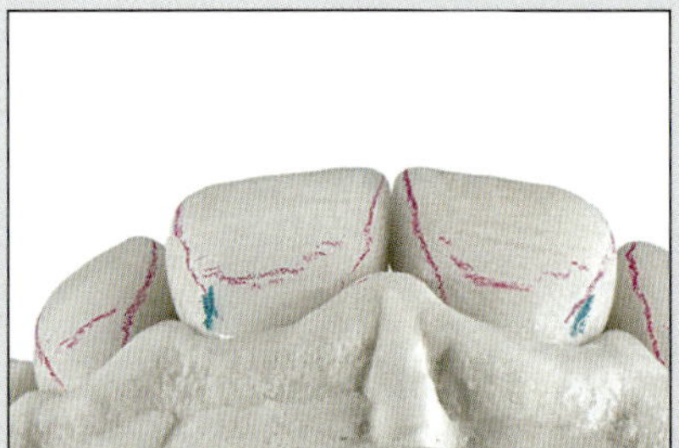

9k

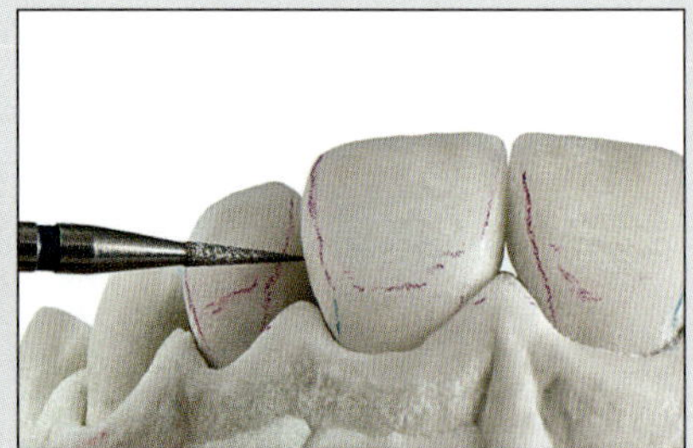

9l

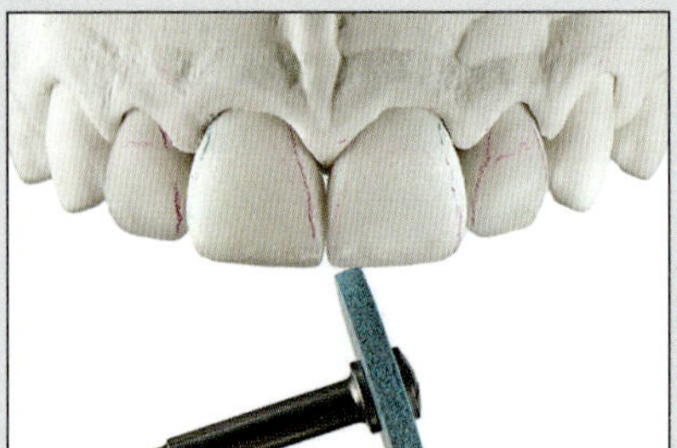

9m

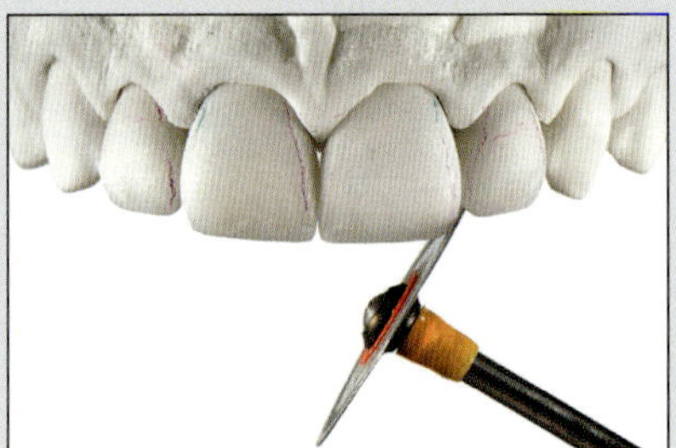

9n

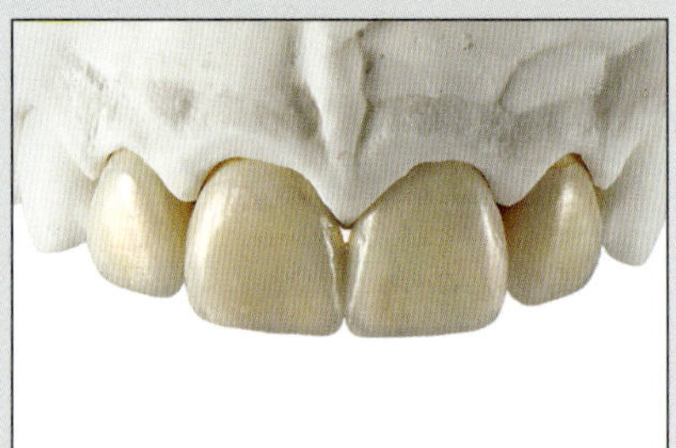

9o

Fig 9m Adjustment of the tooth length and incisal edge.

Fig 9n Adjustment of the incisal embrasures.

Fig 9o After glazing, the veneers are removed from the refractory and adjusted in the cast.

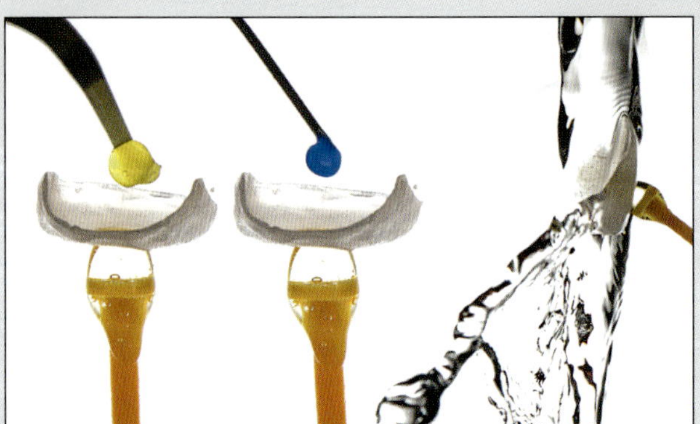

10a

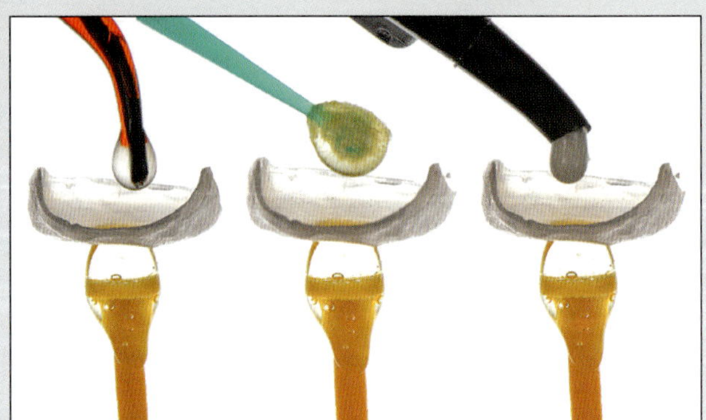

10b

Fig 10a *(left)* Etching with hydrofluoric acid for 20 seconds (Porcelanite, 3M ESPE). *(center)* Application of phosphoric acid for 30 seconds to remove the debris after ceramic etching (Power Etching, BM4). *(right)* Rinsing of the ceramic etched surfaces for 60 seconds.

Fig 10b *(left)* Application of silane (Monobond, Ivoclar Vivadent) and hot air drying for 60 seconds. *(center)* Application of the bonding agent (Excite, Ivoclar Vivadent). *(right)* Application of the luting agent (Variolink II, Ivoclar Vivadent).

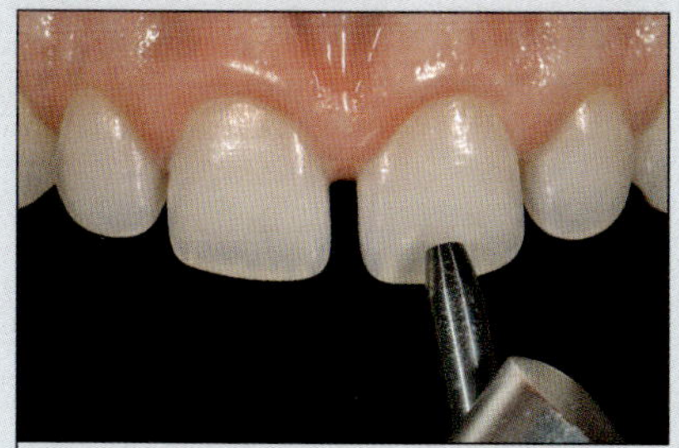

11a

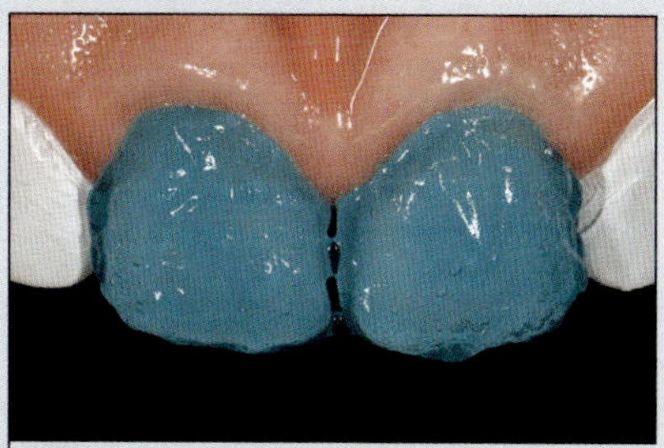

11b

Fig 11a Prophylaxis of enamel surfaces before bonding with pumice slurry and sandblasting with Rocatec (3M ESPE).

Fig 11b Enamel etching for 15 seconds (Power Etching, BM4).

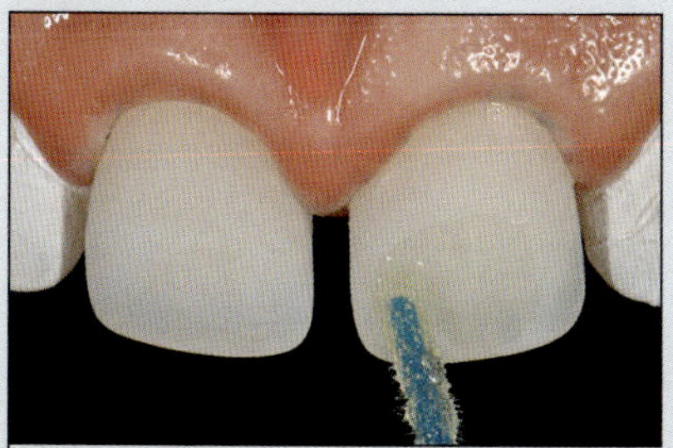

11c

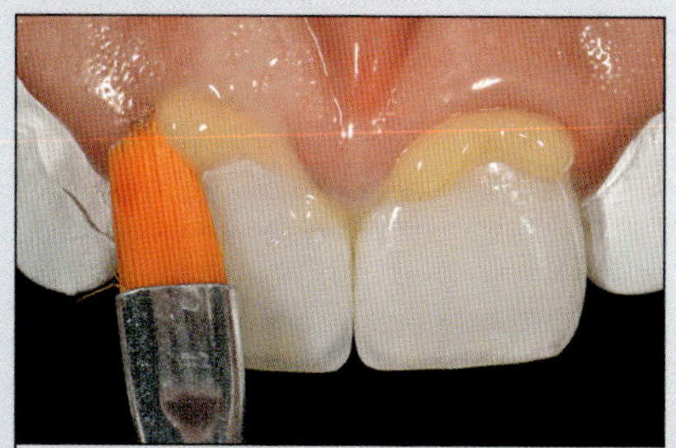

11d

Fig 11c Application of a two-step etch-and-rinse adhesive (Excite, Ivoclar Vivadent).

Fig 11d Removal of excess resin cement with a special artist brush.

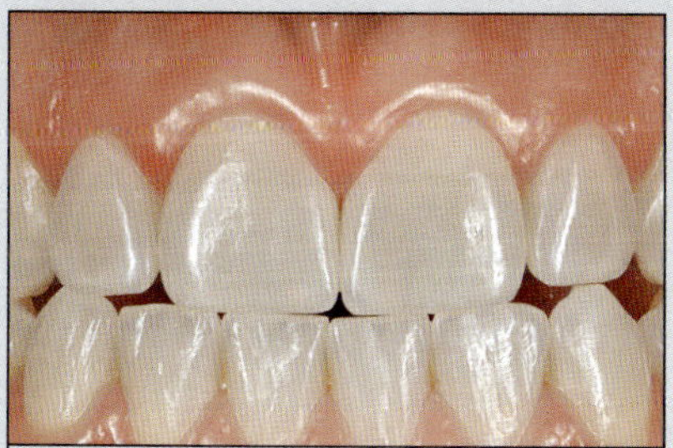

12a

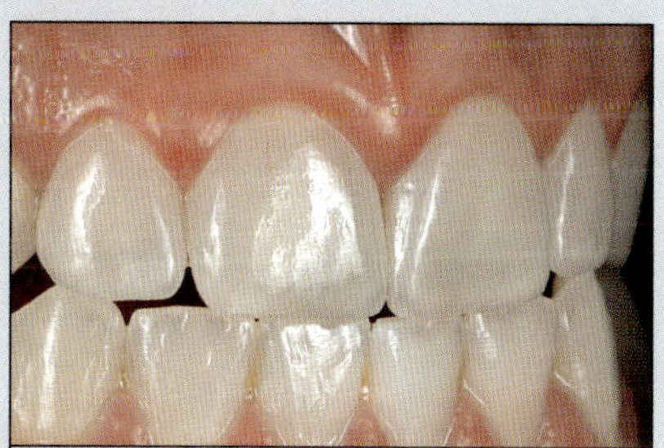

12b

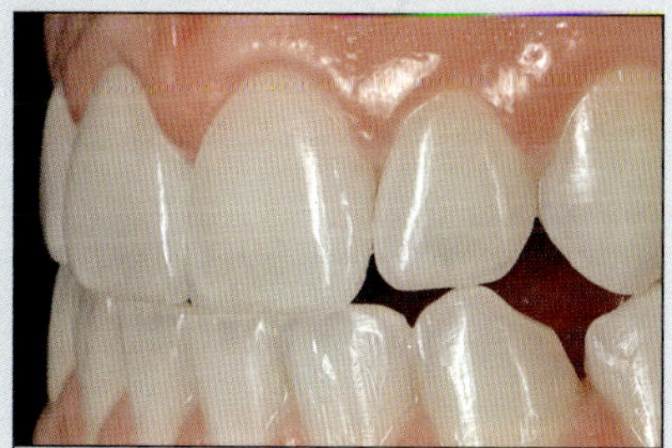

12c

Figs 12a to 12c Intraoral view after cementation. The shade, contour, form, and occlusion were restored.

The cementation technique plays a crucial role in the survival rate of ceramic restorations. Following are the steps used for surface treatment and bonding:

1. Etching with hydrofluoric acid (Porcelain Etch, 3M ESPE) for 20 seconds followed by copious rinsing with tap water.
2. Additional etching with 35% phosphoric acid (BM4) for 30 seconds for the removal of debris.
3. Rinsing of the etched ceramic restorations in an ultrasonic bath using 90% alcohol for 5 minutes.
4. Silane application for 60 seconds (Monobond, Ivoclar Vivadent), followed by hot air/drying for 20 seconds.
5. Adhesive application (Excite, Ivoclar Vivadent).
6. Luting using resin cement (Variolink II, Ivoclar Vivadent) (Fig 11).[10]

The teeth were then isolated and cleaned with a sandblasting device, subsequently etched with 37% phosphoric acid (BM4) for 15 seconds, followed by a 30-second rinsing, application of a two-step etch-and-rinse adhesive (Excite, Ivoclar Vivadent), and cementation (Fig 12).

The occlusion was checked, and the patient was dismissed. The final result and clinical follow-up after 24 months are shown in Figs 13 and 14.

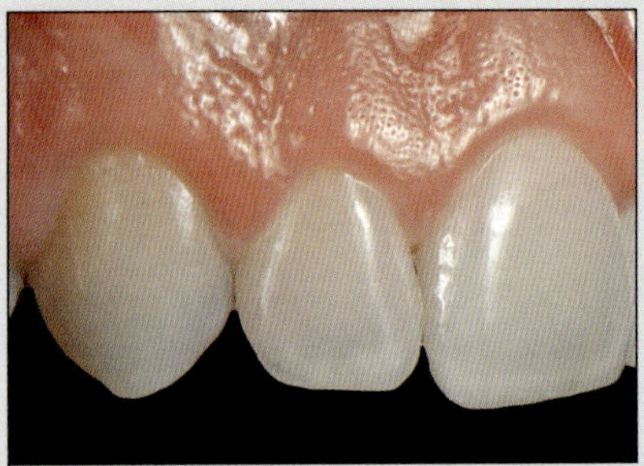

13a

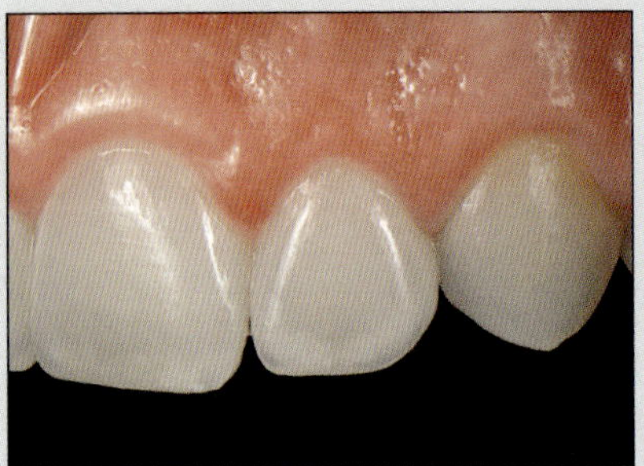

13b

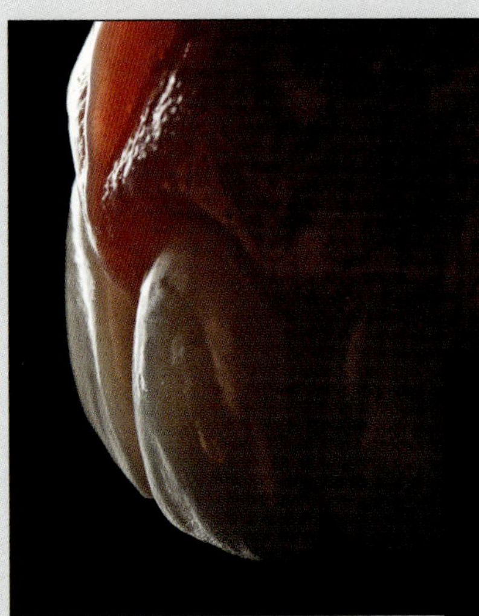

13c

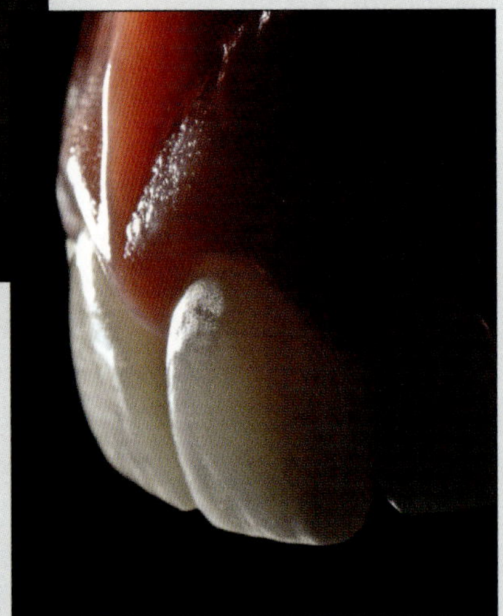

13d

Figs 13a to 13d Clinical follow-up after 24 months.

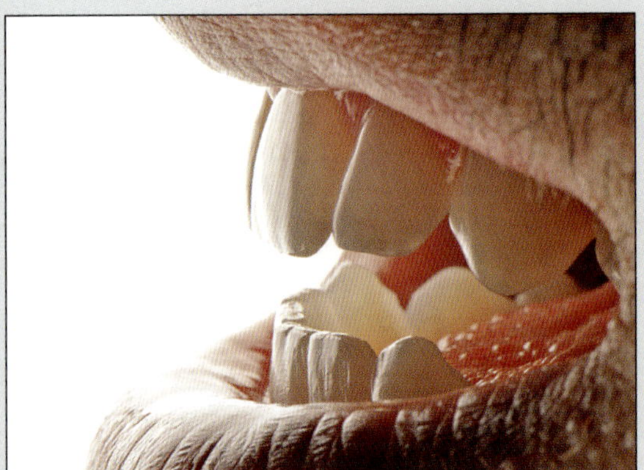

14a

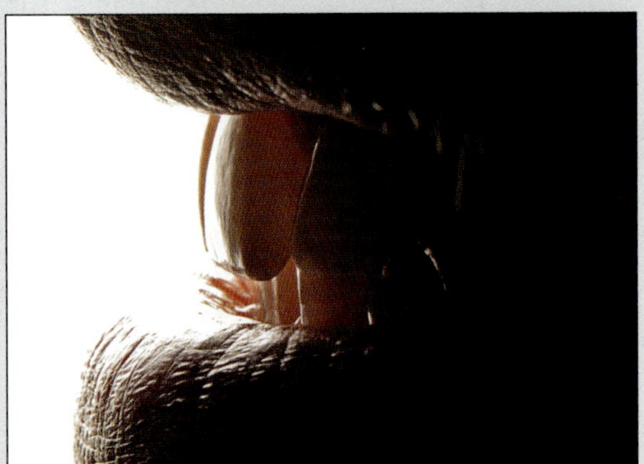

14b

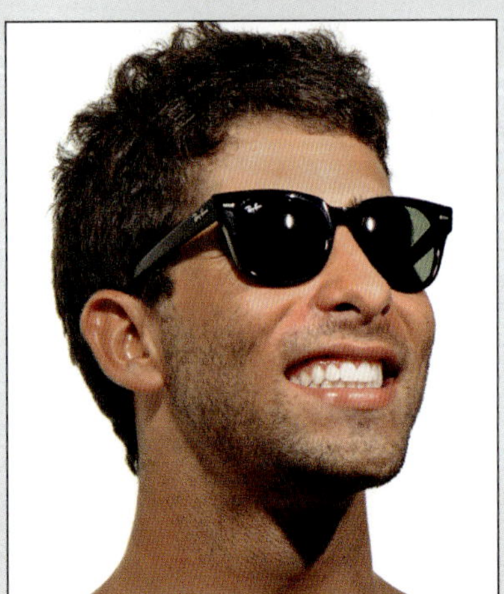

14c

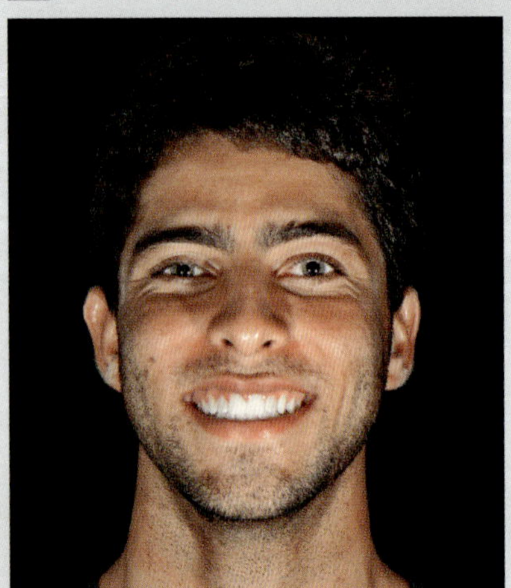

14d

Figs 14a to 14d Final result.

DISCUSSION

The treatment planning for esthetic crown lengthening should take into account the necessity for the associated prosthetic rehabilitation. In clinical situations where veneers or crowns are required, the future prosthetic margins should match the contours of the gingival margin, which will eventually provide the needed orientation for the extent of the osteotomy. In such cases, root exposure is not of concern, since restorations will cover these areas. There should be sufficient time for healing of the soft tissues before the definitive tooth preparation and impression. The gingival sulcus will appear to be completely stabilized after 3 months, although complete healing of the tissues can take up to a year, dependent on the characteristics of the initial surgery[11] and the amount of osteotomy and osteoplasty. When a restoration is not anticipated, the reference for an eventual osteotomy is the cementoenamel junction.

Treatment planning is the key for treatment success.[12] Using a combination of two different treatments, ie, flapless surgery and nonprep veneers, the tooth structures can be preserved, especially considering the noninvasive procedures and latest advances in adhesive techniques, guaranteeing the clinical success of this type of restoration.[13]

CONCLUSIONS

The flapless approach is a safe, easy, and predictable procedure with considerable clinical advantages. When the proper indications for this procedure are respected, it can achieve stable and esthetic outcomes. A multidisciplinary approach provides patients with high-quality noninvasive treatment, resulting in superior esthetics.

REFERENCES

1. Garber DA, Salama MA. The aesthetic smile: Diagnosis and treatment. Periodontol 2000 1996;11:18–28.
2. Campelo LD, Camara JR. Flapless implant surgery: A 10-year clinical retrospective analysis. Int J Oral Maxillofac Implants 2002; 17:271–276.
3. Harrel SK, Rees TD. Granulation tissue removal in routine and minimally invasive procedures. Compend Contin Educ Dent 1995;16:960–964.
4. Becker W, Goldstein M, Becker BE, Sennerby L, Kois D, Hujoel P. Minimally invasive flapless placement: Follow-up results from a multicenter study. J Periodontol 2009:80:346–352.
5. Carvalho PFM, da Silva RC, Joly JC. Aumento de coroa clinica estético sem retalho: Uma nova alternative terapéutica. Rev Assoc Paul Cir Dent 2010;ed esp 1:26–33.
6. Joly JC, Carvalho PFM, Silva RC, Flapless esthetic crown lengthening: A new therapeutic approach. Rev Mex Periodontologia 2011;2:103–108.
7. Gurel G. The Science and Art of Porcelain Laminate Veneers. Chicago: Quintessence, 2003.
8. Scopin de Andrade O, Romanini J, Hirata R. Ultimate ceramic veneers: A laboratory-guided ultraconservative preparation concept for maximum enamel preservation. Quintessence Dent Technol 2012;34:103–119.
9. Adolfi D. Functional, esthetic, and morphologic adjustment procedures for anterior teeth. Quintessence Dent Technol 2009; 32:153–168.
10. Magne P, Magne M, Magne I. Porcelain jacket crowns. Back to the future through bonding. Quintessence Dent Technol 2010; 33:89–96.
11. Müller HP, Könönen E. Variance components of gingival thickness. J Periodontal Res 2005;40:239–244.
12. Malik K, Tabiat-Pour S. The use of diagnostic wax set-up in aesthetic cases involving crown lengthening—A case report. Dent Update 2010;37:303–304,306–307.
13. Gresnigt M, Ozcan M, Kalk W. Esthetic rehabilitation of worn anterior teeth with thin porcelain laminate veneers. Eur J Esthet Dent 2011;6:298–313.

Sergio R. Arias, DDS, MS[1]
Aram Torosian, MDC, CDT[2]
Somkiat Aimplee, DDS, MS[1]
Jimmy Londono, DDS[3]
Gerard Chiche, DDS[4]

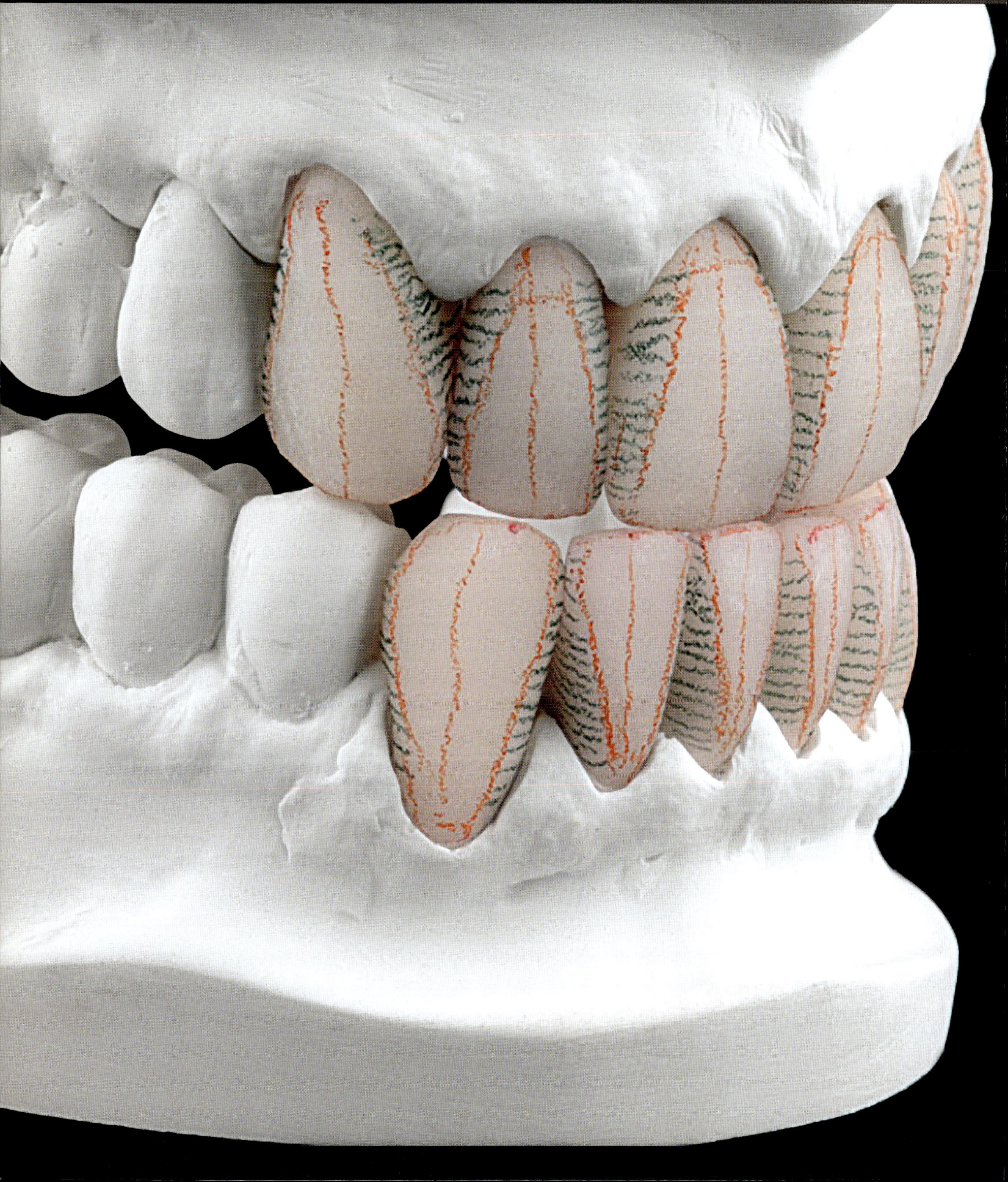

Mastering Esthetic and Functional Rehabilitation of the Severely Worn Dentition

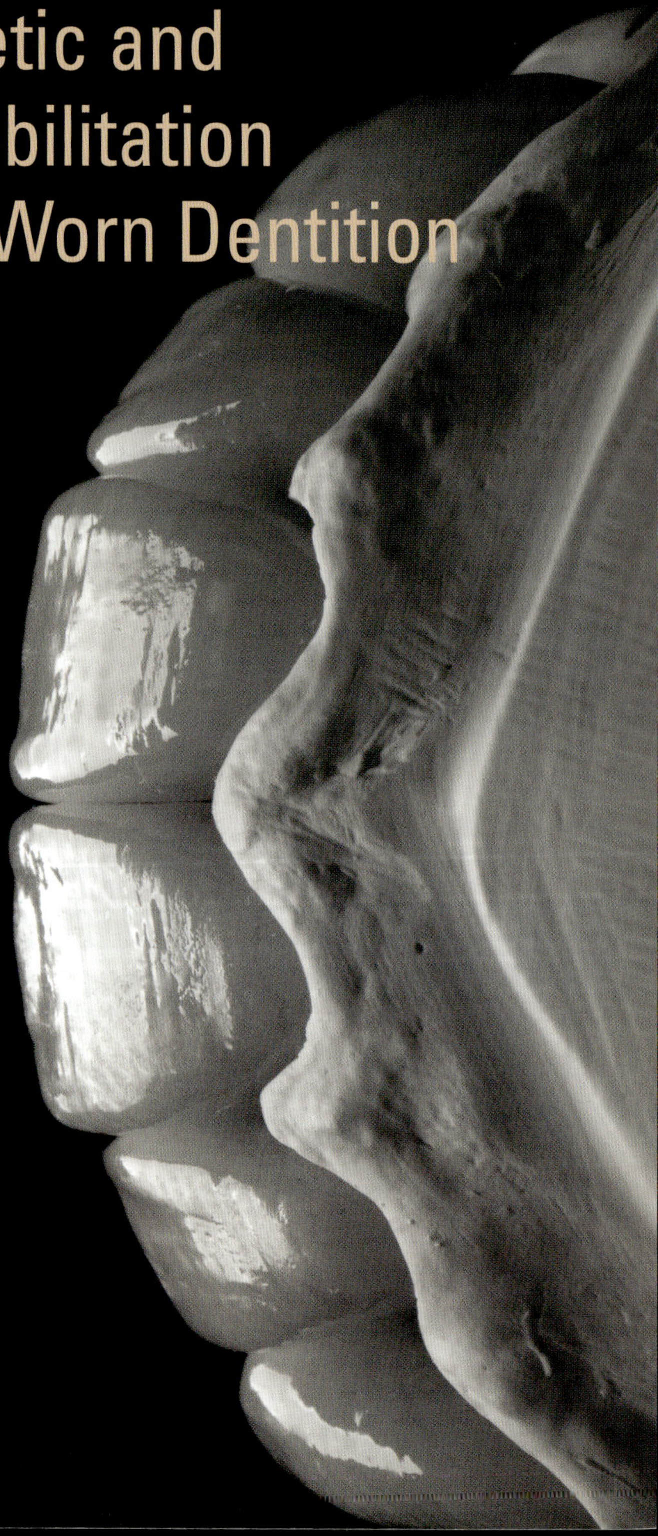

[1]Esthetic and Implant Fellow, Ronald Goldstein Center for Esthetic and Implant Dentistry, Georgia Regents University, College of Dental Medicine, Augusta, Georgia, USA.

[2]Master Dental Ceramist, Ronald Goldstein Center for Esthetic and Implant Dentistry, Georgia Regents University, College of Dental Medicine, Augusta, Georgia, USA.

[3]Assistant Professor, Ronald Goldstein Center for Esthetic and Implant Dentistry, Georgia Regents University, College of Dental Medicine, Augusta, Georgia, USA.

[4]Director, Ronald Goldstein Center for Esthetic and Implant Dentistry, Georgia Regents University, College of Dental Medicine, Augusta, Georgia, USA.

Correspondence to: Dr Sergio R. Arias, College of Dental Medicine, Georgia Regents University Augusta, 1430 John Wesley Gilbert Dr, Augusta, GA 30912. Email: drarias@gmail.com

With advances in all-ceramic systems, adhesive resin cements, implant dentistry, and computer-aided design/computer-assisted manufacture (CAD/CAM) technology, numerous treatment options are available for the fixed prosthetic rehabilitation. These alternatives increase the quality and predictability of dental treatment. A systematic and organized approach is essential in order to evaluate, diagnose, and resolve esthetic and functional problems predictably in a complex restorative case.[1]

The following case is presented to illustrate the use of these treatment options in the management of a patient with a severely worn dentition.

CASE PRESENTATION

A 70-year-old male patient presented for treatment at the Ronald Goldstein Center for Esthetic and Implant Dentistry at Georgia Regents University, College of Dental Medicine. The patient was in good general health, and his medical history was noncontributory. His main concern was "My front teeth are getting thin and keep chipping. They don't look natural." The clinical extraoral evaluation revealed a deviated facial midline, a slanted incisal plane, and a retrusive maxillary incisal profile (Fig 1).

Intraoral evaluation revealed significant generalized incisal wear caused by parafunction and erosion, with loss of posterior support and excessive anterior vertical overlap.[2] In addition, the patient had multiple failing restorations with poor marginal adaptation, and there was an occlusal plane discrepancy caused by supraeruption of maxillary first and second molars into the mandibular edentulous sites. Finally, the central incisors had a narrow tapered appearance and inadequate proportions due to gingival recession and their irregular gingival outlines (Fig 2).

The patient traveled approximately 4½ hours for appointments; therefore, he preferred a treatment plan that would require a minimal number of visits. For this reason, the patient declined orthodontic treatment and requested to have as few surgical procedures as possible.

Based on the compromised esthetic and functional situation of the case, full-mouth rehabilitation was prescribed to *(1)* correct the occlusal plane discrepancy, *(2)* decrease the vertical overlap after achieving proper tooth length, *(3)* correct the incisal edge position, *(4)* harmonize the anterior guidance, and *(4)* improve the esthetic appearance. A diagnostic occlusal splint was fabricated to enable muscular relaxation and to allow the condyles to seat in centric relation (CR), to protect the teeth from further wear, and to evaluate the patient's tolerance of an increase in vertical dimension of occlusion (VDO).[3]

Esthetic Analysis

The treatment planning started with the esthetic evaluation and proceeded with function, structure, and biology.[4] A seven-step esthetic analysis was performed as described by Chiche and Pinault, which allows for an early detection of "esthetic red flags."[5] The first four steps of the analysis relate to the evaluation of the incisal edge position of the maxillary central incisors; their correct position is the foundation from which the smile is built. When the incisal edge position is set correctly, it serves to determine proper tooth proportion and gingival levels.[1]

Determination of Incisal Edge Position

To improve the incisal display at rest and the irregular incisal edges (see Figs 3a and 3b), a direct composite mock-up was made on the central incisors at the predetermined planned position (Fig 3c). This was done directly facing the patient to reestablish parallelism between the occlusal plane and the interpupillary line and to reestablish verticality of the dental midline (Fig 3d). The composite mock-up was preserved and transferred to the diagnostic stone cast (Fig 3e). The mock-up resembled an inverted "T" effect that followed the interpupillary line perpendicular to the facial midline; it also served as the reference for the diagnostic wax-up (Fig 3f).

A polyvinyl siloxane (PVS) matrix was made of the mock-up seated on the stone cast to record the new incisal edge position (Fig 3g). The matrix was marked and trimmed to outline the incisal edges (Figs 3h and 3i). The matrix was reseated on the cast without the composite resin mock-up, and the space was filled with wax to reproduce the incisal edge position and

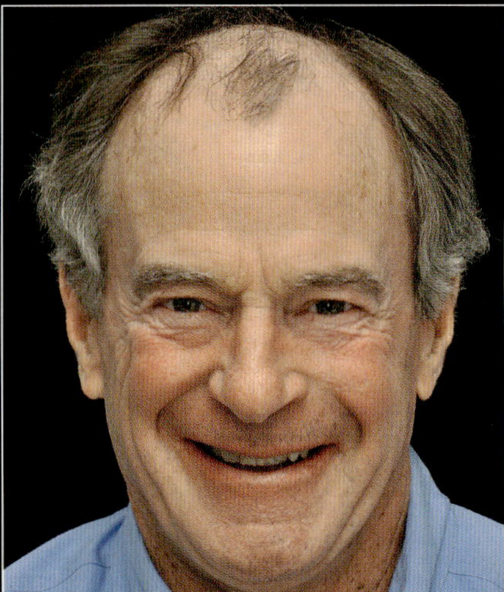
1a

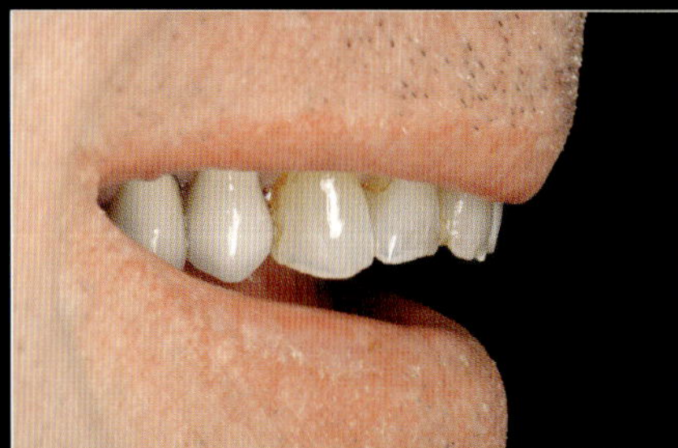
1b

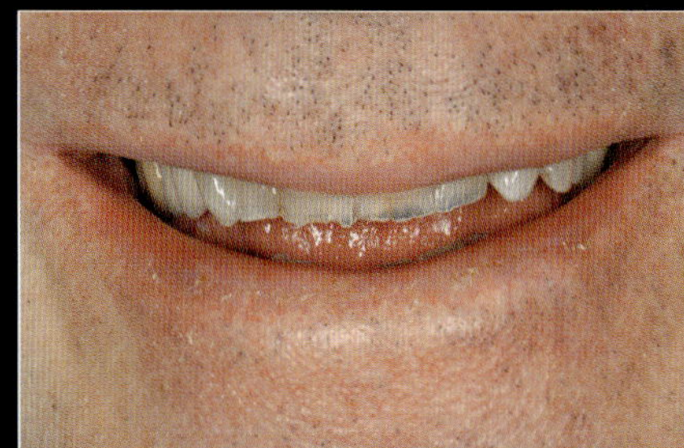
1c

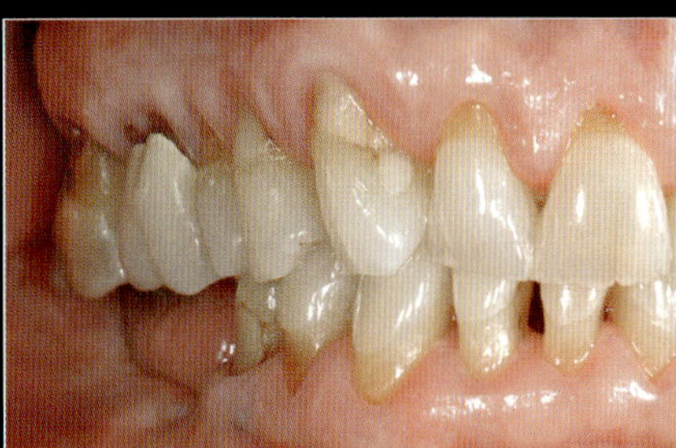
2a

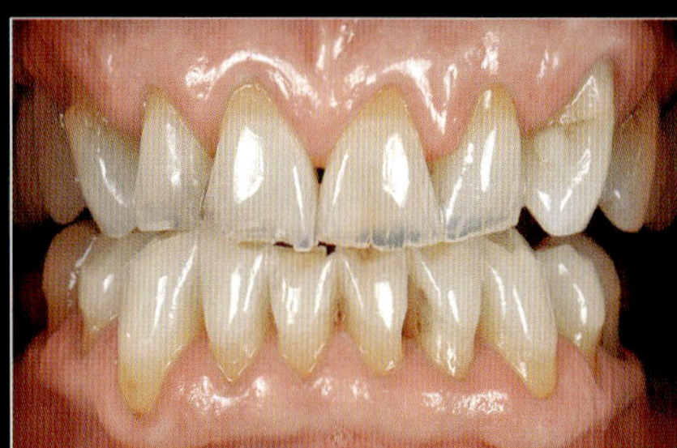
2b

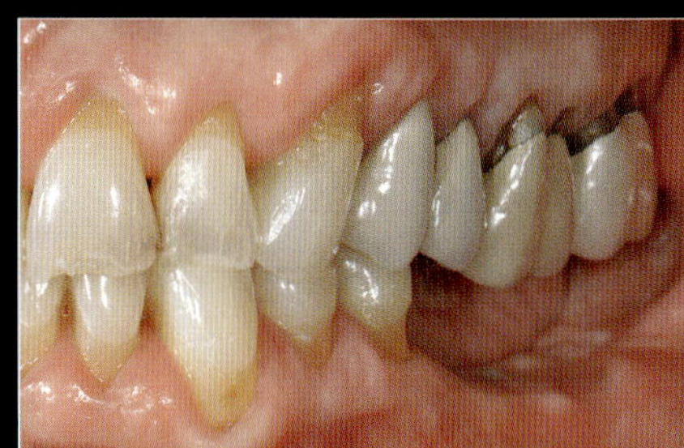
2c

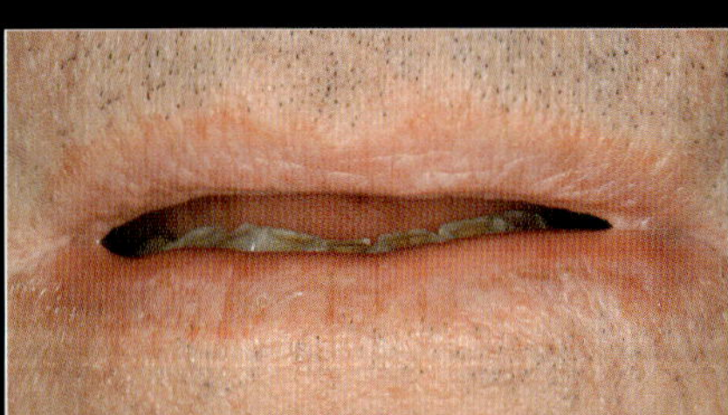
3a

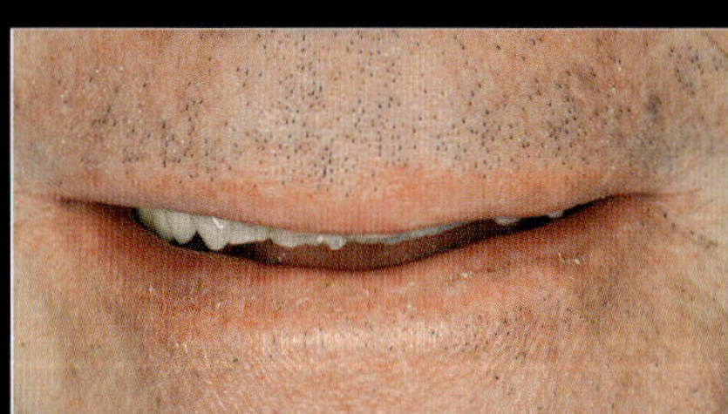
3b

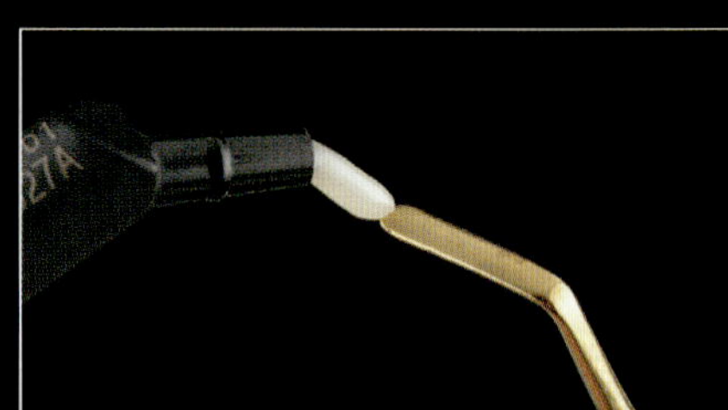
3c

Figs 1a to 1c Preoperative extraoral views.

Figs 2a to 2c Preoperative intraoral views.

Fig 3a Extraoral frontal view of facial lower third at rest.

Fig 3b Moderate smile showing abrasion phenomena on incisal edges of maxillary anterior teeth.

Fig 3c Direct mock-up was performed with composite resin.

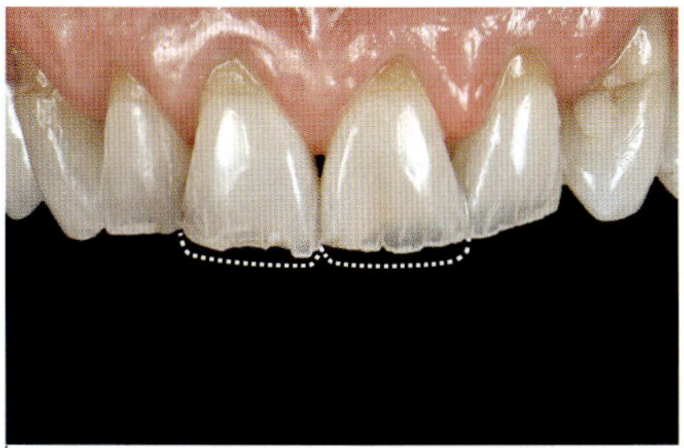

3d

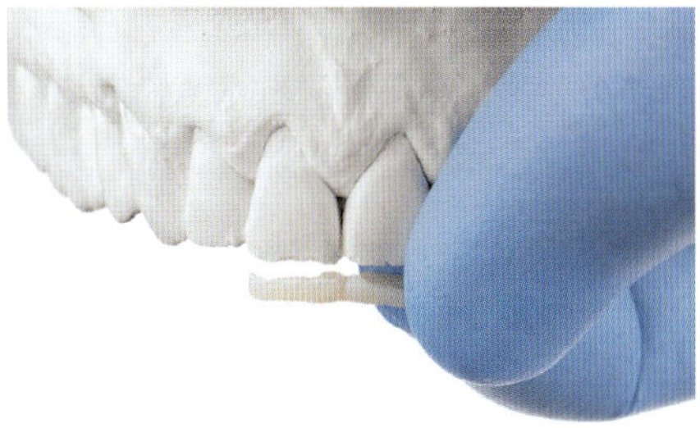

3e

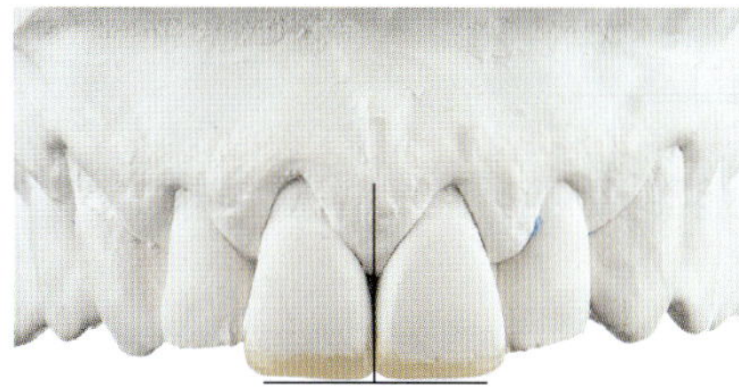

3f

Fig 3d New incisal edge position demarcated by reference line.

Fig 3e Composite mock-up transferred to diagnostic stone cast.

Fig 3f Vertical and horizontal reference lines established with the composite mock-up on the cast.

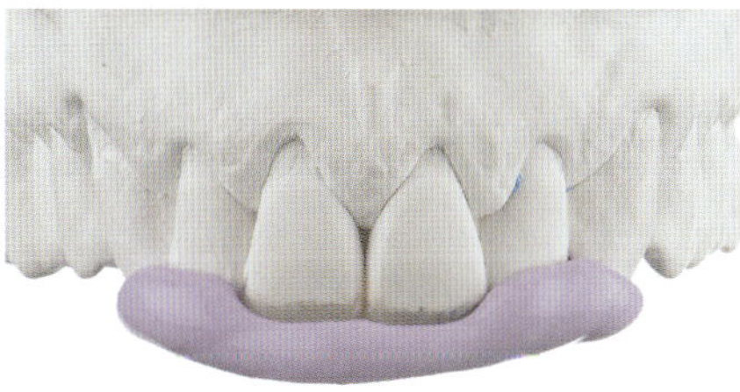

3g

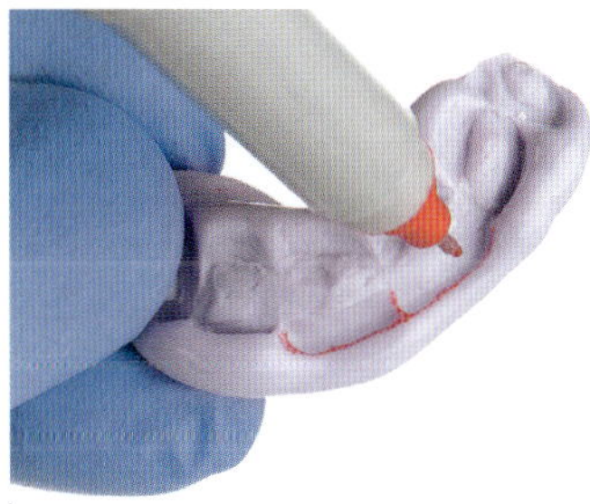

3h

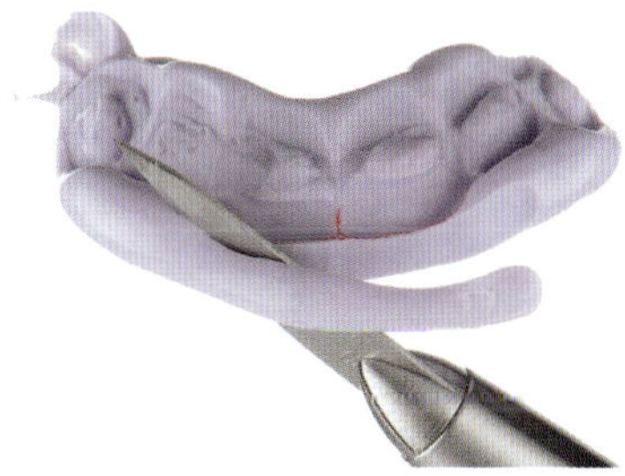

3i

Fig 3g A silicone material is used to record the new incisal edge position.

Fig 3h Silicone matrix is marked for trimming.

Fig 3i Silicone matrix is trimmed at marked level to create space for wax.

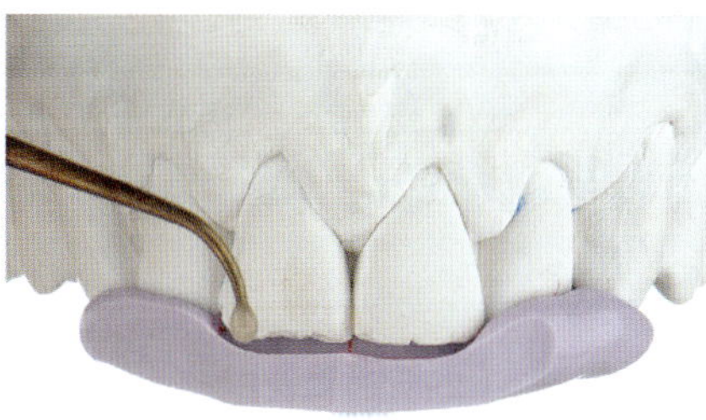

3j

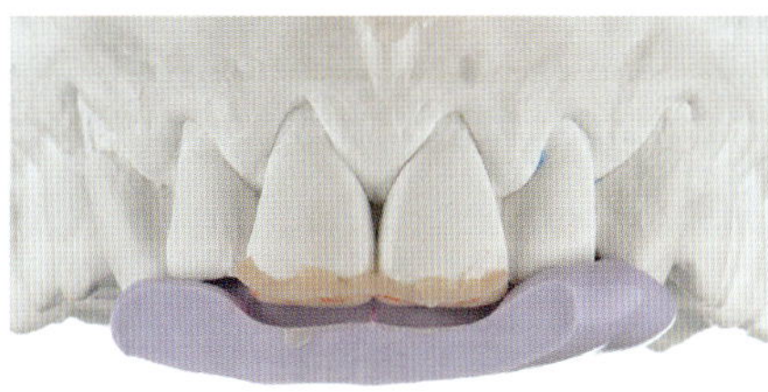

3k

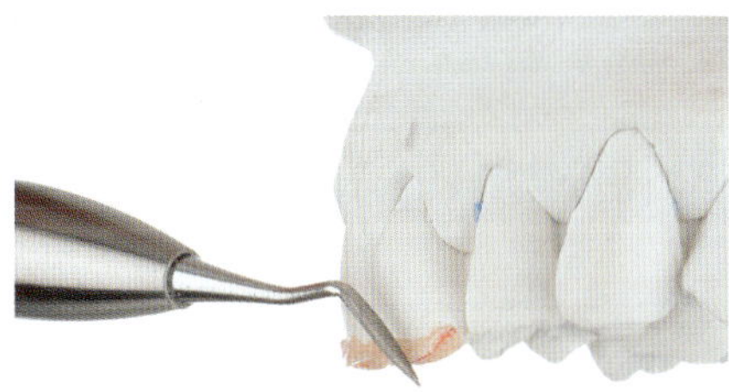

3l

Fig 3j Silicone matrix is filled with wax to transfer the new incisal edge position.

Fig 3k Silicone matrix is removed.

Fig 3l Wax excess is removed.

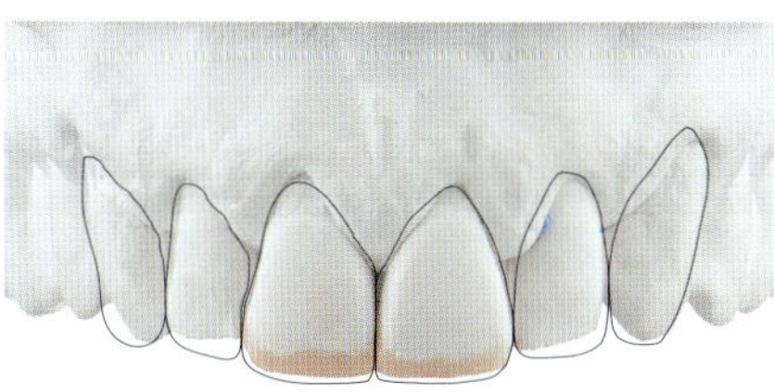

3m

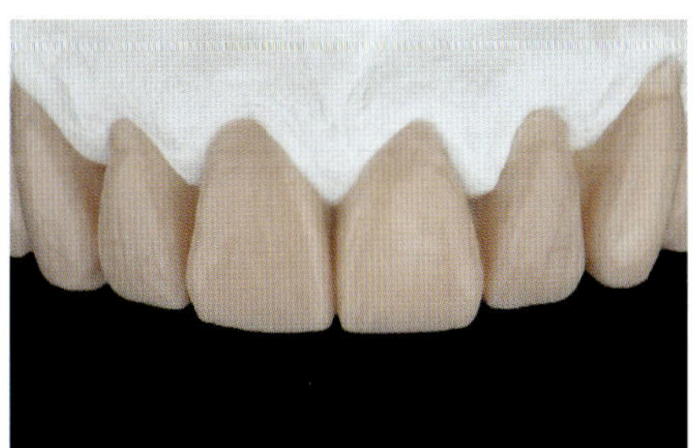

3n

Fig 3m New incisal edge position in wax.

Fig 3n Diagnostic wax-up of maxillary six anterior teeth, completed at the new incisal edge position.

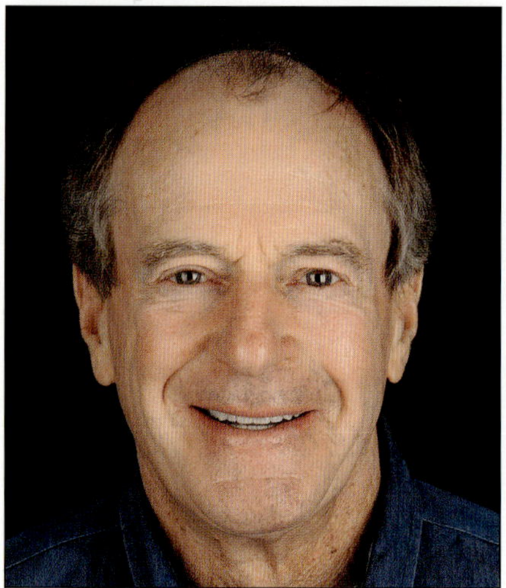
4a

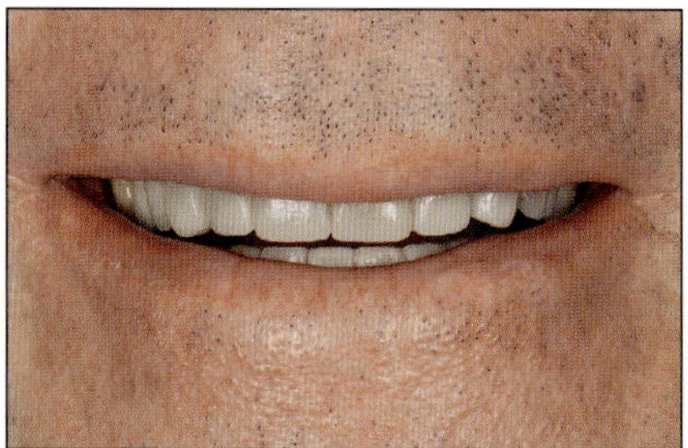
4b

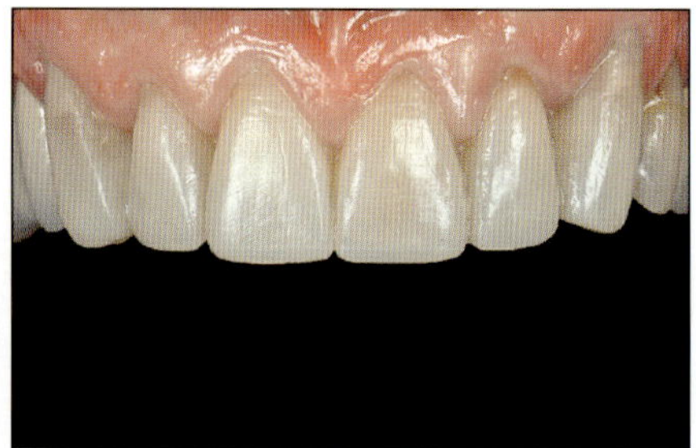
4c

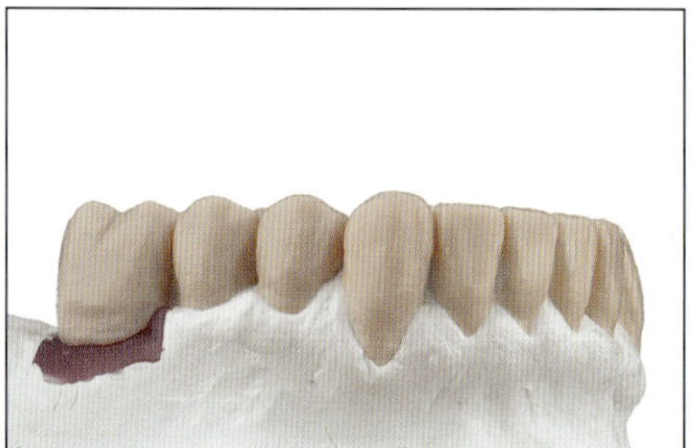
5a

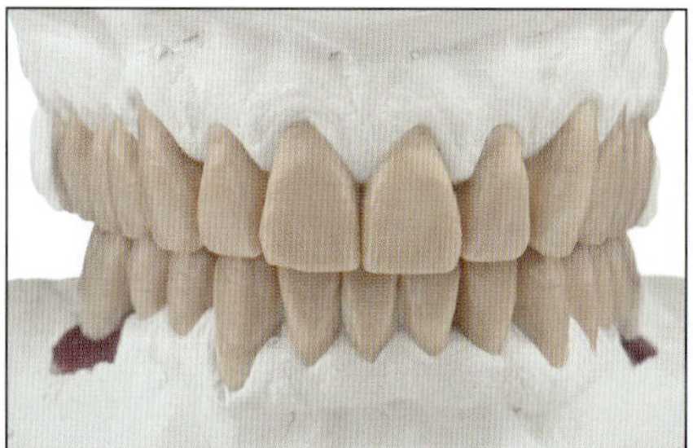
5b

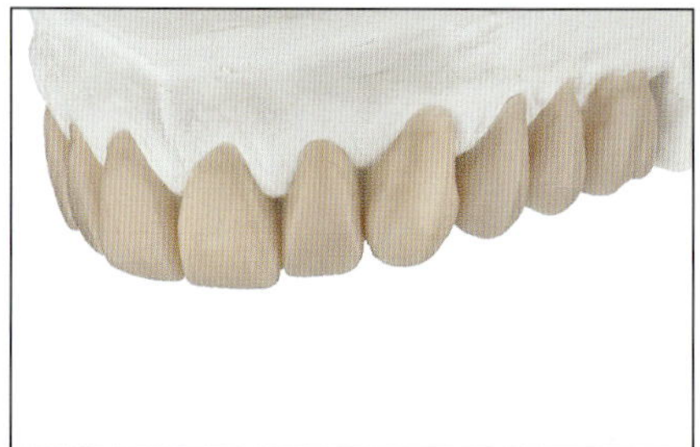
5c

Figs 4a to 4c Intraoral and extraoral views of the esthetic indirect mock-up.
Figs 5a to 5c Full-mouth esthetic wax-up.

midline (Figs 3j and 3k). The flash wax excess was removed with a wax-carving instrument (Fig 3l). The esthetic smile design was planned using the new incisal edge position, creating proper tooth proportions, tooth-to-tooth proportions, and gingival outlines, and fulfilled with the esthetic wax-up[5] (Figs 3m and 3n).

The new esthetic smile design was transferred to the mouth with an indirect mock-up so that it could be reviewed with the patient, and the patient and clinician could get a preview of the new smile (Fig 4). Following the patient's approval, a full-mouth diagnostic wax-up was made that incorporated the following: an increase in VDO to reduce vertical overlap, anterior disocclusion, and a leveled plane of occlusion (Fig 5).

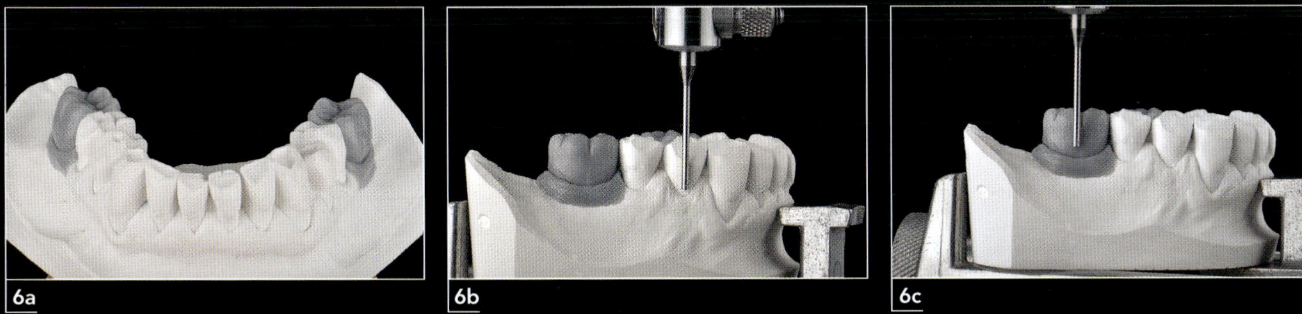

Fig 6a Stone cast with wax-up at future implant sites, mandibular right and left first molars.
Fig 6b Surveyor is aligned with axis of adjacent teeth.
Fig 6c Planned mesiodistal position for right first molar implant.

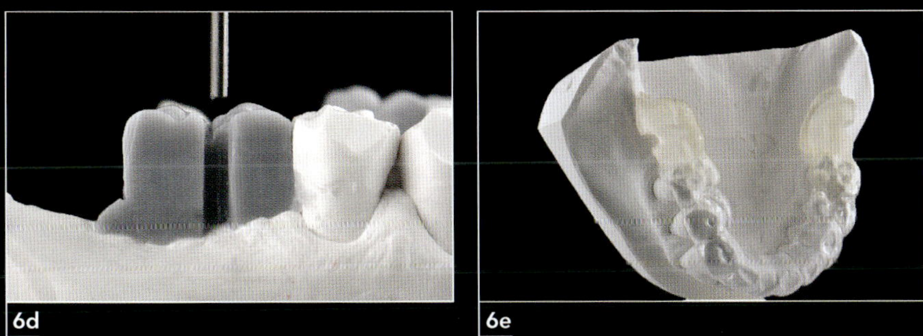

Fig 6d Wax prototype for surgical guide.
Fig 6e Surgical guide generated from the wax-up utilizing a vacuum-formed thermoplastic template and orthodontic acrylic resin.

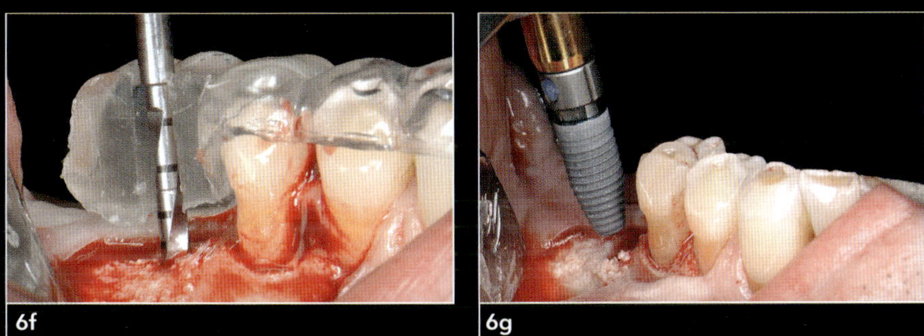

Fig 6f Osteotomy preparation using the surgical guide.
Fig 6g Implant placement.

Surgical Guide Fabrication and Implant Placement

The correct three-dimensional (3D) implant placement into an adequately prepared site is imperative to achieve an optimal esthetic and functional implant restoration. There are three recommended 3D parameters: *(1)* apicocoronal: the implant position should be 2 to 4 mm apical to the expected gingival margin position; *(2)* faciolingual: 2 mm of facial bone is recommended to prevent the loss of facial tissue; and *(3)* mesiodistal: there should be 2 mm between an implant and adjacent teeth and 3 mm between implants.[6-8] Following these recommendations a diagnostic wax-up was made for planning future implant placement in the positions of the mandibular right and left first molars (Fig 6a). The diagnostic cast with wax-up was mounted in a surveyor for planning implant angulations and positions (Figs 6b to 6d). A surgical guide was generated from the wax-up utilizing a vacuum-formed thermoplastic template and orthodontic acrylic resin (Fig 6e). The surgical guide was seated during osseous preparation, and two 5 × 11-mm implants were placed in the first molar sites (Nobel Replace Tapered, Nobel Biocare) (Figs 6f and 6g).

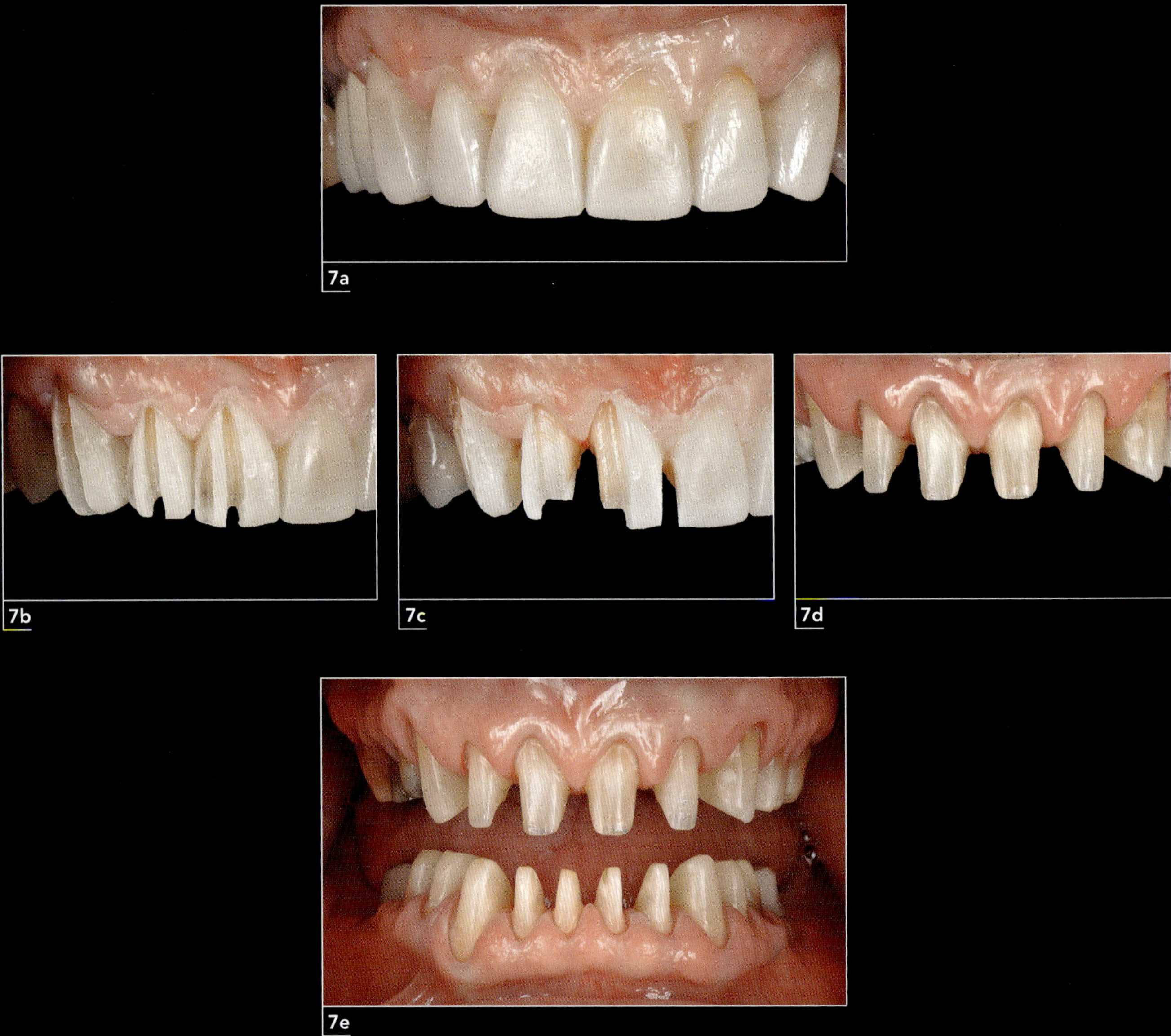

Fig 7a Indirect mock-up used as a tooth-reduction guide.
Fig 7b Calibrated depth cuts.
Fig 7c Adjacent teeth used as preparation references.
Fig 7d Maxillary anterior preparations completed.
Fig 7e Full-mouth preparations completed.

Tooth Preparation Sequence

The mock-up was made again and used as a reduction guide for tooth preservation, a technique that has been described for laminate porcelain veneer prepa- sal depth cuts were made and connected by preparing half of the tooth on adjacent teeth; this helped to maintain the correct axis and orientation between preparations (Figs 7b and 7c). Final anterior and full-mouth preparations were completed (Figs 7d and 7e).

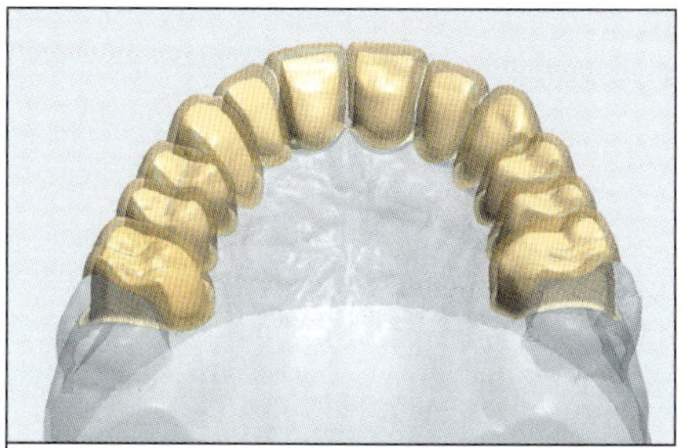

8a

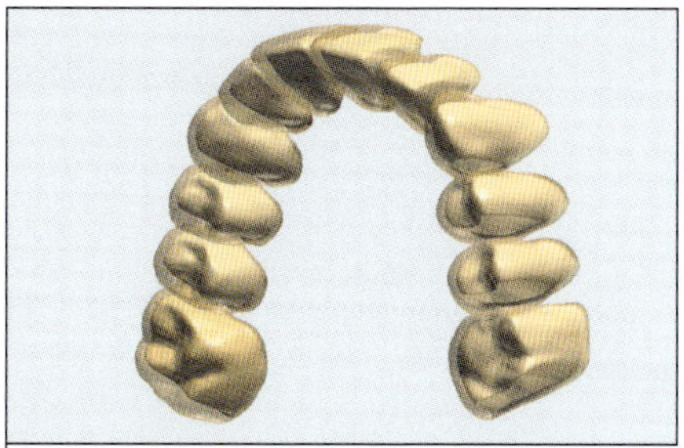

8b

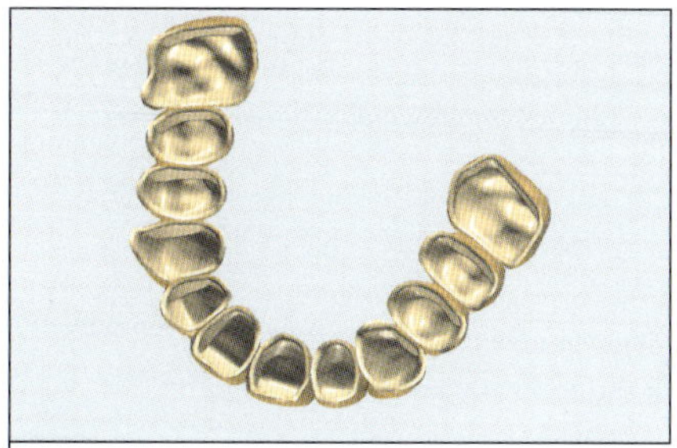

8c

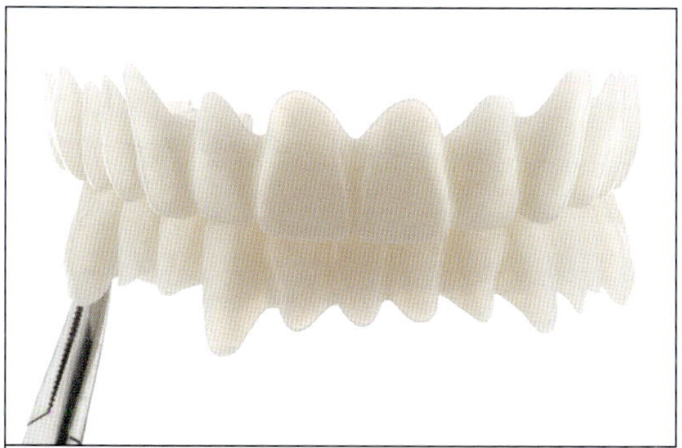

8d

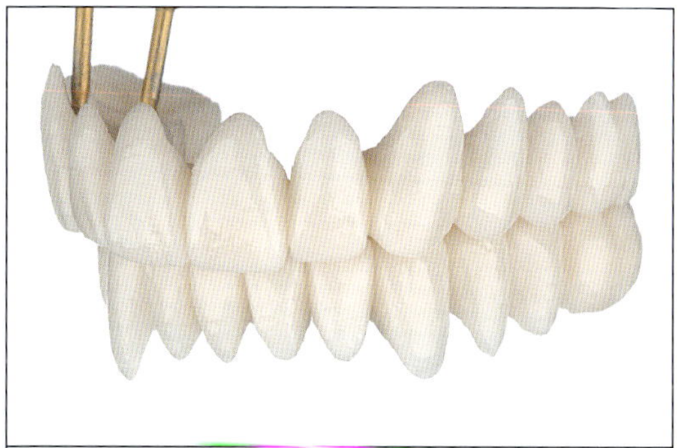

8e

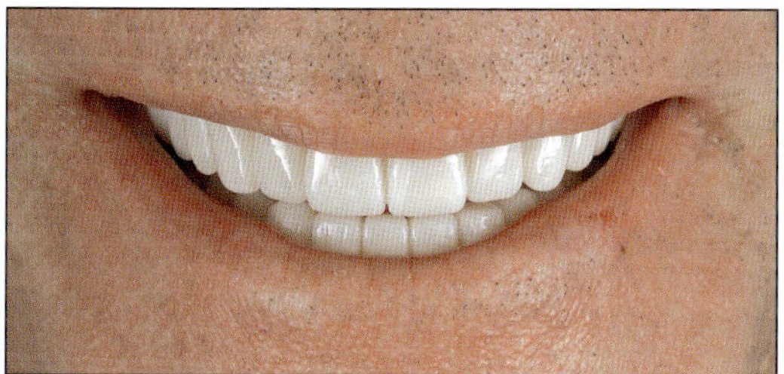

8f

Figs 8a to 8c CAD/CAM provisional shell designs.
Fig 8d Maxillary and mandibular CAD/CAM shells.
Fig 8e Provisionals after relining and polishing.
Fig 8f Smile view with provisionals.

CAD/CAM Provisional Restorations

The interim restoration plays an essential role in the process of full-mouth rehabilitations. It is considered the blueprint for fabrication of the definitive restoration and should be identical in all respects except for the materials from which it is fabricated.[10,11] For this patient, a CAD/CAM provisional was fabricated using the shell technique. There are several advantages of this treatment modality: *(1)* high strength due to less porosity, *(2)* the material is long lasting, and *(3)* chairside time is devoted to relining, reducing, and polishing the cervical areas with minimal occlusal adjustment.[12]

The full-mouth wax-up was scanned for fabrication of CAD/CAM shells (Figs 8a to 8c). Note the accuracy of the maxillary shell in occlusion against the mandibular shell (Fig 8d). Provisional restorations were relined, finished, polished, and delivered (Figs 8e and 8f).

Evaluation of Provisionals

The patient tolerated the provisional restorations well over a period of approximately 8 weeks. During this time the occlusion was checked and adjusted to match the planned occlusal scheme of the diagnostic waxing. Prior to final impressions, the provisionals were measured at the occlusal, incisal, and middle thirds with the temporary cement still in place. This allowed the clinician to determine if the teeth had been sufficiently reduced during preparation (Figs 9a to 9c).

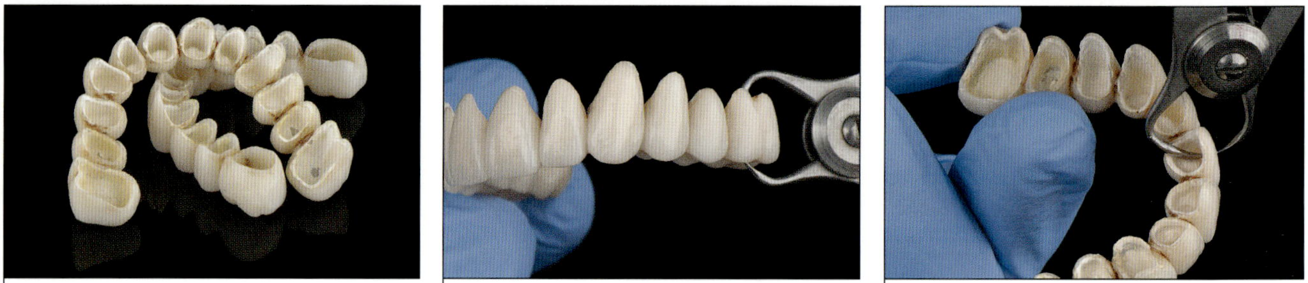

9a 9b 9c

Fig 9a Provisionals with retained temporary cement.
Fig 9b Measuring occlusal thickness.
Fig 9c Measuring facial thickness.

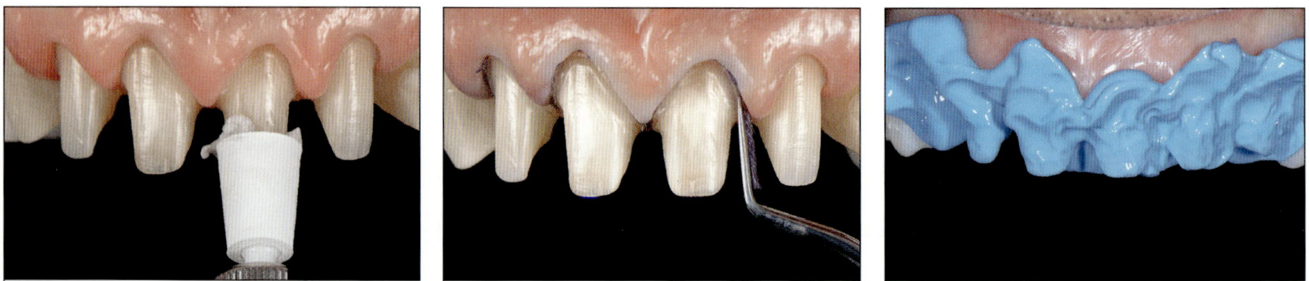

10a 10b 10c

Fig 10a Preparations are cleaned with pumice.
Fig 10b Retraction cord is packed.
Fig 10c PVS impression is made.

Final Impressions

Preparations were cleaned and pumiced, retraction cord was placed, and final impressions were made with a PVS material (Fig 10).

Wax-up and Processing of Pressed Ceramics

Figure 11a shows the wax design of the definitive restorations on the master cast. Wax separator was applied, the margins were sealed with inlay/onlay wax (Schuler-Dental), and the Ivan Ronald Huanca waxing tool was used to finish the margins and to create a pleasing and natural emergence profile (Figs 11b to 11d). Surface texture, irregularities, and unique characteristics were verified to mimic natural morphology (Figs 11e and 11f). The 3-mm wax sprues were attached in the direction of the ceramic flow at the thickest part of the wax-up to allow the smooth flow of the viscous ceramic during pressing (Fig 11g). The anterior segment was pressed utilizing a lithium disilicate glass ceramic ingot in Value 3 (IPS e.max Press, Ivoclar Vivadent). A delicate divesting process was carried out using fine glass beads (Renfert).

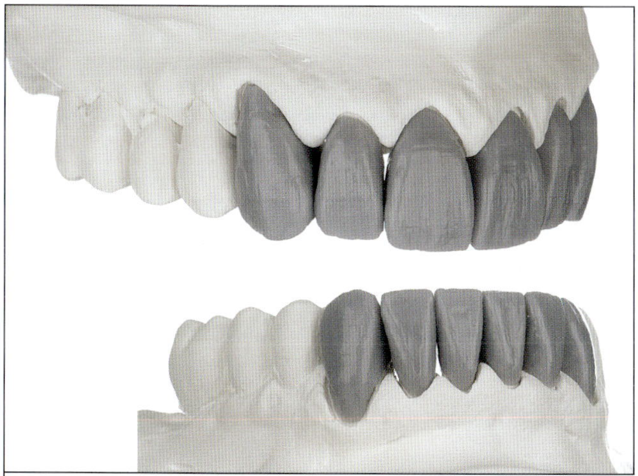
11a

Fig 11a Final wax-up of anterior teeth.
Fig 11b Application of separator.
Fig 11c Sealing the margin.
Fig 11d Finishing the wax margin and completing the emergence profile.

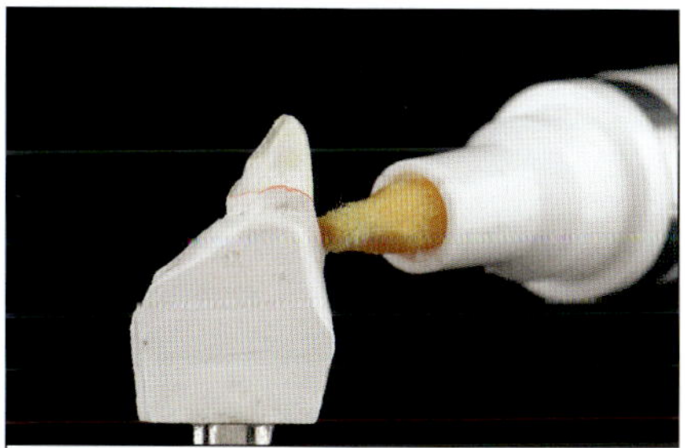
11b

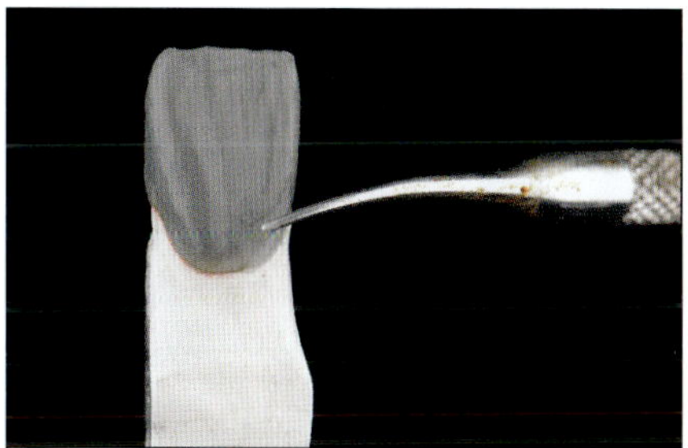
11c

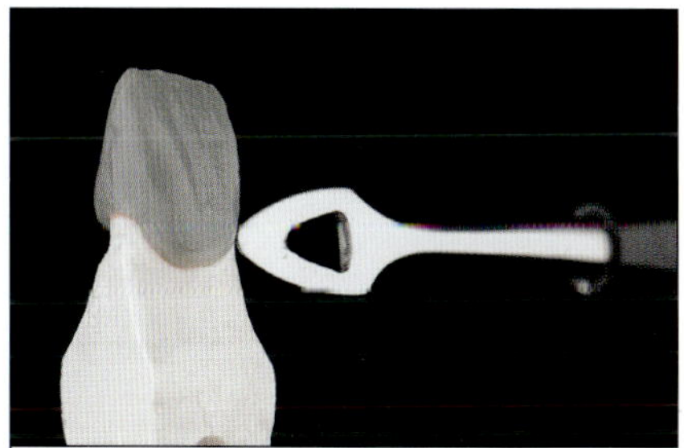
11d

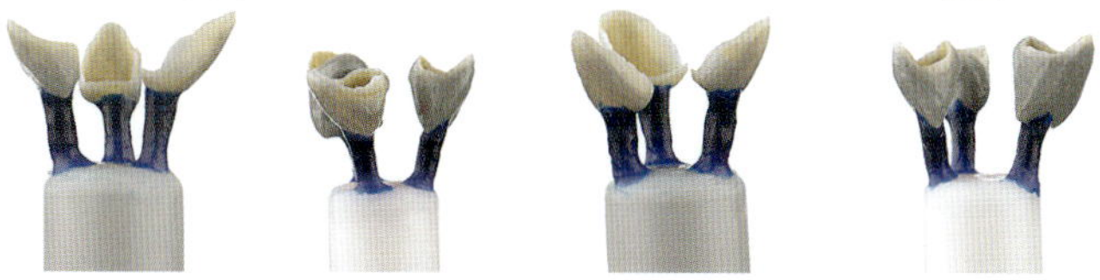

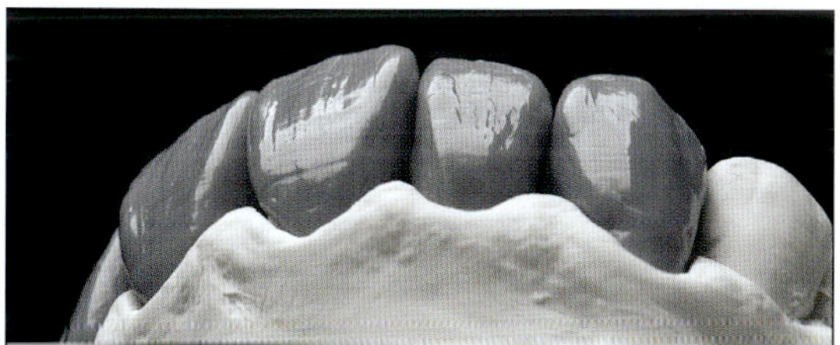
11e

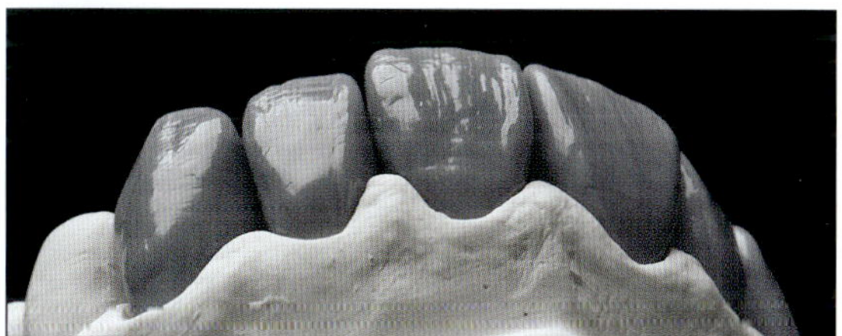
11f

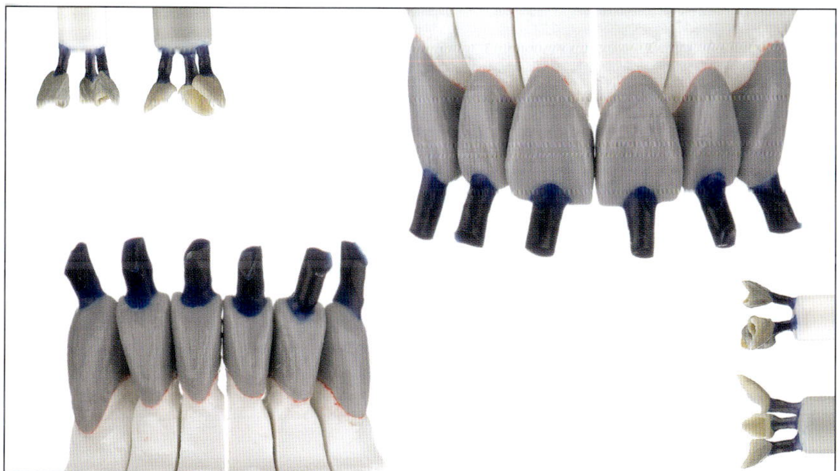
11g

Figs 11e and 11f Texture verification.
Fig 11g Maxillary and mandibular wax-ups with sprues.

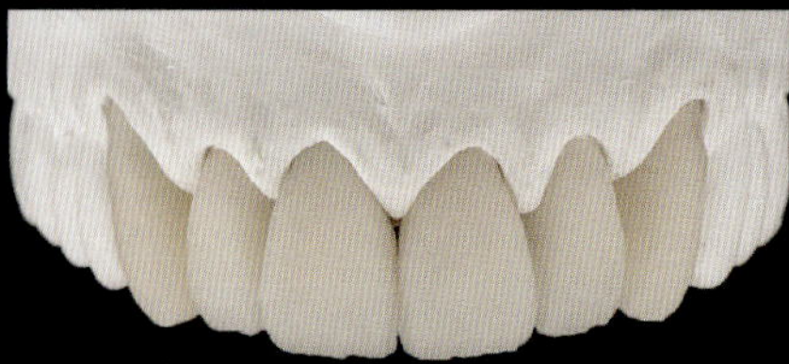
12a

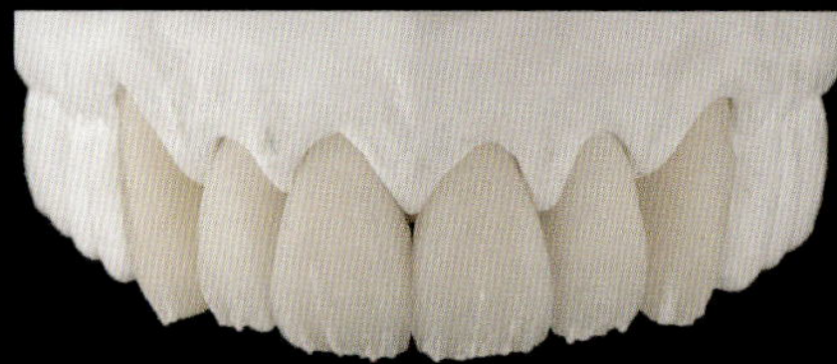
12b

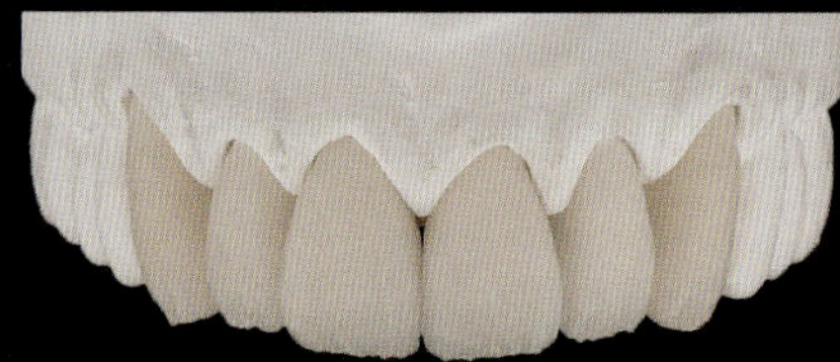
12c

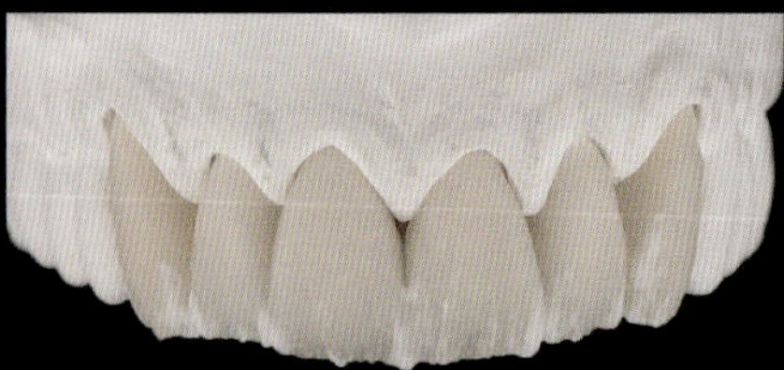
12d

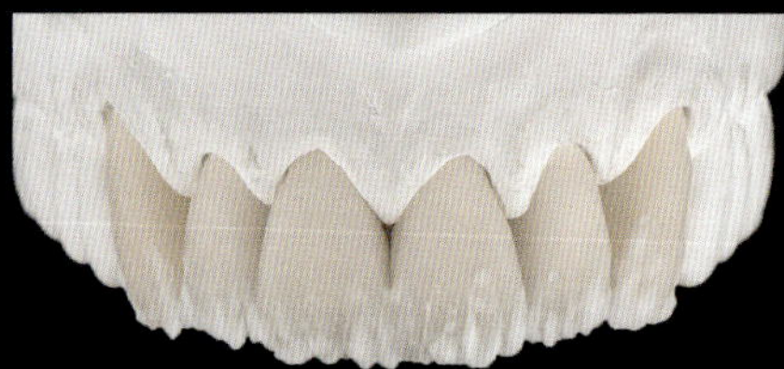
12e

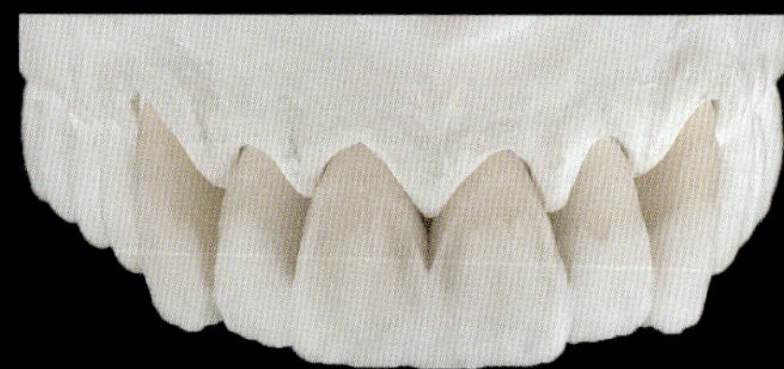
12f

Fig 12a Pressed IPS e.max restorations on cast, minimally cut back at facial third.

Fig 12b First bake: Application of the stain and powder for a bonding layer as well as some internal mamelon-structure effects.

Fig 12c Assessment of wash bake for color and effects.

Fig 12d Second bake: Opal Effect (OE) 1 Ceram material in the interproximal areas.

Fig 12e Segmental ceramic stratification of opalescent and enamel powders, OE 1 on corners, OE 2, OE 3, Bleach incisal, BL4 dentin, and mamelon powders to create contrasts and high- and low-value areas.

Fig 12f Initial ceramic stratification covered by a thin layer of mixed OE 1 and T1.

Ceramic Layering Procedures

The crowns were seated on the master solid cast. The crowns were airborne-particle abraded in the laboratory with glass beads to improve the bond between the pressed and the veneering ceramics. An initial wash firing using a combination of Essence stains and opalescent and mamelon powders was used to enhance the bond between the lithium disilicate and veneering ceramic (IPS e.max Ceram, Ivoclar Vivadent) (Figs 12a to 12c). In the second bake, a combination of Opal Effect 1, Opal Effect 2, Opal Effect 3, BL4 dentin, B1 dentin, and mamelon powders were used segmentally to create subtle contrasts, translucency, and mamelon effects mimicking a natural tooth. The entire build-up was covered with a thin layer of Opal Effect 1/Bleach Incisal to filter the internal stucture while maintaining opalescence (Figs 12d to 12f).

Morphologic Contouring Procedures

After fitting the crowns to the master dies, the contacts must be verified and perfected on the solid cast in a systematic manner starting from the mesial of the central incisors and moving to the distal of the canines. Articulating paper was used to disclose interproximal contact interferences for each and every tooth. Larger interference marks were adjusted first (Fig 13). The morphology of each tooth was outlined in the facial, cervical, and interproximal areas. This provides an overall preview of the final proportions and form of the teeth. It is during this stage that fine adjustments were made to visualize the changes while using the marked outlines as guides to make the necessary morphologic modifications (Fig 14a).

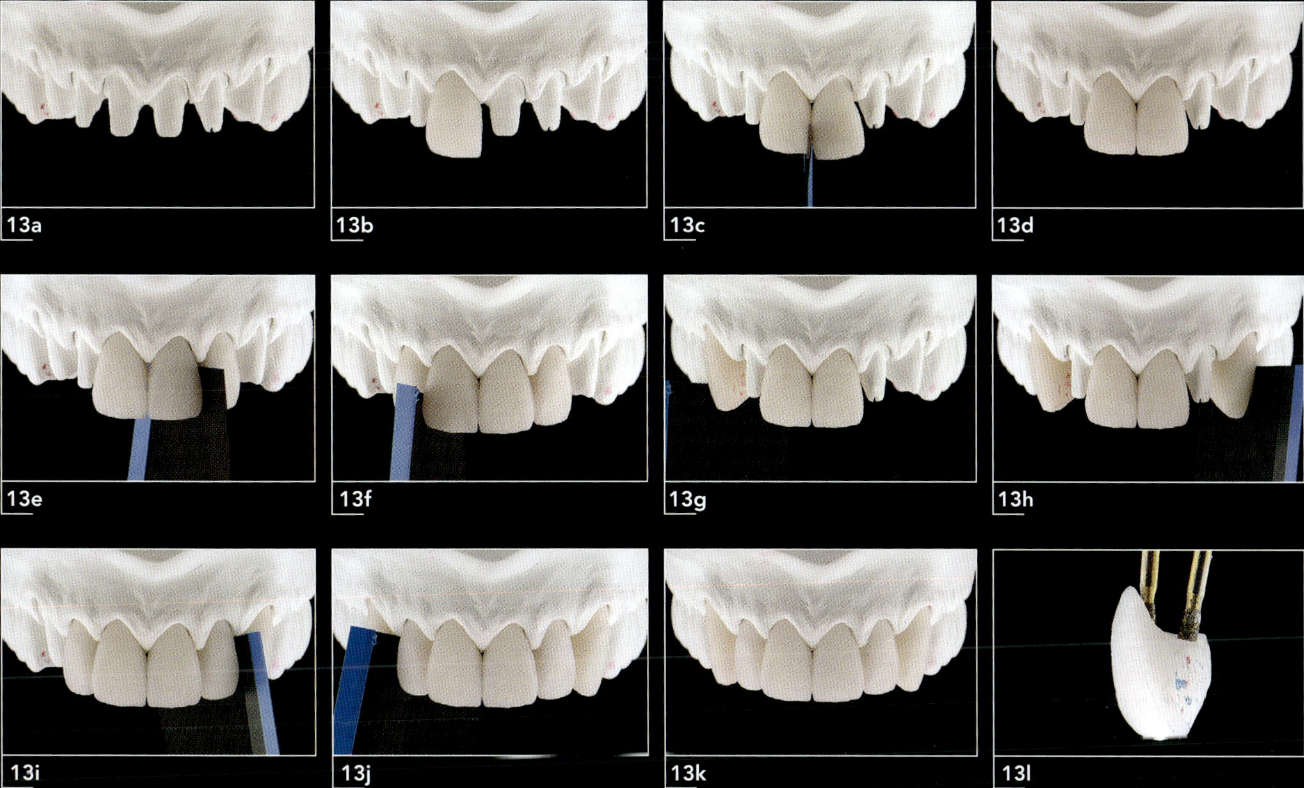

Fig 13a Solid cast.
Fig 13b Start with central incisors when adjusting interproximal contacts.
Fig 13c Identify the interproximal contact interference with articulating paper between the two central incisors.
Fig 13d Tight contact between proximal surfaces.
Figs 13e to 13j Steps in adjustment of the interproximal contacts.
Fig 13k Proper interproximal contacts.
Fig 13l It is important to adjust interferences that cause larger marks.

Staining and Finishing

To achieve a lifelike characteristic with the ceramic, subtle external stain was used on the surface prior to glazing. A simple staining approach was utilized to achieve this look: blue stain in the incisal area, white stain mixed with a cervical shade for the mamelons, and cervical color for the basic hue of the target shade. Pure white should be applied in the incisal area but in specific spots using different intensities. After staining the effects, a fixation firing is carried out to freeze all the stains in place, followed by glaze paste application and hand polishing with silicone wheels and fine pumice. Morphology and surface characteristics are shown in Figs 14b to 14d, and definitive anterior restorations on the solid cast in Fig 14e.

Posterior Segment Finishing Procedures

Figure 15 shows the wax designs of the restorations in the posterior segments. Completed lithium disilicate and monolithic screw-retained zirconia crowns were placed on the solid casts (Fig 16). The milled monolithic zirconia implant crown was cemented to the NT Trading Titanium Base (Custom Automated Prosthetics) using a dual-curing resin cement (Panavia SA, Kuraray). The titanium base was airborne-particle abraded with aluminum oxide to prepare the surface and to enhance the bond to the zirconia. The screw channel was blocked with wax to prevent residual cement from blocking the screw head. The crown was airborne-particle abraded with aluminum oxide, coated with ceramic primer, and loaded with the resin cement.

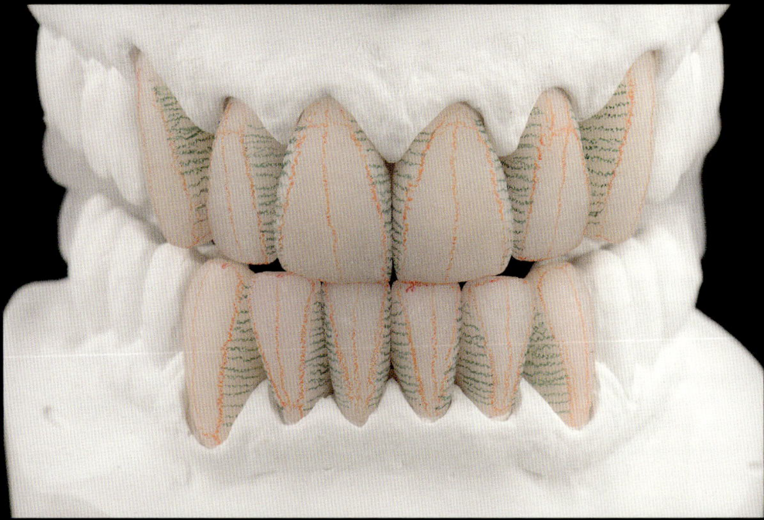

14a

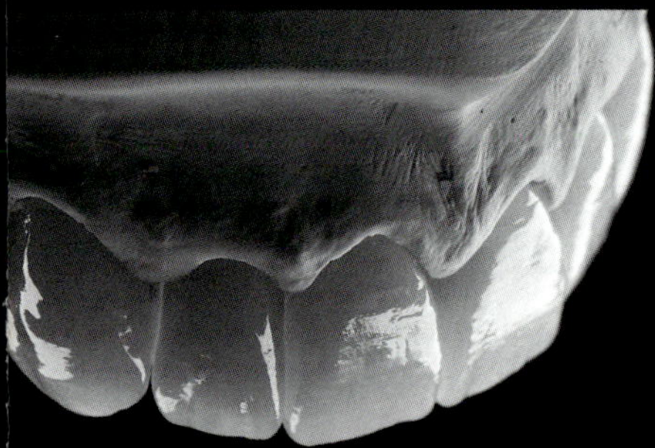

14b

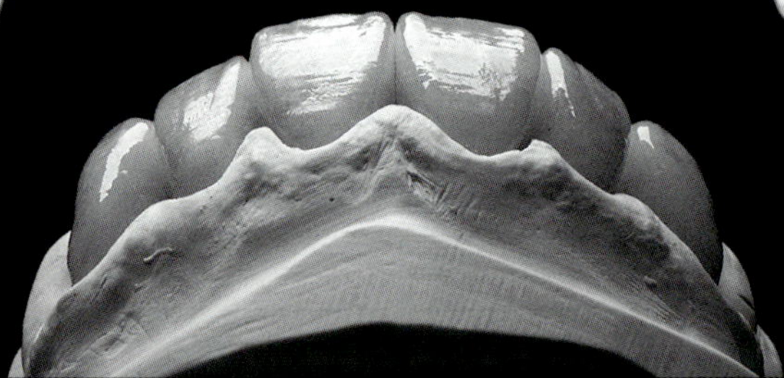

14c

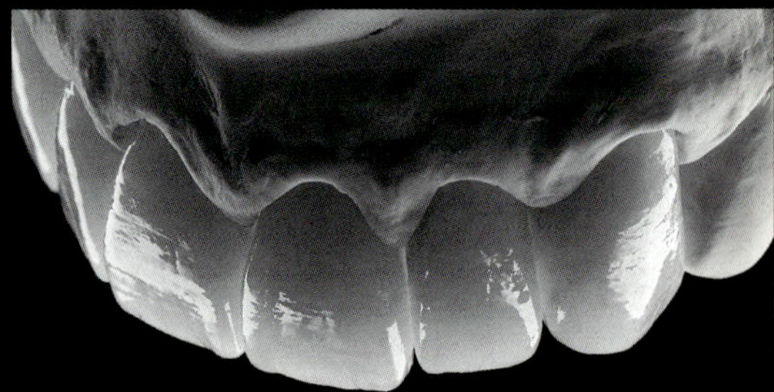

14d

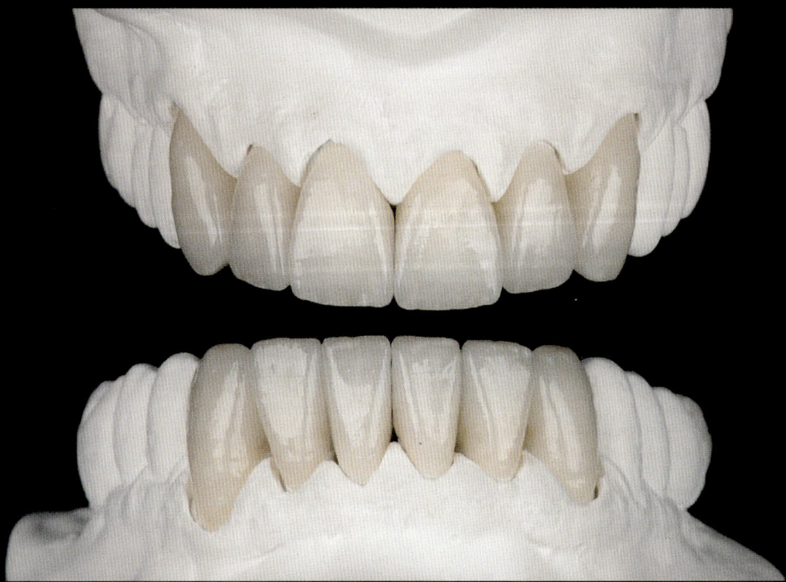

14e

Fig 14a Outline of morphology and surface characteristics to replicate natural teeth.
Figs 14b to 14d Morphology and surface characteristics.
Fig 14e Completed all-ceramic restorations on solid casts.

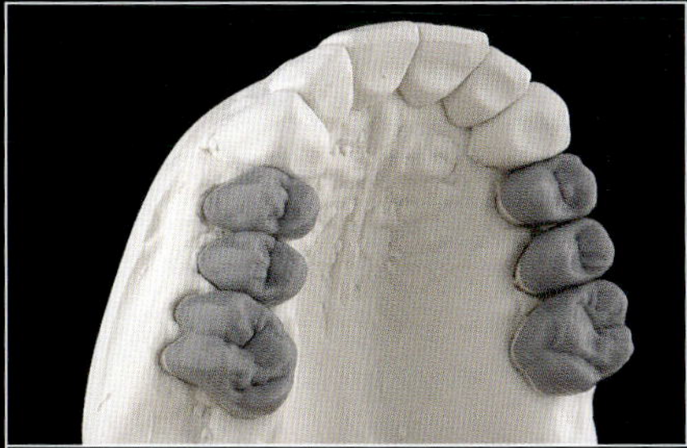

15a

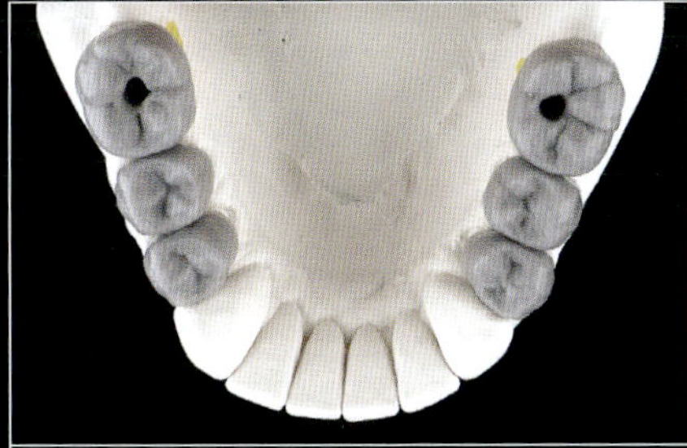

15b

Fig 15a Maxillary wax-up.
Fig 15b Mandibular wax-up.

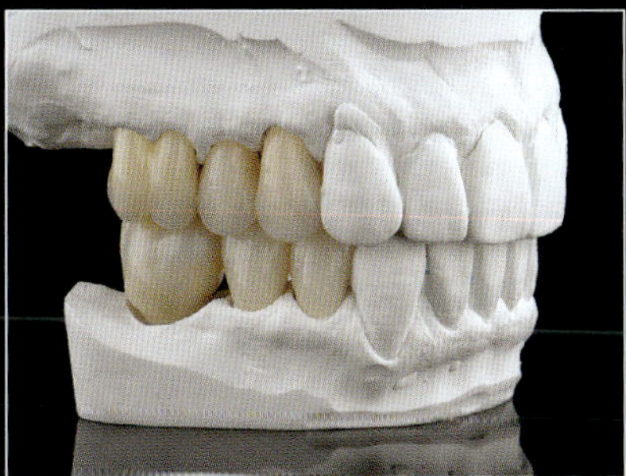

16a

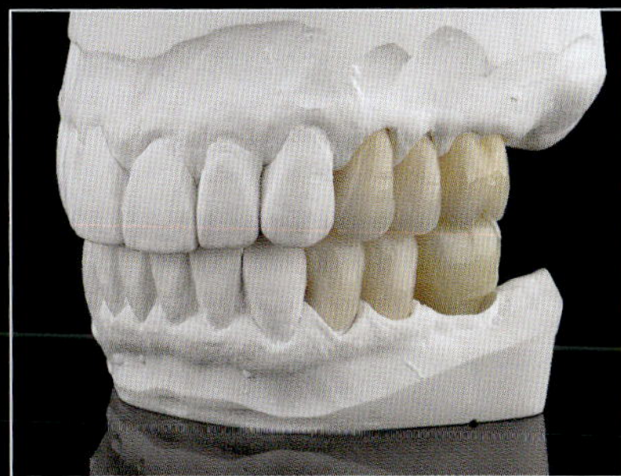

16b

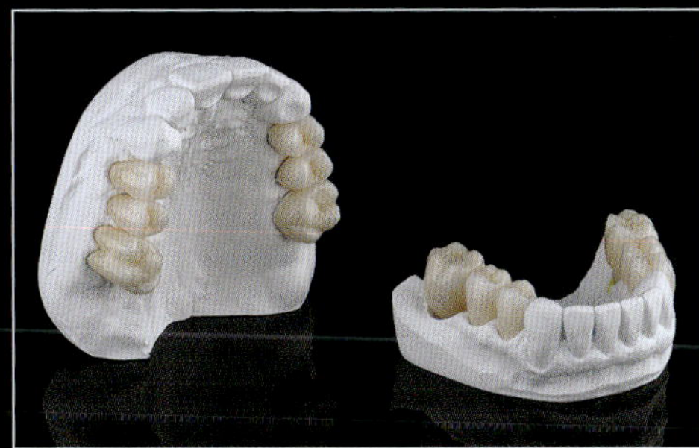

16c

Figs 16a to 16c Completed all-ceramic and screw-retained crowns on solid casts.

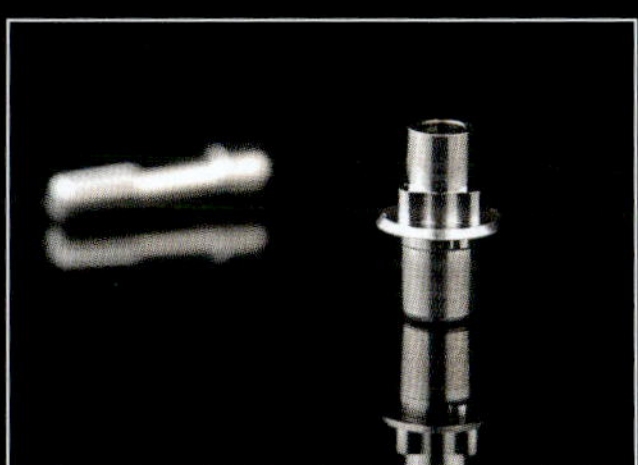

17a

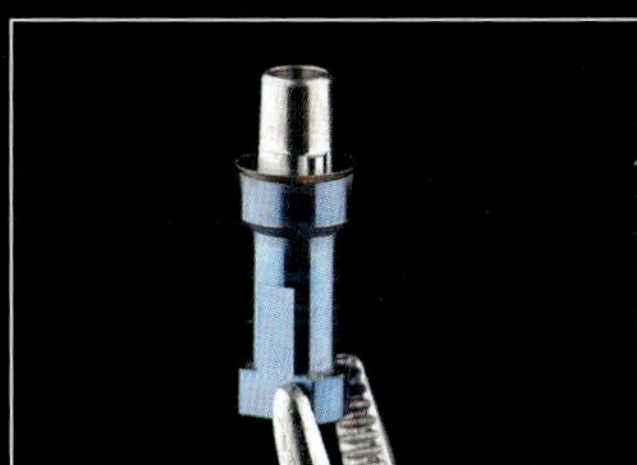

17b

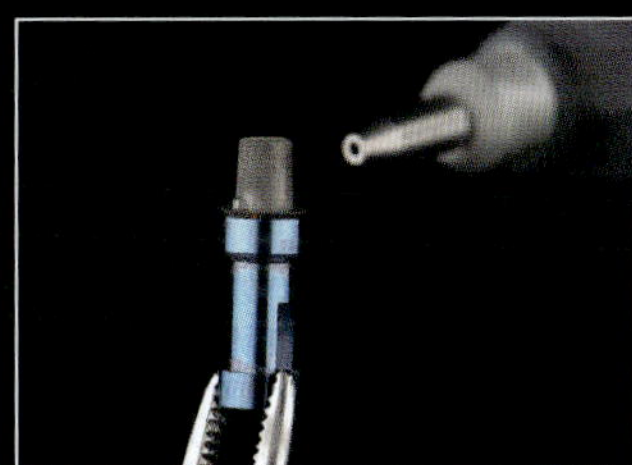

17c

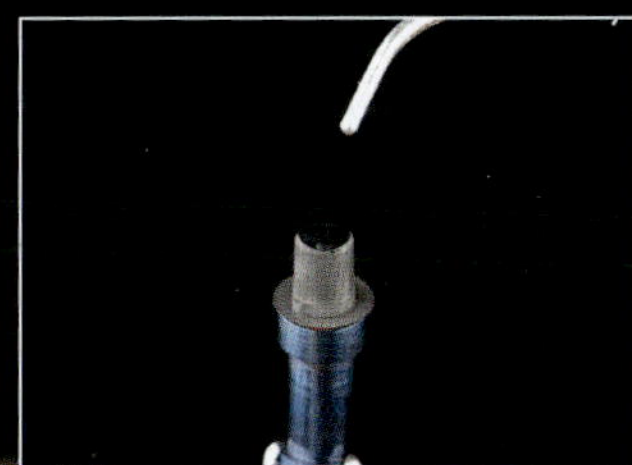

17d

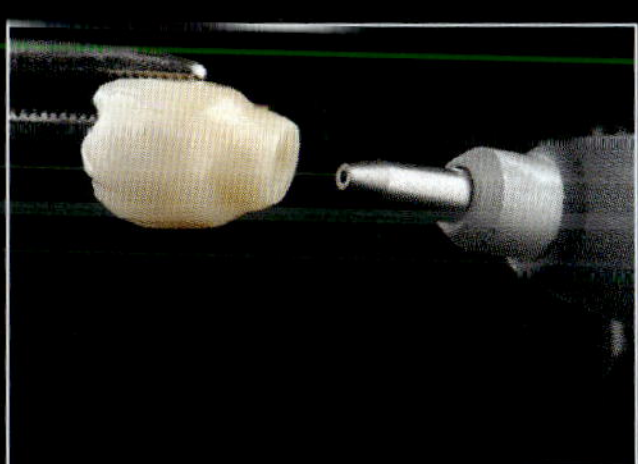

17e

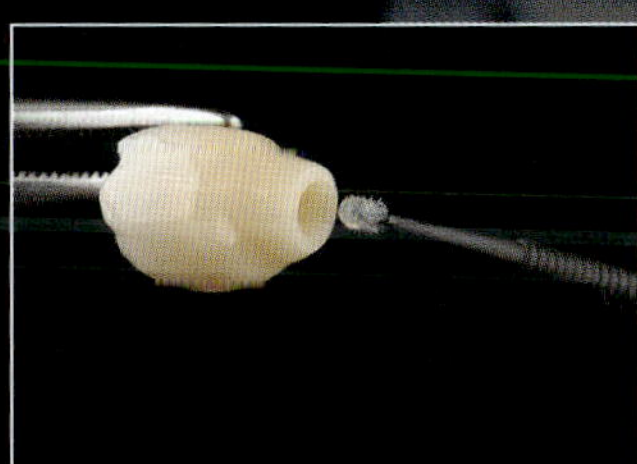

17f

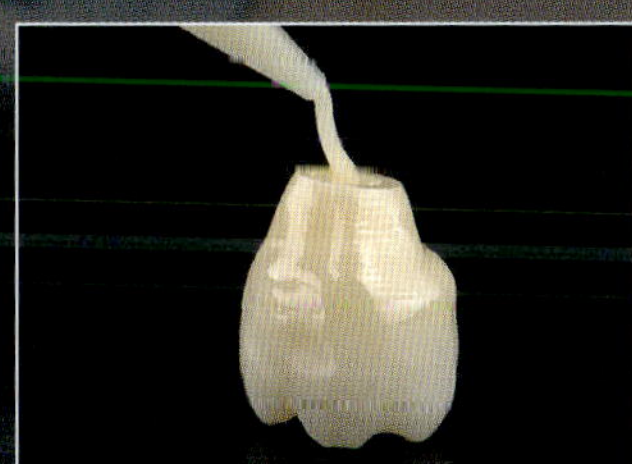

17g

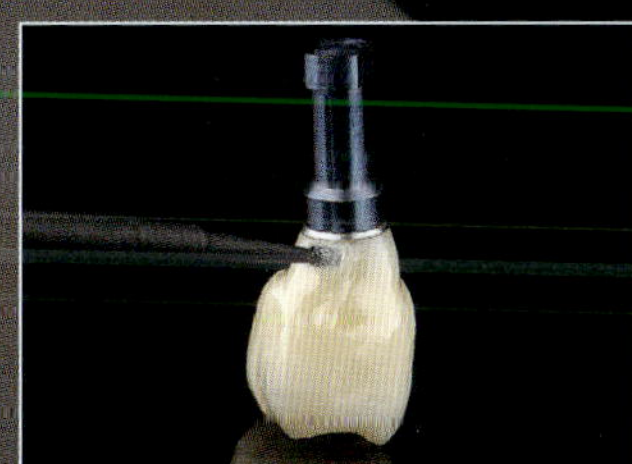

17h

Fig 17a NT Trading Titanium Base and screw for the screw-retained monolithic crown.
Fig 17b Titanium base on implant analog.
Fig 17c Airborne-particle abrasion at 2 bar pressure with aluminum oxide.
Fig 17d Wax added to the access hole to protect the screw.
Fig 17e Airborne-particle abrasion of inside the zirconia crown at 2 bar pressure to prepare the surface.
Fig 17f Application of Clearfil ceramic primer (Kuraray).
Fig 17g Application of Panavia SA resin cement (Kuraray).
Fig 17h Removing excess cement.

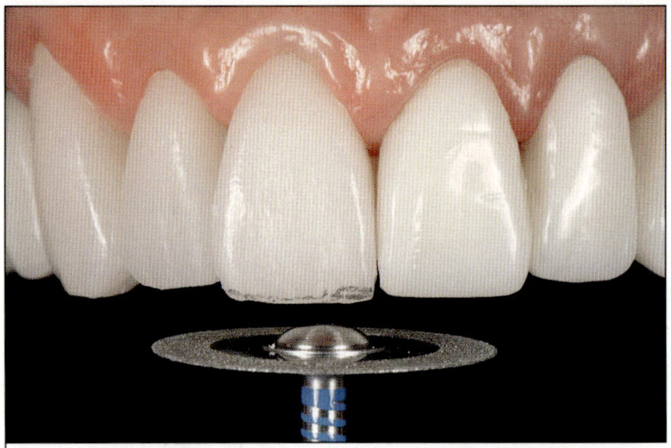

18

Fig 18 Try-in of definitive restorations against provisionals: adjusting the length of definitive restoration.

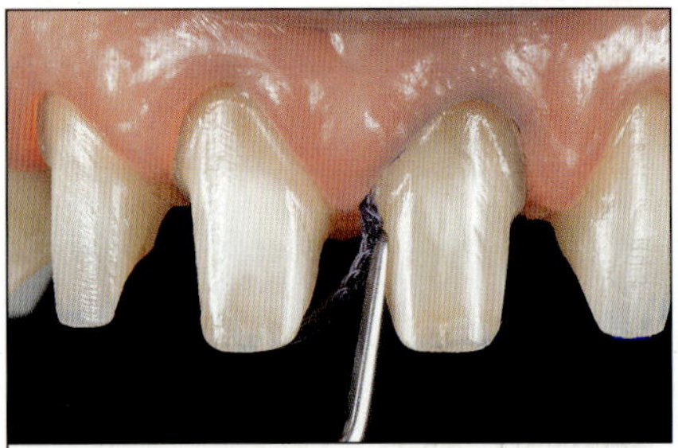

19a

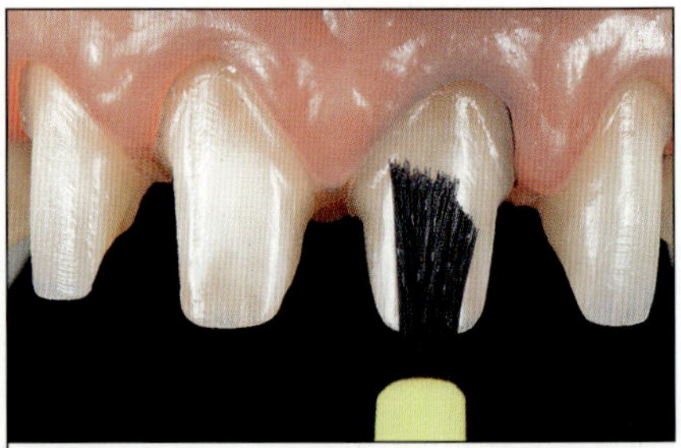

19b

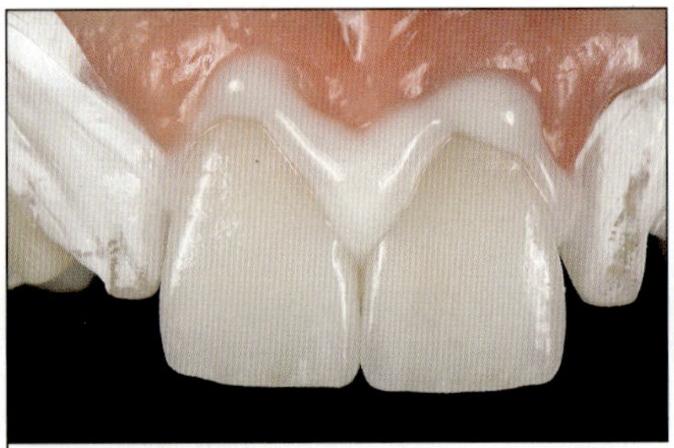

19c

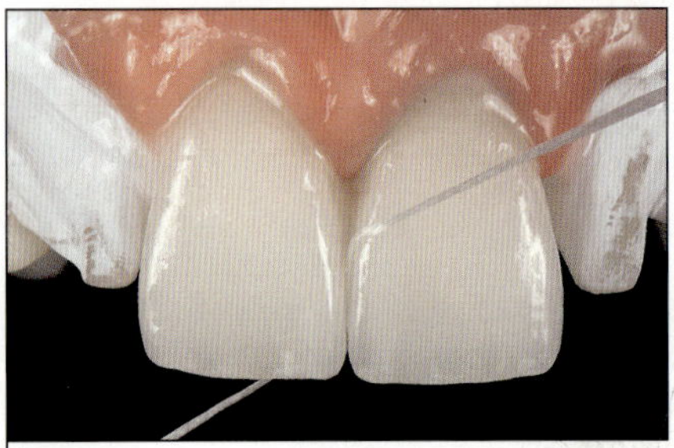

19d

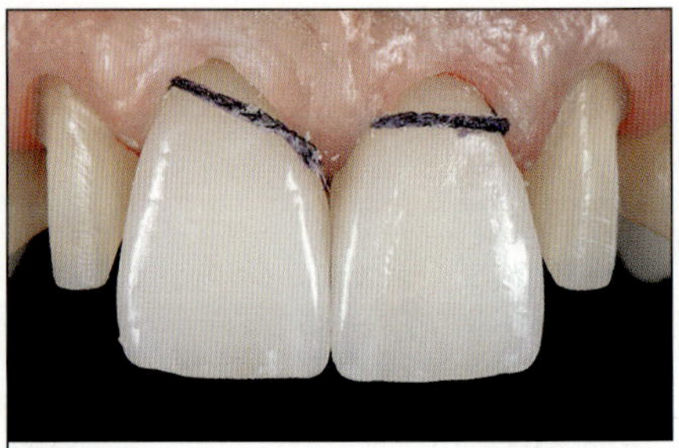

19e

Fig 19a Retraction cord is placed to control cement flow.

Fig 19b Adhesive is applied to the prepared tooth.

Figs 19c to 19e Excess cement cleaned and retraction cords removed.

The crown was seated on the titanium base, and excess cement was removed with a microbrush prior to light curing (Fig 17).

Try-In and Bonding of All-Ceramic Definitive Restorations

The all-ceramic materials selected for the case were monolithic zirconia crowns, stained and glazed, for the maxillary first molars; monolithic zirconia screw-retained implant crowns, stained and glazed, for the mandibular first molars; and pressed monolithic lithium disilicate crowns, stained and glazed, for the anterior teeth and premolars. The completed restorations were examined for accuracy of contacts, fit, contour, and esthetics. Anterior restorations were seated and compared to adjacent provisional restorations to evaluate length and anterior guidance. Adjustments were made as necessary (Fig 18).

The crowns were prepared for bonding, prepared teeth were cleaned, retraction cord was placed (Ultradent), and adhesive was applied (Scotch Bond Universal, 3M ESPE). The crowns were loaded with dual-curing resin cement and seated (RelyX Ultimate, 3M ESPE), and excess cement was removed with a brush and floss. After light curing for 40 seconds per surface, a no. 12 scalpel blade was used to remove excess cement, and the retraction cords were removed (Fig 19).

Figs 20a to 20i Postdelivery intraoral views of definitive restorations.

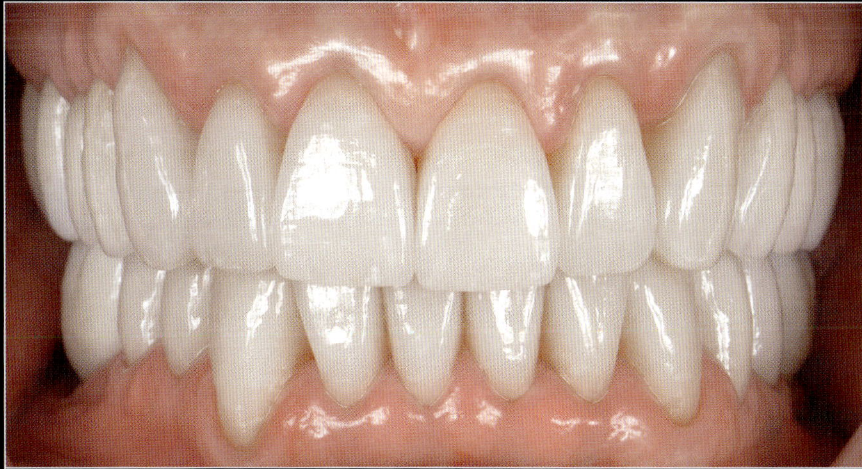

20a

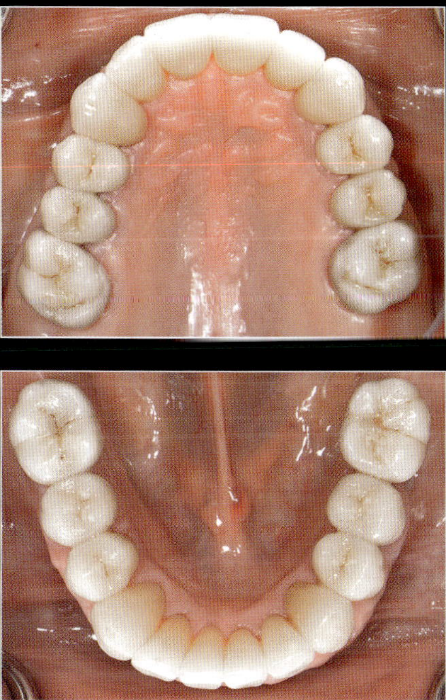

20b, c

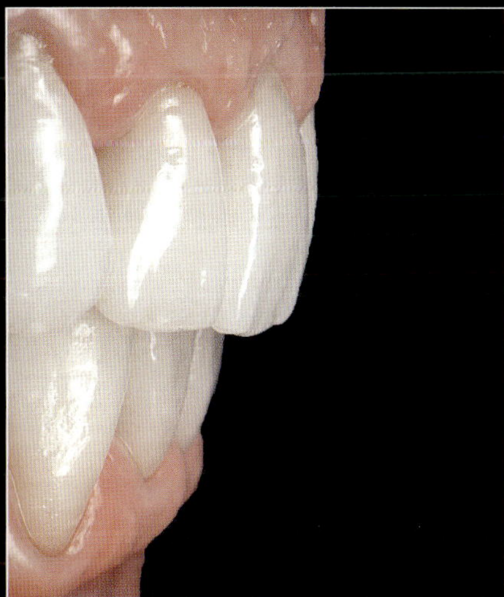

20d

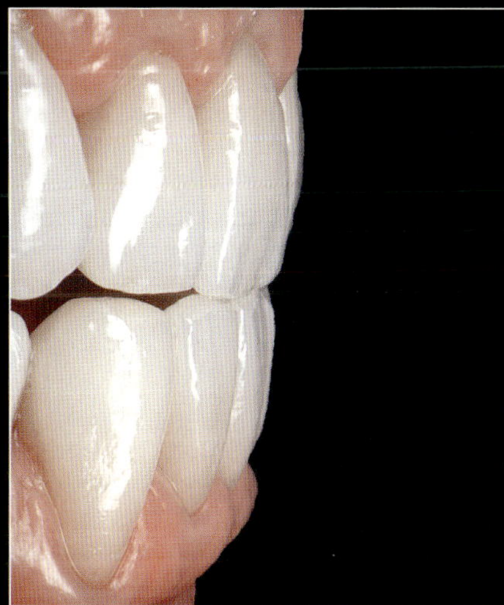

20e

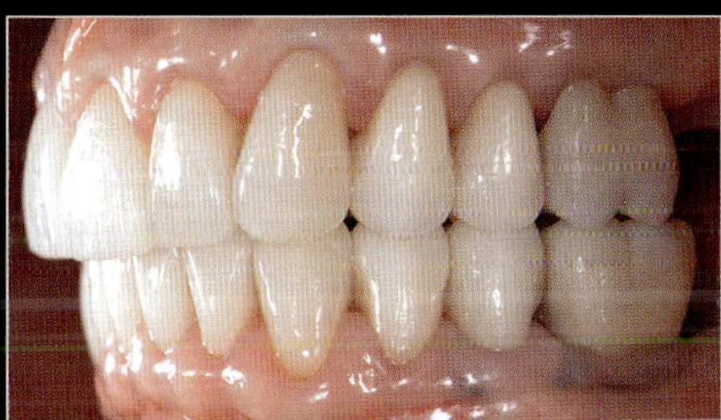

20f

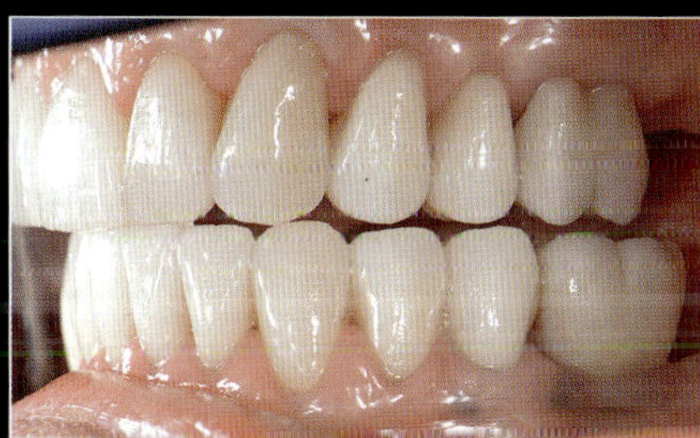

20g

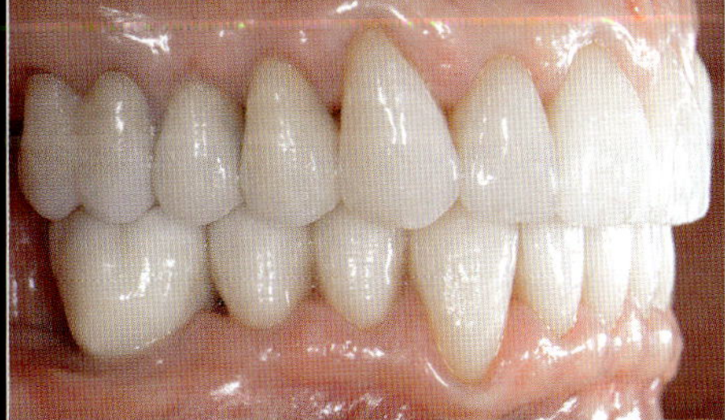

20h

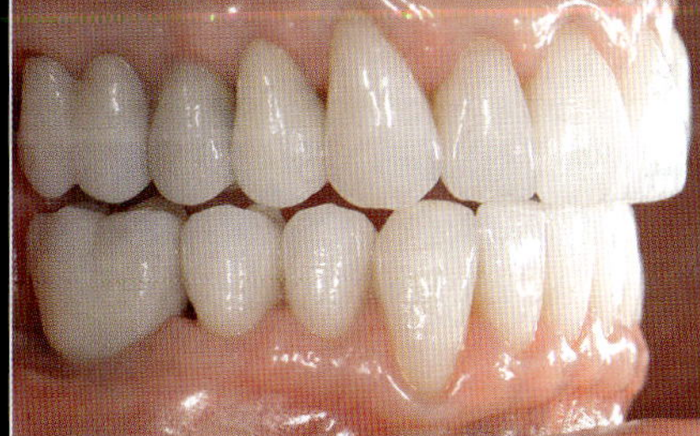

20i

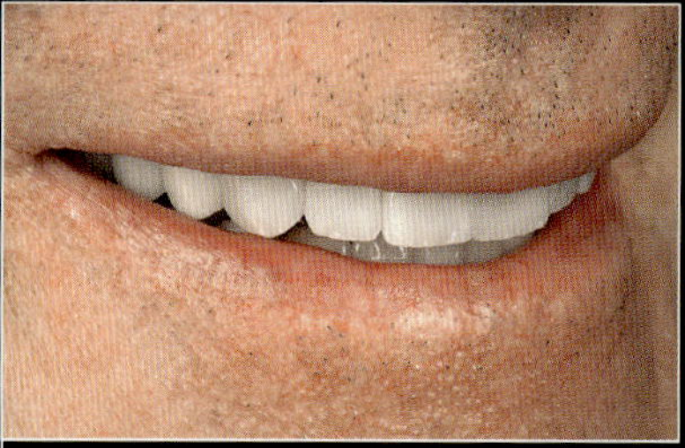

21a

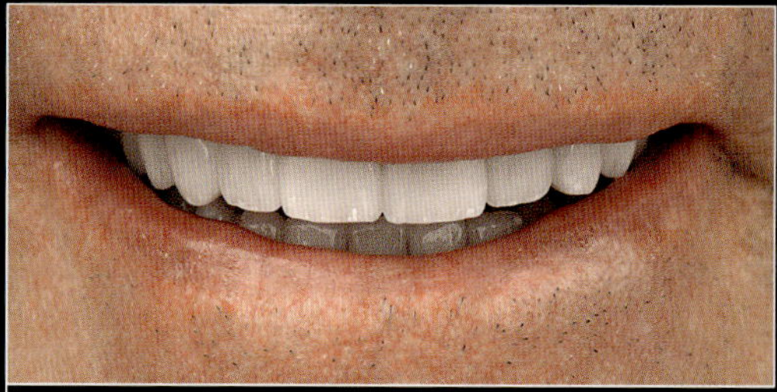

21b

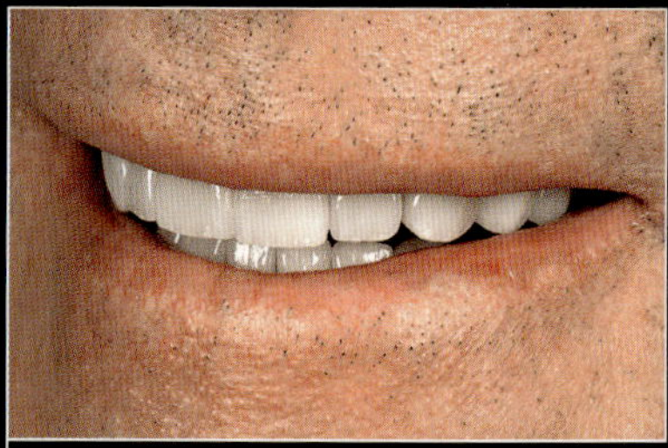

21c

Figs 21a to 21c Extraoral lower-third views.

Fig 21d Portrait frontal view.

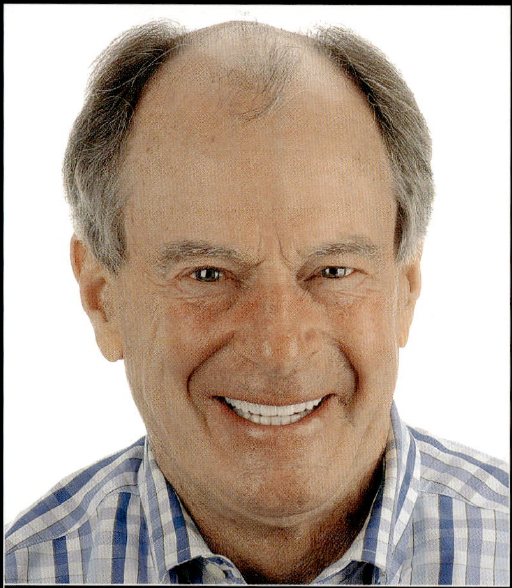

21d

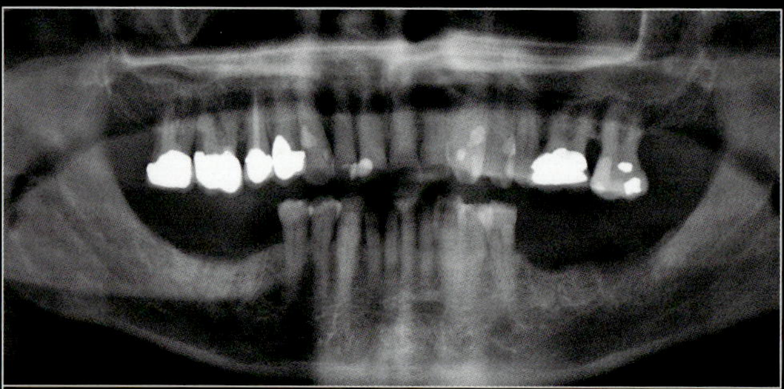

22a

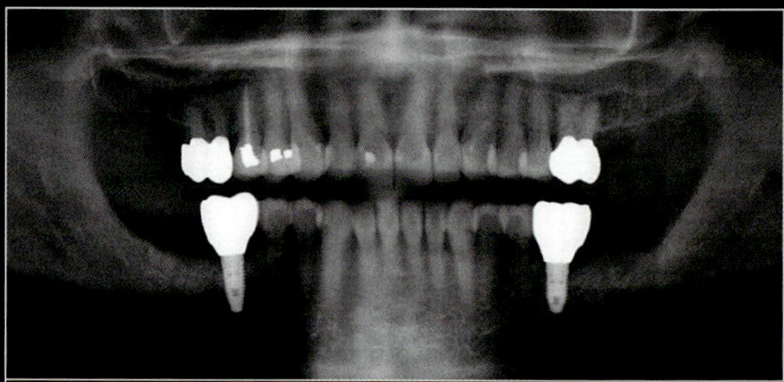

22b

Figs 22a and 22b Initial and posttreatment panoramic radiographs.

CONCLUSIONS

The procedure described in this article is a full-mouth rehabilitation completed with all-ceramic systems, which restored the patient to an excellent esthetic outcome as well as a stable and functional occlusion (Fig 20). Close-up views of the smile and portrait views of the final restorations are shown in Fig 21. The initial and final panoramic radiographs showed a stable bone condition (Fig 22).

ACKNOWLEDGMENTS

The authors thank Nobel Biocare and The Georgia Regents University Center for Excellence for their support in this case. Dr Jae Seon Kim is also thanked for his assistance in sharing his unique expertise with the treatment of the patient.

REFERENCES

1. Chiche G, Pinault A. Esthetics of Anterior Fixed Prosthodontics. Chicago: Quintessence, 1993:202.
2. Carlsson GE, Egermark I, Magnusson T. Predictors of bruxism, other oral parafunctions, and tooth wear over a 20-year follow-up period. J Orofac Pain 2003;17:50–57.
3. Dylina TJ. A common-sense approach to splint therapy. J Prosthet Dent 2001;86:539–545.
4. Spear FM, Kokich VG. A multidisciplinary approach to esthetic dentistry. Dent Clin North Am 2007;51:487–505,X–XI.
5. Chiche G. Proportion, display, and length for successful esthetic planning. In: Cohen M (ed). Interdisciplinary Treatment Planning: Principles, Design, Implementation. Chicago: Quintessence, 2008.
6. Tarnow DP, Cho SC, Wallace SS. The effect of inter-implant distance on the height of inter-implant bone crest. J Periodontol 2000;71:546–549.
7. Salama H, Salama MA, Garber D, Adar P. The interproximal height of bone: A guidepost to predictable aesthetic strategies and soft tissue contours in anterior tooth replacement. Pract Periodontics Aesthet Dent 1998;10:1131–1141.
8. Davarpanah M, Martinez H, Tecucianu JF. Apical-coronal implant position: Recent surgical proposals. Technical note. Int J Oral Maxillofac Implants 2000;15:865–872.
9. Gürel G. Predictable, precise, and repeatable tooth preparation for porcelain laminate veneers. Pract Proced Aesthet Dent 2003;15:17–24.
10. Torosian A, Arias S. Provisionalization of dental implants in the esthetic zone: A Blueprint for Success. Labline 2013;3(1):116–123.
11. Higginbottom FL. Quality provisional restorations: A must for successful restorative dentistry. Compend Contin Educ Dent 1995;16:442, 444–447.
12. Chiche G. Improving marginal adaptation of provisional restorations. Quintessence Int 1990;21:325–329.

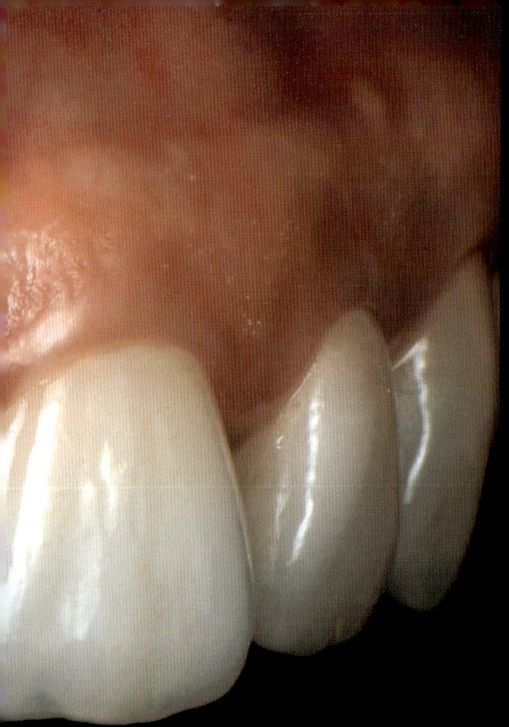

Biologic Esthetics by Gingival Framework Design:

Part 1. Factors for Achieving Biologic and Esthetic Harmony

Yuji Tsuzuki, RDT[1]

Biologic esthetics means genuine oral esthetics, which is the result of the biologic harmony of the prosthesis. The cervical design of the prosthesis is as important as the coronal design in achieving the most favorable esthetic result. All factors—esthetics, biology, function, and structure—need to be satisfied to lead to successful prosthetic treatment. Each clinical and laboratory step should be performed well to achieve the treatment goal (Fig 1).

Factors for achieving biologic and esthetic harmony are presented in this article. The potential and the limitations of prosthetic treatment are presented and discussed through clinical cases.

[1]Dental Technician, Kyoto, Japan.

Correspondence to: Yuji Tsuzuki, Ray Dental Labor, Elitz Yamashina Building 3F, 18-8 Takehanatakenokaidocho Yamashina-ku, Kyoto City, Kyoto, Japan. Email: ray710@camel.plala.or.jp

KNOWLEDGE OF SURROUNDING PERIODONTAL TISSUES

Clear Understanding of Healthy Periodontal Tissue

If the prostheses are to obtain biologic harmony with periodontal tissues, control of inflammation is an important factor (Fig 2). Prosthetic considerations for controlling gingival inflammation include *(1)* marginal fit, *(2)* morphologic control (subgingival morphology), and *(3)* surface texture (Figs 3 to 5). Subgingival prosthetic morphology is designed according to the periodontal environment, which is quite different in the natural dentition from that which surrounds an implant. The prosthetic treatment result will be affected by the periodontal condition, including hard and soft tissue. Greater care must be paid as the prosthesis is extended more subgingivally. It is critical to have a thorough knowledge of healthy periodontal tissue and to be able to recognize how it differs around a natural tooth and an implant (Fig 6). Consideration given to periodontal tissues in different prosthetic environments is presented in Figs 7 to 10.

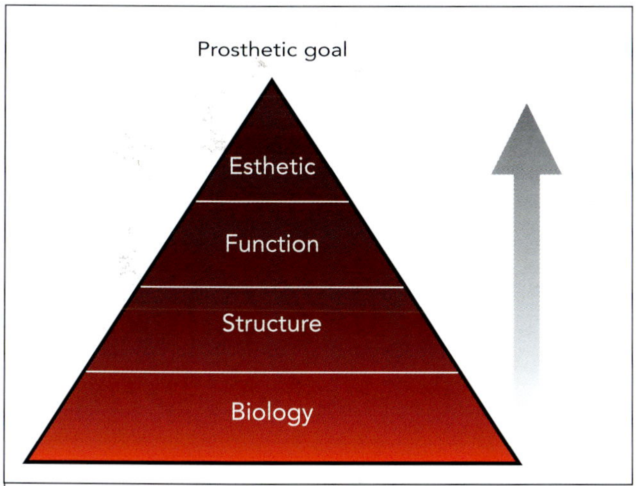

1

Fig 1 When the "prosthetic triangle concept" is applied, the prosthesis should first be designed to eliminate biologic risk and create a biologically stable environment. Second, the prosthesis should be structurally sound for long-term stability. Third, function is guaranteed on a solid structure. Even though esthetics and function are considered two sides of the same coin, esthetics still should be considered after creating a sound foundation. All factors are equally important, and requirements have to be fulfilled to achieve a harmonious prosthesis.

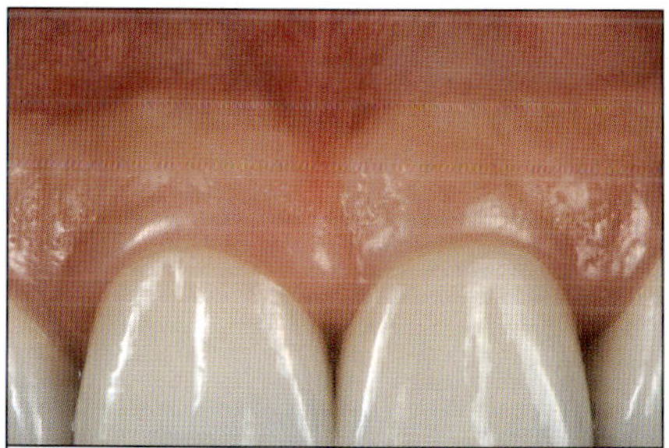

2

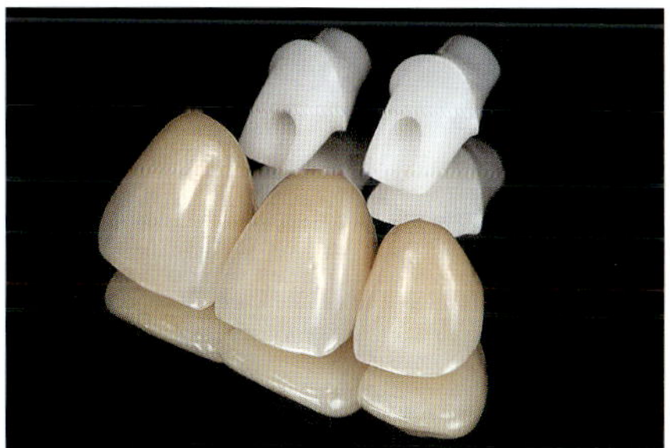

3

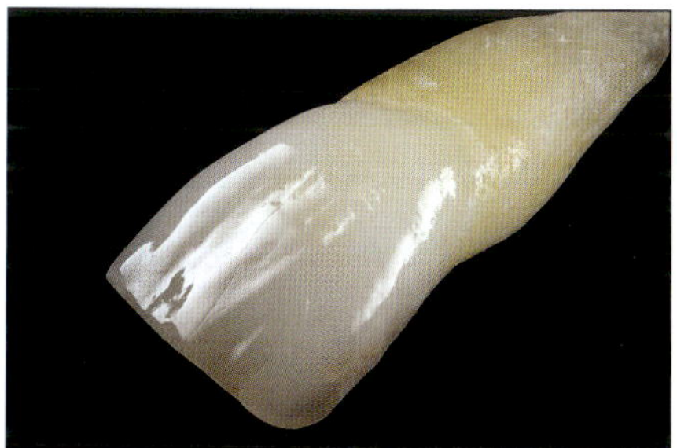

4

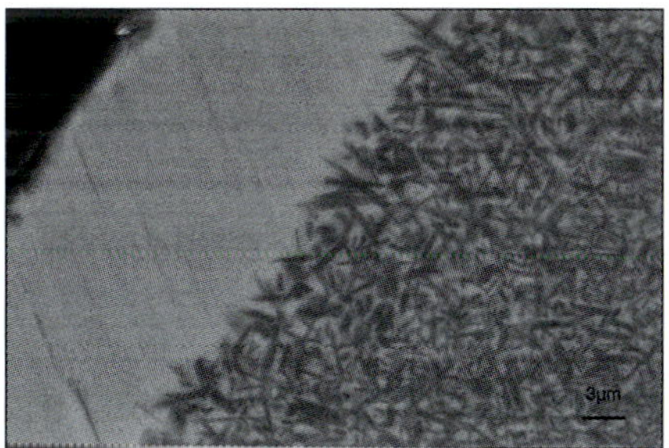

5

Fig 2 Prosthesis with proper subgingival contour on the left central incisor reflects biologic harmony.

Fig 3 Importance of subgingival contour, or the harmonization of the prosthesis with periodontal tissue, is illustrated by this implant-supported fixed dental prosthesis.

Fig 4 Smooth surface texture of the enamel of a natural tooth.

Fig 5 Sectional view of IPS e.max CAD lithium disilicate glass-ceramic material and IPS e.max Ceram Glaze Paste (Ivoclar Vivadent) as seen under an electron microscope. Note the fine, smooth surface of the Glaze Paste. The area of a crown that contacts the gingiva is not finished with a self-glaze, but instead with Glaze Paste to improve gingival tissue response.

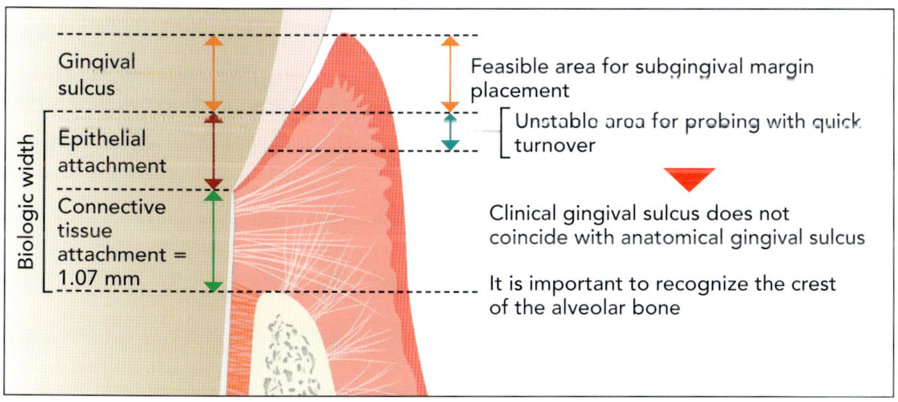

Fig 6 Concept of biologic width (Tsuchiya, 2010). (Illustration from Yamazaki, 2004. Reprinted with permission.)

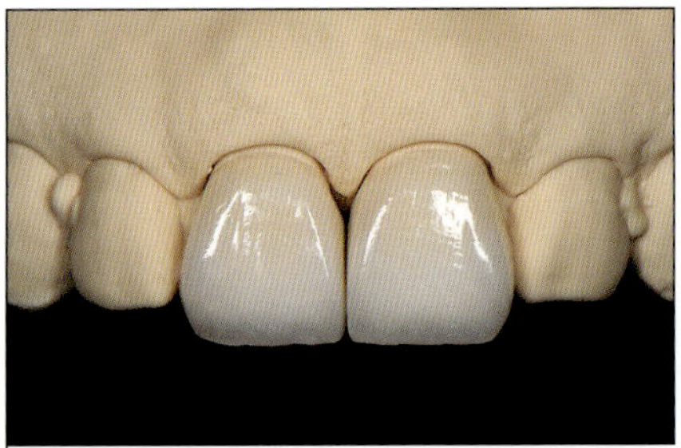
7a

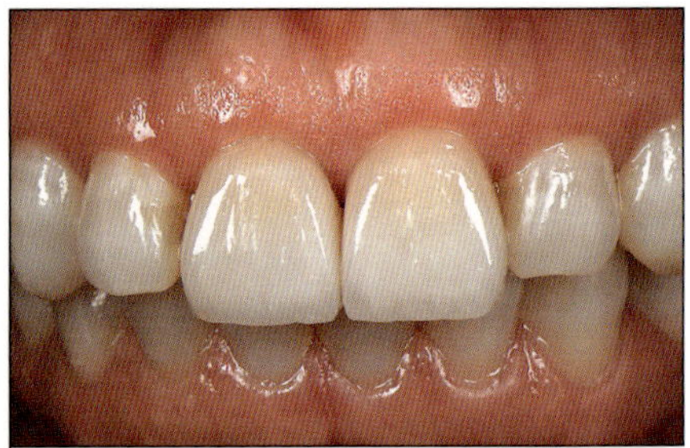
7b

Fig 7a Porcelain laminate veneer restorations on the maxillary central incisors. Particular consideration for periodontal tissues is not necessary when the margin is placed supragingivally.

Fig 7b Veneers after insertion. Gingival tissue health around the restorations as well as around adjacent natural teeth is maintained. (Courtesy of Dr Takashi Ueno, Ito Dental Clinic, Japan.)

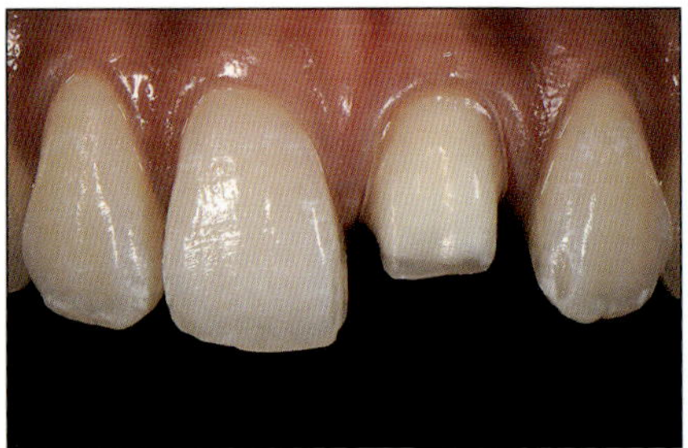
8a

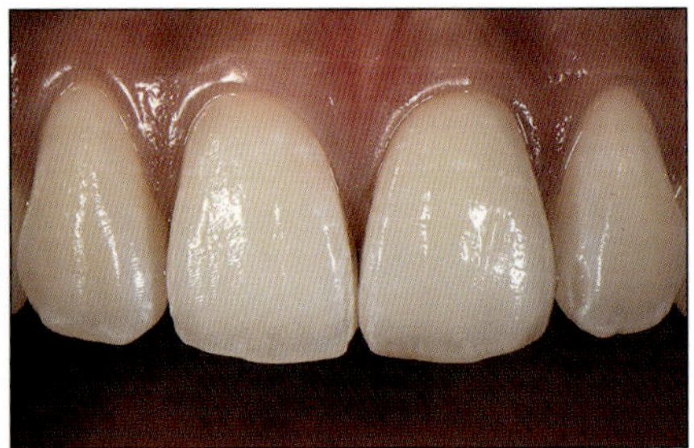
8b

Fig 8a Fractured maxillary left central incisor due to trauma prepared for an all-ceramic restoration. The preparation was minimally invasive with margins placed at the gingival level.

Fig 8b Greater attention can be paid to esthetic elements such as color and surface texture during crown fabrication when minimal consideration to gingival tissues is necessary. (Courtesy of Dr Tsutomu Kubota, Kubota Dental Clinic, Japan.)

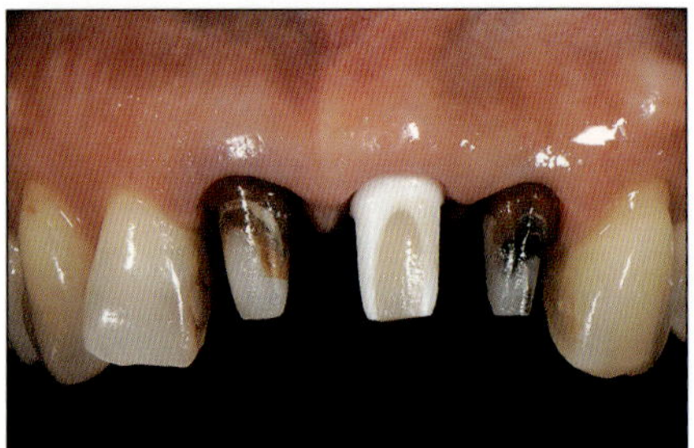
9a

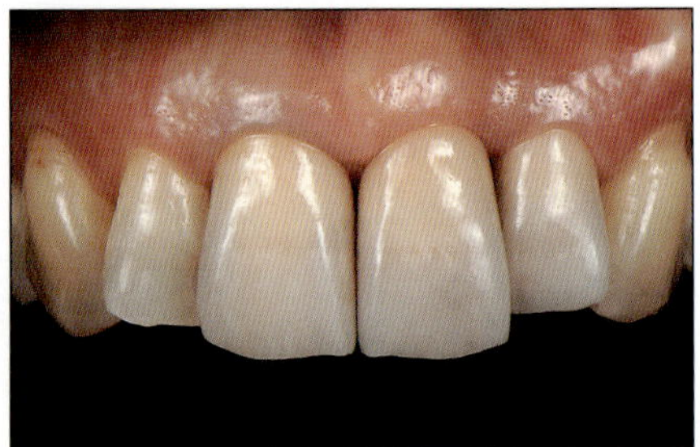
9b

Figs 9a and 9b Combination of prostheses on natural teeth and on an implant. The subgingival prosthetic morphology differs along with differing prosthetic conditions. With advanced surgical techniques and materials, a highly esthetic result including gingival margin areas can be obtained.

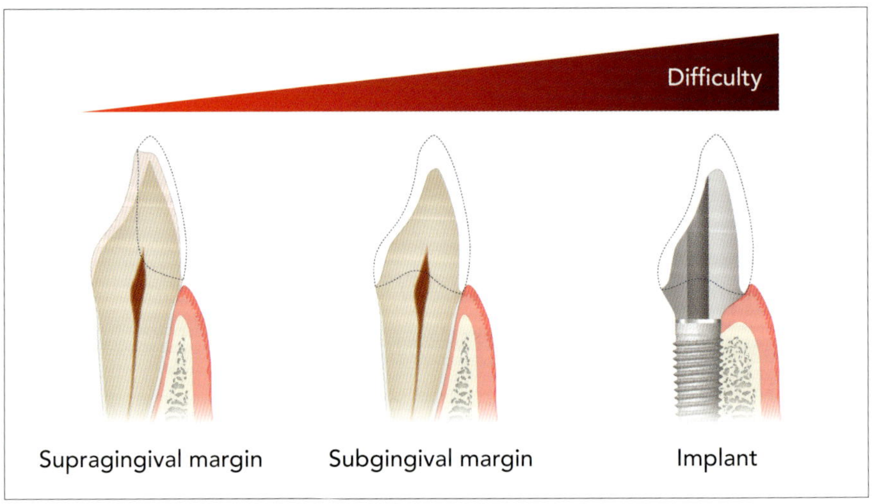

Fig 10 Illustration of degree of difficulty according to the prosthetic condition. The difficulty in achieving biologic harmony increases as treatment involves a more subgingival area.

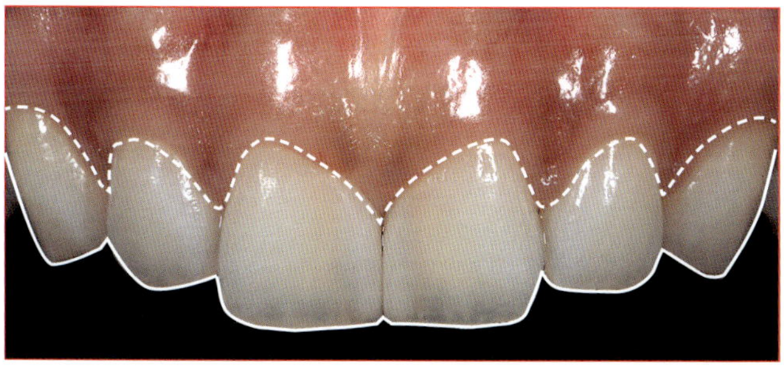

Fig 11 Gingival framework *(dotted line)* and incisal framework *(solid line)* of the dentition. Symmetry and harmonized continuity are factors for an esthetic result.

CASE 1 *Management of the Gingival Margin with a Provisional Restoration*

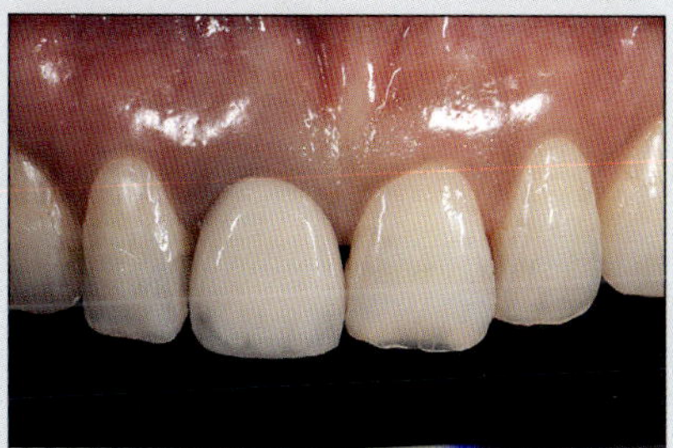

12a

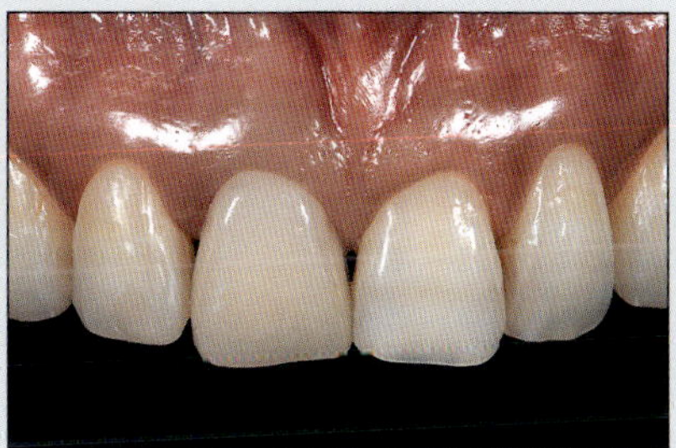

12b

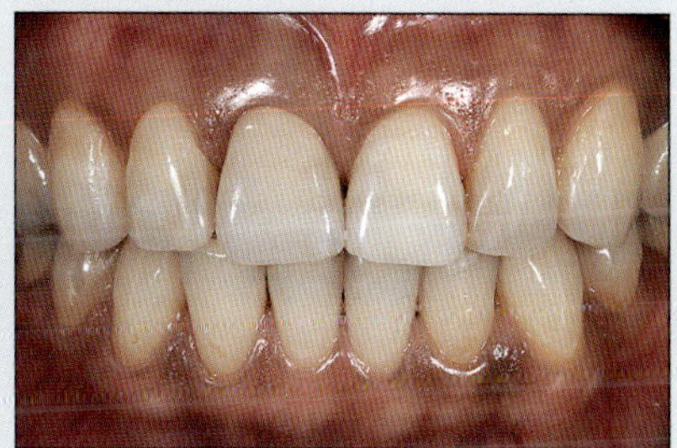

12c

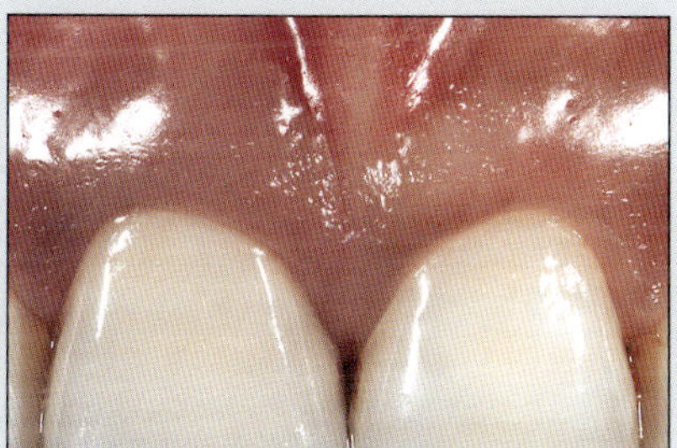

12d

Fig 12a The patient presented with a gingival discrepancy and undesirable color and shape of the crown on the maxillary right central incisor. The gingival discrepancy was corrected by subgingival contouring of the prosthesis without a surgical procedure.

Fig 12b Provisional restoration. Several adjustments were performed, bringing the finish line subgingivally to modify the gingival architecture to the ideal condition. Once a harmonized gingival framework was established by the provisional restoration, the final prosthesis was fabricated.

Fig 12c Definitive prosthesis (IPS e.max Press, Ivoclar Vivadent). The gingival line was corrected by duplicating the gingival contour of the provisional restoration. A thorough examination and diagnosis are mandatory to determine if surgical intervention is indicated.

Fig 12d Two weeks after insertion. The harmonized gingival adaptation can be appreciated because of proper prosthetic contouring and biocompatibility of the ceramics. (Courtesy of Dr Hiroyuki Takino, Takino Dental Clinic, Japan.)

Gingival Framework and Incisal Framework as Evaluation Criteria

Recovery and maintenance of healthy gingival tissue is the major premise for esthetic restorative treatment. A comprehensive approach including surgical and orthodontic treatment in addition to the prosthetic treatment is indicated to improve the prosthetic condition and to achieve a highly esthetic result.

Proper tooth alignment is an absolute requirement when composing an esthetic and functional dentition. Continuity and symmetry of the gingival line (the gingival framework [Tsuchiya, 2010]) are as important as continuity and symmetry of the incisal line (the incisal framework [Tsuchiya, 2010]) in producing esthetics that achieve harmony with the lips. In esthetic restorations, the gingival/incisal framework (defined as the esthetic framework in this article) is an important evaluation criterion in the design of a prosthesis with a harmonized esthetic result (Fig 11).

An example of managing the gingival framework using a prosthetic approach is shown in Case 1 (Fig

CASE 2 *Improvement of the Gingival Framework Using a Half-Pontic Technique*

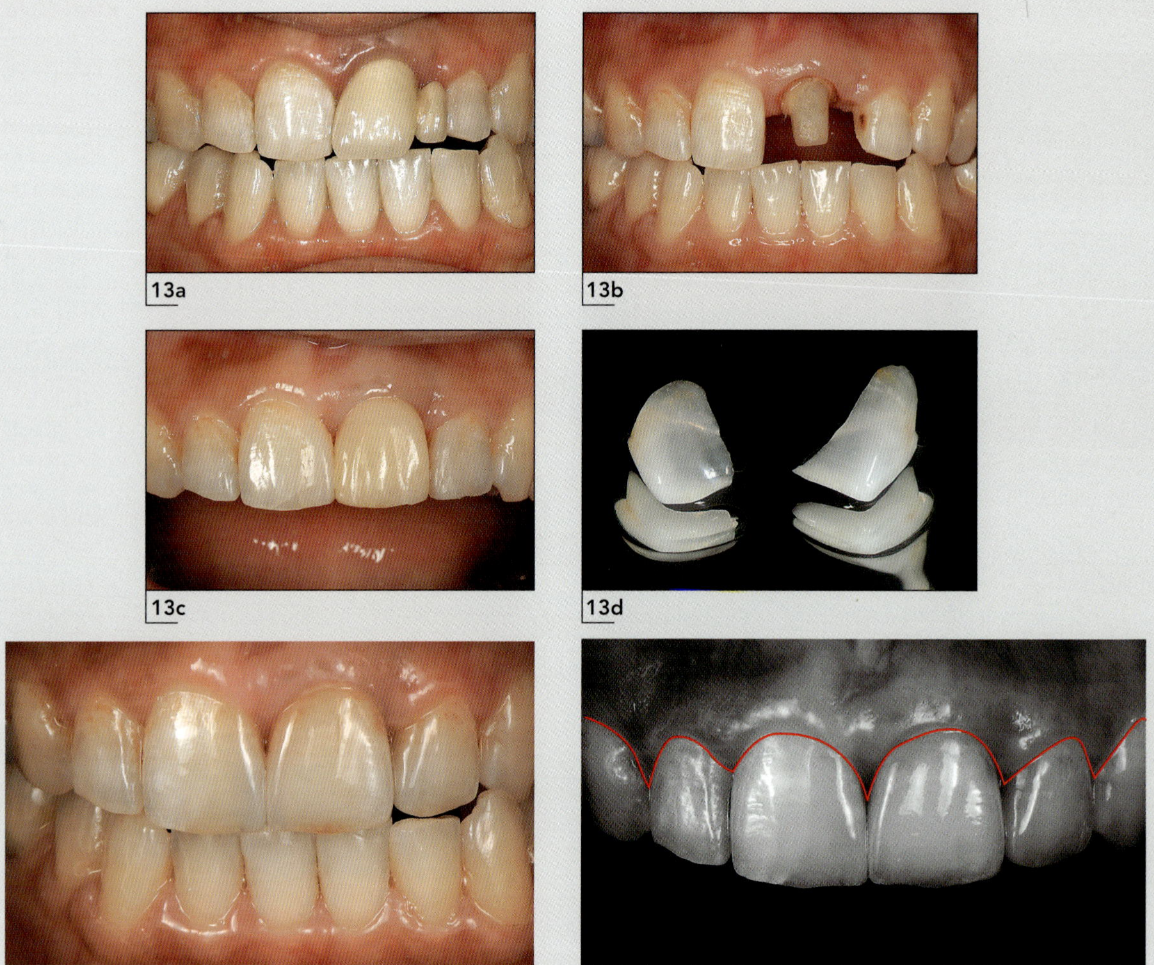

Fig 13a Preoperative photograph. The interproximal space between the maxillary left central and lateral incisors is restored with a crown on the central incisor and a distal pontic. There is a size discrepancy with the contralateral teeth.

Fig 13b Dentition after removal of the existing restoration.

Fig 13c Direct composite resin was added to the right central and left lateral incisors as a diagnostic step to balance the width of the anterior teeth. It is performed within the normal limit of natural teeth with the patient's consent.

Fig 13d Porcelain partial laminate veneer restorations for the right central and left lateral incisors.

Fig 13e Postoperative view of the porcelain partial laminate veneers and an all-ceramic crown on the left central incisor (IPS e.max Press). The veneers were fabricated using the staining method and the all-ceramic crown using the cut-back method.

Fig 13f The gingival framework was harmonized with the rest of the dentition using a half-pontic technique, and balanced width of the dentition was also restored. (Courtesy of Yamaba Dental Clinic, Japan.)

12). The chief complaint of this patient, a female in her 40s, was the color of the crown on the maxillary right central incisor, which did not match the contralateral tooth.

Case 2 describes the half-pontic technique, another method of using a prosthetic approach to manage the gingival framework (Fig 13). The patient, a female in her 40s, was dissatisfied with the esthetics of her anterior crown. Her chief complaint was resolved with treatment of the maxillary right and left central incisors and left lateral incisor.

Table 1 Prosthetic Approaches to Treatment with Limitations and Risks

Approach	Challenge	Objectives	Tool	Limitations	Risks
Add-on technique 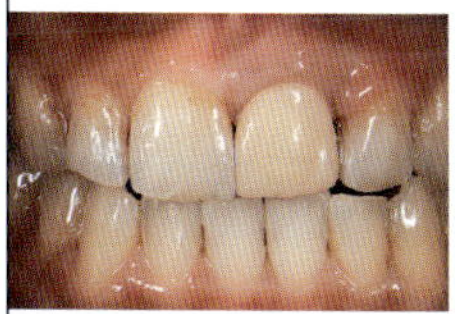	• Interproximal space • Abnormal or unesthetic shape of clinical crowns • Black triangles	• Adjustment of mesiodistal prosthetic space • Correction of crown shape • Closure of black triangles	• Guiding shell for composite resin direct bonding • Additional laminate veneer • Laminate veneer	• Approach depends on bonding • Limitations on the region and thickness for functional and mechanical reasons	• Inevitable discoloration of the composite resin • Risk to the underlying tooth structure (generally, a limited risk)
Subgingival preparation 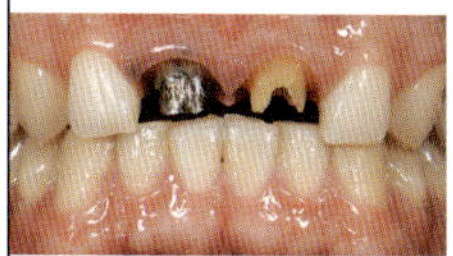	• Short clinical crown • Discolored abutment • Not enough mechanical structure of the abutment	• Elongation of the abutment • Mitigation of the color of the abutment • Improvement of retention and resistance of the abutment • Securing ferrule	• Consideration to subgingival contour of the prosthesis • Preparation guide model	• Biological factors must be considered when the treatment involves the gingival sulcus	• Biological risk increases as subgingival preparation is involved • Prosthetic difficulty increases in aspects of preparation, impression, fit check, and cement removal
Reshaping 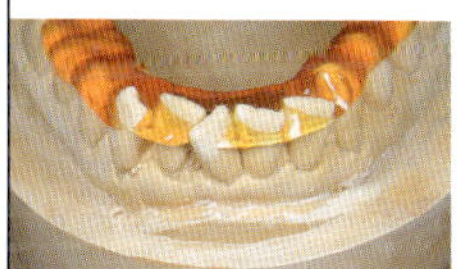	• Lack of mesiodistal prosthetic space due to tooth alignment • Esthetic or functional restriction from adjacent or opposing teeth • Functional occlusal interference	• Expansion of mesiodistal prosthetic space • Correction of crown shape • Improvement of interdental relationship (esthetic and functional aspects) • Occlusal adjustment	• Reshaping guide • Study model for diagnosis of occlusion	• Adjustment should be within enamel	• Certain risks (secondary caries, hypersensitivity) could arise after adjustment
Gingiva-colored material 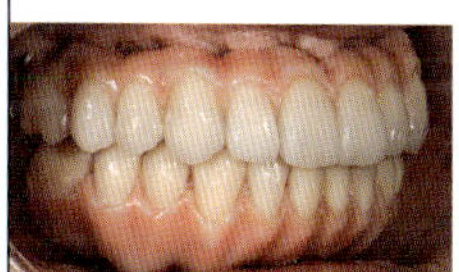	• Excessive ridge resorption • Discrepancy between proper anatomical tooth shape and given prosthetic space	• Adjustment of crown length • Achievement of anatomically correct crown shape • Closure of black triangles • Improvement of hygienic properties (adjustment of buccolingual depth of interproximal space)	• Gingiva-colored porcelain • Gingiva-colored composite resin	• Prosthetic space is limited by the shape and degree of resorption of the ridge	• Consideration to hygienic properties and stress control on the mucosa is important as the contact area of the prosthesis to alveolar mucosa increases • Retrievable design of the prosthesis is recommended

CASE 3 *Refusal of Orthodontic Treatment*

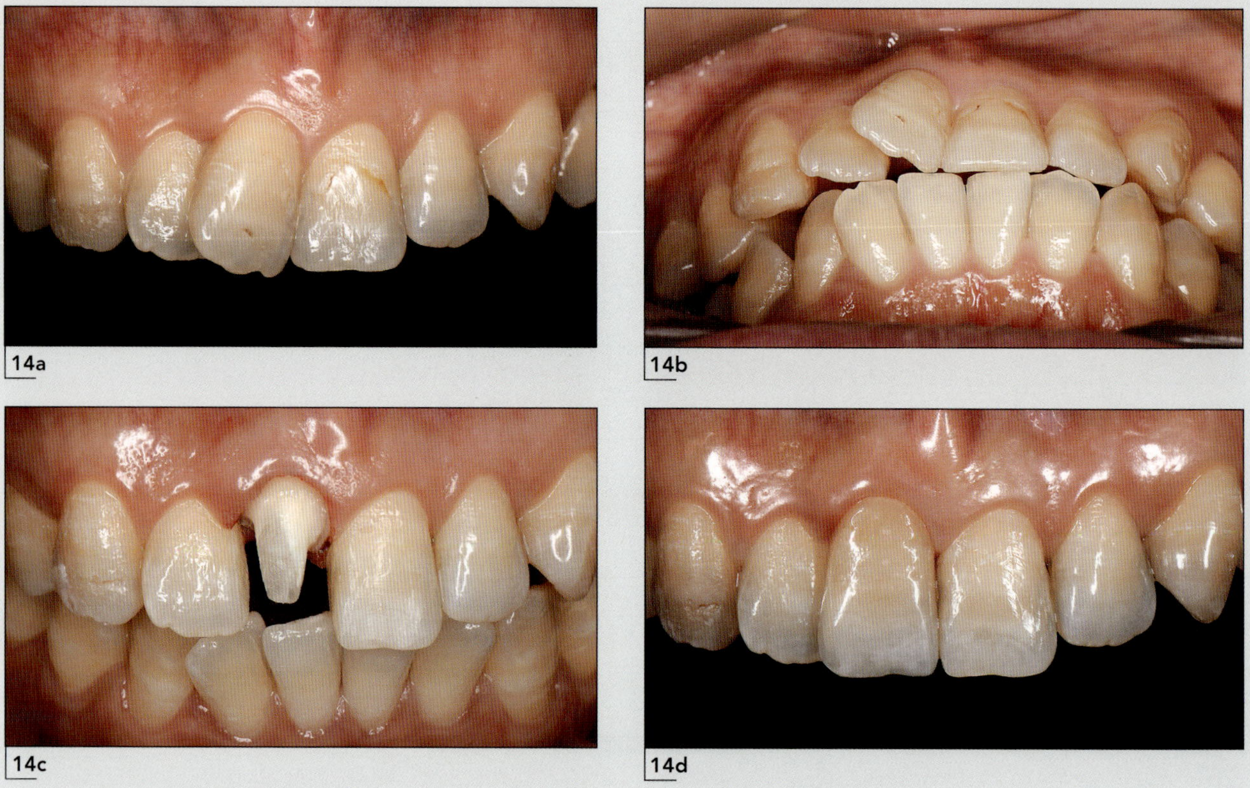

Figs 14a to 14d Even though orthodontic treatment was indicated and recommended to treat the malaligned maxillary and mandibular dentition, the patient refused it. The case was managed only by prosthetic treatment. Root canal therapy and a crown (IPS e.max Press) on the maxillary right central incisor and enameloplasty of the maxillary left central incisor were indicated as a consequence.

POTENTIAL AND LIMITATIONS OF PROSTHODONTIC TREATMENT

In prosthodontic treatment, the dental technician should be involved at the treatment-planning stage so that constructive suggestions can be made to organize an effective and well-thought-out treatment plan and goal. It is also important to recognize limitations of prosthodontic materials and techniques. There are treatment obstacles that a prosthodontic approach cannot overcome. An interdisciplinary approach is important to set a reasonable treatment goal and to construct the treatment plan. The prosthetic approach to improving the prosthetic condition is described in Table 1.

Cases 3 and 4 show how the limitations of prosthodontic treatment affected the patients' therapy. The patient in Case 3 did not accept the proposed orthodontic treatment for her malaligned maxillary right central incisor. The chief complaint of the patient, a female in her 40s, was "I am not happy with the color of my front crown" (Fig 14). Case 4 presents the treatment of a male patient in his 50s with the chief complaint of being unhappy with the esthetics of his anterior fixed dental prosthesis. Fabrication of a new fixed dental prosthesis from the maxillary left central incisor to the left canine was accompanied by reshaping of the right central incisor (Fig 15).

CASE 4 *Esthetic Rehabilitation with Remaining Functional Risk*

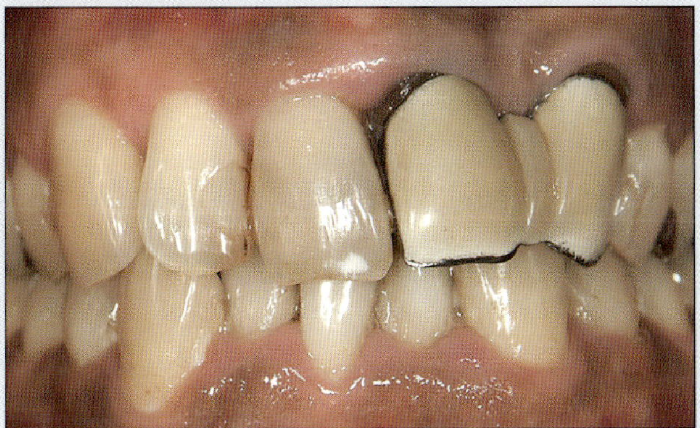

15a

Fig 15a Orthodontic treatment was indicated to improve function and esthetics. However, the patient refused the recommended treatment because of time restrictions. The case was managed only by prosthodontic treatment.

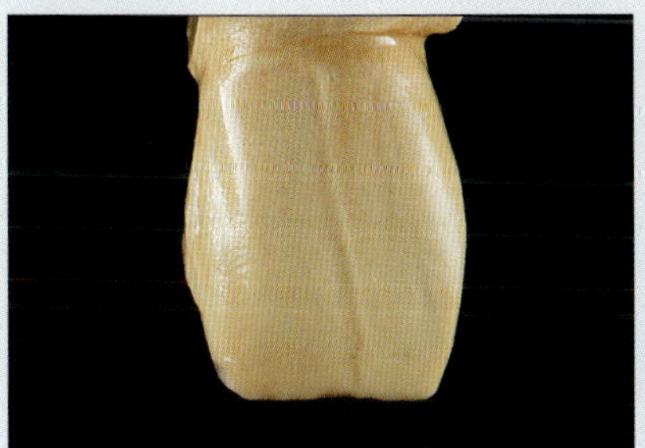

15b

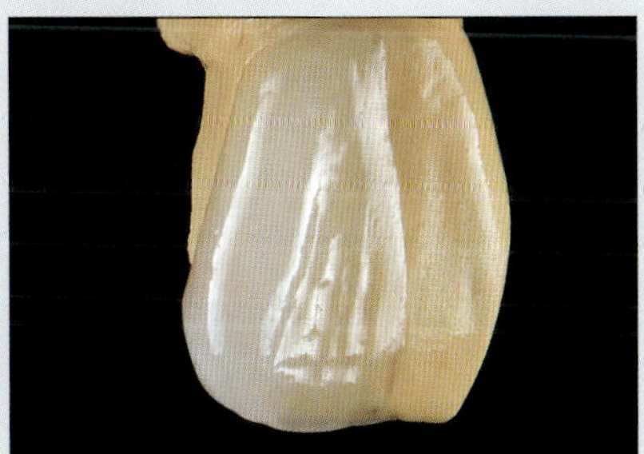

15c

Figs 15b and 15c Lack of prosthetic space was identified as being due to the mesial tilt of the maxillary right central incisor. It was adjusted by *(1)* reshaping its mesial aspect (enameloplasty at the incisal edge area and additive composite resin at the cervical area) and *(2)* placing a partial laminate veneer restoration on the distal aspect. The size and long axis of the tooth were corrected at the clinical crown level.

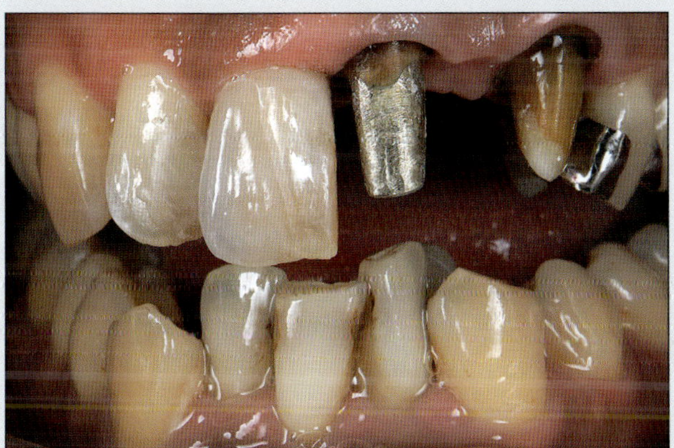

15d

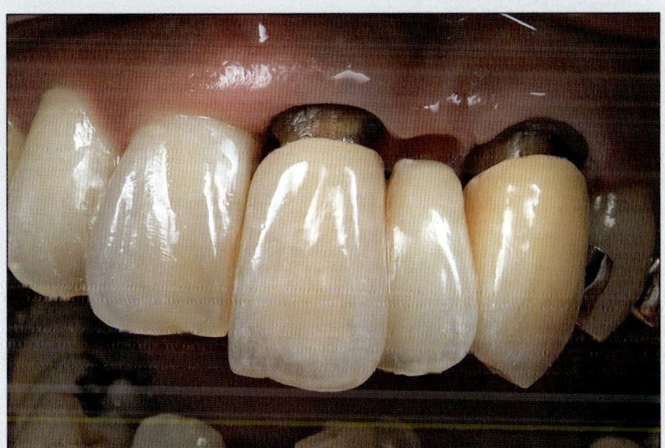

15e

Figs 15d and 15e The available prosthetic space and shape of the fixed partial denture from the left central incisor to the left canine were improved by reshaping the right central incisor. As a result, the esthetics of the maxillary anterior area was dramatically improved. However, the fundamental functional problem was not resolved.

CASE 5 *Improvement of Gingival Levels by Controlling Subgingival Contour*

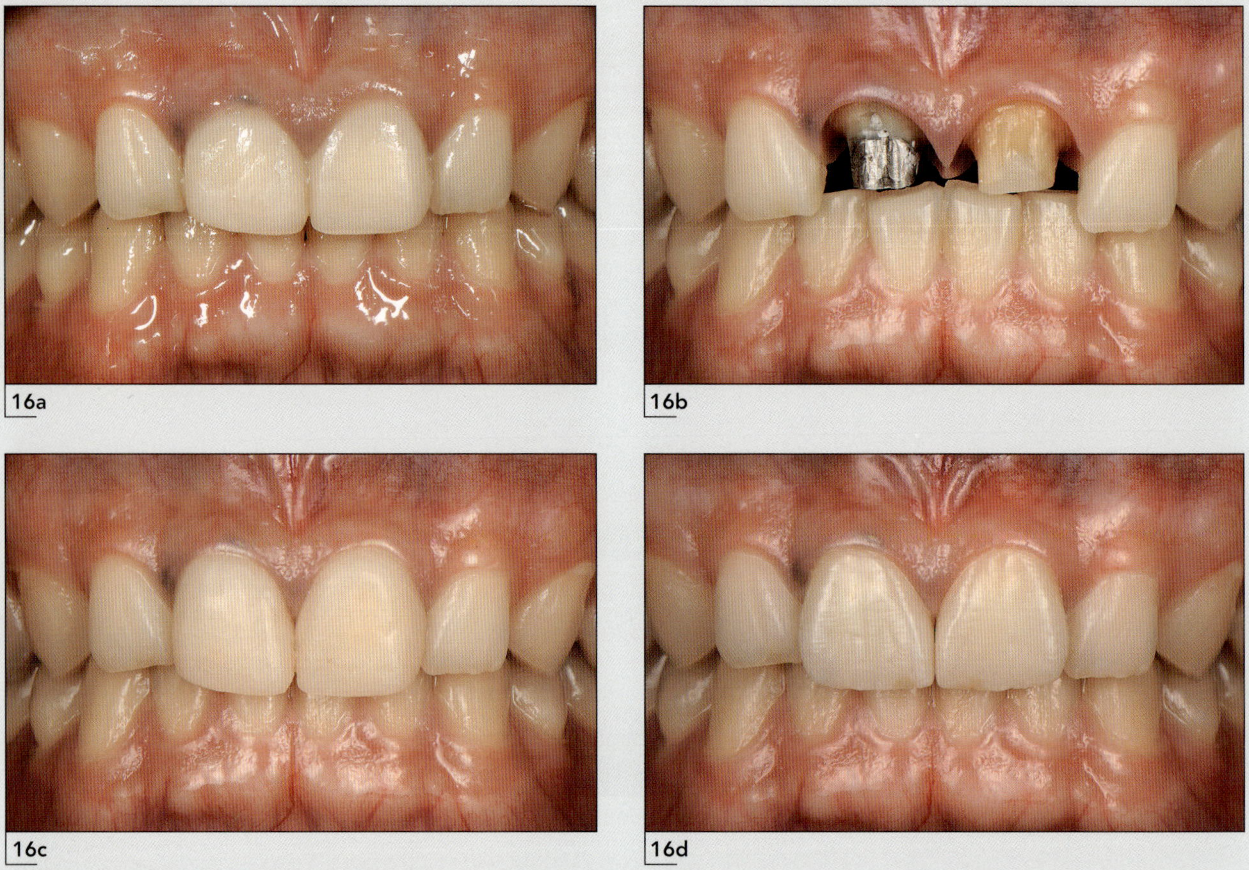

Figs 16a to 16d The patient presented with two short clinical crowns and an unbalanced gingival framework. The gingival level was corrected by controlling the subgingival contour of the prostheses without surgical treatment. When the subgingival area is involved, priority is given to biologic compatibility of the prosthesis and periodontal tissue. Prosthetic treatment is still effectively utilized after proper diagnosis and treatment procedure (IPS e.max Press). *(a)* Pretreatment; *(b)* abutment preparation; *(c)* provisional restoration; *(d)* definitive restoration. (Courtesy of Dr Tsutomu Kubota, Kubota Dental Clinic, Japan.)

Case 5 illustrates the potential of prosthodontic treatment to improve gingival levels by controlling subgingival contour. The patient, a male in his 20s, complained of dissatisfaction with the color of the two crowns on his maxillary central incisors (Fig 16).

Diagnostic Tools + Orthodontic/Implant Treatment

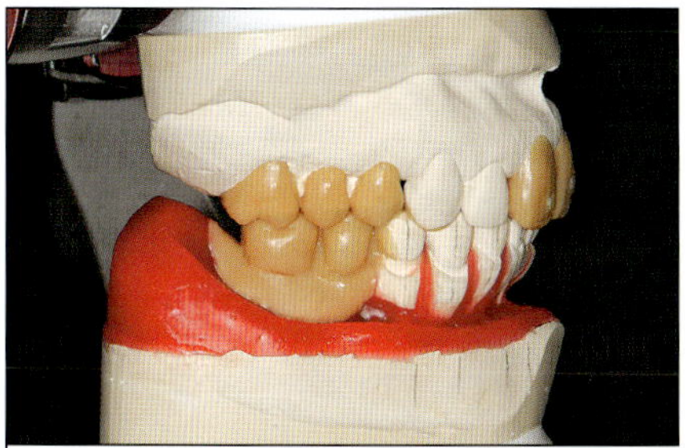

17a

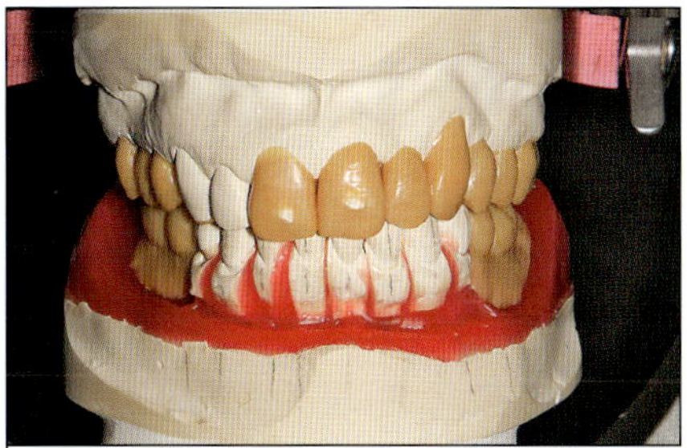

17b

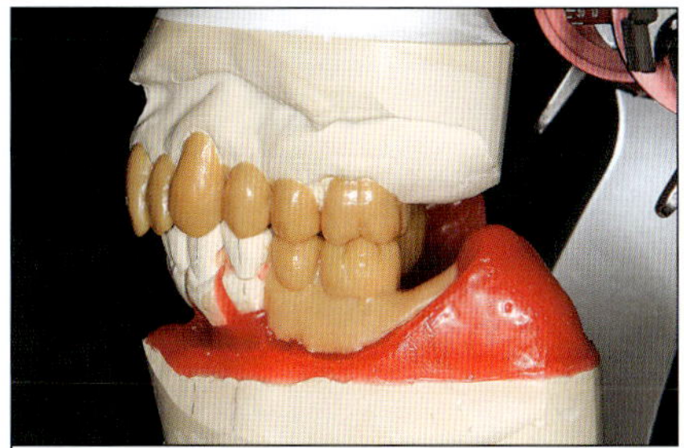

17c

Figs 17a to 17c Orthodontic and implant combined case. Diagnostic tooth alignment and wax-up on the articulator simulates the final occlusion, implant position, and prosthesis.

Diagnostic Tools + Surgical Treatment

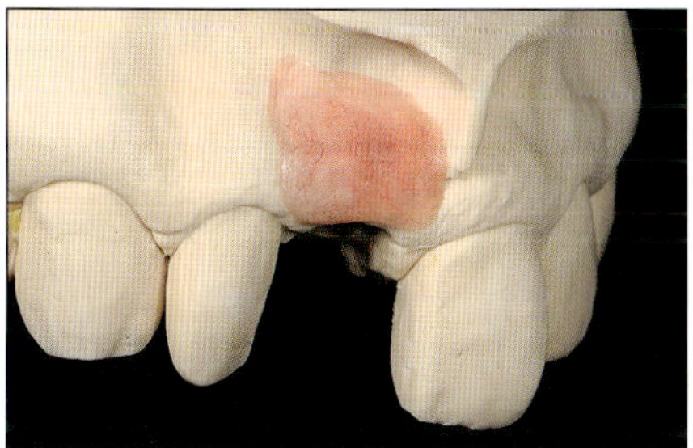

18a

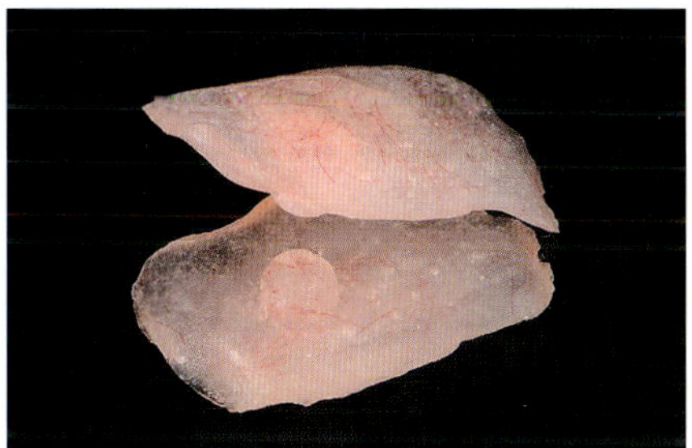

18b

Figs 18a and 18b Study cast with simulation of gingival graft. Gingival graft model is fabricated of self-curing resin to make it retrievable. The dentist can easily estimate the size of the graft with the removable tissue model.

IMPORTANCE OF A TEAM APPROACH

As mentioned before, prosthetic treatment has its limitations and it is impossible to manage all cases by a prosthetic approach alone. The technician should have enough understanding and knowledge of other treatment options to be able to offer appropriate suggestions that can contribute to the development of the treatment goal and plan accordingly.

The importance of a comprehensive team approach is illustrated in Figs 17 to 20. Two examples of the use of diagnostic tools combined with surgical or orthodontic treatment are shown in Figs 17 and 18. Other treatment options can be combined with surgical and orthodontic treatment in improving the gingival framework. The results of a treatment plan combining orthodontics and prosthodontics are shown in Fig 19. Periodontal plastic surgery and prosthodontics are also often integrated with excellent results (Fig 20).

Orthodontics + Prosthodontics

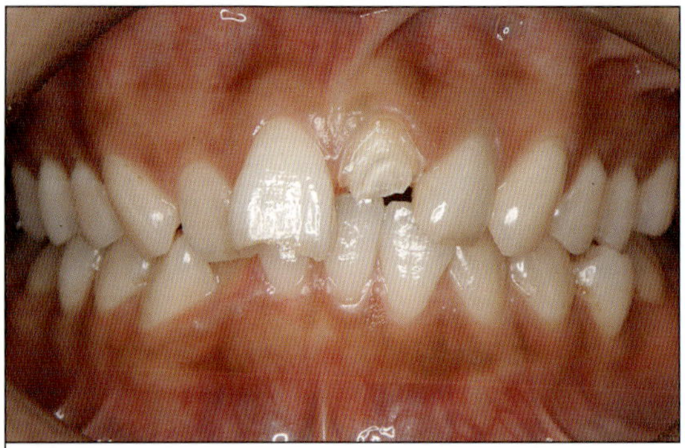
19a

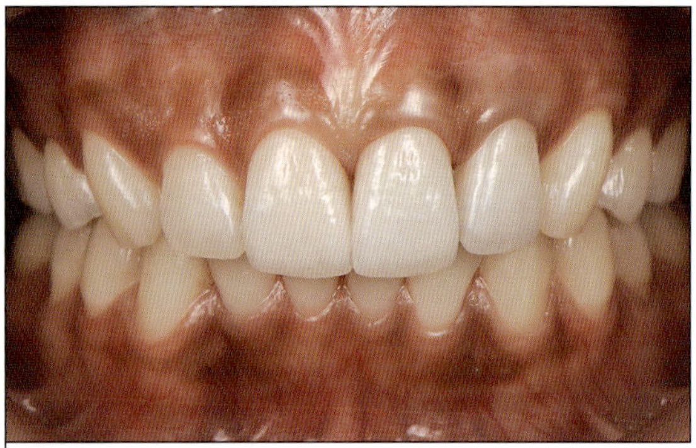
19b

Figs 19a and 19b The purpose of orthodontic treatment is to improve function and esthetics by realigning teeth into their proper positions. The condition of the periodontal tissue (both hard and soft tissues) may improve along with orthodontic tooth movement. As a result, the prosthodontic condition improves as well. In this case, proper prosthetic space and gingival framework were achieved by orthodontic expansion of the dentition (crowns, IPS e.max Press). (Courtesy of Dr Hiroyuki Takino, Takino Dental Clinic, Japan.)

Periodontal Plastic Surgery + Prosthodontics

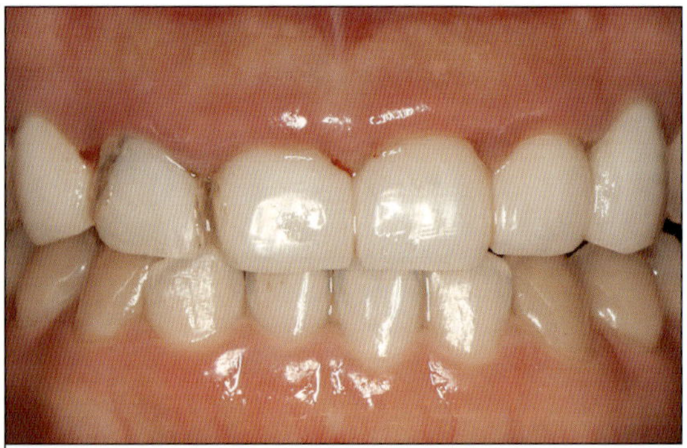
20a

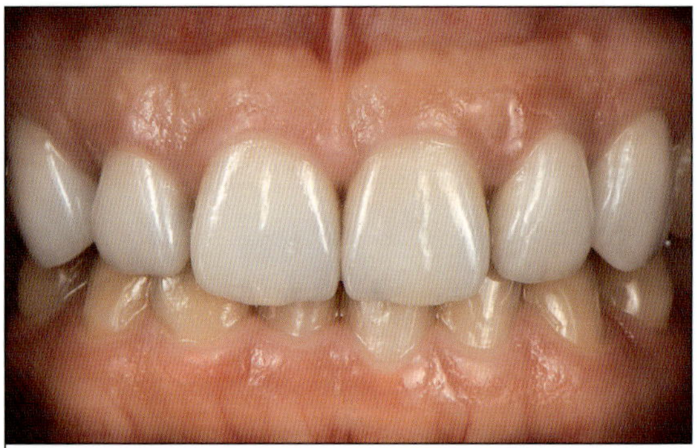
20b

Figs 20a and 20b A crown-lengthening procedure was combined with prosthodontic treatment in this patient who presented with persistent inflammation and violation of biologic width. A surgical approach was indicated. Periodontal surgery was performed prior to prosthodontic treatment to obtain predictable biologic compatibility. Proper contour and prosthetic materials play important roles in maintaining the health of the periodontal tissue (crowns, IPS e.max Press). (Courtesy of Dr Kotaro Nakata, Nakata Dental Clinic, Japan.)

CONCLUSIONS

This article has discussed and illustrated the importance of periodontal tissue consideration and gingival design for successful prosthetic treatment. There are close correlations between esthetics and biology. The combination of proper preprosthetic and prosthetic treatment plays an important role in obtaining esthetic and predictable results. It is not possible to achieve these goals with a prosthetic approach alone.

BIBLIOGRAPHY

Chiche GJ, Aoshima H. Smile Design. Chicago: Quintessence, 2004.

Fradeani M. Esthetic analysis for prosthodontic treatment. In: Yamazaki M (ed). Esthetic Rehabilitation, vol 1. Tokyo: Quintessence, 2006.

Hayashi N. Tooth Preparation Design. Communication tool: Preparation guide. In: Yamazaki M, Chiba T, Komine F (eds). Clinical Prosthodontics Supplement. All Ceramics: Preparation, Theory and Clinical Steps for Abutment Preparation. Tokyo: Ishiyaku, 2010:72–85.

Hidaka T, Minami M (eds). Clinical Prosthodontics Supplement: Basics, Prosthodontic Treatment. Tokyo: Ishiyaku, 2002.

Ide Y, Kuwata M, Nishikawa Y. Dental Laboratory Supplement: Biological Crown Contour, Biologically Harmonized Crown Shape. Tokyo: Ishiyaku, 2008.

Ito Y (ed). The Provisional Restorations in the Quest for Function: Esthetics of the Prosthesis. Tokyo: Quintessence, 2006.

Kataoka S. Harmony, Texture. Tokyo: Quintessence, 2005.

Kataoka S, Mutobe Y. Harmony with nature: Part 4. In: QDT Supplement Year Book 2000. Tokyo: Quintessence, 2000.

Kataoka K, Nishimura Y. Nature's Morphology [in Japanese]. Tokyo: Quintessence, 2003.

Kina S, Bruguera A. Dental Laboratory Supplement. Invisible: Esthetic Ceramic Restorations. Clinical and Laboratory Steps for Ceramic Restorations Harmonizing with Natural Teeth. Shinya A (trans). Tokyo: Ishiyaku, 2010.

Kois JC. Altering gingival levels: The restorative connection. Part 1: Biological variables. J Esthet Restor Dent 1994;6:3–9.

Kobayashi A, Kobayashi T, Funato A. Chairside information the laboratory wants and should know: Periodontal treatment [in Japanese]. QDT 2007;32(7):17–36;32(8):13–42.

Magne P, Belser U. Bonded Porcelain Restorations in the Anterior Dentition: A Biomimetic Approach. Chicago: Quintessence, 2002.

Matsumoto K. Periodontal tissue and abutment preparation. In: Yamazaki M, Chiba T, Komine F (eds). Clinical Prosthodontics Supplement. Preparation for All-Ceramic Restoration: Theory and Clinical Steps for Abutment Preparation. Tokyo: Ishiyaku, 2010:52–64.

Mutobe Y. Basic concept of periodontal tissue and its clinical significance for esthetic prosthodontics of the anterior area: Margin placement and crown morphology [in Japanese]. QDT 1999;25(2):28–48.

Obama T. Anterior Esthetic Rehabilitation: Implant, Prosthetic Guideline and Surgical Treatment Strategy According to the Treatment Purpose. Tokyo: Quintessence, 2007.

Obama T. Esthetic Restoration for Anterior Teeth for Natural Teeth: Differential Diagnosis According to Difficulties and Its Treatment Strategy [in Japanese]. Tokyo: Quintessence, 2007.

Obama T. The role of the dental technician in dentistry. Part 1: Clinical decision criteria for crown shape [in Japanese]. QDT 1999;24(11):32–42.

Obama T, Chiba K, Terakado M. Anterior esthetic restorations: Keys to clinical success [in Japanese]. QDT 2007;32(4):19–44.

Obama T, Uebayashi K. The role of the dental technician in dentistry. Part 2: Clinical decision criteria [in Japanese]. QDT 1999;24(12):28–45.

Ogura K, Sasaki S. Nature's balance. Part 2: A way of approach to cervical contour of the prosthesis (transitioning area to periodontal tissue) [in Japanese]. Quintessence Dent Technol 2008;33(9):17–33.

Okawa M, Kataoka S. Clinical Prosthodontics Supplement, Anterior 6 White & Pink Esthetics. Tokyo: Ishiyaku, 2013.

Okawa M, Onishi K, Otake A, et al. Esthetic of Dental Technology. Part 3: Examination, Diagnosis and Laboratory Steps. QDT Supplement 2004. Tokyo: Quintessence, 2004.

Palacci P, Ericsson I (eds). Implant Esthetic Dentistry: Soft and Hard Tissue Management. Chicago: Quintessence, 2000.

Saadoun AP, LeGall M, Touati B. Selection and ideal tridimensional implant position for soft tissue aesthetics. Pract Periodontics Aesthet Dent 1999;11:1063–1072.

Shigeno K. Periodontal plastic surgery manual for prosthodontic treatment [in Japanese]. Clin Prosthodont 2000;33(1–6):74–82, 190–191, 288–297, 396–405, 526–541, 643–652.

Takahashi K. Team approach in esthetic restorative treatment [in Japanese]. QDT 2008;33(7–8):17–36, 13–42.

Tarnow DP, Magner AW, Fletcher P. The effect of the distance from the contact point to the crest of bone on the presence or absence of the interproximal dental papilla. J Periodontol 1992;63:995–996.

Townsend C. Prerestorative periodontal plastic surgery. Creating the gingival framework for the ideal smile. Dent Today 2004;23:130–133.

Tsuchiya K. Comprehensive Treatment Strategy for Successful Prosthetic Treatment. Tokyo: Ishiyaku, 2010.

Tsuzuki Y. Clinical approach for success in esthetic prosthetic treatment. In: Hayashi N, Takahashi K (eds). Dental Laboratory Supplement. Prosthetic Laboratory Technique and Collaboration Method for Successful Esthetic Rehabilitation. Tokyo: Ishiyaku, 2012:76–82.

Tsuzuki Y, Ito Y. Masterpiece/The biological esthetics: Ceramic work with biological harmony and balance. QDT 2010;35(6):115–122.

Yamazaki M. Dental Esthetics. Part 4: Theory and Clinical of Cutting Edge Approach to Esthetic Restoration [in Japanese]. In: Quintessence Year Book 2002. Tokyo: Quintessence, 2002.

Yamazaki M. Esthetic Classifications: Management of Difficult Esthetic Prosthetic Treatment. Tokyo: Quintessence, 2009.

Yamazaki M, Minami M. Requirement of a crown contour is support of gingivae [in Japanese]. Clin Prosthodont 2001;34(6):638–657.

Yamazaki M, Obama T, Seto N. Crown preparation. In: To Be a Clinical Expert. Vol 1: Conventional Restoration. Tokyo: Ishiyaku, 2004.

Maintaining the Esthetics of Anterior Teeth with a Flapless Single-Tooth Immediate Implant Placement

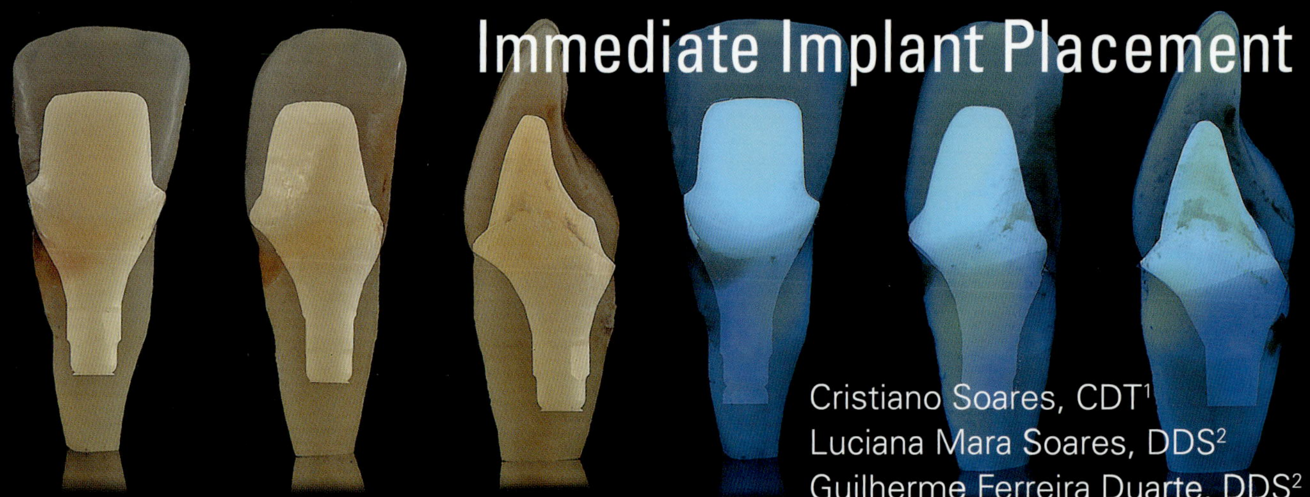

Cristiano Soares, CDT[1]
Luciana Mara Soares, DDS[2]
Guilherme Ferreira Duarte, DDS[2]
Neimar Sartori, DDS, MS, PhD[3]

The majority of patients today are looking for esthetic dental treatments. One of the biggest esthetic challenges is the restoration of a single anterior tooth with an implant-supported prosthesis. In this treatment it is important to mimic all lost structures—such as bone level, soft tissue, and clinical crown—as closely as possible to those of the contralateral tooth.[1] The final results are influenced by the shape and position of the implant, soft tissue management during the surgery, design of the provisional restoration, type of abutment, and characteristics of the definitive restoration.

Predictable esthetic results can be achieved when the oral situation is correctly diagnosed, followed by the execution of an adequate treatment plan. Therefore, some details must be assessed before implant placement, such as integrity of the bony walls, quantity of apical bone, gingival recession, periodontal biotype, and absence of acute infection. The skills of the clinician and technician are also important in achieving predictable results.

A crucial factor for the esthetic outcome of the definitive restoration is the emergence profile, which must be defined initially by the provisional restoration. Moreover, the materials and techniques selected for both the abutment and restoration influence the final result. In some cases, a customized abutment must be fabricated to guarantee an esthetically adequate definitive restoration.

The improvement of implant techniques associated with modern restorative materials has allowed the development of other options to create customized implant-supported crowns. Therefore, the aim of this article is to describe, through a clinical case report, how to esthetically customize a prefabricated zirconia abutment with an adequate emergence profile.

[1]Dental Technician, Campinas, São Paulo, Brazil.
[2]Private Practice, Campinas, São Paulo, Brazil.
[3]Assistant Professor, Division of Restorative Sciences, Ostrow School of Dentistry, University of Southern California, Los Angeles, California, USA.

Correspondence to: Cristiano Soares, Street Germano Casellatto 60, Campinas, São Paulo, Brazil, CEP: 13084-776.
Email: protesecristiano@gmail.com

CASE REPORT

Diagnosis and Treatment Planning

A 34-year-old female patient, healthy and a nonsmoker, came to the authors' clinic complaining of mobility and extrusion of the maxillary left central incisor (Fig 1). Clinical examination indicated that the mobility was due to a subgingival horizontal fracture of the root. Radiographic evaluation (Fig 2) showed a satisfactory endodontic treatment, absence of intraradicular retainers, and an increase in the periodontal ligament space without a radiolucent lesion in the periapical area.

Clinical examination with a periodontal probe (15 UNC Color-Coded Probe, Hu-Friedy) revealed that the probing depth did not exceed 3 mm in any of the examined areas (Fig 3). The subgingival root fracture, approximately 4 mm from the gingival margin, was confirmed during the periodontal examination. However, no fracture of the buccal plate of bone was detected. Neither acute infectious process nor gingival recession was observed during the clinical examination. The oral hygiene of the patient was satisfactory, with only minor accumulation of plaque and supragingival calculus.

It was also observed that the patient had a flat and thick periodontal biotype, with an excellent profile of gingival tissue and preservation of the proximal alveolar crests. A cone beam computed tomography (CBCT) scan confirmed that the buccal bone plate was preserved and revealed an adequate amount of apical bone available for the implant placement.

Based on clinical, radiographic, and CBCT scan examinations, the best treatment option for this patient was extraction of the tooth followed by immediate implant placement and provisionalization using the patient's own natural crown.

Immediate Implant Surgery

To maintain the integrity of bone and gingival tissue around the maxillary left central incisor, the crown was removed using a forceps for primary teeth without touching the gingiva (Fig 4). The remaining tooth root was then prepared for the use of a device for mechanical vertical atraumatic root extraction (Benex-Control Professional Root Extraction System, Meisinger) (Fig 5). The main goal of using this device is to decrease the forces on the socket walls, providing a conservative and minimally traumatic extraction.

The extraction socket was carefully curetted to confirm the integrity of the bony walls. An implant (4.1 × 10-mm Bone Level RC-SLA, Straumann) was placed in its ideal three-dimensional position (Fig 6). The platform of the implant was placed 4 mm below the future gingival margin of the prosthetic crown, which would permit the creation of an ideal emergence profile for the future abutment[2] (Fig 7). Good primary stability (approximately 25 Ncm) of the implant was achieved but was not adequate for immediate provisionalization. A 0.5-mm closure screw (Straumann) was then placed.

The gap between the implant and facial socket bony wall (Fig 8) was filled with an anorganic bovine bone matrix (Bio-OSS, Geistlich) (Fig 9) to compensate for the natural reduction of the socket that occurs after tooth extraction.[3–5] Because the patient had a thick tissue biotype, it was unnecessary to place a connective tissue graft.[6] A gingival graft with a similar shape as the socket and with approximately 2 mm of thickness was placed and stabilized by four interrupted sutures[7] (Fig 10). This suture technique aims to seal and protect the bone graft and implant and prevents the collapse of the gingival margins and papillae that occur after extraction.

CASE REPORT

Fig 1 Initial intraoral view of the maxillary anterior teeth.

Fig 2 Periapical radiograph of the maxillary central incisor.

Fig 3 Periodontal examination indicated that there was no fracture of the bone around the fractured tooth.

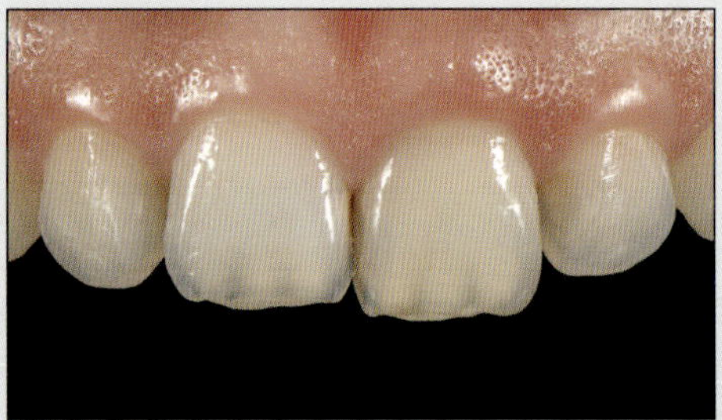
1

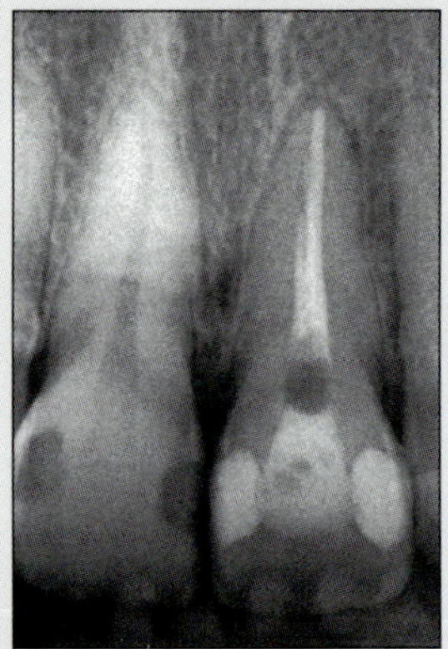
2

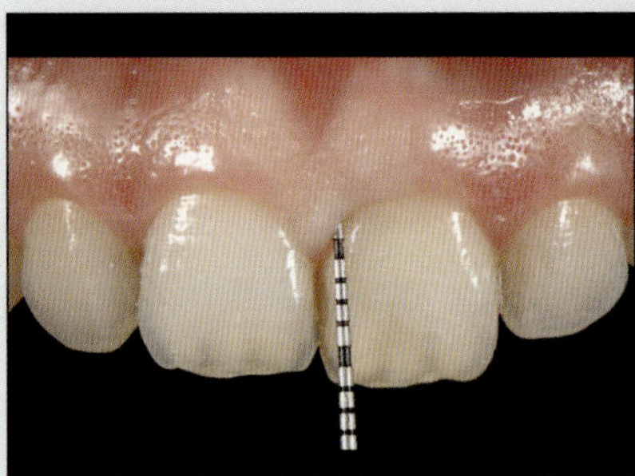
3a

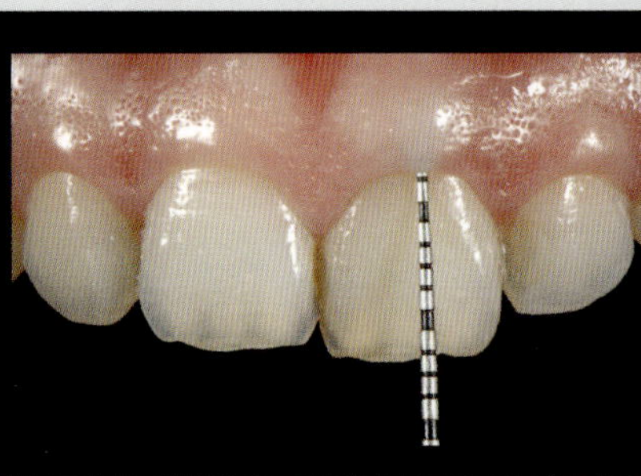
3b

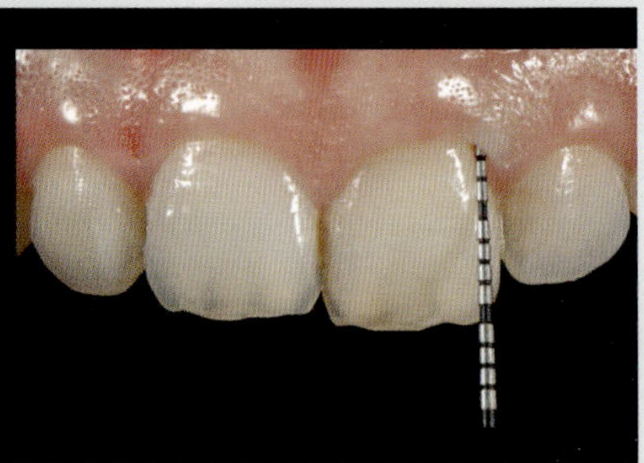
3c

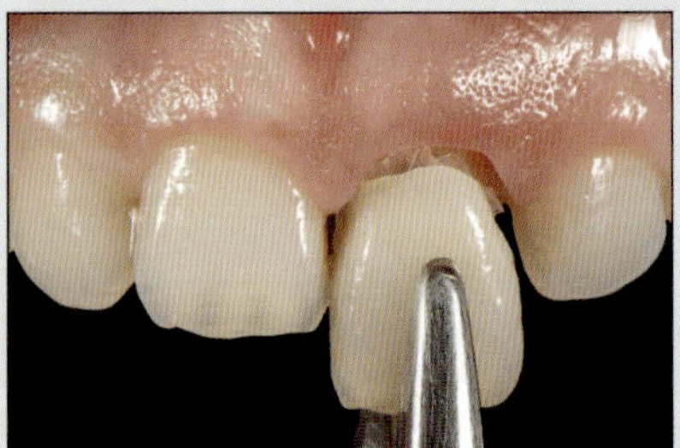
4

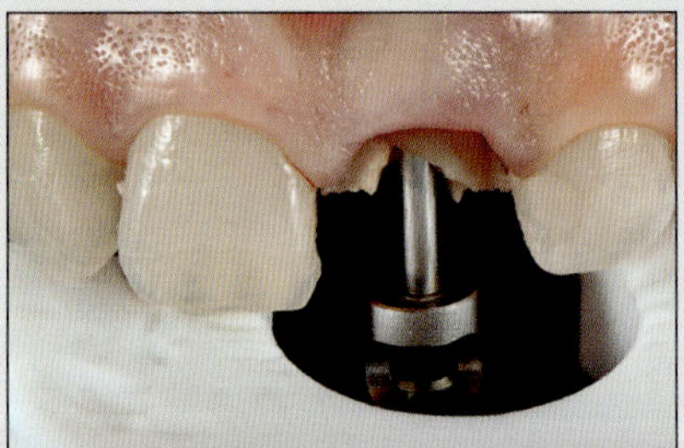
5a

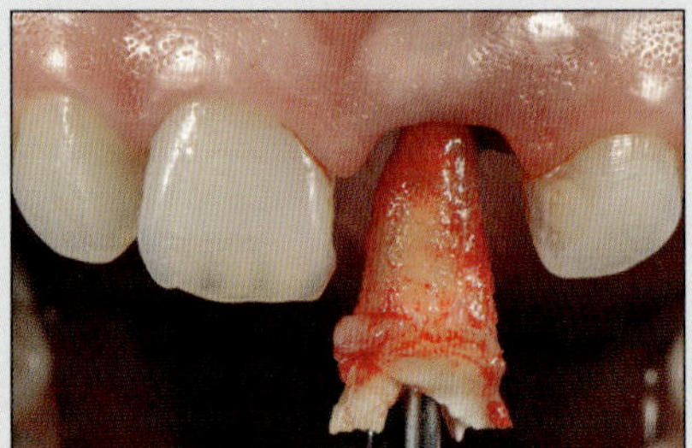
5b

Fig 4 Tooth crown extraction using a forceps for primary teeth.

Figs 5a and 5b Atraumatic root extraction.

Fig 6 Flapless implant placement.

Fig 7 Implant placed at 4 mm below the gingival margin and confirmed using a periodontal probe.

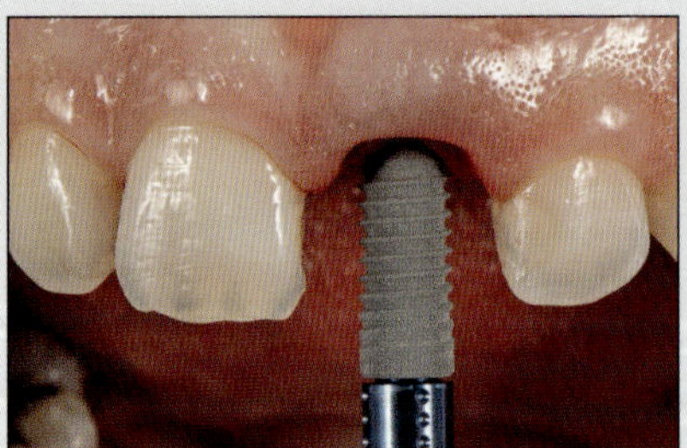
6

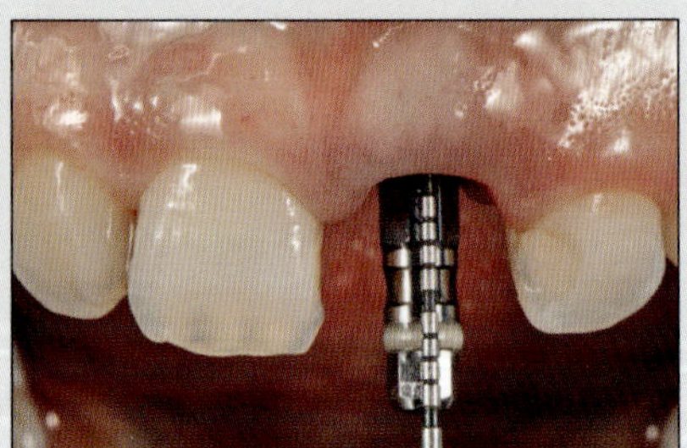
7

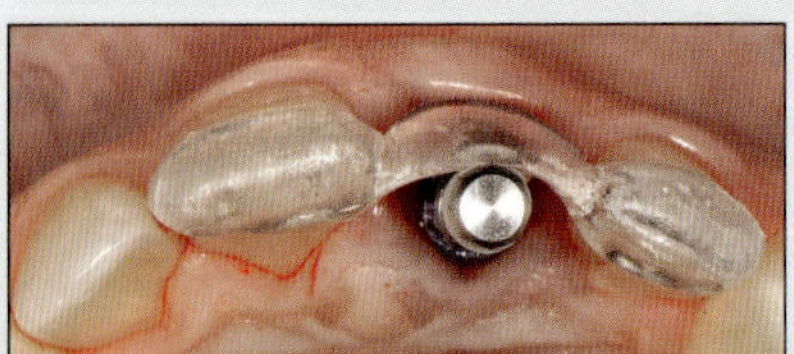
8

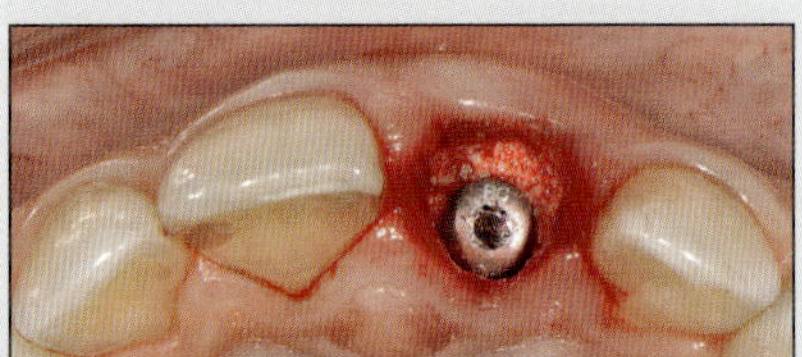
9

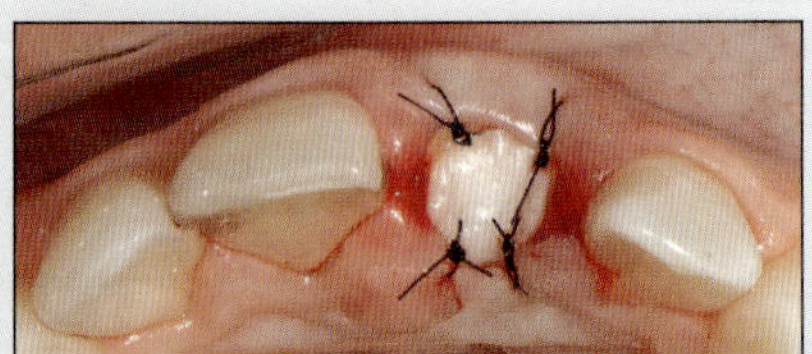
10

Fig 8 Best position for the implant.

Fig 9 The gap was filled with anorganic bovine bone matrix.

Fig 10 Free gingival graft placed and stabilized with four interrupted sutures.

Provisionalization with Patient's Natural Crown

The patient's extracted crown was first stored in saline solution and, after the implant placement, used to fabricate the provisional restoration. The pulpal chamber of the patient's crown was cleaned using a coarse diamond. The pulpal chamber was then etched with 35% phosphoric acid for 15 seconds. It was rinsed and dried, and an adhesive system was applied, which was light cured for 20 seconds. The chamber was filled with a flowable composite (Sinfony, 3M ESPE) to build the correct shape of the cervical area (Fig 11). The contours of the provisional restoration were finished and polished using flexible aluminum oxide abrasive disks (Sof-Lex Finishing and Polishing System, 3M ESPE) to create an adequate restoration emergence profile (Fig 12). The proximal surfaces of both the provisional restoration and adjacent teeth were etched, rinsed, and coated with primer and bonding agent. The provisional restoration was placed in an adequate position, bonded to the adjacent teeth using composite resin (Filtek Supreme Ultra, 3M ESPE), and light cured for 40 seconds (Fig 13). The occlusion of the patient was checked, leaving the prosthesis free of contacts with the opposing teeth.

The patient was instructed to suspend dental brushing in that region and to rinse her mouth with 15 mL of 0.12% chlorhexidine solution for 1 minute every 12 hours for 14 days. The sutures were removed 15 days after surgery. Thirty days after implant placement, a favorable esthetic outcome, contours, and symmetry of the gingival tissue were observed (Fig 14).

Screw-Retained Provisionalization

Four months after the implant placement, bone levels and gingival contours were in an adequate position. Because a sufficient amount of soft tissue was available, an incision slightly shifted toward the lingual was performed to expose the cover screw (Fig 15). The cover screw was removed, a prefabricated titanium abutment (Straumann) was screwed into position, and the implant shoulder was prepared prior to provisional repositioning and adjustment.

The internal portion of the patient's natural crown was prepared to fabricate a screw-retained provisional restoration. The internal portion of the crown was cleaned and etched followed by rinsing, drying, and adhesive system application. The prepared crown was repositioned and connected to the prefabricated titanium abutment in the mouth using a flowable composite resin (Sinfony) (Fig 16). The voids were filled using the same composite resin, and proper contouring and polishing were carried out in the laboratory (Fig 17). After the final adjustments, the provisional restoration was screwed into position to support the soft tissue, creating a gingival emergence profile and contour similar to the contralateral maxillary central incisor.

At the 30-day follow-up examination, adequate contour and position of the gingiva, guided by the correct shape of the subgingival portion of the provisional restoration, were noted (Figs 18 and 19). The emergence profile of the provisional restoration should contain two specific areas: one is concave, about 1 mm subgingival and continuing for 360 degrees around all margins of the provisional restoration, to provide a nonsurgical increase in tissue thickness and long-term stability; the interproximal subgingival area of the provisional restoration should be convex to support the papillae. Furthermore, excellent finishing and polishing of the emergence profile of the provisional restoration is indispensable for precise soft tissue management.[8,9]

Shade Selection

The use of digital photographs for shade selection is essential for correct visual communication with the dental technician. This protocol for shade selection with digital photographs is quite simple and effective; however, some factors should be respected. To correctly select the hue, chroma, and value, a photograph should be taken with four shade guides (Vita Classical Lumin Vacuum shade guide, VITA) similar to the tooth shade and positioned at the same level as the teeth (Fig 20).

A close-up photograph with a black background should be taken to evaluate details such as mamelons, translucence, opalescence, incisal halo, regions with higher and lower value, and presence of staining. The photograph can be manipulated using photo-editing software to increase its contrast and sharpness and to decrease the brightness to highlight these characteristics[6] (Fig 21).

Fig 11 The pulpal chamber of the extracted crown was filled with a flowable composite resin.

Fig 12 Provisional restoration finished and polished with an adequate emergence profile.

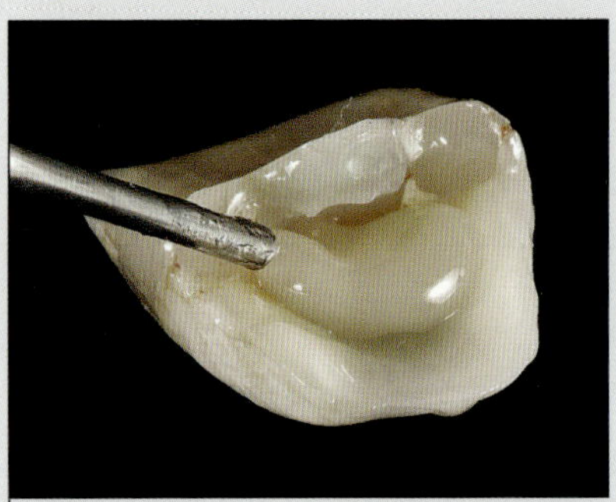

11

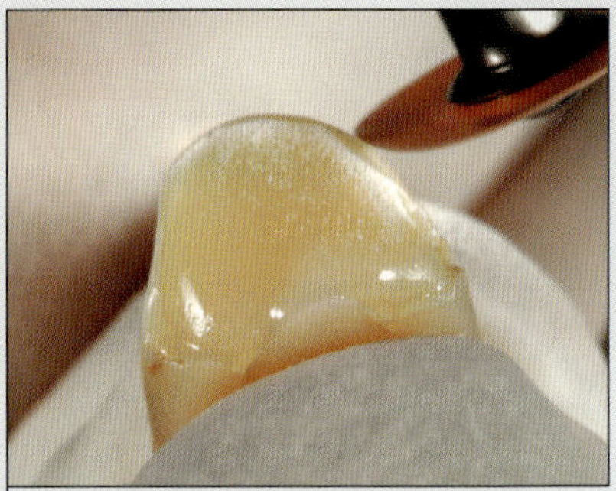

12

Fig 13 Provisional restoration bonded to the adjacent teeth using composite resin.

Fig 14 Clinical appearance 30 days after implant placement.

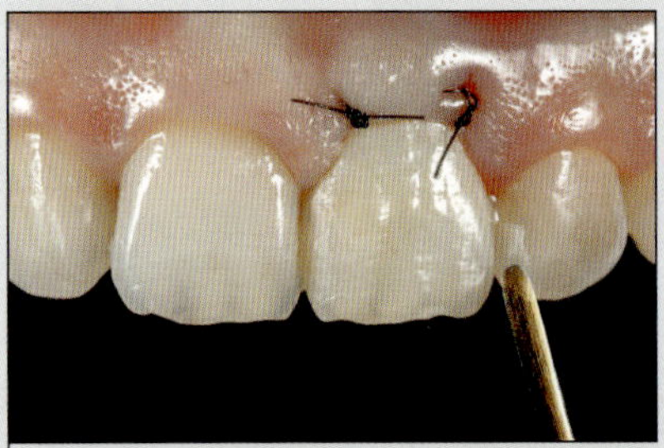

13

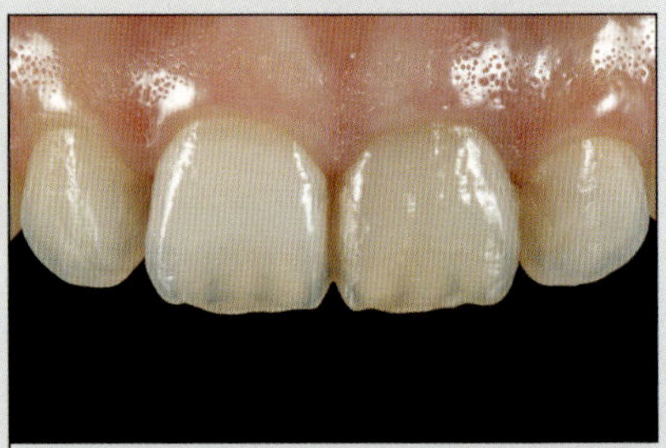

14

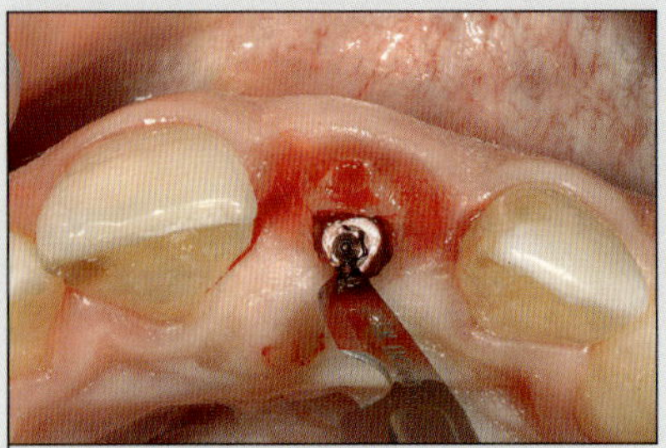

15

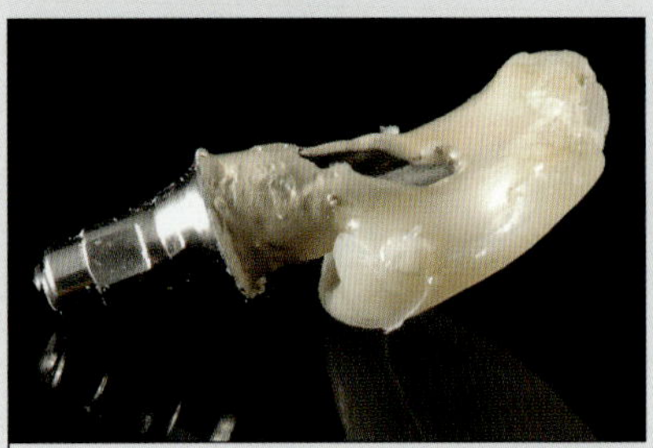

16

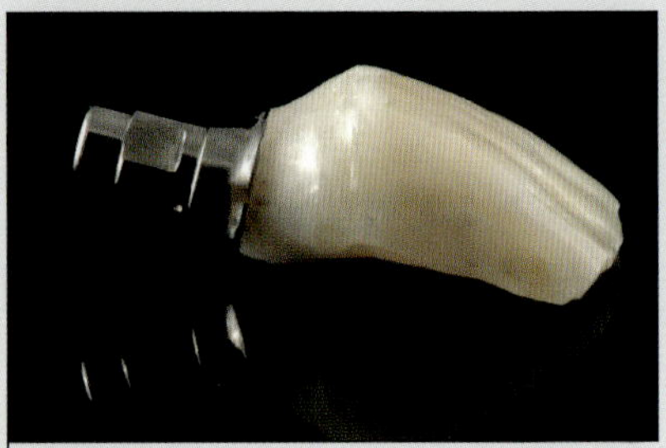

17

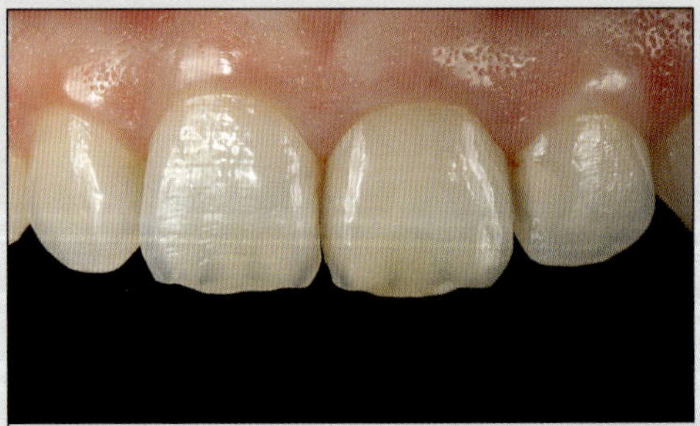

18

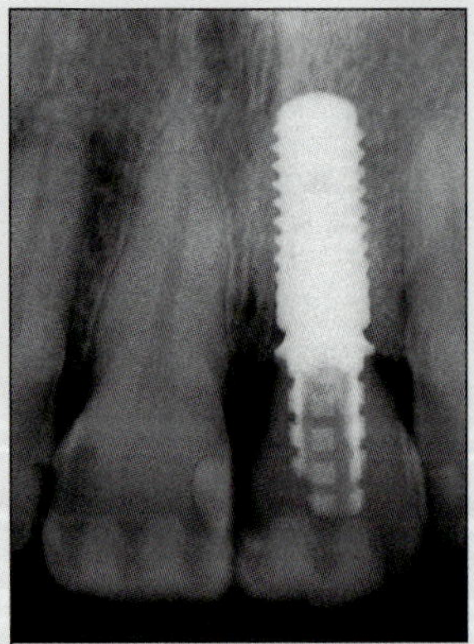

19

Fig 15 Exposure of the cover screw.

Fig 16 The patient's own crown was adapted to a prefabricated titanium abutment with flowable composite resin.

Fig 17 View of the screwed-retained provisional restoration after filling voids with composite resin, finishing, and polishing.

Fig 18 Clinical appearance 30 days after placement of the screw-retained provisional restoration.

Fig 19 Periapical radiograph of the maxillary central incisors.

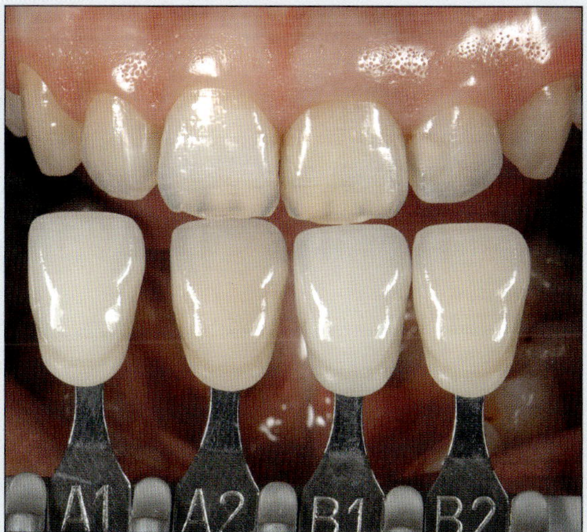

20

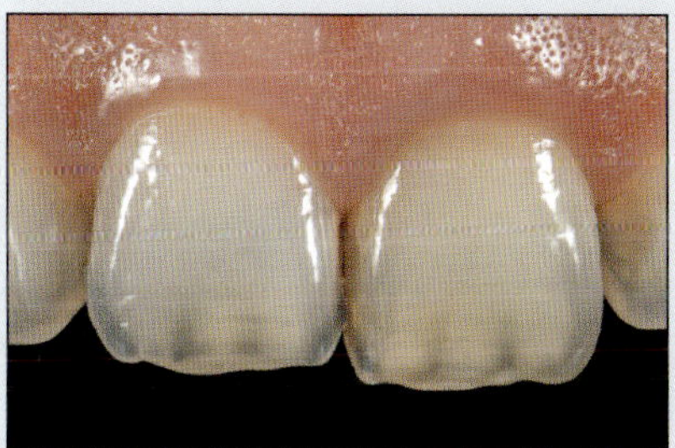

21

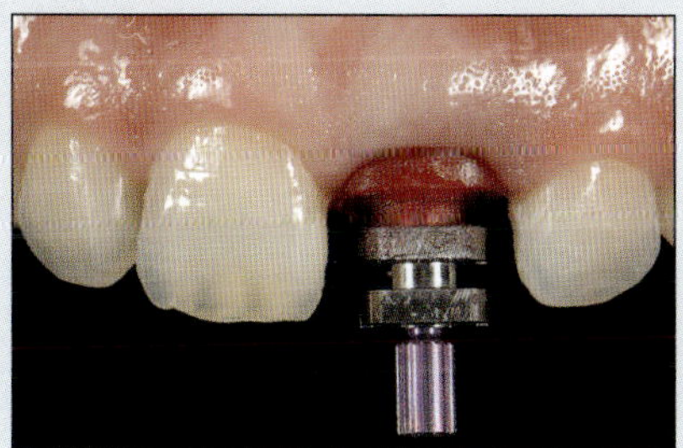

22

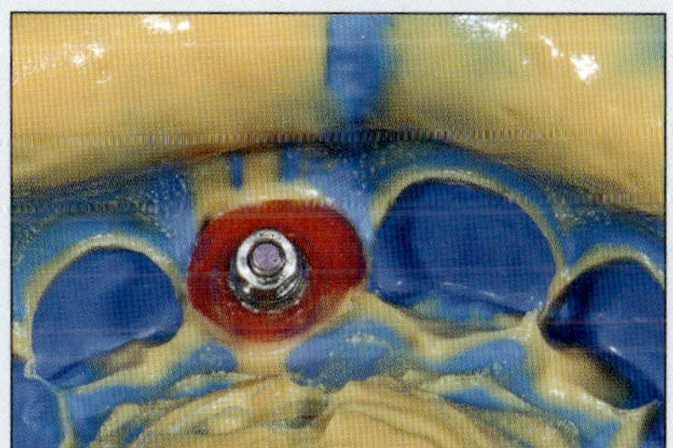

23

Fig 20 Shade selection using digital photography of the anterior maxillary teeth.

Fig 21 Close-up photograph of the maxillary central incisors with increased contrast and reduced brightness for better visualization of the tooth details.

Fig 22 Customized impression post connected to the implant to transfer the provisional subgingival contours.

Fig 23 Impression with the customized impression post in position.

Final Impression Using a Customized Impression Post

After obtaining an adequate emergence profile, it is important to customize the impression post to transfer the provisional subgingival contours along with the implant position. The most common method of transferring the provisional contours and preventing gingival tissue collapse is to use putty and acrylic resin.

The provisional restoration was removed and connected to a laboratory analog, and an impression of the subgingival contours of the provisional restoration was taken using condensation silicone laboratory putty (Zetalabor, Zhermack). The provisional was removed from the laboratory analog, and the impression post (RC Impression Post, Straumann) was connected to the laboratory analog. The space between the impression post and the putty was then filled with a self-curing acrylic resin (Pattern Resin LS, GC America).

After acrylic resin polymerization, the customized impression post was connected to the implant. A previously fabricated custom-made impression tray was placed in position and perforated to allow the impression post to stick out, which is necessary for the open-tray impression technique (Fig 22). A single-step impression was taken using a vinyl polysiloxane (VPS) impression material (Virtual XD, Ivoclar Vivadent). After VPS polymerization, the screw was uncovered and loosened before removal of the impression from the patient's mouth (Fig 23).

Laboratory Phase

Master Cast Fabrication

The implant laboratory analog was placed and attached to the impression post to accurately replicate the implant orientation and position on the master cast. The soft tissue surrounding the implant was duplicated using a resilient addition silicone developed for gingival reproduction on models (Gingifast Rigid, Zhermack). The excess soft tissue was trimmed, and the master cast was poured with stone (Noritake Super Rock EX, Kuraray) (Fig 24). The removable soft tissue

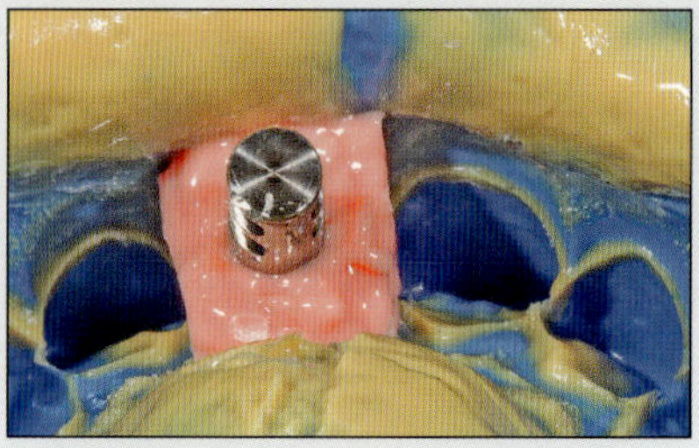

Fig 24 Fabrication of the emergence of the abutment and crown with a removable soft tissue analog.

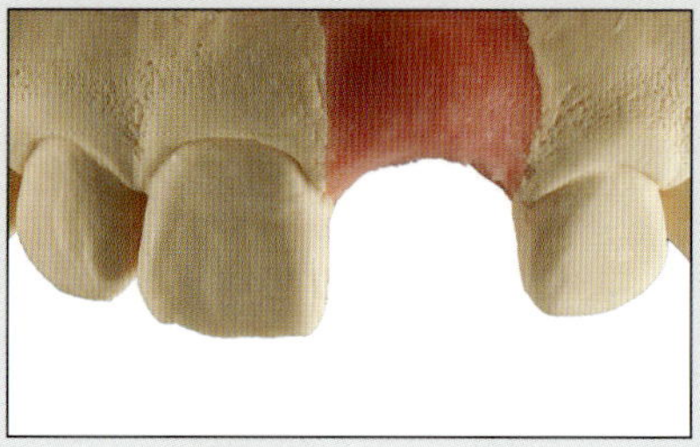

Fig 25 Facial view of the master cast with the removable soft tissue.

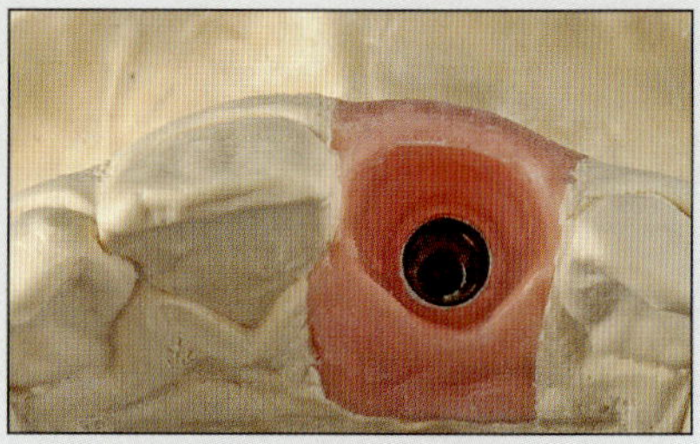

Fig 26 Incisal view of the master cast with the removable soft tissue.

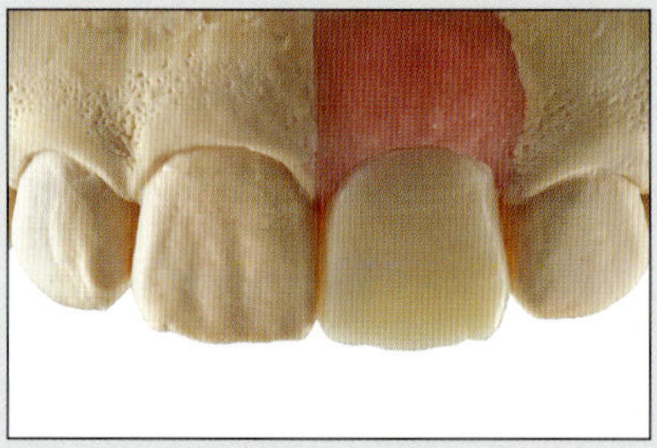

Fig 27 Facial view of the master cast with the definitive wax-up.

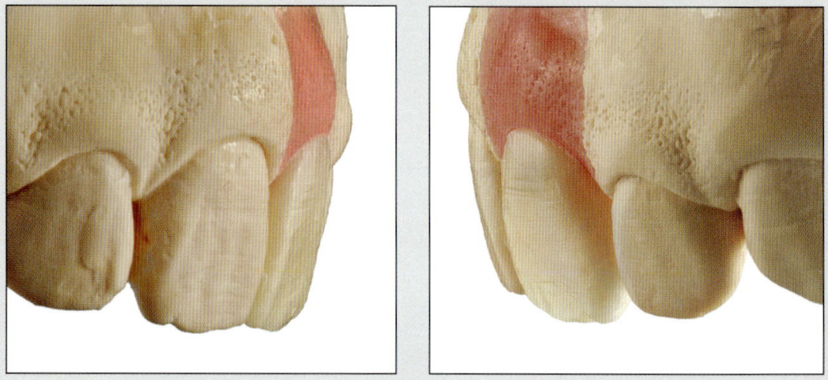

Figs 28a and 28b Left and right profile views of the definitive wax-up.

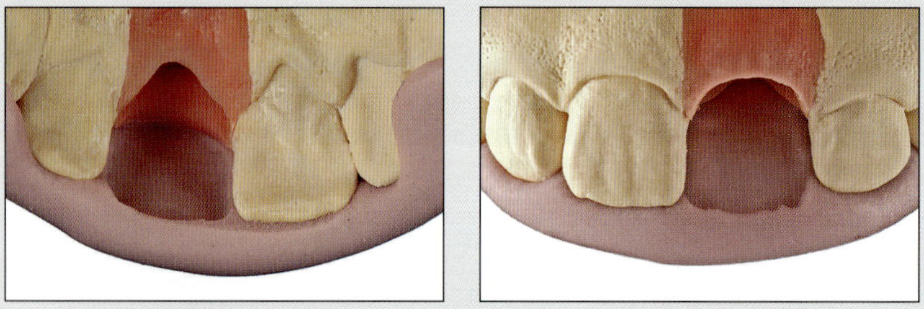

Figs 29a and 29b Silicone indices pressed against the master cast after removing the waxed crown.

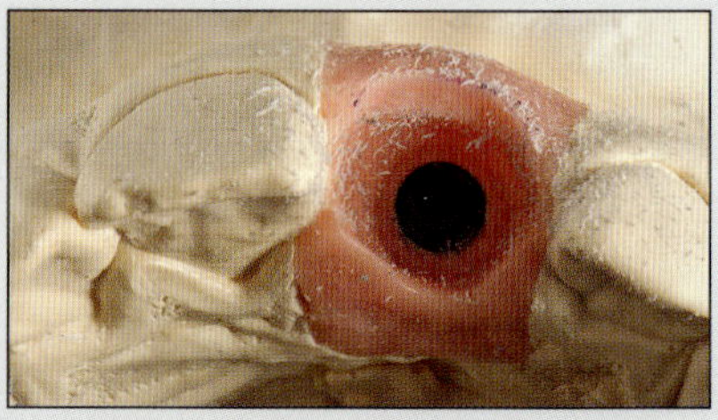

Fig 30 Gingival reshaping with a round diamond-coated bur to create an adequate emergence profile for the definitive restoration.

ensures that the emergence profile of the abutment and crown has an optimal contour (Figs 25 and 26).

Wax-up and Laboratory Correction of the Gingival Asymmetry

The wax-up of the definitive restoration must replicate the height, volume, and contours of the contralateral maxillary right central incisor (Figs 27 and 28). After finishing the wax-up of the definitive restoration on the master cast, two silicone indices, one from the labial and another from the palatal surface, were made with condensation silicone laboratory putty (Zetalabor). The waxed crown was then removed from the master cast to expose the soft tissue analog. A line marking the ideal transition position between the crown (based on the definitive wax-up) and the soft tissue was drawn on the indices using a blue pencil.[10] The indices were pressed against the master cast to indicate the correct gingival margin position of the maxillary left central incisor[11] (Fig 29). The gingival margin was then reshaped using a round diamond-coated bur (Fig 30).

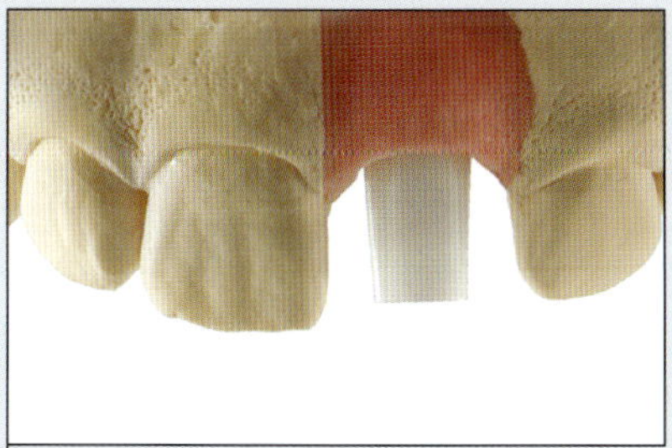

31

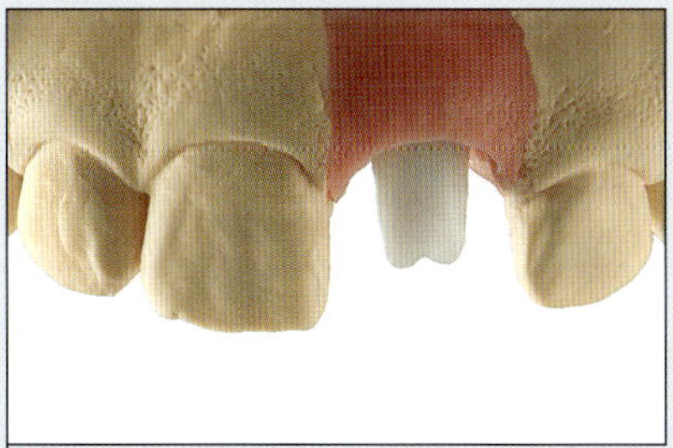

32

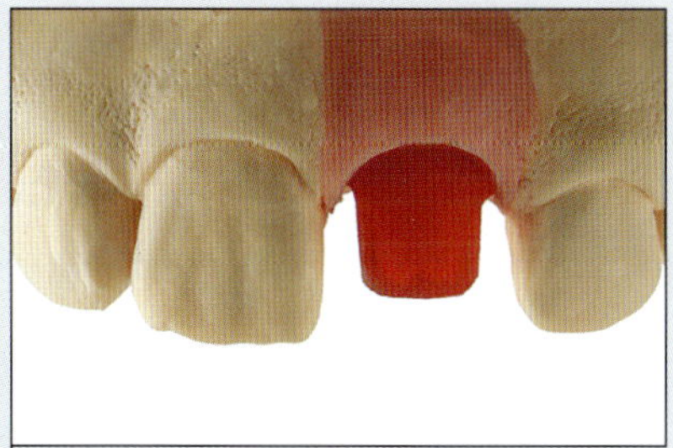

33

Fig 31 Prefabricated anatomically shaped zirconium oxide abutment in position.
Fig 32 Abutment reshaped to create adequate space to accommodate the veneering ceramic.
Fig 33 Abutment customization with acrylic resin.

Customization of the Implant Abutment

A prefabricated anatomically shaped zirconium oxide abutment (Straumann Anatomic/IPS e.max Abutment, Straumann) was selected and connected with the laboratory analog (Fig 31). The abutment was customized using abrasive instruments under light grinding pressure (Fig 32). The emergence profile and the final shape of the abutment were modified with acrylic resin (Pattern Resin LS) to meet the requirements of the material for cementation of the definitive restoration (Fig 33). The customized abutment was invested with phosphate-bonded investment material (IPS PressVEST Speed, Ivoclar Vivadent), and subsequently a fluorapatite glass-ceramic ingot (IPS e.max ZirPress, Ivoclar Vivadent) was pressed onto the zirconium oxide following the manufacturer's instructions (Fig 34).

The main goal of using a customized abutment is to properly restore both the shape and the optical properties, such as color, translucency, opacity, and fluorescence, of the lost tooth structure[12] (Figs 35 and 36). The abutment design should provide excellent adaptation as well as biologic stability of peri-implant soft tissues. It was possible to create an abutment emergence profile with gentle curves with the margin located 1 mm subgingival because the implant was placed 4 mm from the buccal gingival margin (Fig 37).

Ceramic Application

A lithium disilicate coping (IPS e.max Press, Ivoclar Vivadent) was fabricated using the press technique to support the layering ceramic. The coping was sandblasted with type 100 Al_2O_3 at 1 bar (15 psi) pressure and then cleaned with a steam jet to remove any dirt and grease. The definitive restoration was then fabricated using a nanofluorapatite layering ceramic (IPS e.max Ceram, Ivoclar Vivadent).

A thin layer of IPS e.max Ceram Build-up Liquid was first applied in the coping for the wash firing. A layer of DD A1 was applied on the cervical area to reproduce the deep dentin, followed by a layer of D A1 + 20% D BL2 on the middle third to restore the superficial dentin (Fig 38). After the dentin stratification, the positions of the mamelons were defined to create a restoration with a natural incisal third (Fig 39). Vertical layers of ceramic D A1 + 20% D BL2, extending from the labial to the lingual surface, were applied to give a natural appearance to the crown (Fig 40). The space among the mamelons and the incisor proximal contours were filled with E1 + 10% T blue, and a layer of MM salmon was applied over the mamelons to adequately replicate the incisal third. Finally, two horizontal bands of ceramic E 03 were applied to the cervical and middle third, as well as stripes of White Stain to the incisal third (Fig 41). The restoration was then fired according to the firing parameters to stabilize the ceramic layers in the correct position (Fig 42).

After firing, a second layer of ceramic was reapplied to compensate for the shrinkage, complete the missing areas, and enhance the natural appearance of the definitive restoration. A layer of ceramic CT Orange was applied on the cervical, and E 01 + E 02 mixed 1:1 and TS2 on the middle third. The application of ceramic on the mamelons and incisal third was repeated as aforementioned (Fig 43). The restoration was submitted to a third firing cycle (Fig 44).

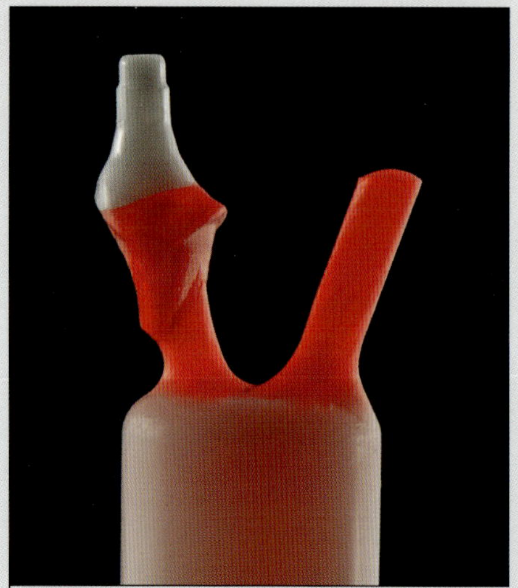

34a

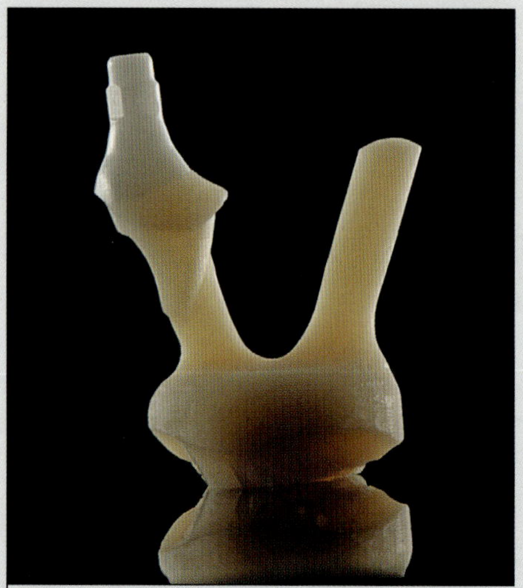

34b

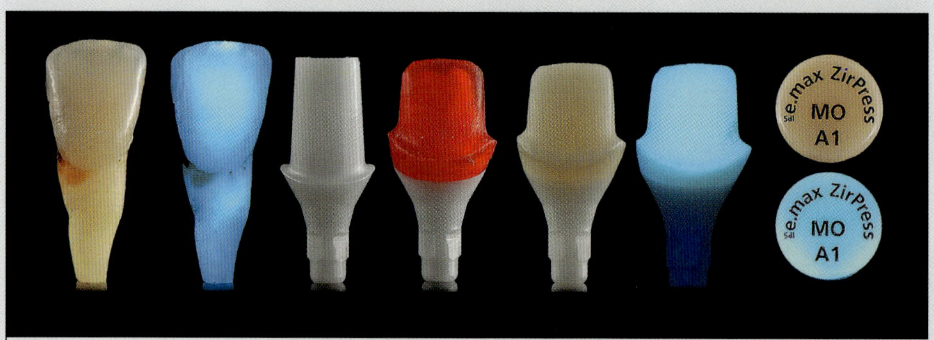

35

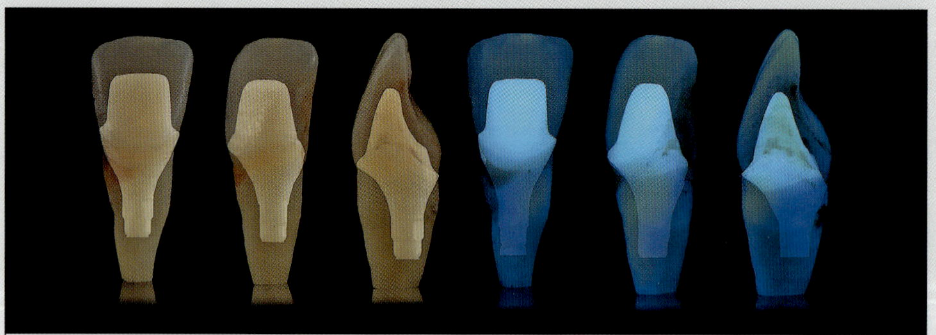

36

Figs 34a and 34b Customized abutment before and after pressing a fluorapatite glass-ceramic ingot onto the prefabricated zirconium oxide abutment.

Fig 35 Sequence of abutment customization based on the natural central incisor root morphology.

Fig 36 Image of the customized abutment superimposed on a natural central incisor tooth.

Fig 37 Customized abutment final shape.

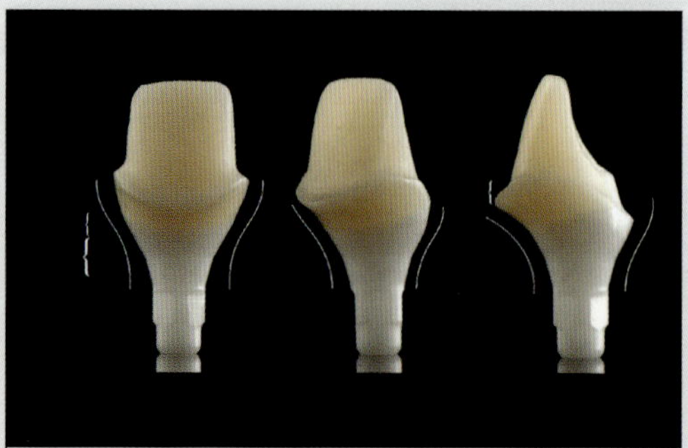

37

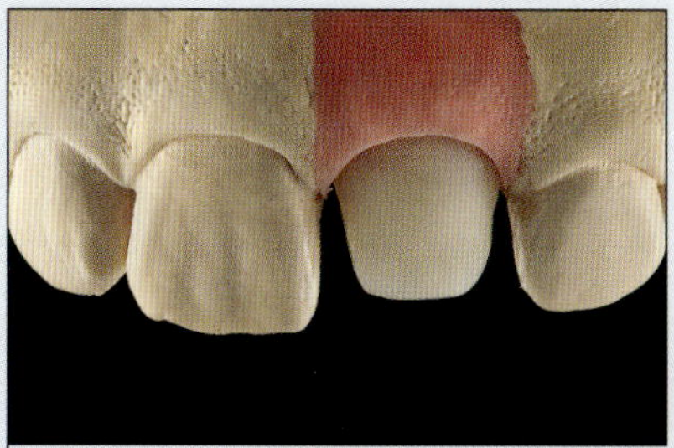
38

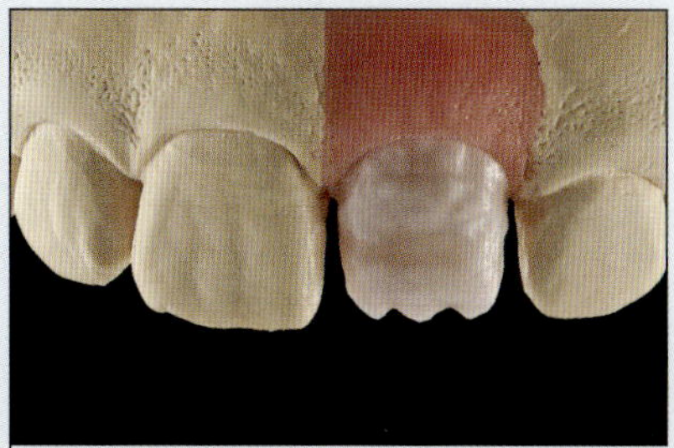
39

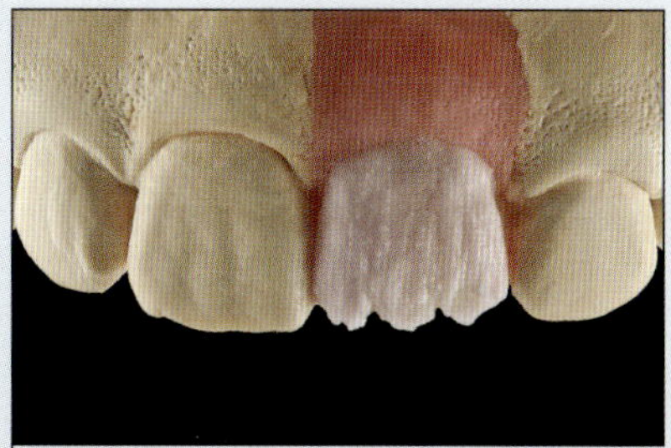
40

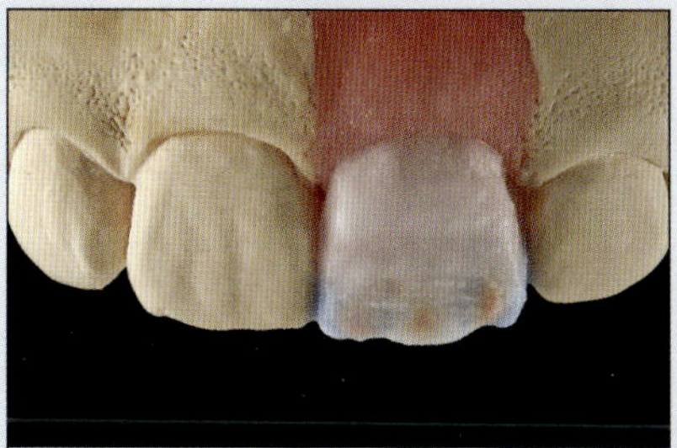
41

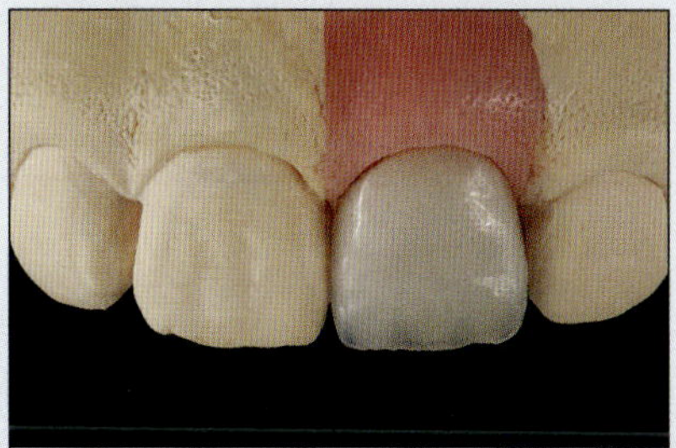
42

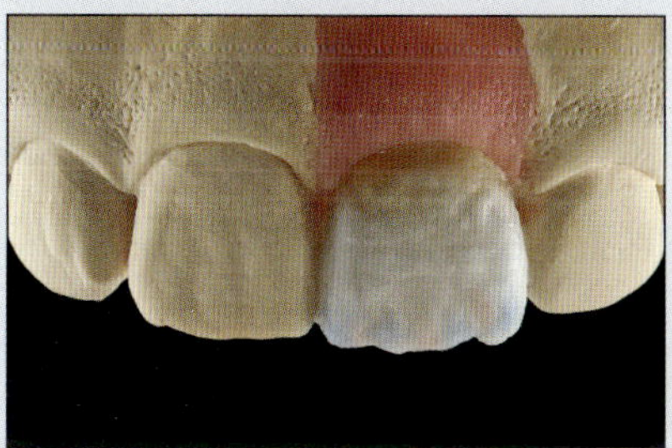
43

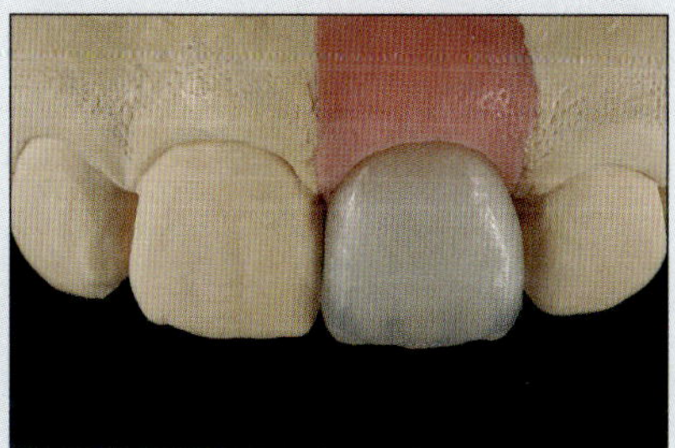
44

Fig 38 Lithium disilicate coping after the wash firing and application of the deep and superficial dentin.

Fig 39 Application of the ceramic using the stratification technique.

Fig 40 Ceramic cutback to define the mamelon positions.

Fig 41 Creating the incisal optical properties.

Fig 42 Appearance of the restoration after the second firing.

Fig 43 Application of the ceramic to create the correct contour of the restoration.

Fig 44 Appearance of the restoration after the third firing.

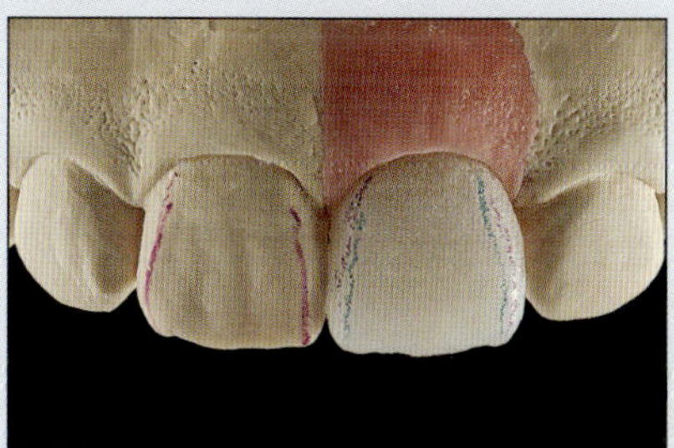
45a

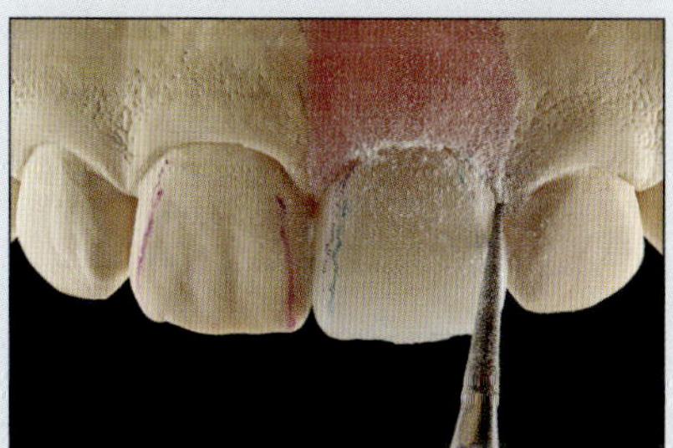
45b

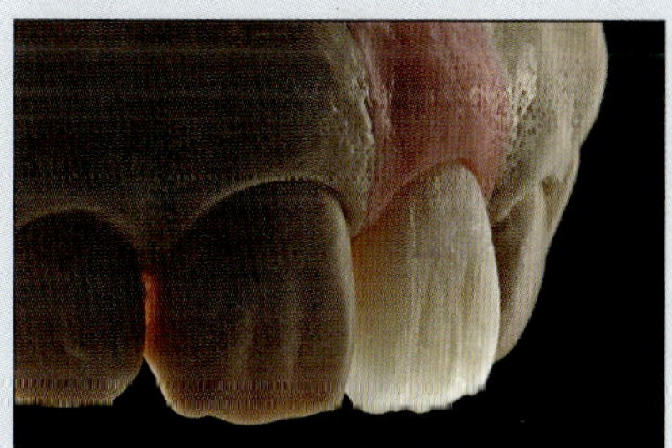
46

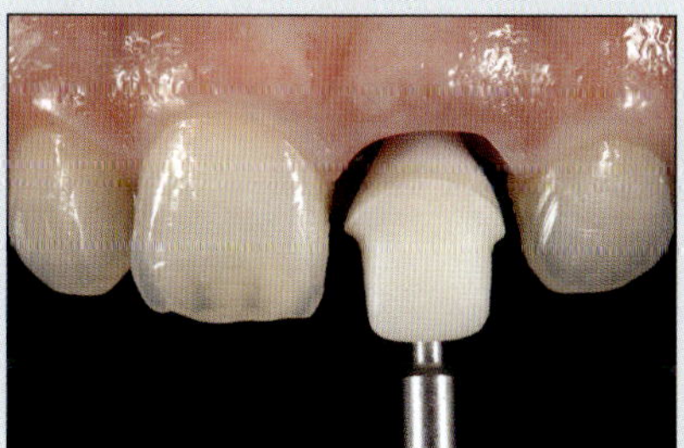
47

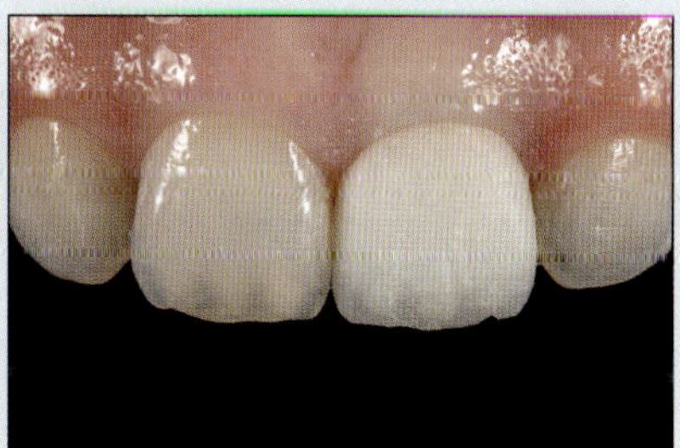
48

Figs 45a and 45b Defining and correcting the position of the mesial and distal line angles.

Fig 46 Facial surface texture of the restoration.

Fig 47 Placing the abutment in position.

Fig 48 Trying in the restoration without glaze for final adjustment of the gingival zenith, as well as shape and color corrections.

Fig 49 Light curing the dual-curing resin cement.

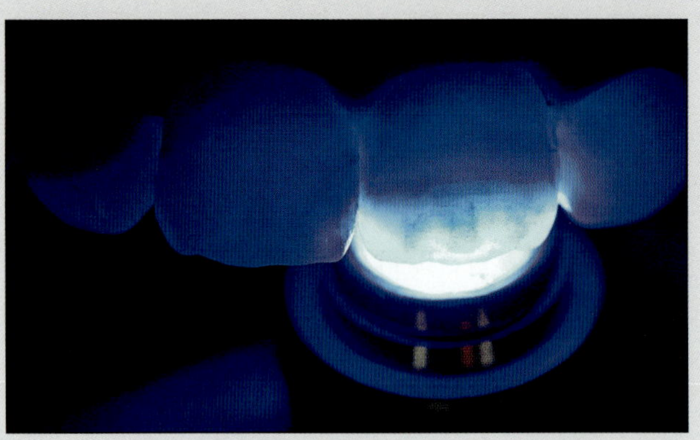

Creation of Adequate Surface Texture

After finishing the firing cycle, the first step to replicate the morphology of the contralateral tooth is to roughen the entire crown with a fine-grained diamond bur. Next, the position of the mesial and distal line angles were marked with purple, and the ideal position of the line angles, based on the adjacent central incisor, were marked with a green pencil (Fig 45a). The ideal position of the line angles, shape, and superficial texture were then created using the patient's maxillary right central incisor as reference (Figs 45b and 46).

The crown was placed in position without any glaze (Figs 47 and 48). The shape of the restoration, superficial texture, position of the contact points, and gingival zenith were checked and adjusted during the try-in of the restoration. Any needed shade corrections can be done with external characterization before glazing. After glazing, the luster of the restoration was adjusted using polishing abrasive rubber points (Exa Cerapol, Edenta).

Restoration Cementation

After confirming the adequate position of the restoration, both abutment and restoration were cleaned with the steam jet. The abutment (external surface) and the crown (intaglio surface) were etched with 5% hydrofluoric acid (IPS Ceramic Etching Gel, Ivoclar Vivadent) for 20 seconds.[13] The etching agent was rinsed off under running water for 60 seconds and then placed in an ultrasonic bath for 5 minutes to remove any residual etching agent. The restoration and abutment were dried with a stream of air, a universal primer for conditioning glass ceramic restoration (Monobond Plus, Ivoclar Vivadent) was applied for 60 seconds, and any remaining excess primer was dispersed with a strong stream of air.[13]

Because of the stability of the soft tissue, the abutment was tightened with a final torque of 35 N. The screw access hole of the abutment was sealed with polytetrafluoroethylene tape and composite resin. A retraction cord (Ultrapack, Ultradent) was inserted subgingivally around the torqued abutment to inhibit any contamination by gingival fluid and to prevent penetration of composite resin cement between the abutment and gingiva.

The restoration was then cemented with dual-curing resin cement (Variolink 2, Ivoclar Vivadent). After the crown was seated in position, the excess cement was removed with artistic brushes; after 1 minute, the cord was removed. All margins were checked, and any remaining cement was removed before the final polymerization of each surface for 60 seconds (Fig 49).

At the 11-month follow-up examination, the restoration had a natural appearance, with excellent biologic, optical, and esthetic integration. Moreover, the gingival position was adequate in level and shape, without any black triangles (Figs 50 to 53).

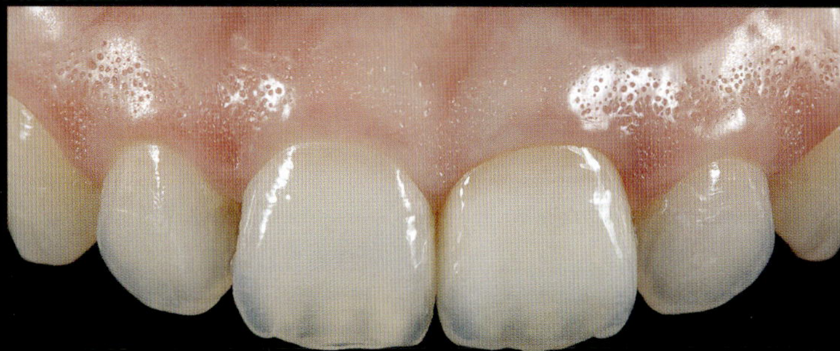

50

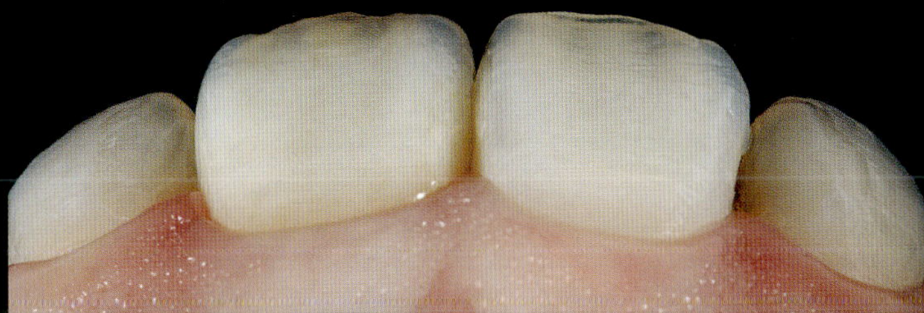

51

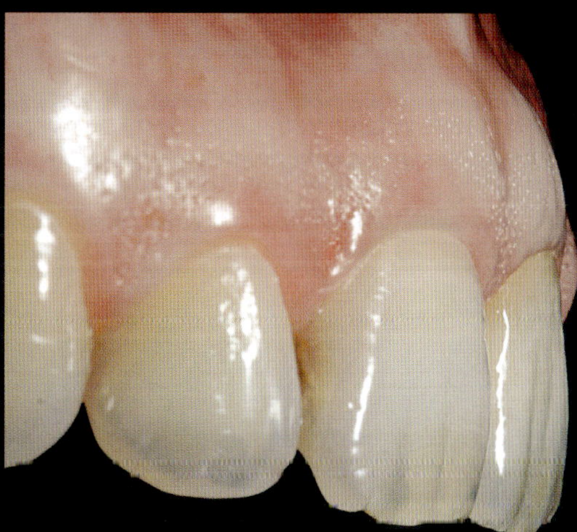

52

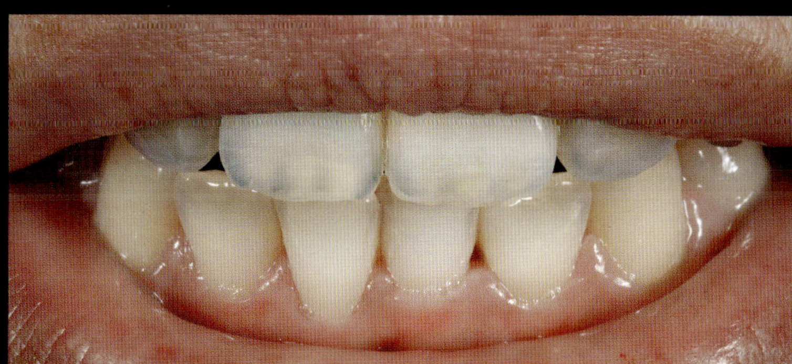

53

Fig 50 Intraoral view of the maxillary anterior teeth with the definitive restoration at 11-month follow-up.

Fig 51 Optical properties of the ceramic restoration are similar to those of the natural tooth.

Fig 52 Superficial texture of the restoration and tissue volume can be observed.

Fig 53 Incisal third of the restoration is similar to that of the natural tooth.

CONCLUSIONS

The excellent outcome is directly associated with the correct tissue management during the surgery, anatomical screw-retained provisional restoration, and customization of the abutment for the definitive restoration. The correct choice of biocompatible materials allows the fabrication of crowns with adequate dental esthetics and a natural appearance.

REFERENCES

1. Marinello CP, Meyenberg KH, Zitzmann N, Luthy H, Soom U, Imoberdorf M. Single-tooth replacement: Some clinical aspects. J Esthet Dent 1997;9:169–178.
2. Saadoun AP, LeGall M, Touati B. Selection and ideal tridimensional implant position for soft tissue aesthetics. Pract Periodontics Aesthet Dent 1999;11:1063–1072.
3. Araujo MG, Lindhe J. Dimensional ridge alterations following tooth extraction. An experimental study in the dog. J Clin Periodontol 2005;32:212–218.
4. Araujo MG, Sukekava F, Wennstrom JL, Lindhe J. Ridge alterations following implant placement in fresh extraction sockets: An experimental study in the dog. J Clin Periodontol 2005;32:645–652.
5. Araujo MG, Linder E, Lindhe J. Bio-Oss collagen in the buccal gap at immediate implants: A 6-month study in the dog. Clin Oral Implants Res 2011;22:1–8.
6. Clavijo VGR, Carvalho PFM, Calgaro M, Silva RC, Joly JC. Integrated esthetic rehabilitation with multiple adjacent implants, periodontal reconstruction, and ceramic restorations. Quintessence Dent Technol 2014;37:13–31.
7. Landsberg CJ, Bichacho N. A modified surgical/prosthetic approach for optimal single implant supported crown. Part I—The socket seal surgery. Pract Periodontics Aesthet Dent 1994;6:11–17.
8. Lemongello GJ. Customized provisional abutment and provisional restoration for an immediately-placed implant. Pract Periodontics Aesthet Dent 2007;19:419–424.
9. Su H, Gonzalez-Martin O, Weisgold A, Lee E. Considerations of implant abutment and crown contour: Critical contour and subcritical contour. Int J Periodontics Restorative Dent 2010;30:335–343.
10. Dooren EV, Soares C, Bichacho N, Giordani G, Clavijo V, Bocabella L. Model-guided soft tissue augmentation. Quintessence Dent Technol 2014;37:49–58.
11. Bichacho N, Landsberg CJ. Single implant restorations: Prosthetically induced soft tissue topography. Pract Periodontics Aesthet Dent 1997;9:745–752.
12. Glauser R, Sailer I, Wohlwend A, Studer S, Schibli M, Scharer P. Experimental zirconia abutments for implant-supported single-tooth restorations in esthetically demanding regions: 4-year results of a prospective clinical study. Int J Prosthodont 2004;17:285–290.
13. Tian T, Tsoi JK, Matinlinna JP, Burrow MF. Aspects of bonding between resin luting cements and glass ceramic materials. Dent Mater 2014;30:e147–e162.

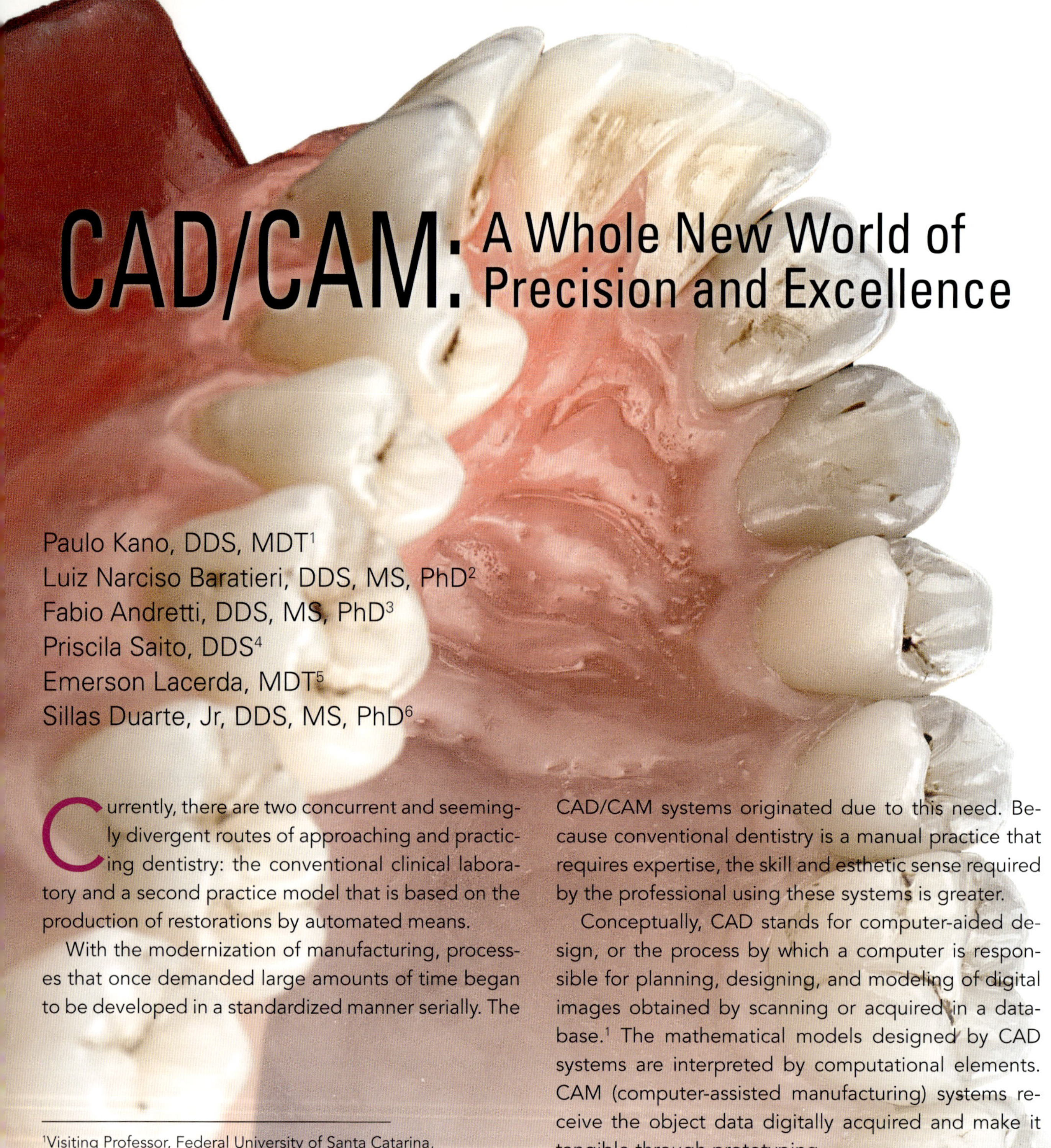

CAD/CAM: A Whole New World of Precision and Excellence

Paulo Kano, DDS, MDT[1]
Luiz Narciso Baratieri, DDS, MS, PhD[2]
Fabio Andretti, DDS, MS, PhD[3]
Priscila Saito, DDS[4]
Emerson Lacerda, MDT[5]
Sillas Duarte, Jr, DDS, MS, PhD[6]

Currently, there are two concurrent and seemingly divergent routes of approaching and practicing dentistry: the conventional clinical laboratory and a second practice model that is based on the production of restorations by automated means.

With the modernization of manufacturing, processes that once demanded large amounts of time began to be developed in a standardized manner serially. The CAD/CAM systems originated due to this need. Because conventional dentistry is a manual practice that requires expertise, the skill and esthetic sense required by the professional using these systems is greater.

Conceptually, CAD stands for computer-aided design, or the process by which a computer is responsible for planning, designing, and modeling of digital images obtained by scanning or acquired in a database.[1] The mathematical models designed by CAD systems are interpreted by computational elements. CAM (computer-assisted manufacturing) systems receive the object data digitally acquired and make it tangible through prototyping.

The CAD/CAM technology is not new; it has been used in several fields for decades. Far afield from dentistry, the first system was developed in 1950 by the defense arm of the United States Air Force Semi-Automatic Ground Environment (SAGE). In 1957, Patrick J. Hanratty developed a system that would become the base code for what we know as CAD/CAM.[2] A few years later, thanks to the spread and standardization of numerical codes, the system could be implemented in various industries, facilitating the production of raw

[1]Visiting Professor, Federal University of Santa Catarina, Florianópolis, Brazil; Private Practice, São Paulo, Brazil.
[2]Professor and Chair, Department of Dentistry, Federal University of Santa Catarina, Florianópolis, Brazil.
[3]Visiting Professor, Federal University of Santa Catarina; Private Practice, Florianópolis, Brazil.
[4]Private Practice, São Paulo, Brazil.
[5]Dental Technician, São Paulo, Brazil.
[6]Associate Professor and Chair, Division of Restorative Sciences, Ostrow School of Dentistry, University of Southern California, Los Angeles, California, USA.

Correspondence to: Dr Paulo Kano, Rua das Pitombeiras 126, São Paulo, SP, 04321-160 Brazil. Email: ipkano@gmail.com

materials. In 1977, Young and Altschuler proposed the use of optical instrumentation to develop a system of surface mapping for an intraoral grid.[3] A short time later, in 1979, Mormann and Brandestini developed a system called CEREC, acronym for ceramic reconstruction, which was the first dental CAD/CAM system. It was initially marketed by Siemens and later by Sirona.[4] In 1984, Francois Duret developed the Duret System, which was marketed as the Sopha BioConcept system in 1992.[5]

The large-scale use of CAD/CAM techniques in the dental environment, however, was not widespread, and it remained very limited for two main reasons: the high cost and the difficulty of copying structures with complex geometry with the highest fidelity.[6]

The scanning mechanism consists of modeling surfaces by creating a geometric model, which may in turn be stored and later used. In addition to generating three-dimensional models from two-dimensional drawings, the file created enables communication with other, different formats of software. The program also calculates the thickness of the produced parts and assemblies, which is important, for example, for predicting the required strength at each region of a prosthetic element.

A major advantage of using CAD/CAM systems is that they allow the production of single-unit restorations (inlays, onlays, crowns, laminate veneers), single- and multiple-unit infrastructures, implant-supported infrastructures, models, and surgical stents without requiring significant prosthetic skills on the part of the operator. The systems can also be classified according to the workplace, as clinical (chairside) or laboratory systems.

The CAD/CAM technology can be used jointly with conventional techniques. Thus, one can enjoy the "best of both worlds" by combining the accuracy and speed of digital systems with the excellence, beauty, and art of conventional dentistry. However, knowing only the hardware and software without mastering specific concepts of dentistry can result in suboptimization of the process. In other words, CAD/CAM systems do not replace the clinical steps but make them more dynamic, predictable, and effective.

For orthodontics, conventional orthodontic treatment has usually involved setup, manual preparation of working models, insertion of appliances, and application of forces based on a treatment plan obtained from cephalometric calculations, with the expectation that the torque and the magnitude of these forces would produce a desired effect. Currently, scanned virtual models and radiographic images may be overlapped by a CAD/CAM system, and the areas, distances, and angles calculated, allowing a simulation of the result of the movements even before inserting the appliance.

For orthognathic and implant dentistry surgeries, a trend is the use of CAD/CAM systems that enable planning and preoperative simulation of procedures by prototyping, with the possibility of integration of image acquisition and milling systems.

In the case of direct and indirect restorations, the digital age does not replace planning, proper case selection, the correct indication of the material, nor the preparation, gingival retraction, and the establishment of appropriate conditions from the periodontal and occlusal points of view. Furthermore, it does not ensure a successful treatment on its own if the steps of cementation, finishing, polishing, and maintenance are neglected. Indeed, digital manufacturing provides precision and time savings in essential laboratory steps that are invisible to the patient, such as fabricating the die, waxing, inclusion, injection, divesting, etc.

When the goal is recreating nature, numerous variables enter the equation. In dentistry, the correct reproduction of shape, texture, translucency, and color are essential to mimic a natural tooth element. The CAD/CAM systems, at this stage, uniquely allow the reproduction of shape and texture of the surfaces to be restored. The aspects relating to the color and translucency vary according to the selected and indicated material.

DEVELOPMENT

This article explains specifically the dental chairside CEREC (Sirona) CAD/CAM system, which has four operation modes or workflows. These can be described as follows: database, mirroring copy, customized digital impression, and three-dimensional application of the adjacent morphology (CEREC Biogeneric patented technology, developed by Sirona).

The simplest way to acquire the images is through a database formed by standard pictures provided by the manufacturer or a software engineer. These shapes may be purely digital, ie, embedded in the CAD system, or obtained by scanning from any physical model. In this type of work, the dentist should simply scan intraorally the tooth preparation and the antagonist teeth. The images are acquired, the virtual model is created by the system, and the operator selects the most appropriate tooth shape from the database. The occlusion with the antagonist teeth is simultaneously checked by the system, the proposed restoration is generated, and the material can be milled. However, this database has a limited amount of shapes. The manufacturer in this case typically provides four basic morphologies (young, adult, elderly, or Asian; these shapes have been developed by Sirona). This often may not be enough to achieve anatomy similar to the adjacent teeth. This first workflow differs from others by the convenience of using previously stored digital images and the degree of standardization.

The second approach is the method of mirroring. The dental arches are scanned in the same manner as in the previous workflow; however, this scan is performed to capture the image of an element homologous to the missing tooth, which in turn can be mirrored to the absent tooth. When using CEREC, this workflow was originally known as Bioreference. Currently, it is called Biogeneric Reference, with the insertion of the Biogeneric function with which the restoration proposal may also be generated from a contralateral or antagonist tooth. However, this tooth should still belong to the same class as the missing tooth.

The workflow for the customized digital impression is called Biocopy (or Correlation Mode, in version 3.8 of the software) and offers the following acquisition options: *(1)* from a wax-up, *(2)* from a provisional restoration, *(3)* from a trial restoration, or *(4)* from the morphology of the patient's own teeth (for teeth requiring only color or alignment changes), copied before the preparation of the teeth. Then, a second scanning of the prepared teeth is obtained. Therefore, this technique is known as the double-scanning technique. The images are digitally superimposed, the restoration proposal is created, and the material is milled. Currently, in the CEREC system this mode is called Biogeneric Copy, and its main function is the preservation of the proposed morphology, obtained from references provided at the first scanning. However, in the latest versions of the software, the Biogeneric technology has been linked to the Biocopy mode, and in some situations it can merge parts of existing surfaces and adjacent anatomical landmarks to the prepared tooth.

The fourth method is the three-dimensional application of the adjacent morphology, called Biogeneric, which is available only in the CEREC system. This is a method that analyzes and uses the anatomy of the adjacent teeth to compose a restoration. In this workflow, the software uses the anatomical landmarks of the patient's other teeth, such as cusps, inclines, slopes, and free surfaces, to calculate the missing part of the element to be restored. Thus, for example, when all molars are absent, it is possible to rebuild them using information from the premolars, considering the occlusion and the functional movements.

WORKFLOW

The following demonstrates the potential of a CAD/CAM system to reproduce nature in detail.

Fabrication and Preparation of the Cast

First, an impression of the natural dentition of a previously selected patient was made with a high-/low-viscosity polyvinyl siloxane impression material (Virtual, Ivoclar Vivadent). The impression was poured with a special stone material (Fujirock EP, GC), which was kept intact. After pouring of the stone material, the technicians waited at least 2 hours before removal of the cast. Next, this cast was replicated twice with high-quality industrial silicone (Poli 400 Polisil, Poli Resinas Indústria Comércio Resinas). In the first duplicated silicone cast, the areas of the main sulci with restorations were corrected or emphasized.

In the second duplicated silicone cast, all teeth were individualized, and dies were fabricated according to the Geller technique. These dies were isolated with petroleum jelly and repositioned in the impression. The spatulated stone material was poured to obtain the cast base. The dies were removed from this cast after 2 hours, and the dies and the base (without dies) were duplicated with industrial silicone.

The impression of the dies was poured again with special stone. Medium-hardness organic wax was poured inside the impression of the cast base, which was fabricated with industrial silicone (red Inowax, Formaden). This wax was poured into the mold in its liquid state after being heated over a flame until its melting point (74°C). After pouring, the assembly was kept in an oven for temperature homogenization of the wax while still in a fluid state (at 74°C). The wax impression was placed in a muffle (at 4 bar pressure) for progressive cooling to room temperature to avoid bubble formation. After this step, the wax cast was carefully removed from the silicone, resulting in a gingival mask. The wax cast obtained was finalized with manual sculpture to define the anatomy of the palatal area and the marginal and inserted gingiva with differently colored waxes.

The duplicated stone dies were prepared for all-ceramic crowns with chamfer margins. After the preparation, the dies were replicated with industrial silicone, and the obtained impression was poured twice: first with stone and a second time with acrylic resin (Ivocron, dentin body and incisal, Ivoclar Vivadent).

The prepared dies were then repositioned in the base of the cast and from this, the scanning process (CAD) was initiated for the fabrication of the ceramic crowns by the CEREC system (Cerec AC, Sirona).

Image Acquisition

Double-Scanning Technique using Biocopy

For the Biocopy technique, images of the stone cast with emphasized sulci were initially acquired with a benchtop scanner (inEos Blue, model D3446, Sirona). This requires a contrast spray to be applied prior to scanning (CEREC OptiSpray, Sirona). Next, image acquisition of the cast with prepared teeth was performed—hence, the name "double-scanning technique," because it seeks to correlate the information of the initial tooth morphology to that of the tooth preparations. Only through this technique is it possible to obtain detailed and accurate information of the morphology found in the cast with emphasized sulci and to transfer this information perfectly to the digitally produced ceramic restorations.

Double-Scanning Technique Using Biogeneric Copy

Importantly, the software version (4.2) used in the present example has a working mode that combines the Biogeneric and Biocopy modes, which were distinct modes in previous versions of the software. The Biogeneric Copy mode sometimes produces defects in regions that are not included in the Copy Line step. To avoid this shortcoming, the outlines, embrasures, and emergence profile of the restoration should be thoroughly determined during the sculpture to avoid lack of continuity of the preparation. Therefore, every effort should be made to preserve the information gathered in the previous step in order to avoid adjustments and modifications of the calculated restorations.

Digital Design

First, the type of the restoration (individual), the design mode (Biogeneric Copy), and the teeth (maxillary third molar to third molar) were determined in the Administration tab of the software, along with the material to be used (IPS Empress CAD Multi, Ivoclar Vivadent; shade: A2; size: C14). Next, under the Acquisition tab, images were acquired of both casts (the nonprepared cast, with emphasized sulci, and the prepared cast) using a benchtop scanner (inEos Blue, model D3446).

After the image acquisition, the software generated the virtual models; in this example, these were a maxillary model and the maxillary Biogeneric Copy model, which were digitally correlated. Using this workflow, the final restoration will represent the external morphologic features of the natural tooth (obtained from the cast with emphasized sulci) correlated to the information obtained from the prepared cast.

It is important to emphasize that the scanning of the opposing arch was not mandatory in the Biogeneric Copy mode, because all the information required was obtained from the initial cast with emphasized sulci. The virtual models were subsequently positioned and aligned in the arch, the areas were trimmed, the preparation margins were virtually drawn, the preparation axis was defined, and the areas to be selected for the correlation were determined (see Fig 9). At this point, the following parameters were set in μm: spacer; oc-

clusal milling offset; proximal, occlusal, and dynamic contact strengths; minimal occlusal and radial thicknesses; and margin thickness. Parameters were also set for resources such as instrument geometry and removal of retentive areas, which were both disabled. Next, the restorations were calculated. Note that the calculated restorations should be preserved as much as possible. Any adjustments that may be necessary later should be limited to the proximal contacts, correction of excessively thin areas, and smoothing of cervical regions, without retouching the anatomy and the morphology of the restorations.

Milling

The milling unit, milling speed (set to Normal), and the block size (C14) were chosen in this step. The restorations were positioned within the ceramic block in the software screen according to the level of saturation required for each tooth, because the chosen blocks were polychromatic or multishade.

Nevertheless, the milling time for each block depends upon the type of material, the volume, the complexity and size of the restorations, and the burs to be used. In this case, where a CEREC milling unit was used, the milling time ranged between 8 and 15 minutes because the unit operates with a pair of motors (one motor uses a cylinder bur positioned to mill the external areas of the restoration and to relieve or compensate external areas, and the other uses a step bur that mills the intaglio surfaces). This arrangement speeds up the process to approximately half the time of other milling systems using only one motor with one bur.

Adjustments, Finishing, and Polishing

The sole adjustment required was the removal of sprues with stones, diamond points, and diamond rubber wheels. The as-milled ceramic restorations showed excellent fit on the preparations. However, although the restorations look matte, lifeless, shallow, lacking texture, and with undefined occlusal morphology, a simple yet careful polishing technique using a diamond paste (Universal Diamond Gloss 2, 3 μm, KG Sorensen) and goat-hair brushes (SUN) revealed the richness of texture and morphology that was faithfully and accurately reproduced by the CEREC system.

Indeed, after milling, the one single maneuver required, in addition to the elimination of sprues, was manually highlighting the main sulci and characterizing them with tints (Universal Stains, IPS Empress, Ivoclar Vivadent). Finally, the pieces were glazed (Universal Glaze Paste, IPS Empress, Ivoclar Vivadent) and again polished manually with goat-hair brushes in a handpiece and diamond polishing paste (Universal Diamond Gloss 2, 3 μm).

These steps, illustrated in Figs 1 to 33, accurately reproduced the texture and the anatomical details exactly as in the natural elements.

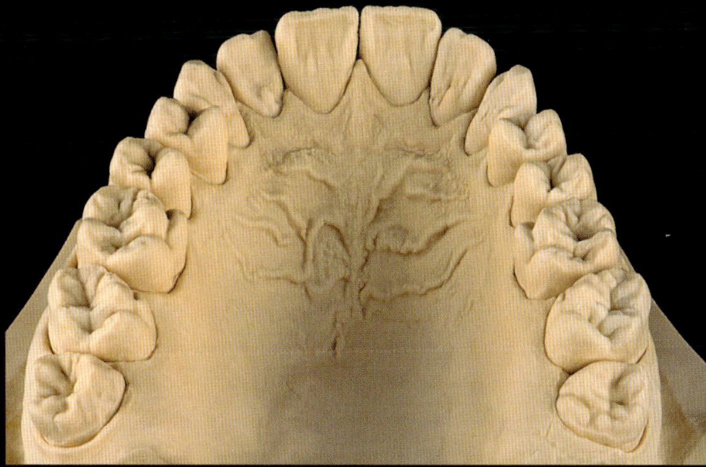

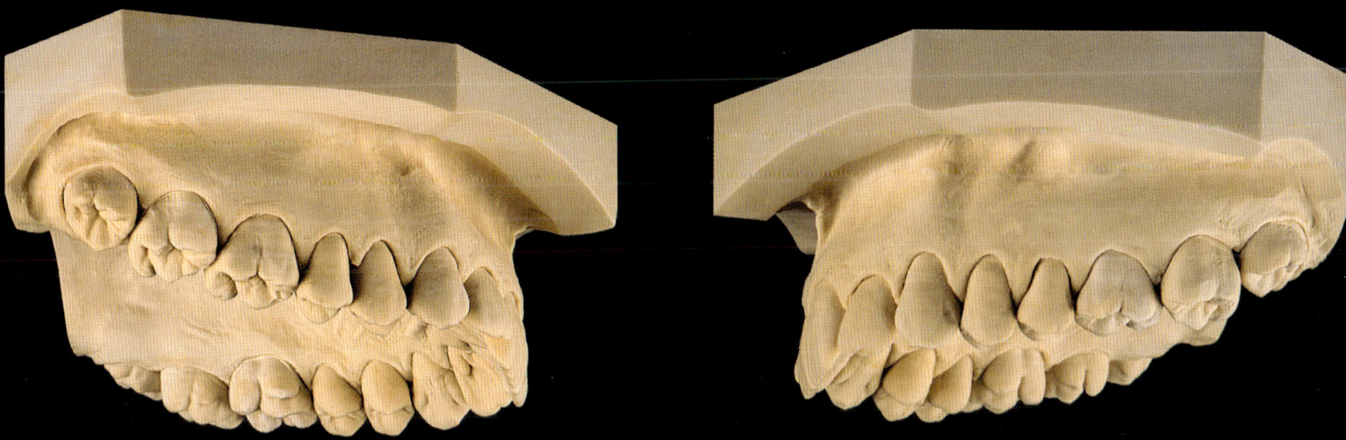

Figs 1a to 1c Occlusal and right and left lateral views of maxillary intact dentition to be used as biocopy.

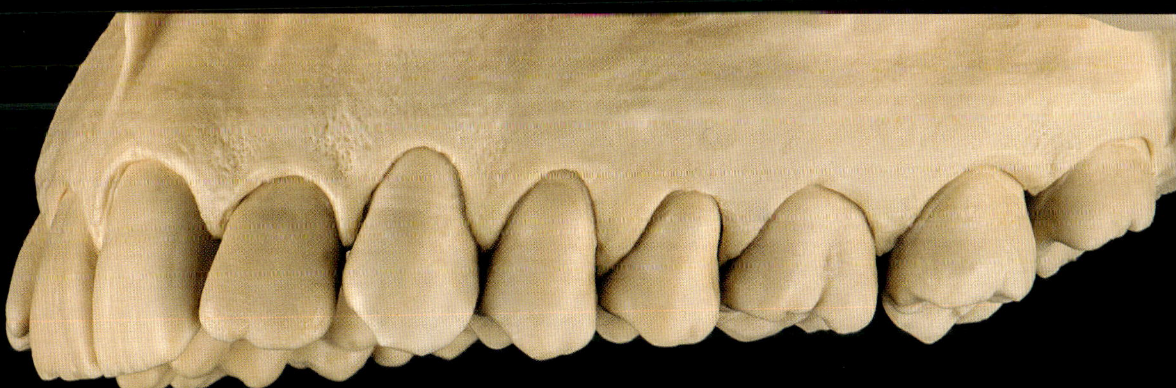

Fig 2 Note the detailed dental morphology to be used as a guide for the definitive replicas.

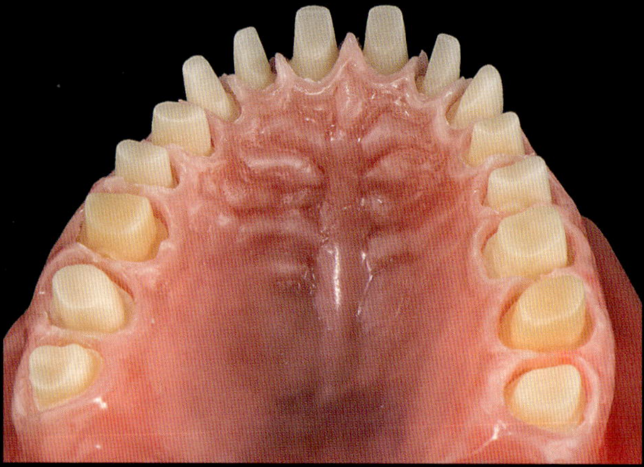

Fig 3a Occlusal view of maxillary arch crown preparations.

Fig 3b Frontal view of maxillary anterior crown preparations.

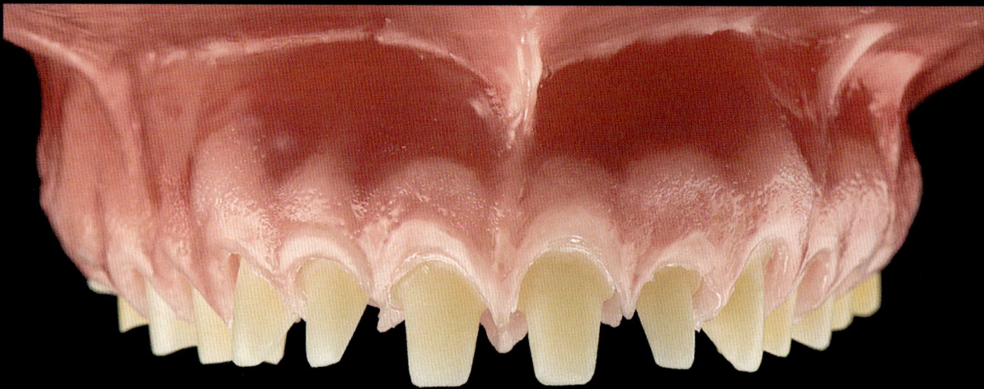

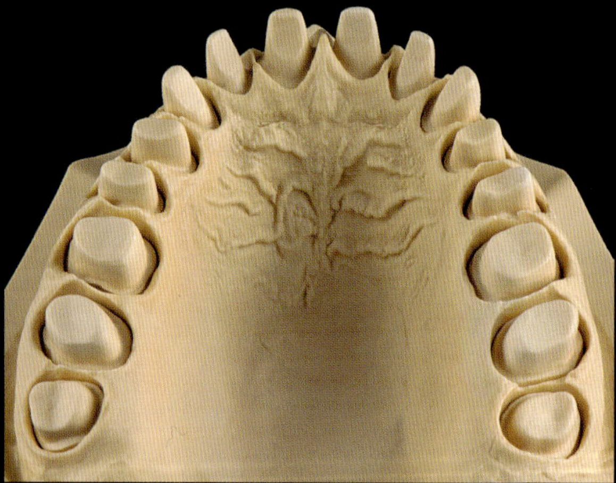

Fig 4a Occlusal view of the cast of the maxillary arch crown preparations.

Fig 4b Frontal view of the cast of the maxillary anterior crown preparations.

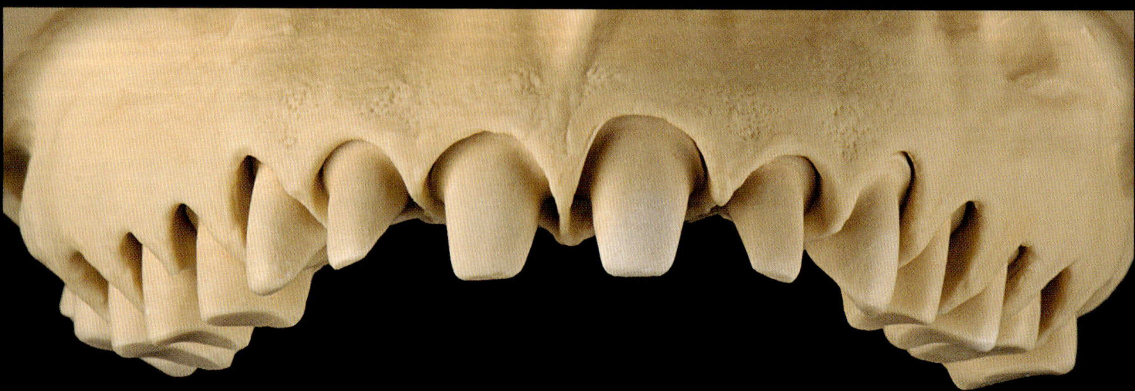

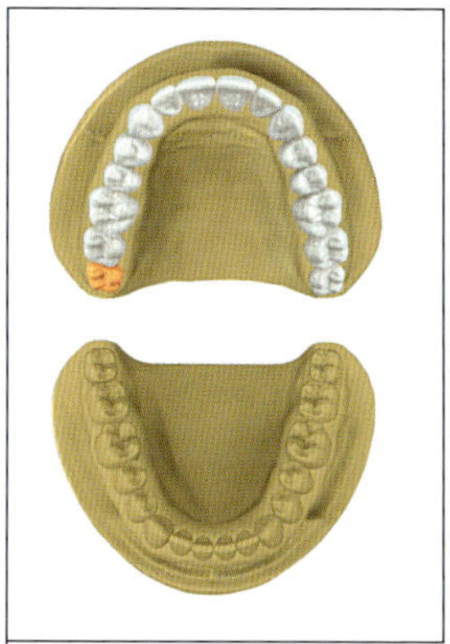

5

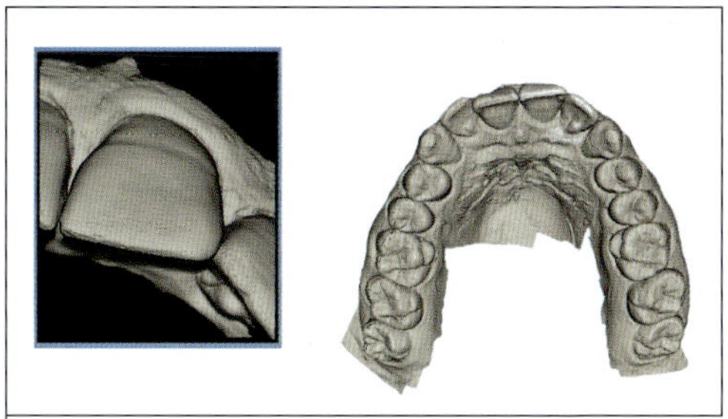

6a

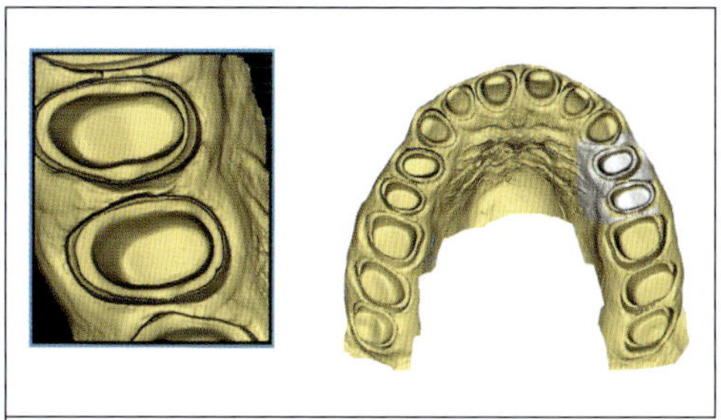

6b

Fig 5 In the CEREC software, under the Administration tab, the tooth to be restored was chosen. Under Design Mode, Biogeneric Copy was selected; the Restoration Type was "crown."

Fig 6a Acquisition (scanning) of the cast of the unprepared teeth for biocopy.

Fig 6b Acquisition (scanning) of the prepared teeth.

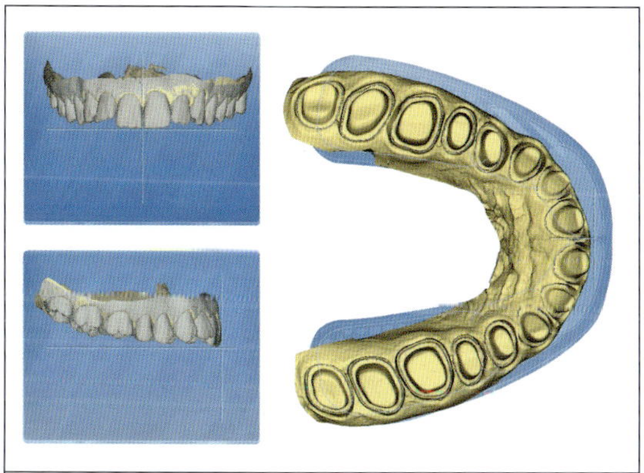

7a

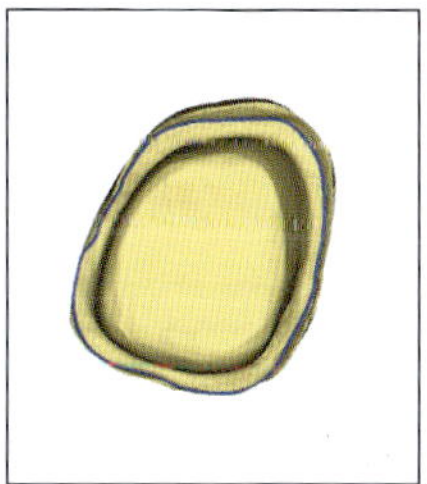

7b

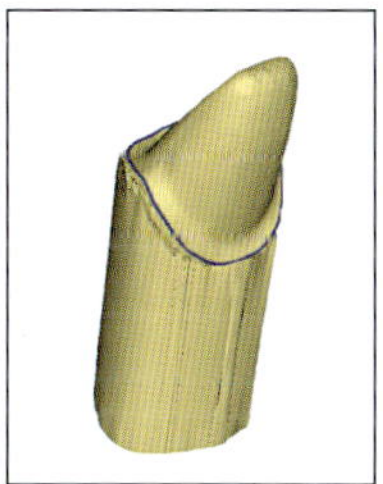

7c

Fig 7a On the Model tab, the model axis was set.

Fig 7b Under the Model tab, the margins of the posterior prepared teeth were drawn.

Fig 7c Under the Model tab, the margins of the anterior prepared teeth were drawn.

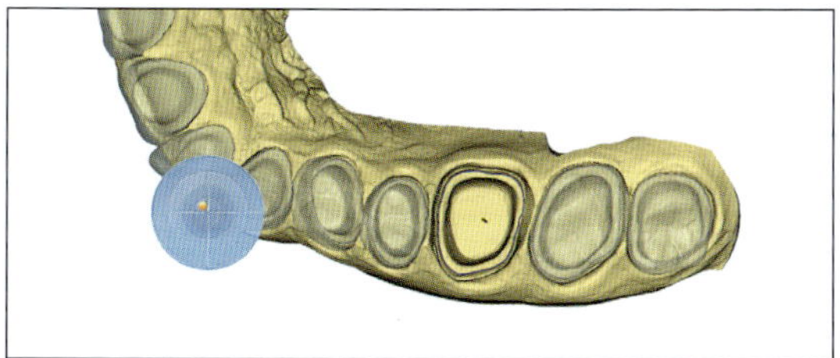

8a

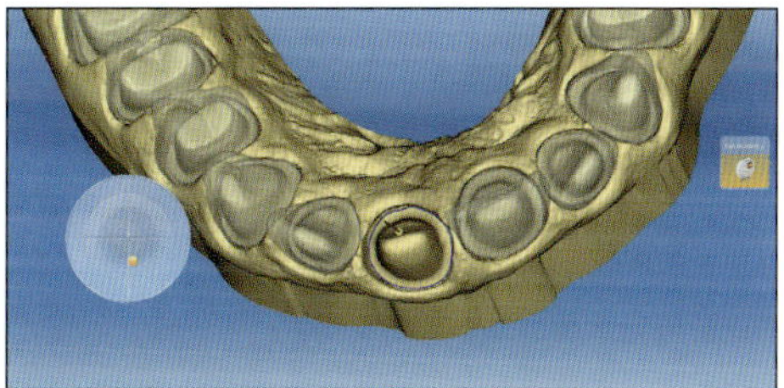

8a

Fig 8a Defining the insertion axis for posterior teeth.

Fig 8b Defining the insertion axis for anterior teeth.

Fig 9 Delimitation of the biocopy line of the maxillary teeth.

Fig 10 Design parameters for the restorations.

Fig 11 Design based on the biocopy.

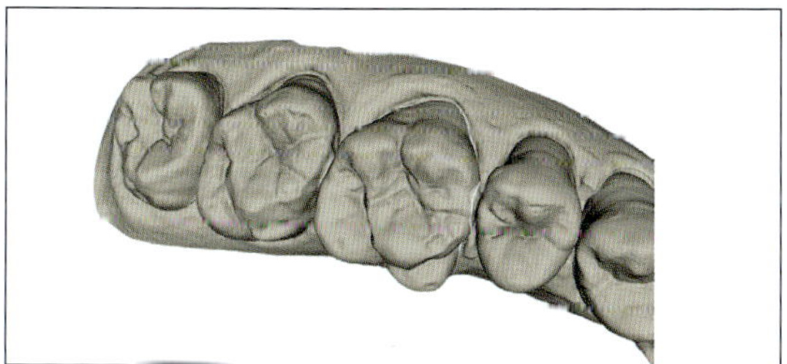

9

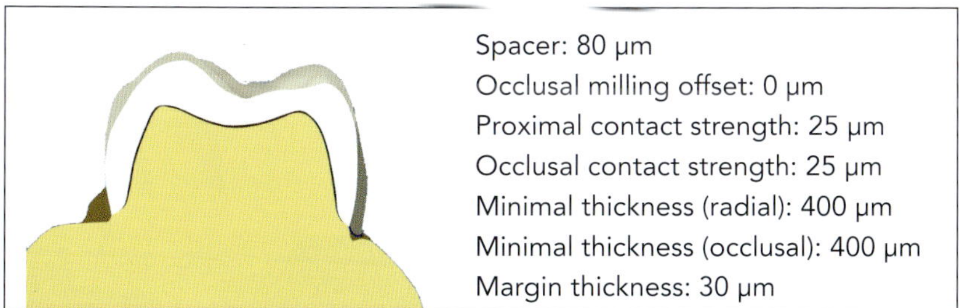

10

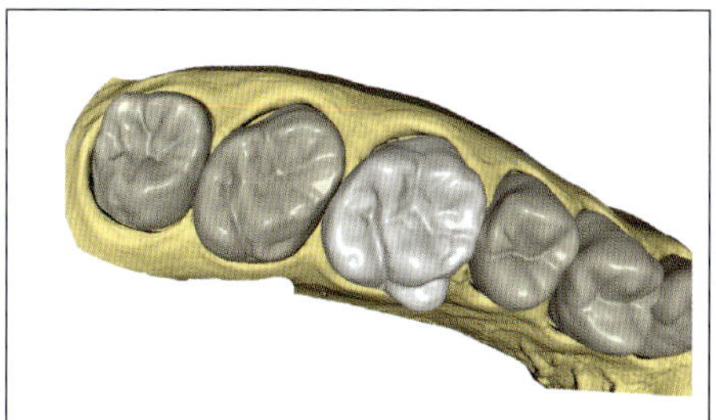

11

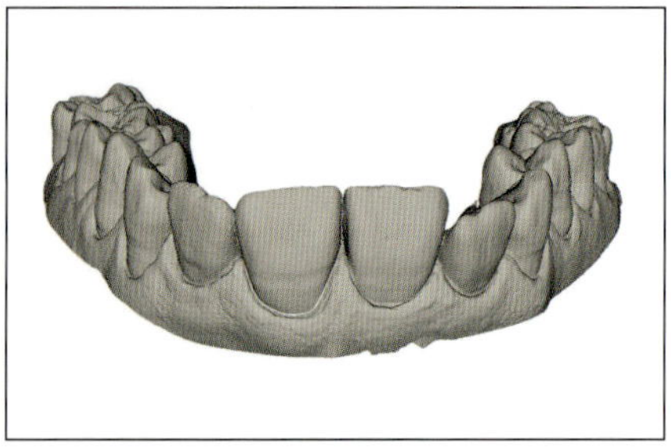

Fig 12a Biocopy line.

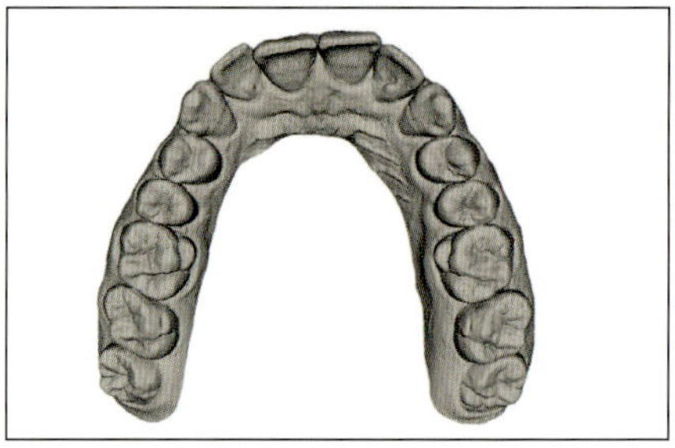

Fig 12b Biocopy model.

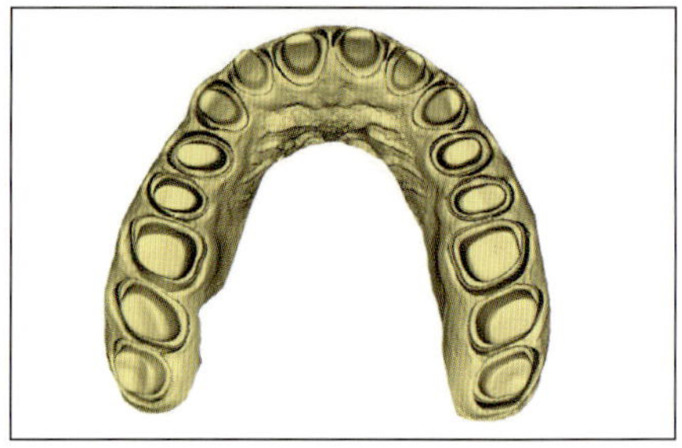

Fig 13a Digital model of the prepared teeth.

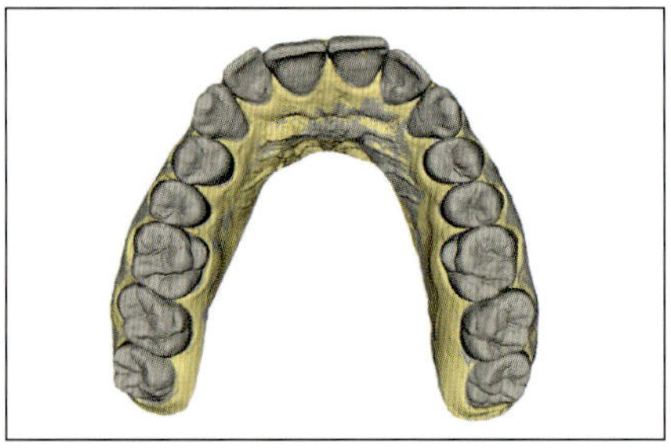

Fig 13b Biocopy model superimposed over the digital model of the prepared teeth (occlusal view).

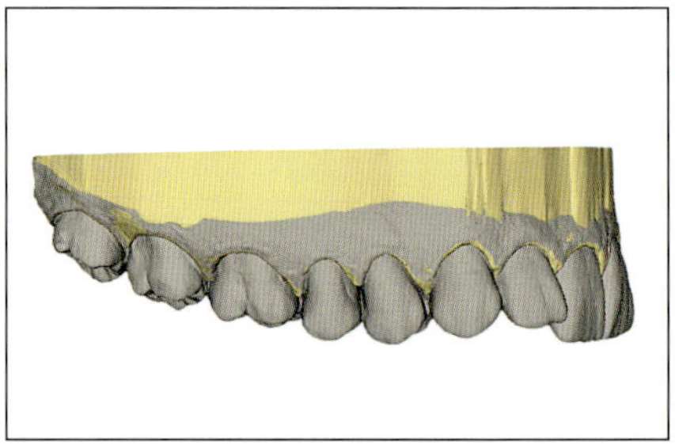

Fig 14a Biocopy model superimposed over the digital model of the prepared teeth (lateral view).

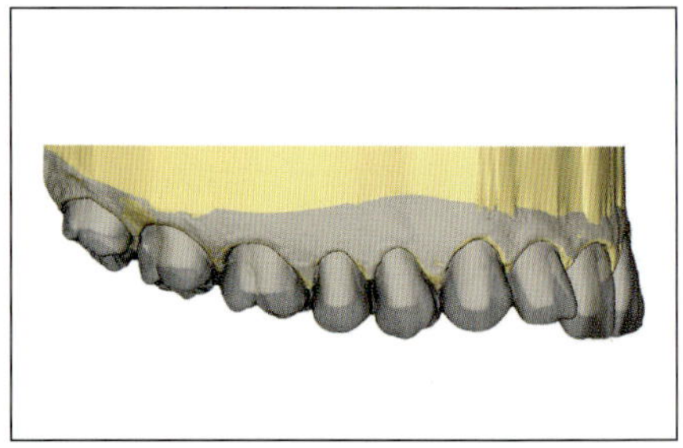

Fig 14b Biocopy model superimposed over the digital model of the prepared teeth (lateral view with transparency).

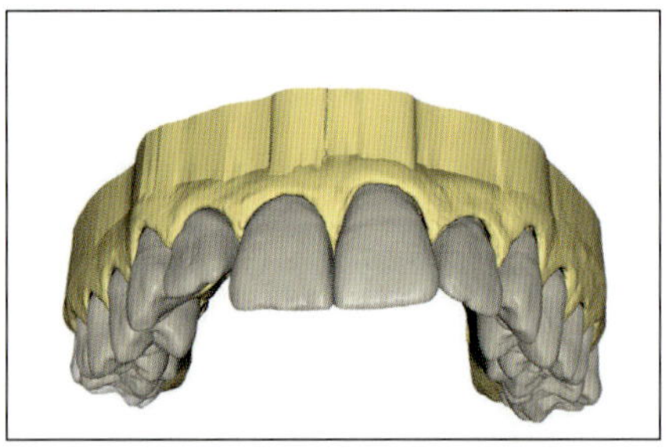

Fig 15a Final design based on the biocopy.

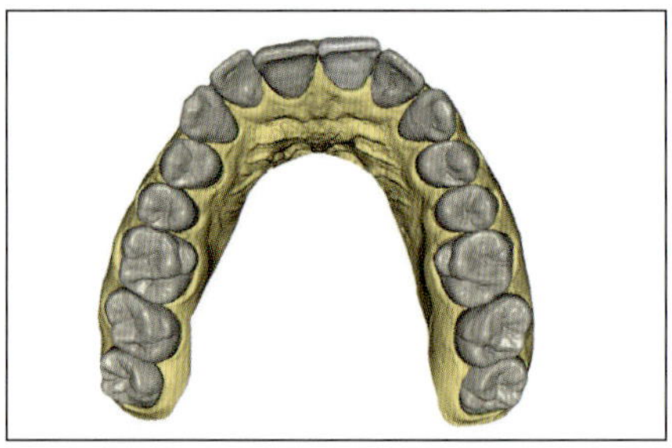

Fig 15b Occlusal view of the final design based on the biocopy.

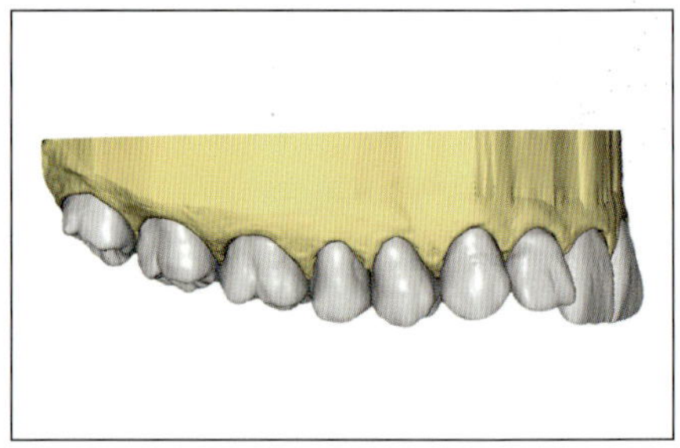

Fig 15c Digital restorations ready for milling.

16

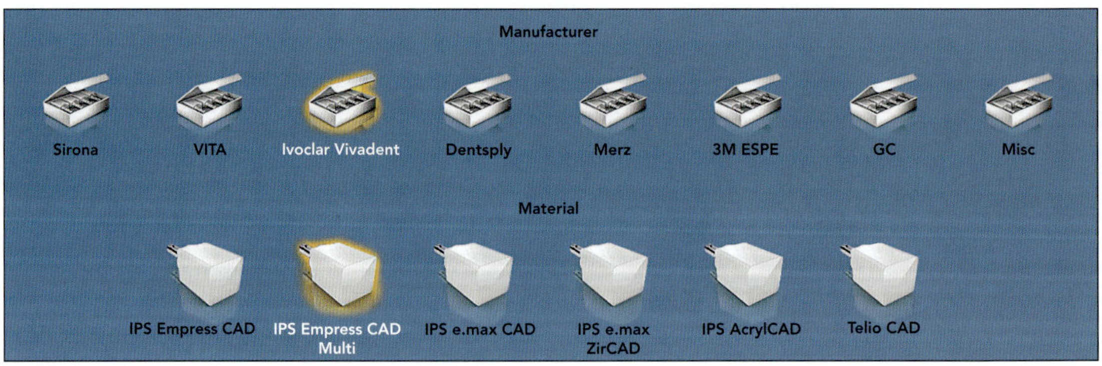

Fig 16 Material selection step.

Fig 17a Digital positioning of an anterior restoration within a multishade block.

Fig 17b Digital positioning of a posterior restoration within a multishade block.

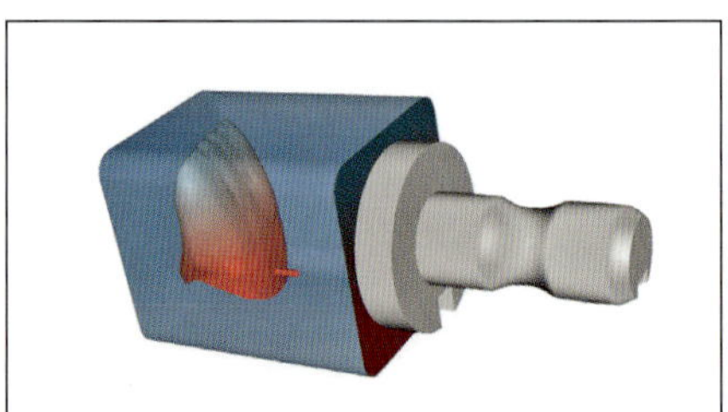

17a

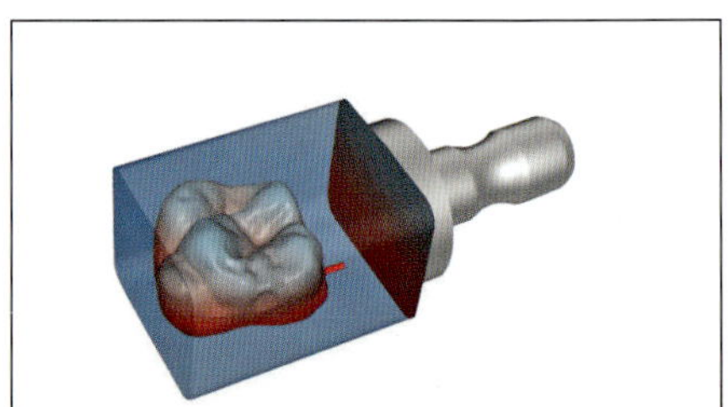

17b

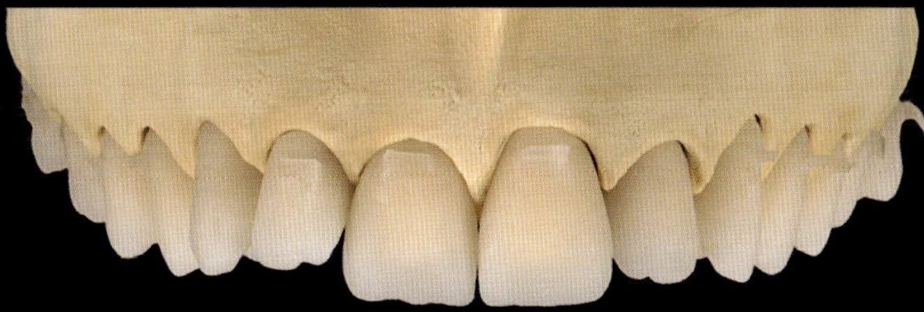

Fig 18a Milled lithium disilicate restorations generated using biocopy.

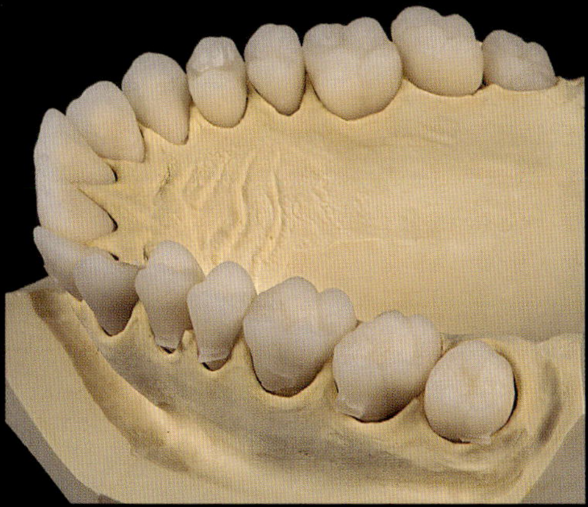

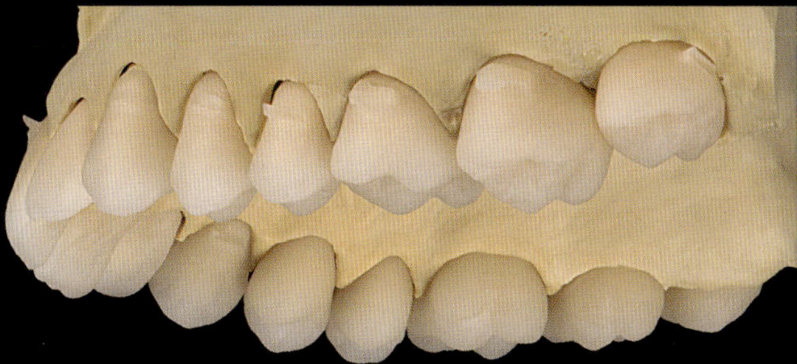

Fig 18b Occlusal view of the milled restorations using biocopy.

Fig 18c Lateral view of the milled restorations using biocopy prior to finishing

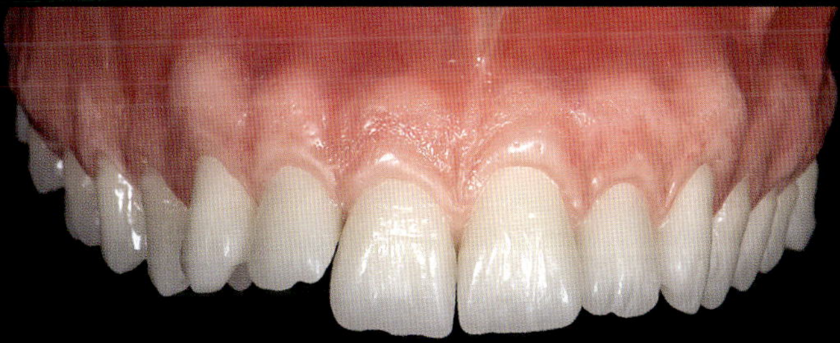

Fig 19a Milled restorations just after initial polishing.

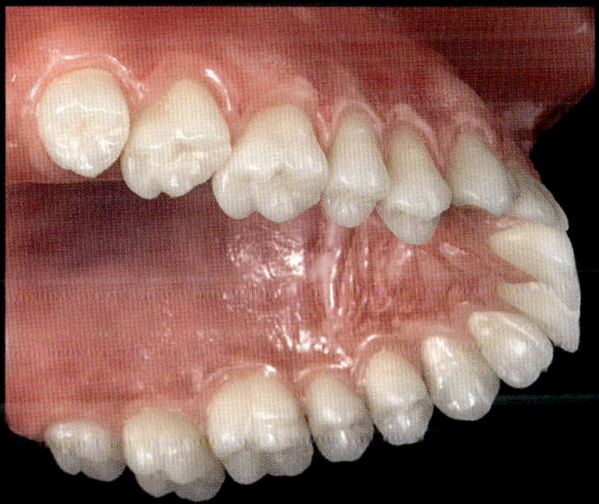

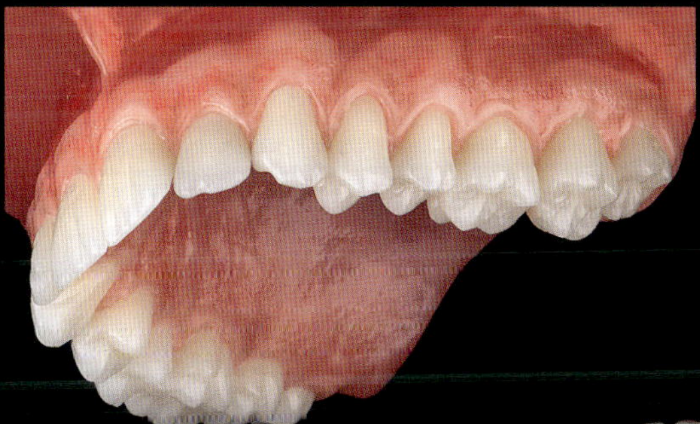

Figs 19b and 19c Lateral occlusal views of the milled restorations after initial polishing.

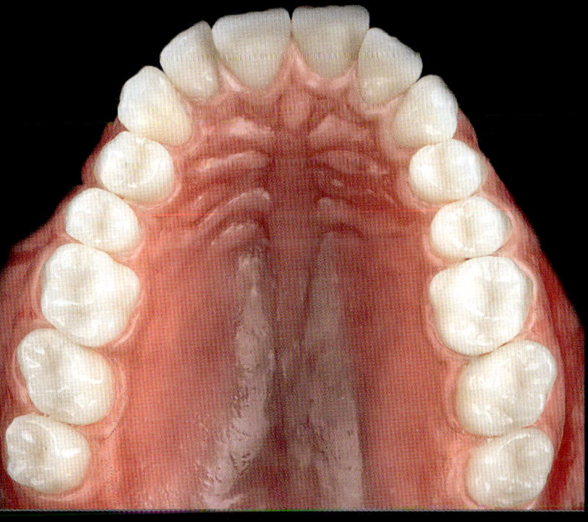

Fig 19d Occlusal view of the milled restorations. Occlusal developmental grooves and fissures were carefully redefined using a low-speed bur.

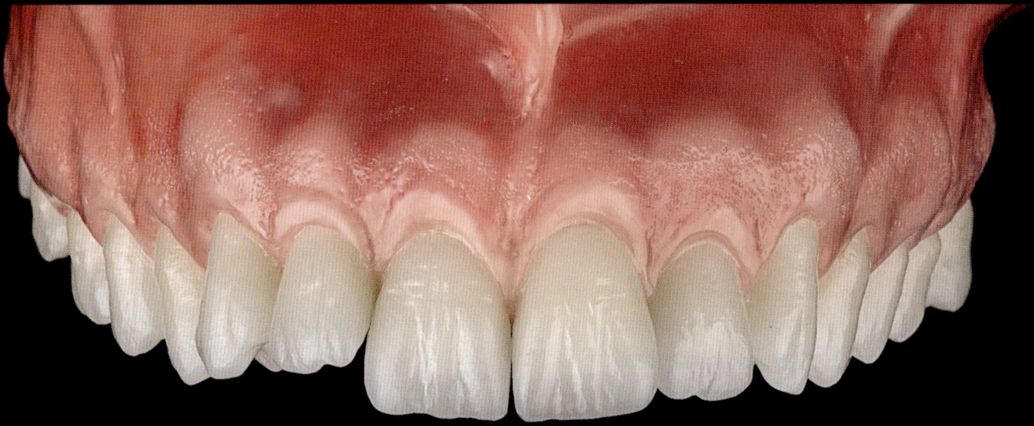

Fig 20 Facial and buccal developmental grooves were carefully highlighted.

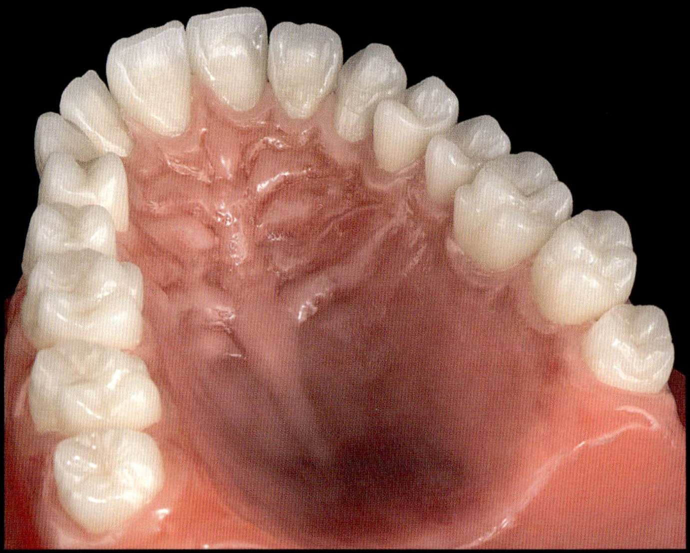

Fig 21 Palatal/occlusal view of the milled restorations.

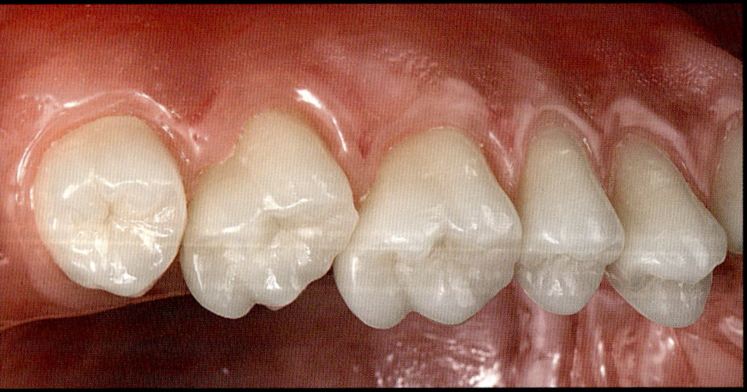

Fig 22a Close-up view of posterior teeth. Note that only the central grooves were slightly redefined.

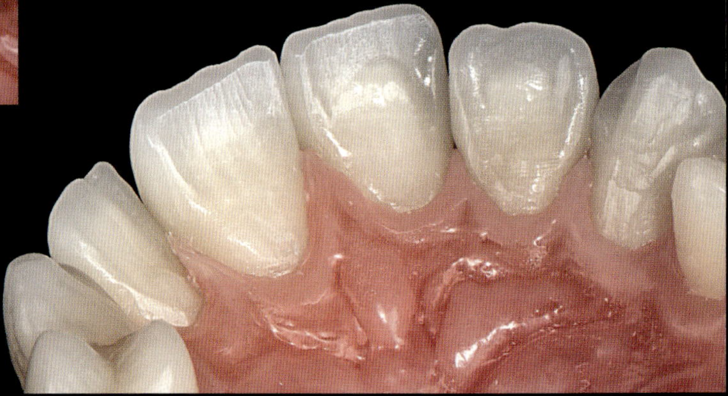

Fig 22b Palatal view of maxillary anterior teeth. Only the marginal ridges were slightly redefined.

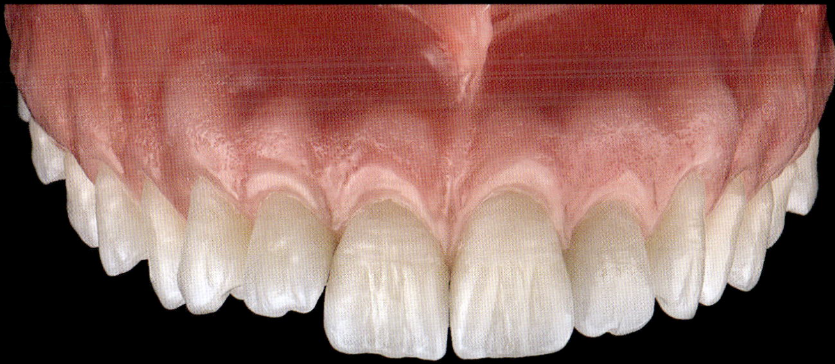

Figs 23a to 23c Mild-intensity characterization was applied onto the buccal gingival third to impart a more natural aspect to the restorations followed by glazing and manual polishing.

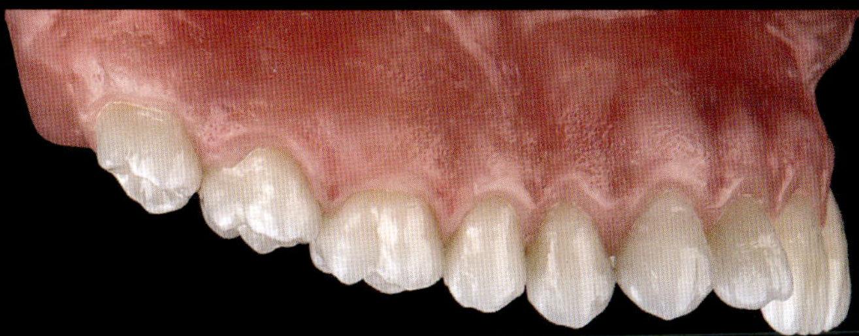

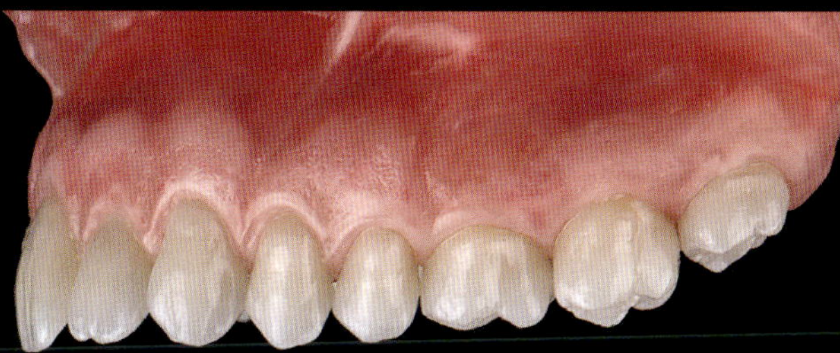

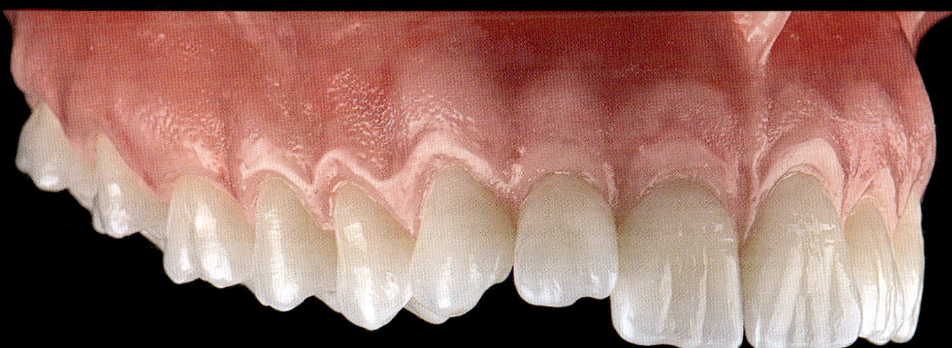

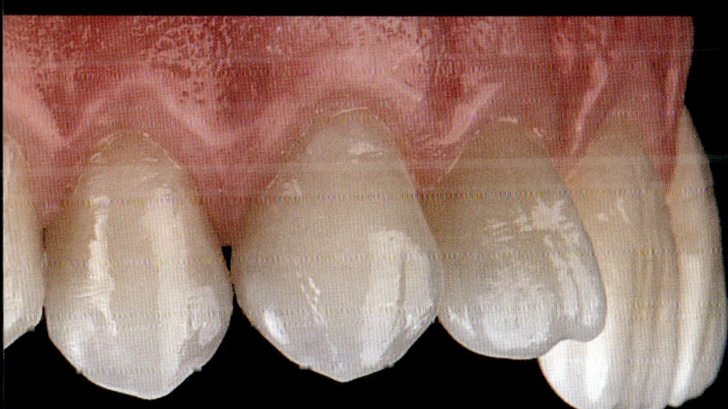

Figs 24a to 24c Lateral and close-up views after mild intensity characterization was used.

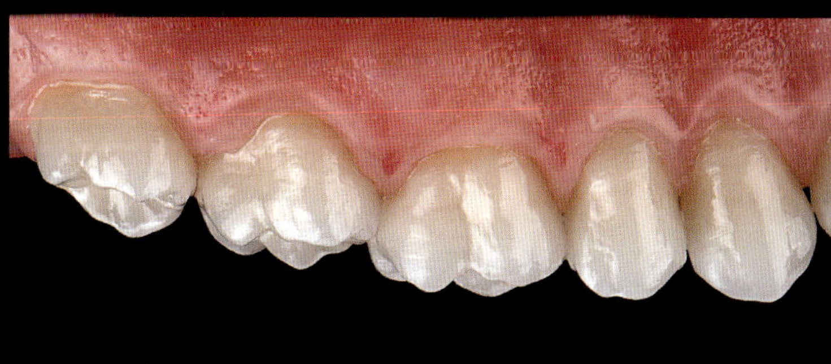

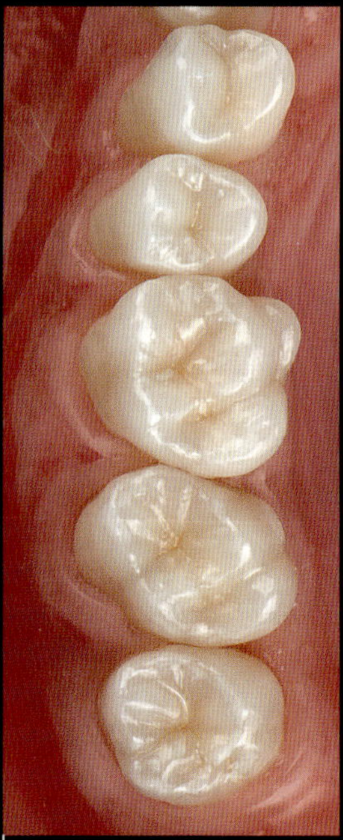

25a

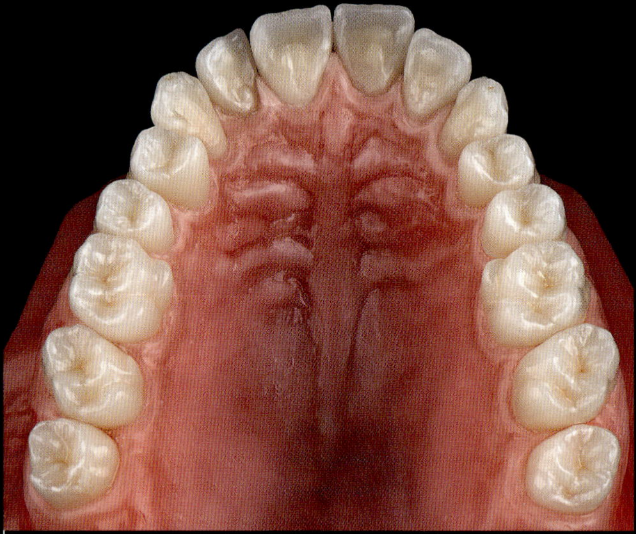

25b

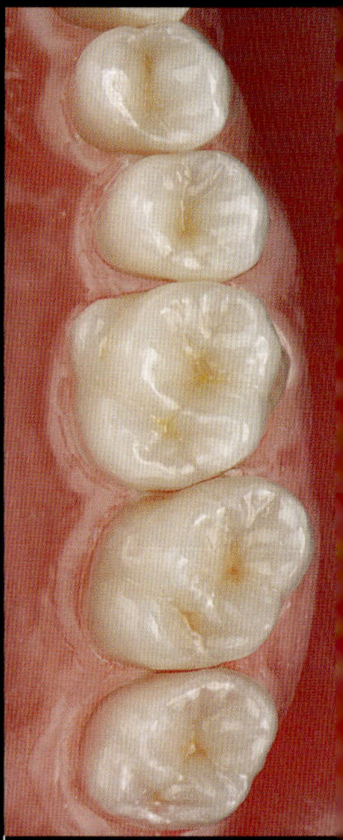

25c

Fig 25a Maxillary right posterior teeth after mild-intensity characterization.

Fig 25b Occlusal view of posterior teeth after mild-intensity characterization.

Fig 25c Maxillary left posterior teeth after mild-intensity characterization. A mixture of ochre and orange was placed internally to increase chroma around the central grooves. Central grooves were carefully stained using the same mixture.

Fig 26 Incisal translucency and halo were added to the maxillary anterior teeth as a mild characterization.

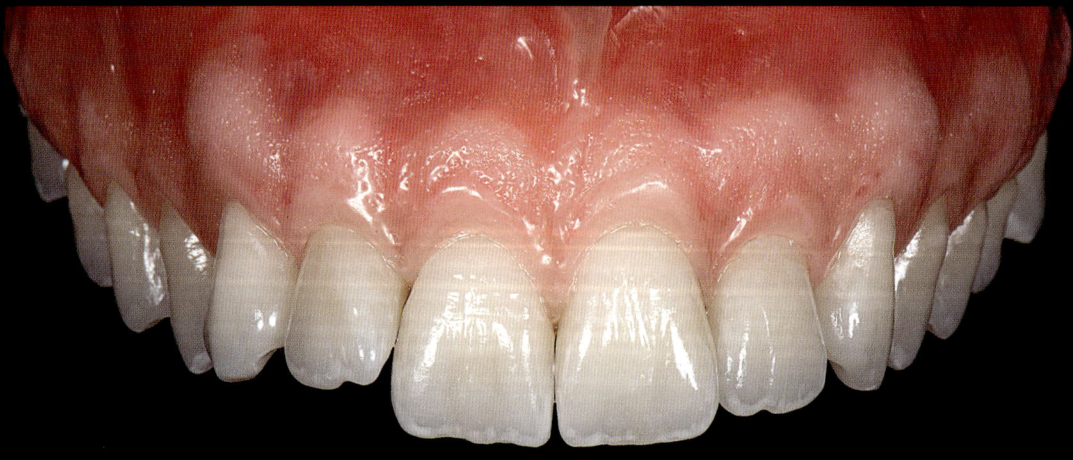

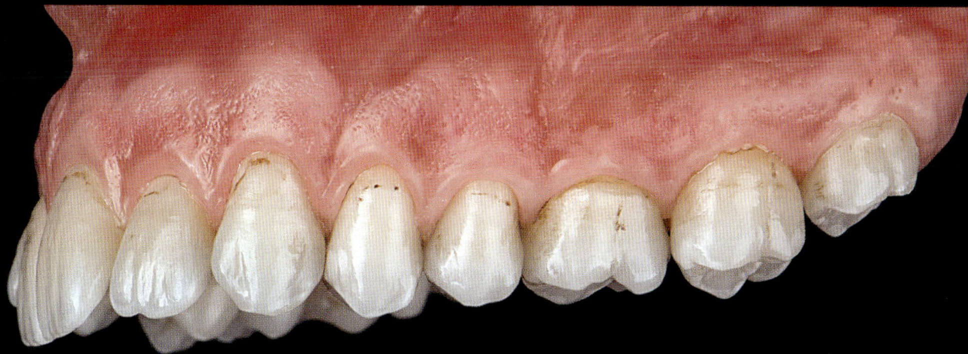

Fig 27 Lateral left side maxillary view of CAD/CAM restorations after intense characterization was used.

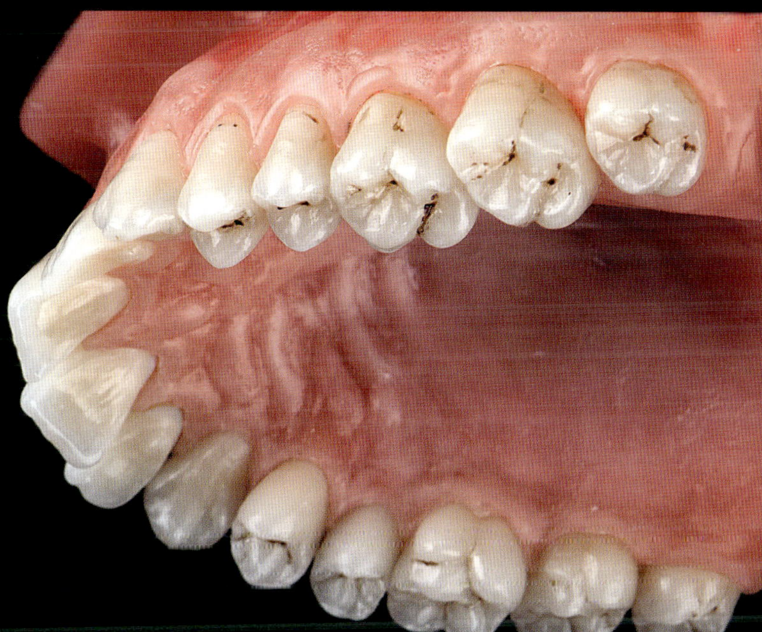

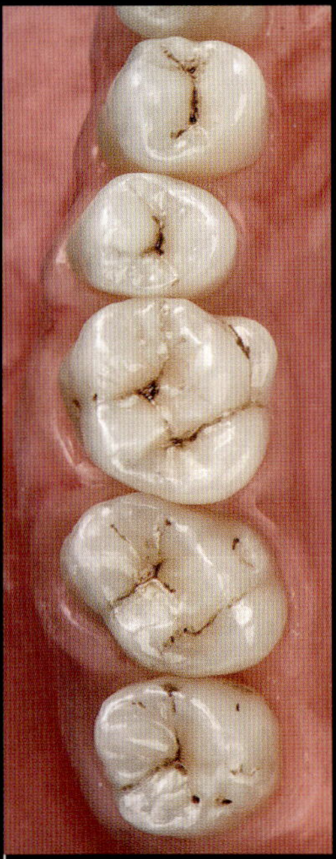
29a

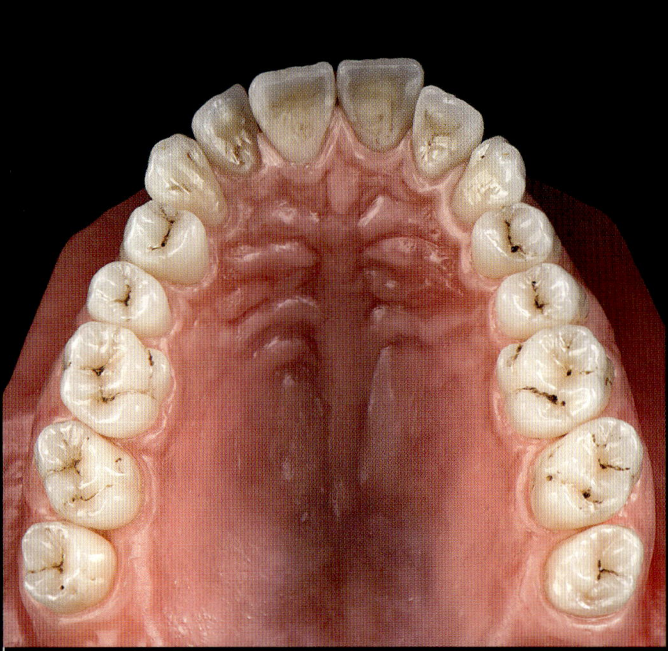
29b

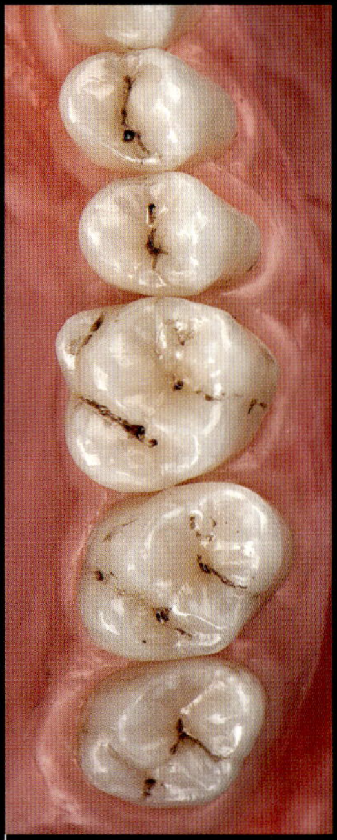
29c

Fig 29a Maxillary right posterior teeth after high-intensity characterization.

Fig 29b Occlusal view of posterior teeth after high-intensity characterization.

Fig 29c Maxillary left posterior teeth after high-intensity characterization. A mixture of ochre and orange was placed internally to increase chroma around the central grooves. Central grooves were carefully stained using brown stains.

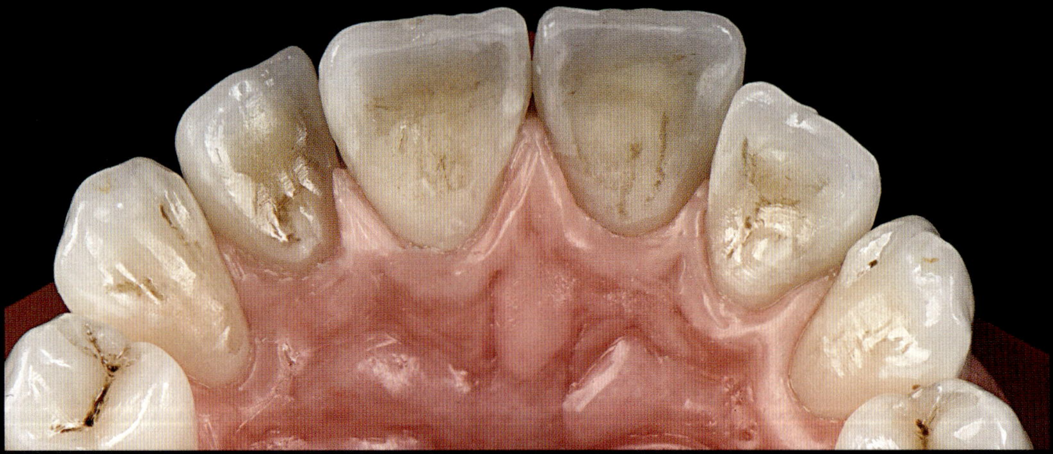

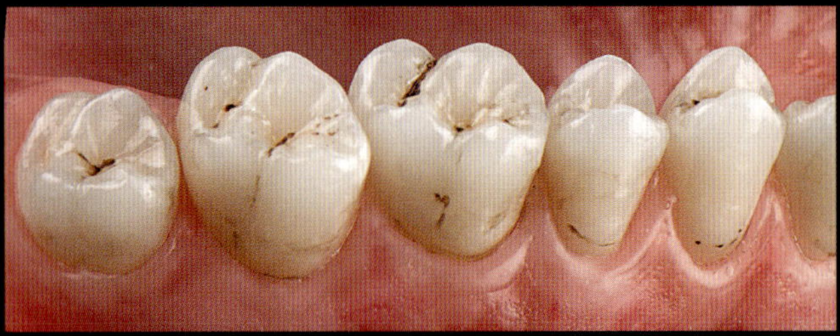

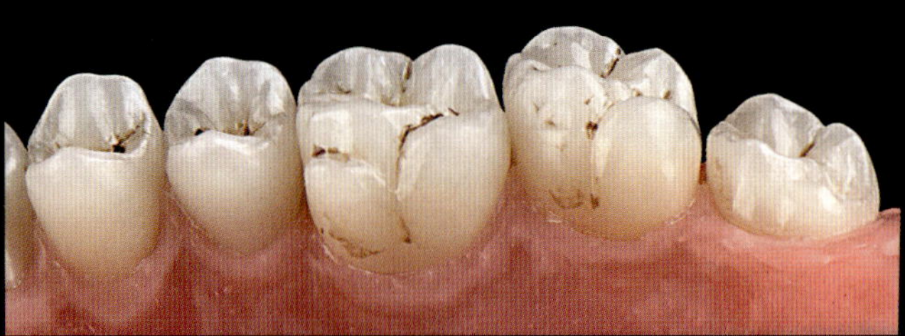

Figs 30a to 30c Palatal, buccal, and lingual views of CAD/CAM restorations after high-intensity characterization.

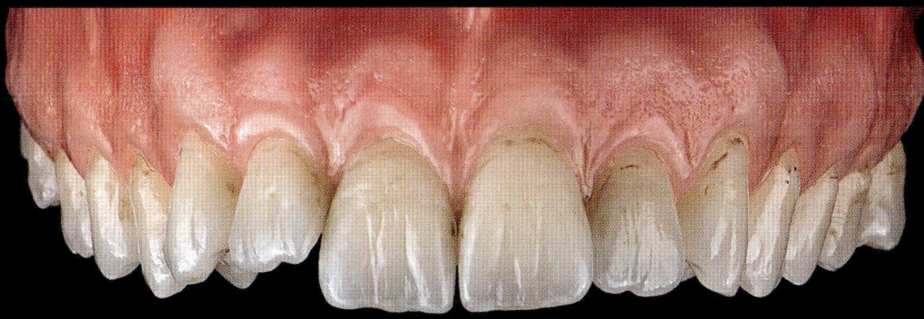

Figs 31a and 31b Maxillary anterior CAD/CAM restorations displaying intense characterization.

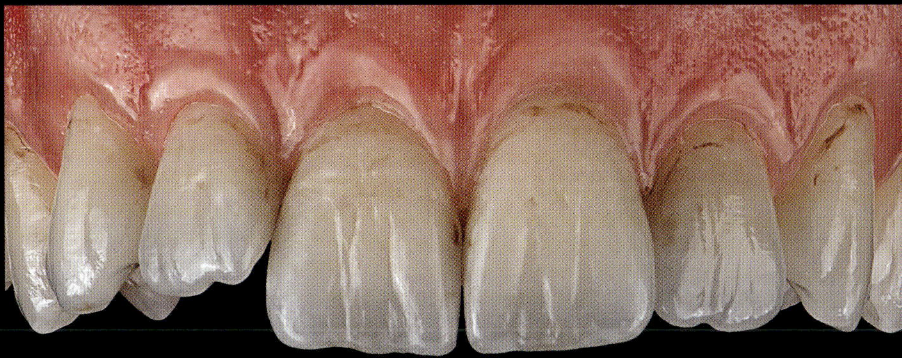

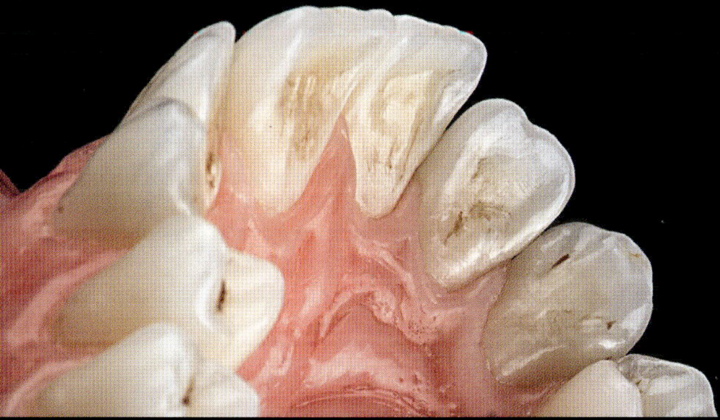

Figs 32a and 32b Palatal views of CAD/CAM restorations displaying intense characterization.

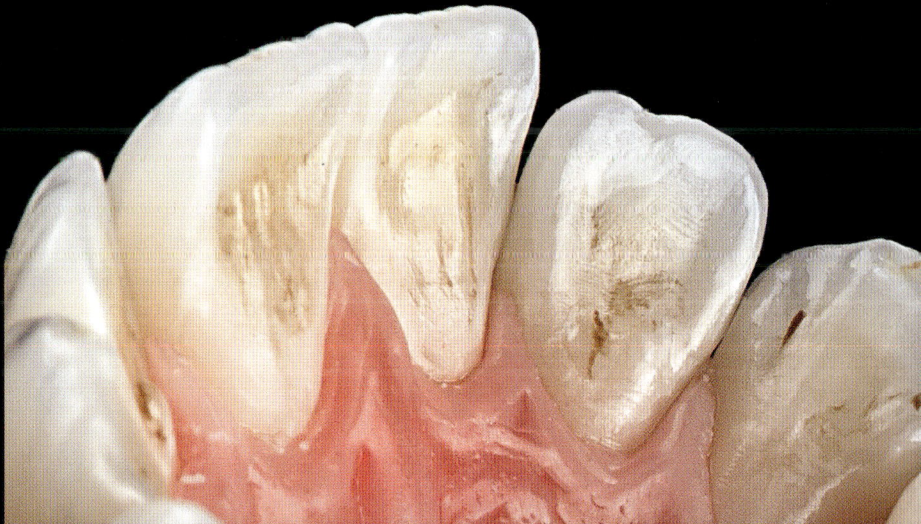

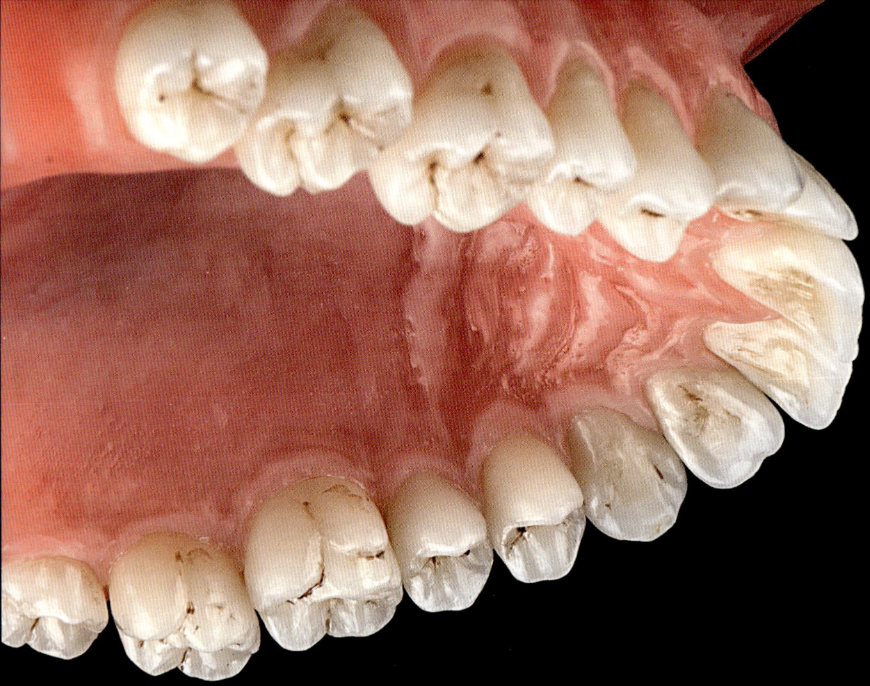

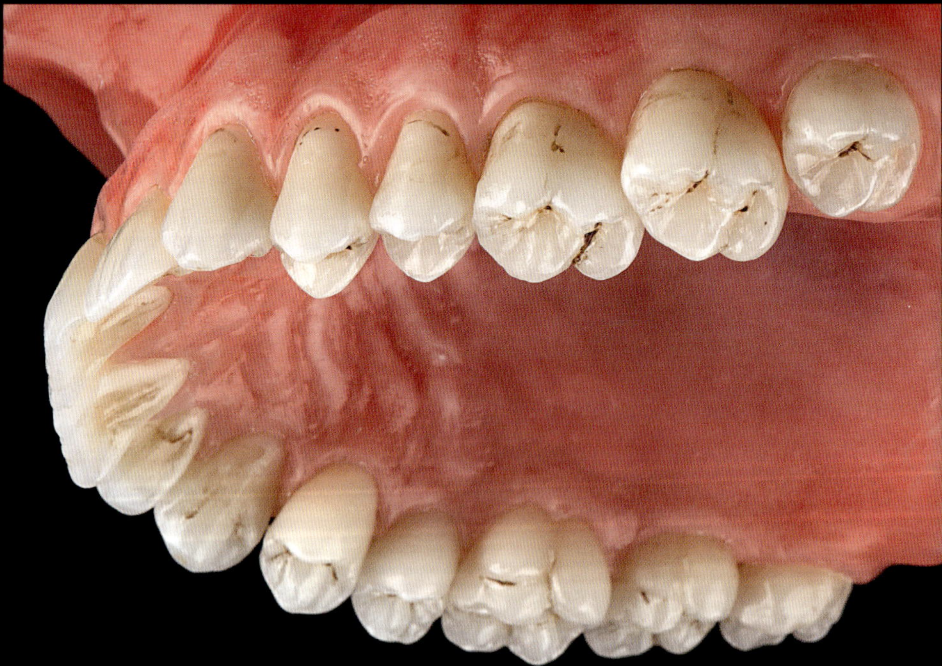

Figs 33a and 33b Characterized CAD/CAM restorations using biocopy.

REFERENCES

1. Lee K. Principles of CAD/CAM/CAE Systems. Boston: Addison-Wesley Longman, 1999.
2. Sanders N. An industry perspective on the beginnings of CAD. SIGCSE Bulletin 2008;40(2):128–156.
3. Young JM, Altschuler BR. Laser holography in dentistry. J Prosthet Dent 1977;38:216–224.
4. Correia ARM, Fernandes JCAS, Cardoso JAP, Silva CFCL. CAD-CAM: A informática a serviço da prótese fixa [in Portugese]. Revista de Odontologia da UNESP 2006;35(2):183–189.
5. Duret F. Chairside creations: The Sopha bioconcept system. Dent Today 1992;11(7):44–47.
6. Ueda RYI, Tsuzuki MDSG. Desenvolvimento de um sistema CAD com suporte a curvas e superficies. Congresso Brasileiro de Engenharia Mecânica [in Portugese]. São Paulo: Escola Politécnica da USP, 1998:15.

BIBLIOGRAPHY

Aoki H, Fujita T, Nishina T. CAD system and NC construction for the automation of dental laboratory. J Dent Technol 1986;14:1495–1526.

Caparroso C, Duque JA. CAD-CAM restorations system and ceramics: A review. Rev Fac Odontol Univ Antioq 2010;22(1):88–108.

Duret F. Occlusal adaptation by CAD-CAM. In: Tsuru H, Preiskel HW, Matsuo E, Moriya Y (eds). Advanced Prosthodontics Worldwide. Hiroshima: WCP Hiroshima, 1991:30–31.

Duret F, Blouin JL, Duret B. CAD-CAM in dentistry. J Am Dent Assoc 1998;117:715–720.

Duret F, Preston JD. CAD/CAM imaging in dentistry. Curr Opin Dent 1991;1:150–154.

Effrosyni A, Tsitrou E, Northeast S, van Noort R. Evaluation of the marginal fit of three margin designs of resin composite crowns using CAD/CAM. J Dent 2007;35:68–73.

Ellingsen LA, Fasbinder DJ. In vitro evaluation of CAD/CAM ceramic crowns [abstract 2640]. J Dent Res 2002;81:331.

Fasbinder DJ. Clinical performance of chairside CAD/CAM restorations. J Am Dent Assoc 2006;137(9, suppl):22S–31S.

Hikita K, Uchiyama Y. Studies on three dimensional measurement and restoration of tooth crown form by CAD/CAM. J Jpn Prosthondont Soc 1989;33(S82):142.

Hotta Y, Ozawa A, Kobayashi Y, Miyazaki T. Development of a dental CAD/CAM system fabricating dental prostheses. J Showa Univ Dent Soc 2001;21:86–91.

Liu PR. A panorama of dental CAD/CAM restorative systems. Compend Contin Educ Dent 2005;26:507–512.

Miyazaka T, Hotta Y, Kunii J, Kuriyama S, Tamaki Y. A review of dental CAD/CAM: Current status and future perspectives from 20 years of experience. Dent Materials J 2009;28(1):44–56.

Mörmann WH. The evolution of the CEREC system. J Am Dent Assoc 2006;137(suppl):7S–13S.

Mörmann WH. The origin of the CEREC method: A personal review of the first 5 years. Int J Comput Dent 2004;7:11–24.

Nakamura T, Dei N, Kojima T, Wakabayashi K. Marginal and internal fit of Cerec 3 CAD/CAM allceramic crowns. Inter J Prosthodontics 2003;16:244–248.

Persson M, Andersson M, Bergman B. The accuracy of a high-precision digitizer for CAD/CAM crowns. J Prosthet Dent 1995;74:223–229.

Reiss B, Walther W. Clinical long-term results and 10-year Kaplan-Meier analysis of Cerec restorations. Int J Comput Dent 2000;3:9–23.

Rekow D. Computer-aided design and manufacturing in dentistry: A review of the state of the art. J Prosthet Dent 1987;58:512–516.

Rekow ED. Dental CAD/CAM systems: What is the state of the art? J Am Dent Assoc 1991;122:43–48.

Rudolph H, Luthardt RG, Walter MH. Computer-aided analysis of the influence of digitizing and surfacing on the accuracy in dental CAD/CAM technology. Comput Biol Med 2007;37:579–587.

Schimitter M, Seydler B. Minimally invasive lithium disilicate ceramic veneers fabricated using chairside CAD/CAM: A clinical report. J Prosthet Dent 2012;107:71–74.

Strub JR, Rekow ED, Witkowski S. Digital design and fabrication of dental restorations: current systems and future possibilities. J Am Dent Assoc 2006;137:1289–1296.

Tinschert J, Natt G, Mautsch W, Spiekermann H, Anusavice KJ. Marginal fit of alumina- and zirconia-based fixed partial dentures produced by a CAD/CAM system. Oper Dent 2001;26:367–374.

Trost L, Stines S, Burt L. Informed decisions about incorporating CEREC into a practice. J Am Dent Assoc 2006;137(9, suppl):32S–36S.

Tsitrou EA, Northeast SE, van Noort R. Evaluation of the marginal fit of three margin designs of resin composite crowns using CAD/CAM. J Dent 2007;35:68–73.

Tsutsumi S, Fukuda S, Tani Y. 3-D image measurements of teeth and alveolar ridge. J Dent Res 1989;68(2, suppl):924.

Williams RJ, Bibb R, Eggber D, Collis J. Use of CAD/CAM technology to fabricate a removable partial denture framework. J Prosthet Dent 2006;96:96–99.

A Challenge to Natural Teeth

MASTERPIECE

Naoki Hayashi, RDT

Ultimate Styles Dental Laboratory
23 Mauchly, Suite 111
Irvine, CA 92618, USA
Email: nao@ultimate-dl.com

Esthetic prosthetic treatment is comprehensive treatment that considers, through examination and diagnosis, many elements that are required for long-term success. The patient's expectations, facial outline, position of the eyes, and shape and movement of the lips are some of the factors that determine the incisal position, length, and width of restorations. The angle and position of each tooth are also determined with consideration of these factors. The author focuses particularly on lip movement ("lip dynamics"), whereby the restoration is fabricated over various examinations and trials so that it looks natural and well-balanced with the shape and in all movements of the lips.

Esthetic prosthetic dental treatment involves restoration of the anterior to premolar teeth, those visible in daily life, to improve esthetics and function healthfully and beautifully. Not as many design elements or creativity is required to restore a single anterior tooth, since the adjacent teeth will be the primary guides. However, elements of esthetics and harmony with the dentition have to be considered when two central incisors are restored.

A natural-looking restoration, one that imitates the natural tooth, is considered the ideal by many dental technicians. However, a patient's subjective view of esthetics and the operator's objective view do not always coincide. Today, the esthetic restoration needs to be balanced between the white teeth often desired by the patient and the natural-looking teeth preferred by the dental technician.

The author has established a classification of restorative treatment into five types based on difficulty. A patient's desires/expectations can be organized using this classification to plan the treatment. Four of the five different types of cases outlined below are presented in this article (Type 1 to Type 4). Each case has a particular treatment goal (pure anatomical reproduction to fulfillment of the patient's desires/expectations). Each restoration has personality to harmonize with the patient's dentition and face as total esthetics.

Classification of Restorative Treatment

Type 0: Basic restorative treatment. Treatment is limited to vital problems (ie, pain, dislodged or damaged previous restoration).

Type 1: Natural restorative treatment. Treatment is limited to a tooth with caries or discoloration. The main treatment goal is to harmonize the color, shape, and function of the treated tooth with that of the adjacent dentition.

Type 2: Enhanced natural restorative treatment. Multiple teeth are involved in the treatment to arrange the entire dentition to look and function naturally.

Type 3: Esthetic treatment. Prosthetic treatment is carried out to improve esthetics of mainly the anterior teeth to harmonize with the face and lip dynamics. Treatment is indicated for purposes of esthetics, not for a functional problem.

Type 4: Esthetic treatment + Total oral rehabilitation. Comprehensive treatment includes orthodontic and surgical treatment in addition to prosthetic treatment. The dentition, including tooth shape and color, are idealized according to the patient's desires/expectations. The facial appearance, lip dynamics, and dentition need to be harmonized for esthetics and function.

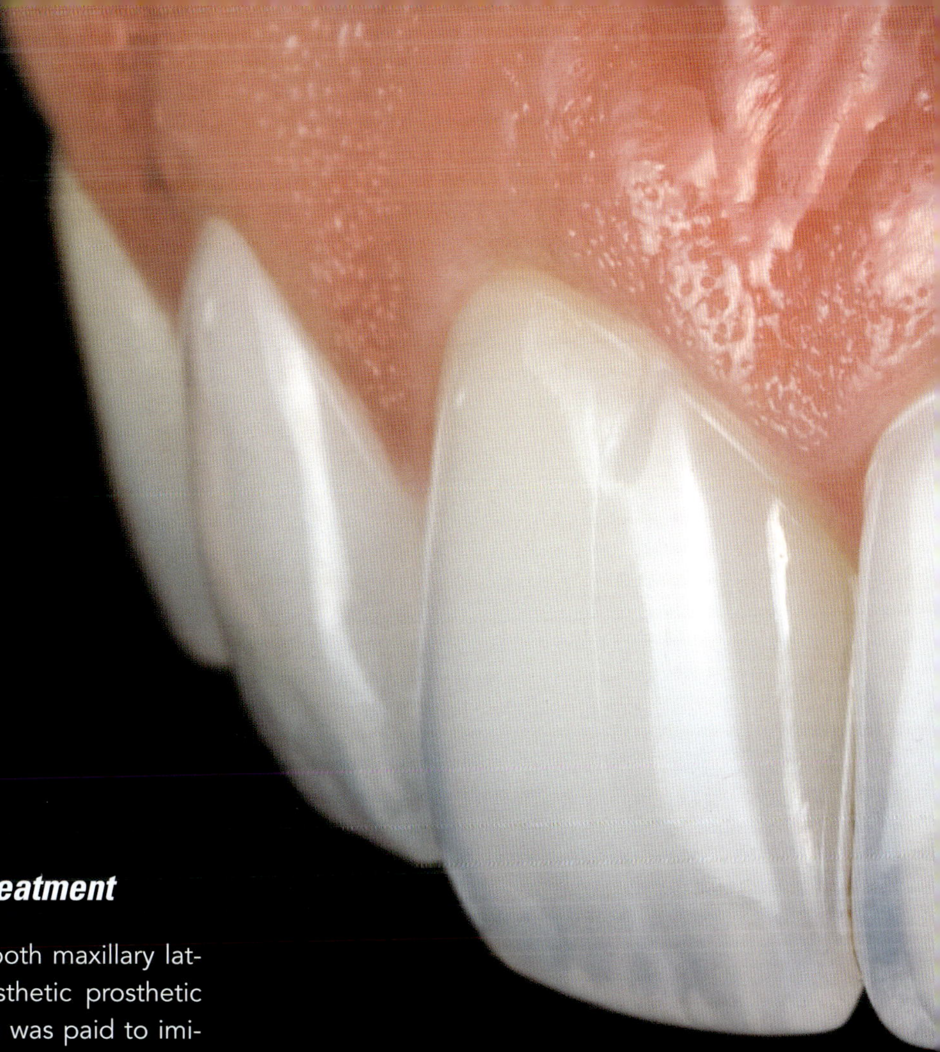

Type 1: Natural restorative treatment

n this typical crown restoration of both maxillary lat-eral incisors, many elements for esthetic prosthetic treatment already existed. Attention was paid to imi-tate the color, shape, surface texture, and gloss of the adjacent teeth to produce a natural-looking dentition. Esthetics was dictated by the character of the patient's natural teeth.

Katana zirconia crowns (Kuraray Noritake Dental). Collaboration with Dr Gianmarco O'Brien.

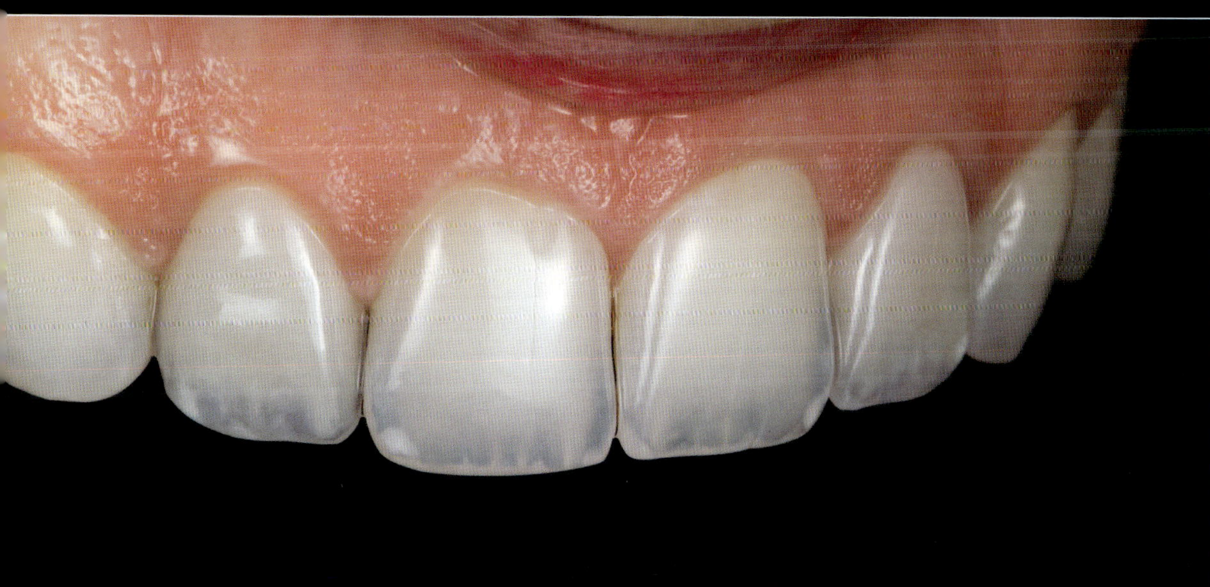

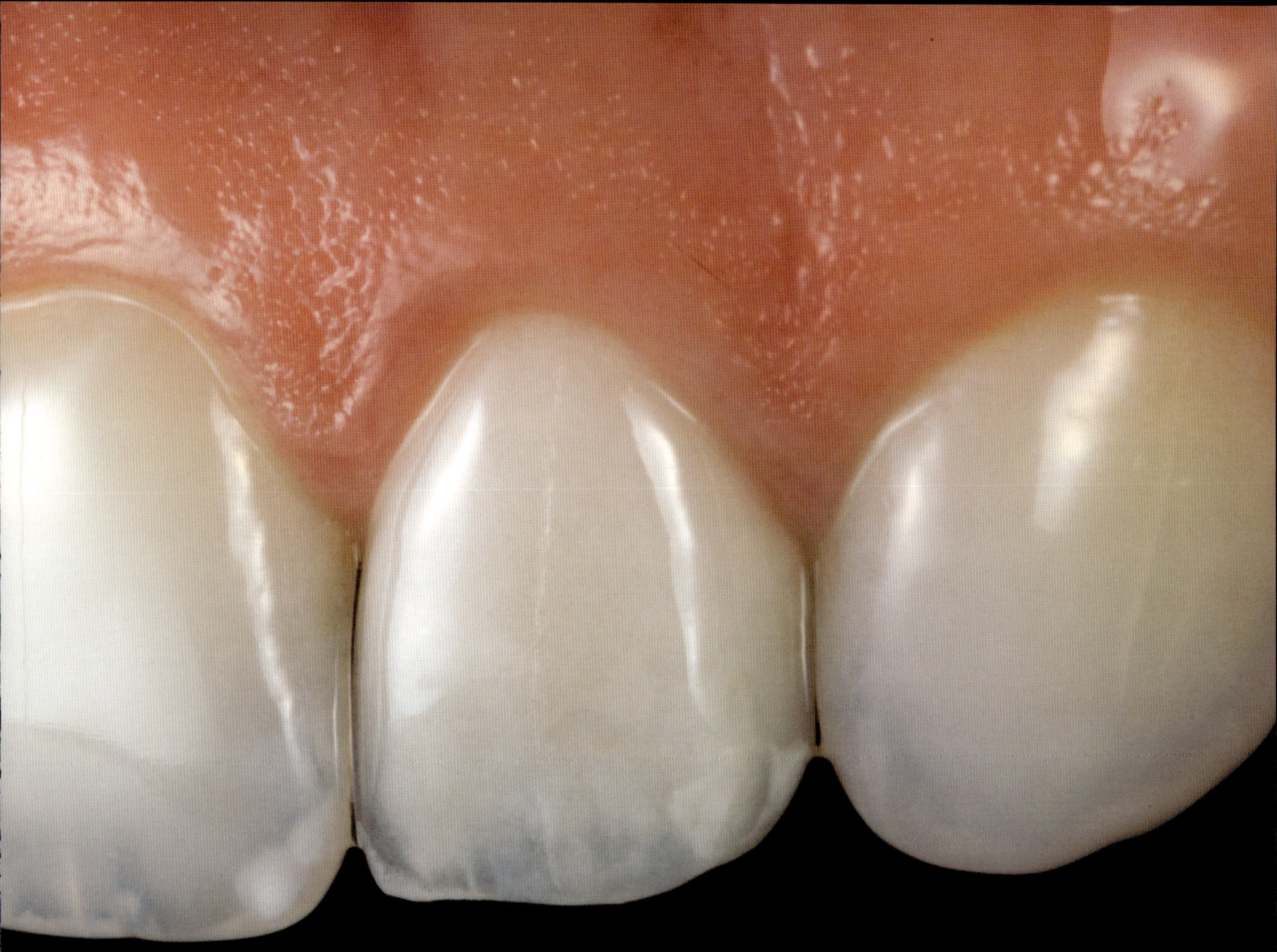

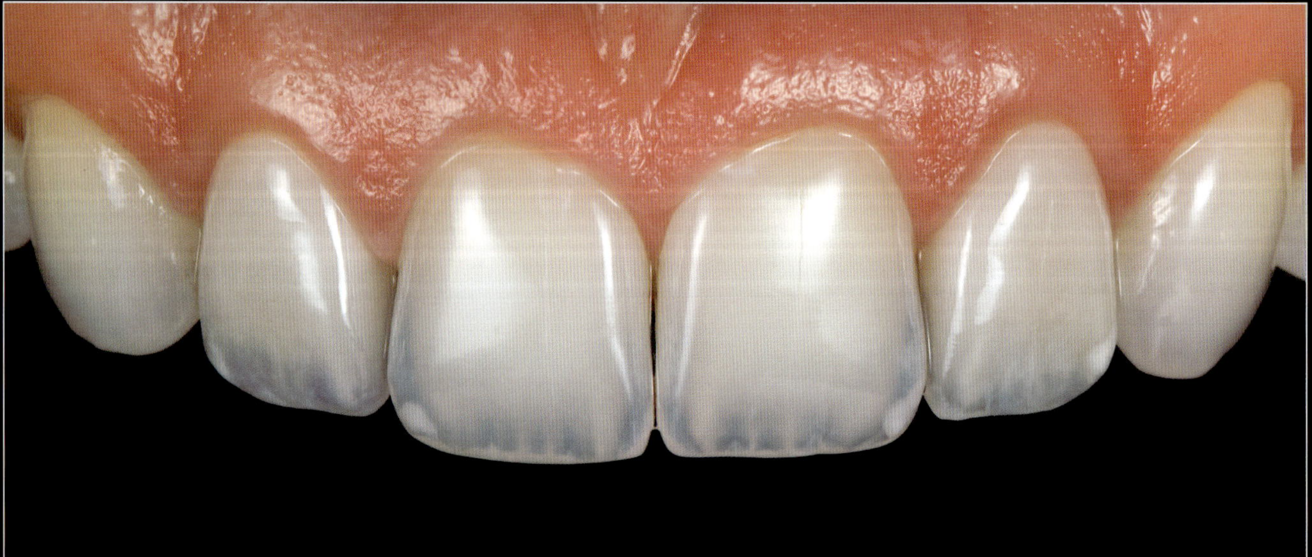

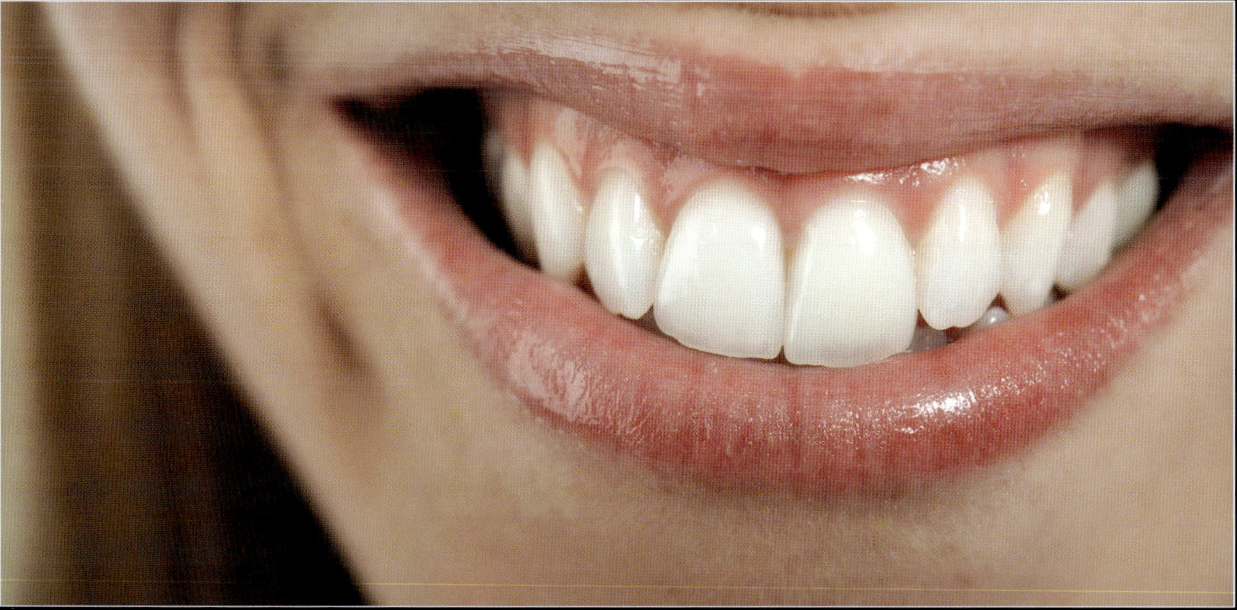

Type 2: Enhanced natural restorative treatment

This case involved prosthetic treatment of the maxillary central incisors, one with a porcelain laminate veneer and the other a zirconia crown. The main purpose was to make these restorations harmonize with the adjacent dentition. However, it was important to design the shape, length, and width of the restorations to harmonize with the patient's facial appearance, entire dentition, and lips as well. The minor rotation of both lateral incisors and the unbalanced incisal and cervical lines were visually managed by making the shapes of the two restorations slightly different. The definitive restorations work to improve the balance of the anterior dentition.

Katana zirconia crown and CZR laminate veneer (Kuraray Noritake Dental). Collaboration with Dr Kurt Schneider

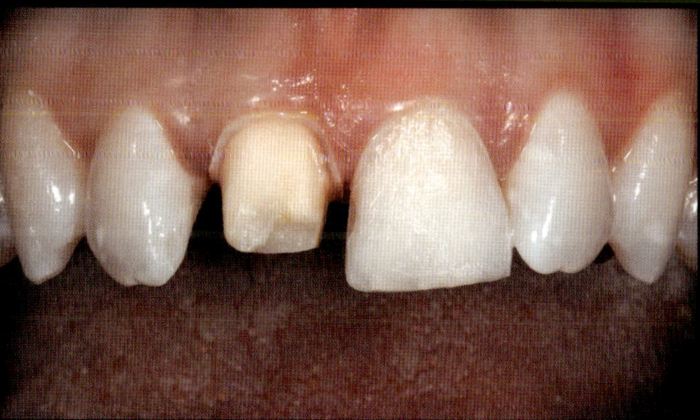

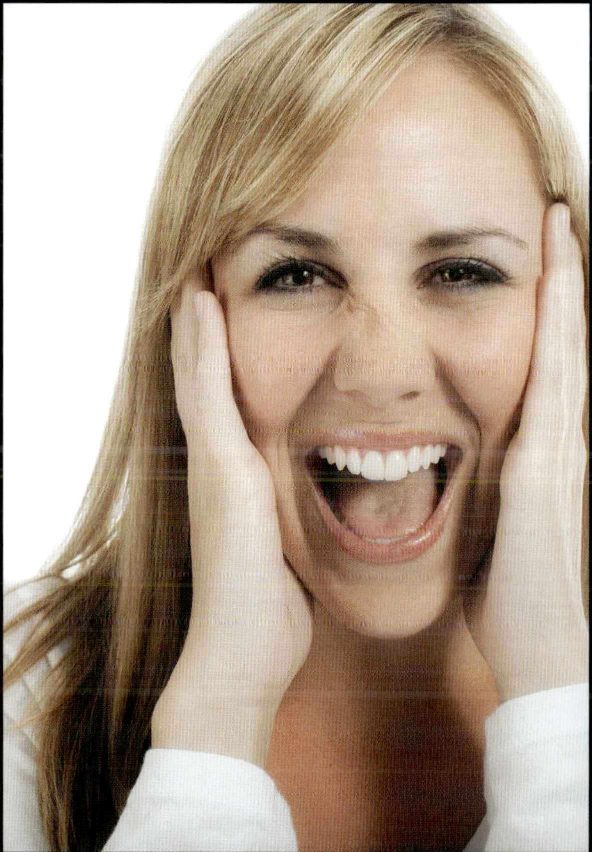

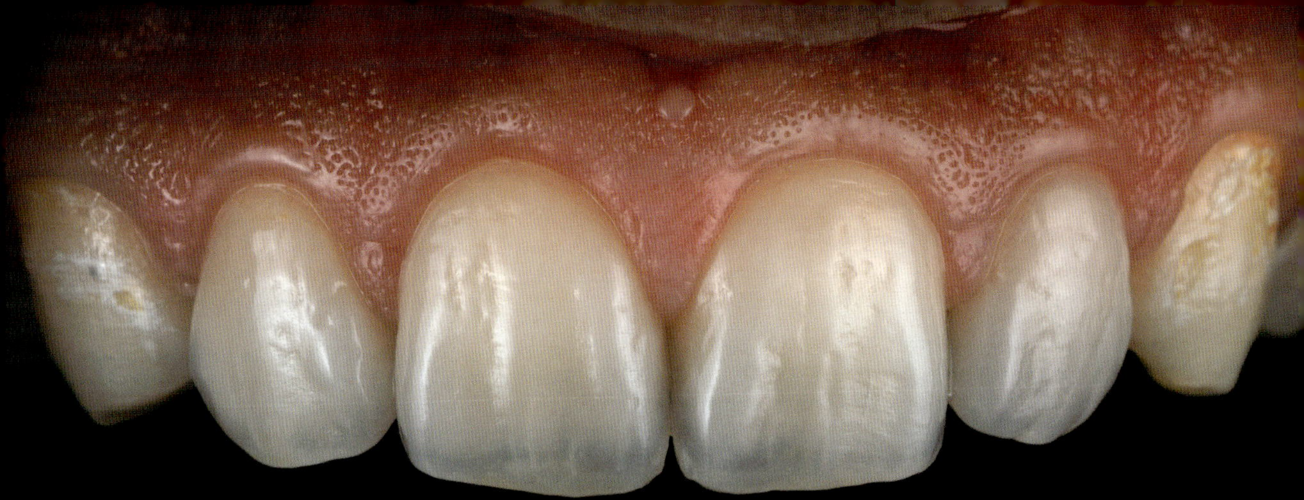

Type 2: Enhanced natural restorative treatment

This patient had multiple facial caries lesions and defective composite resin restorations on the anterior teeth. Noncarious areas were included in the restorative treatment to balance the anterior dentition. The canines were not involved. Crown shape, position, color, and internal characterization were emphasized in the treatment of this patient.

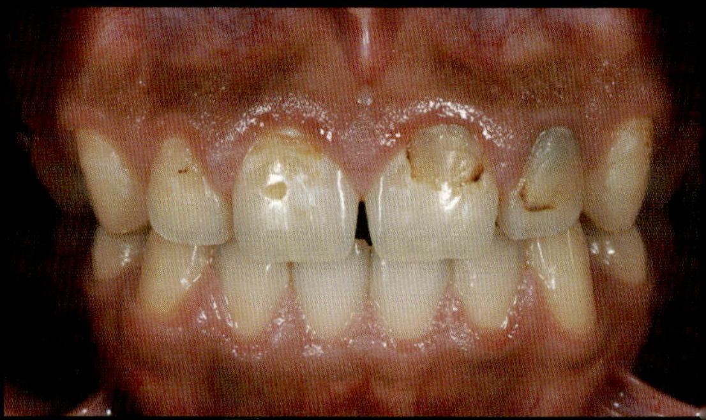

EX-3 laminate veneer (Kuraray Noritake Dental). Collaboration with Dr Shunya Sasaki.

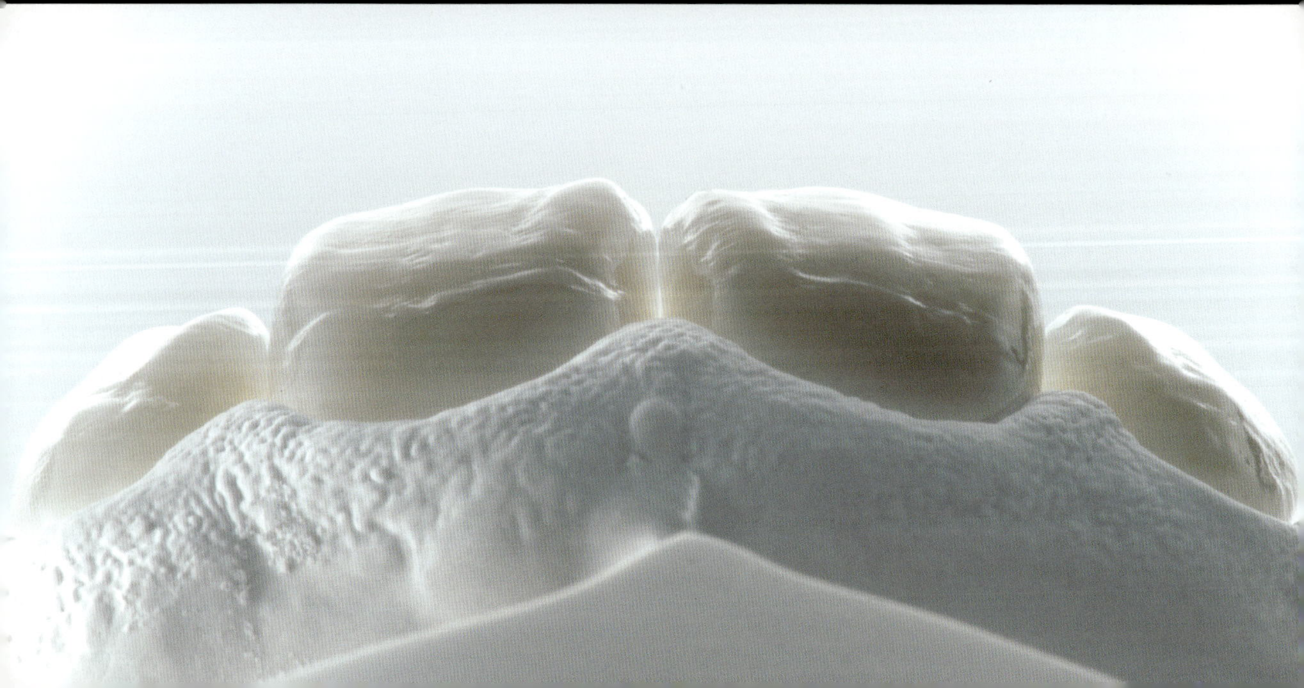

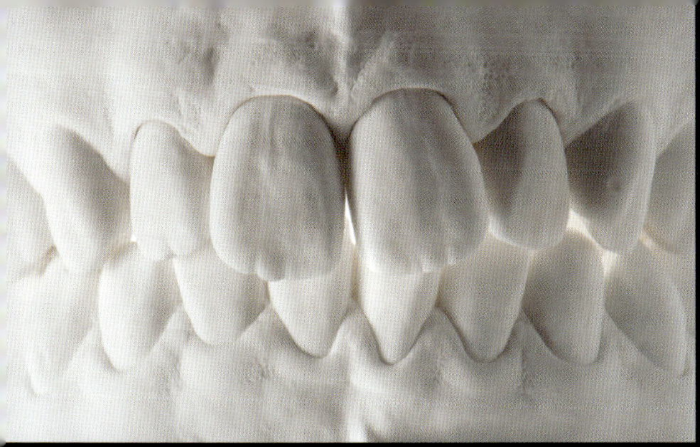

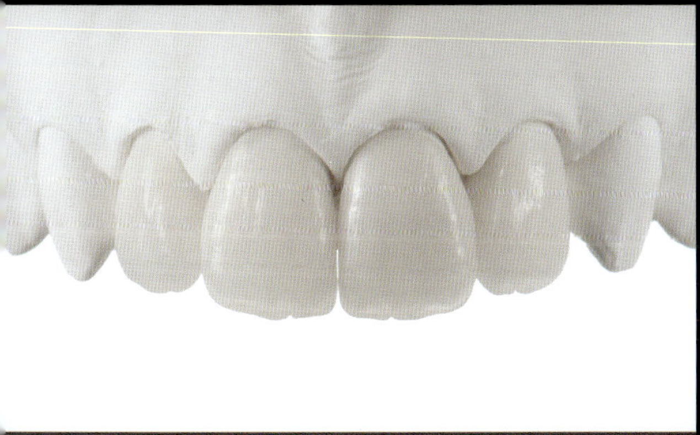

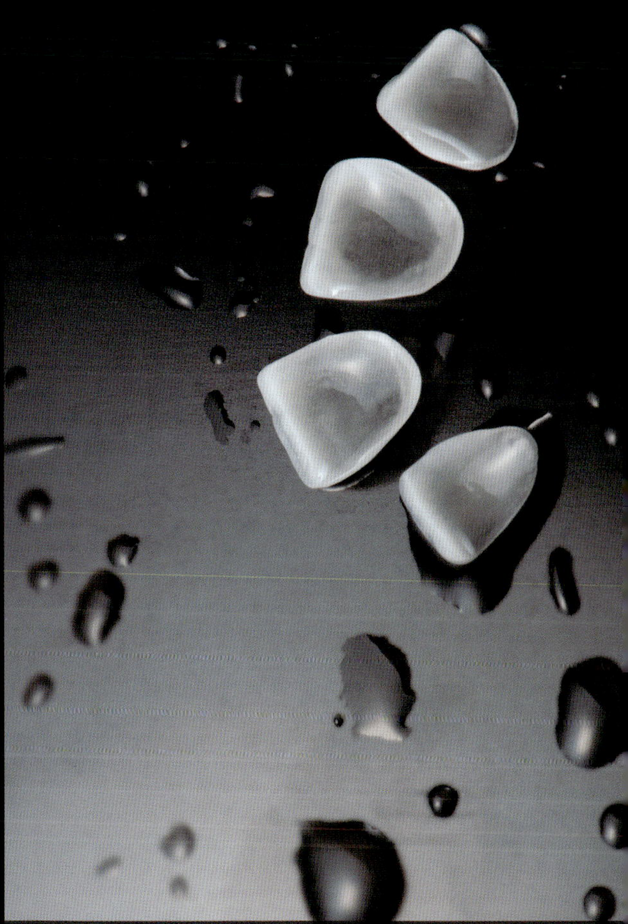

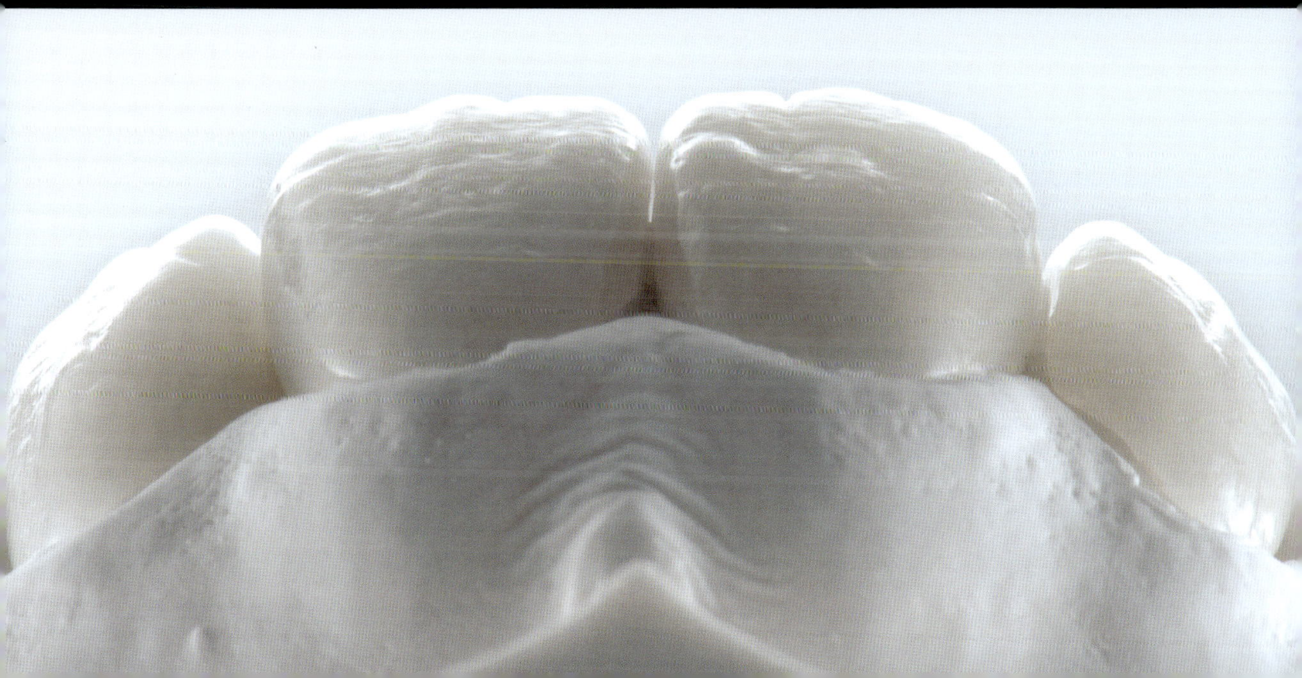

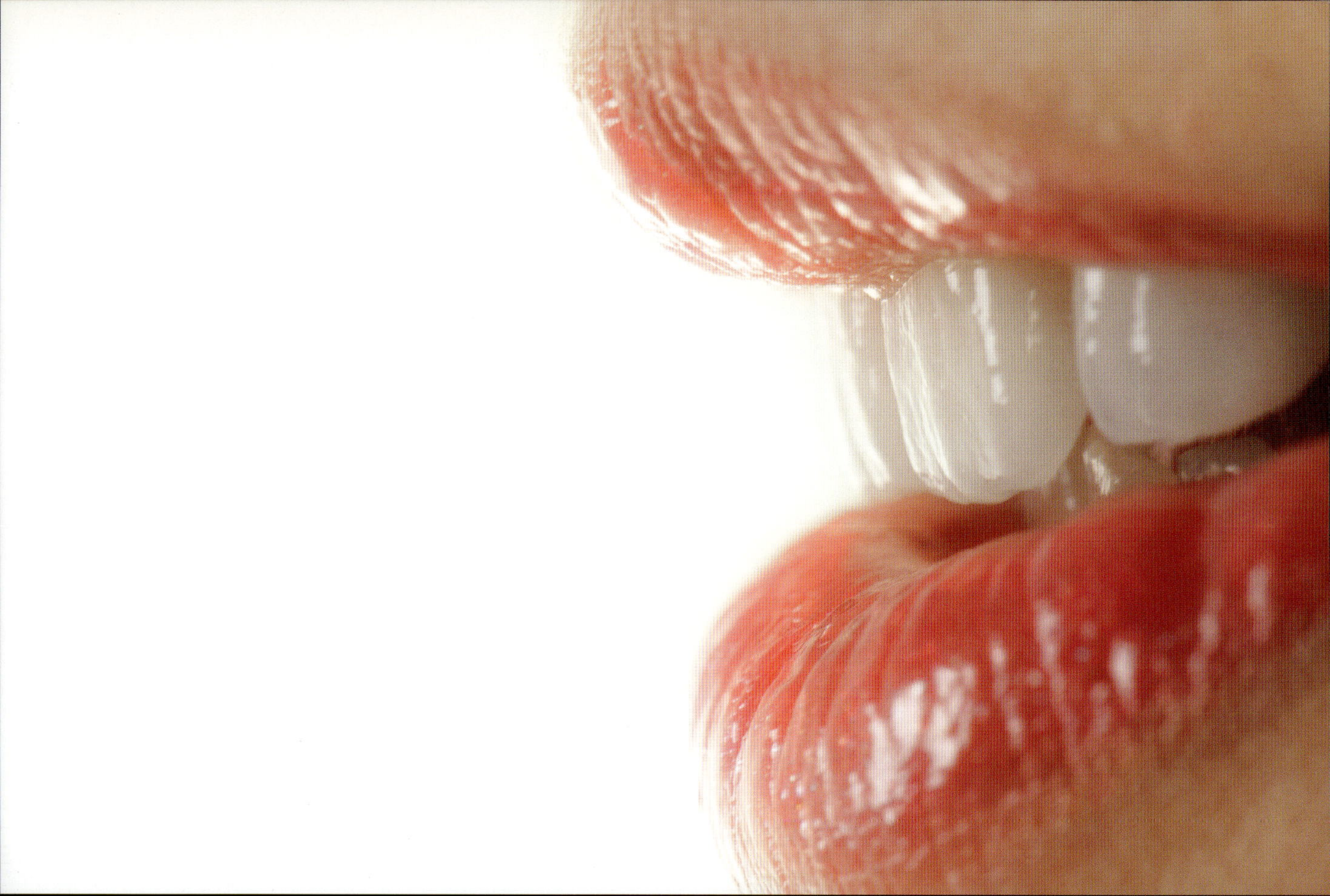

EX-3 laminate veneers (Kuraray Noritake Dental). Collaboration with Dr Ed McLaren.

Type 3: Esthetic treatment

Restorative treatment of four anterior teeth to improve the long axes, inclination, crown shape, and interproximal space was performed without orthodontic treatment. Minimum gingivectomy was required to reduce the patient's gummy smile. The teeth were healthy and so needed only minimal preparation. Because the patient requested that both lateral incisors be brought 1 mm facially, almost no preparation was necessary on these teeth. Harmony of the six anterior teeth and proper balance with the facial appearance and lip dynamics were achieved.

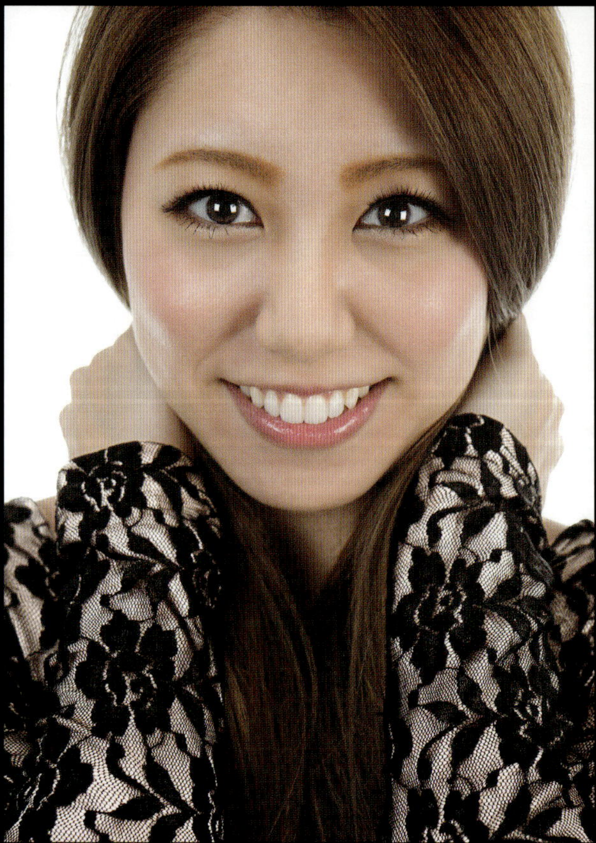

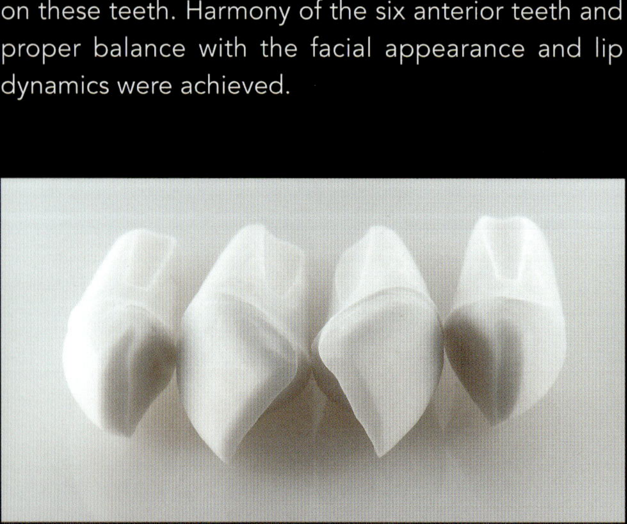

Type 4: Esthetic treatment + Total oral rehabilitation

Comprehensive treatment was performed to fulfill the patient's request for functional esthetic rehabilitation. After multiple periodontal plastic surgical procedures, esthetic prostheses that were well balanced with the patient's facial appearance and lip dynamics were fabricated. Color control was difficult in this case because of the mixed dentition that included a zirconia crown, an implant-supported zirconia crown to restore the right central incisor, and porcelain laminate veneers. The multiple laminate veneer preparations were created first by applying porcelain on zirconia copings. They were tried in the patient's mouth to check the color. A unified color of the zirconia copings and abutments for the laminate veneers was possible by this process. Eventually, color coordination of the different materials was achieved by simply applying the same porcelain on color-adjusted zirconia copings and laminate veneer abutments.

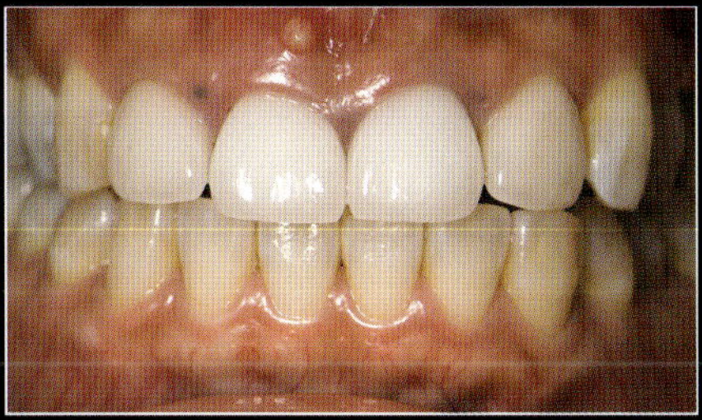

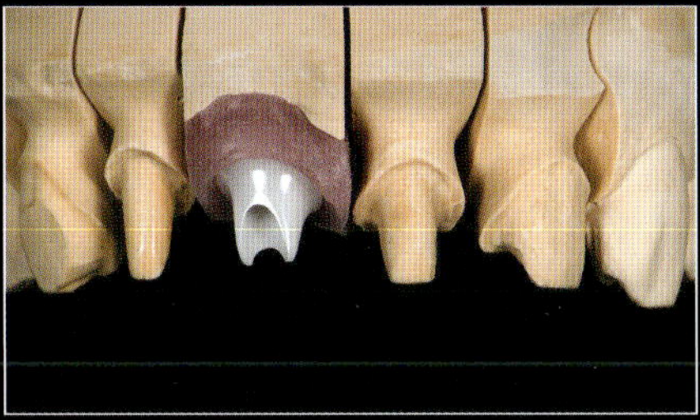

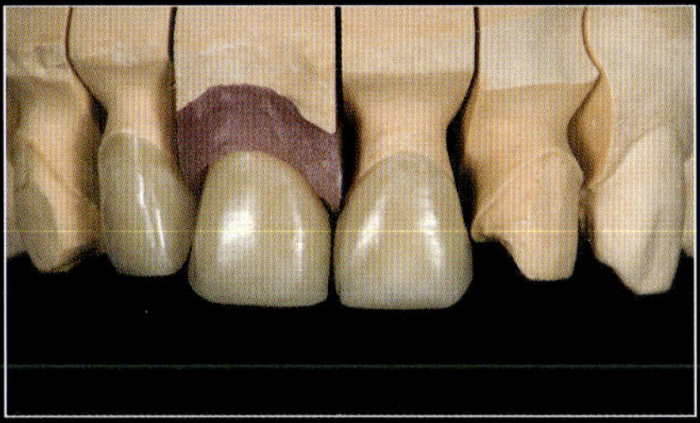

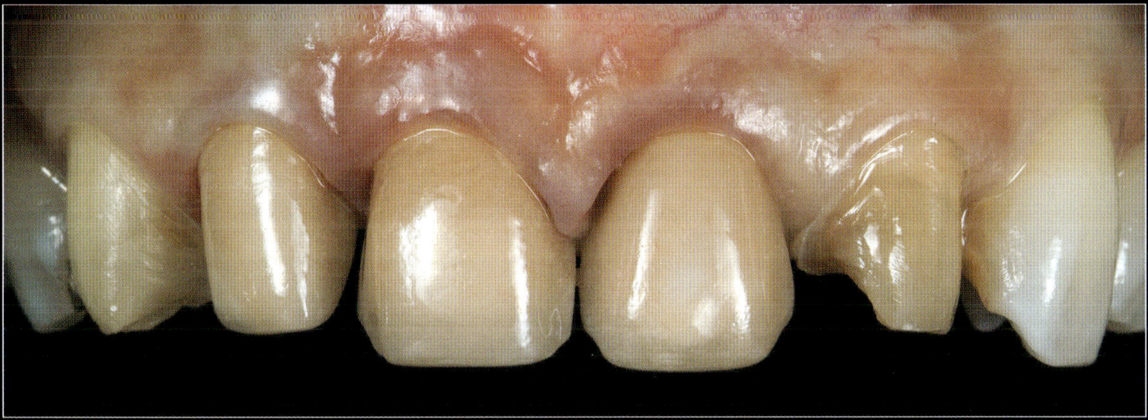

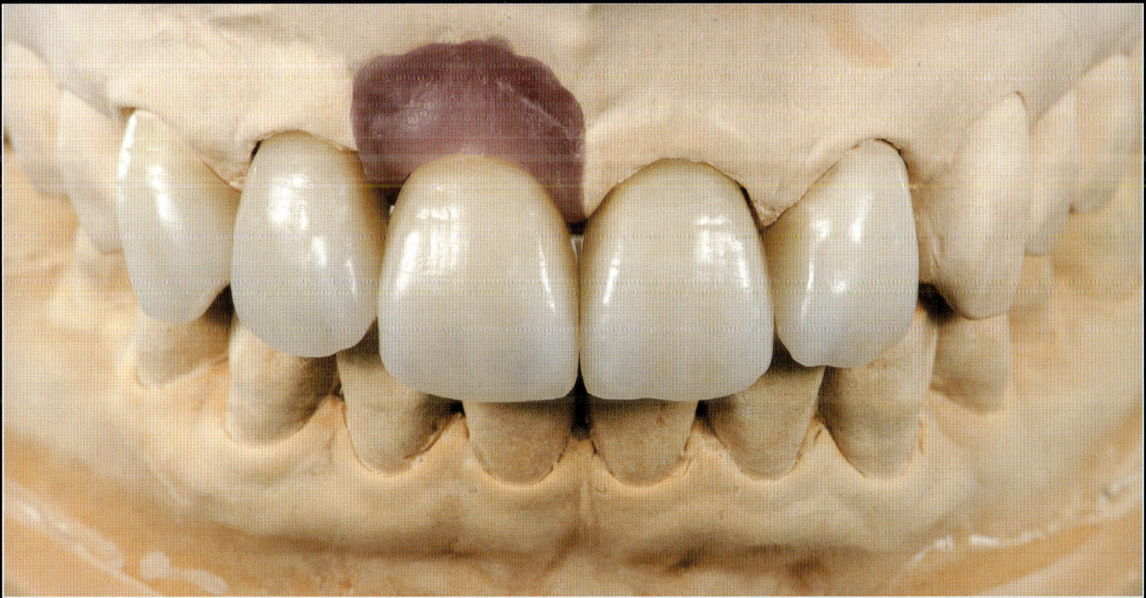

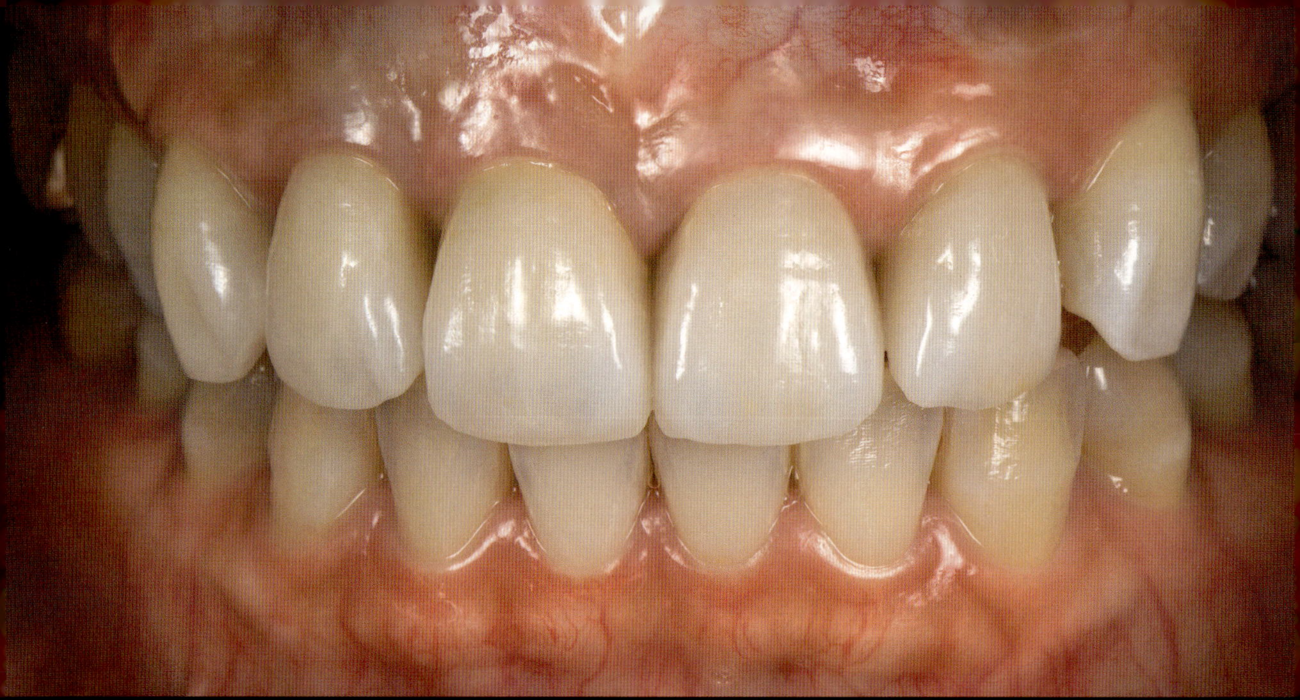

Nobel Active RP (Nobel Biocare); Katana zirconia crown and CZR laminate veneers (Kuraray Noritake Dental
Collaboration with Dr Akitoshi Sato.

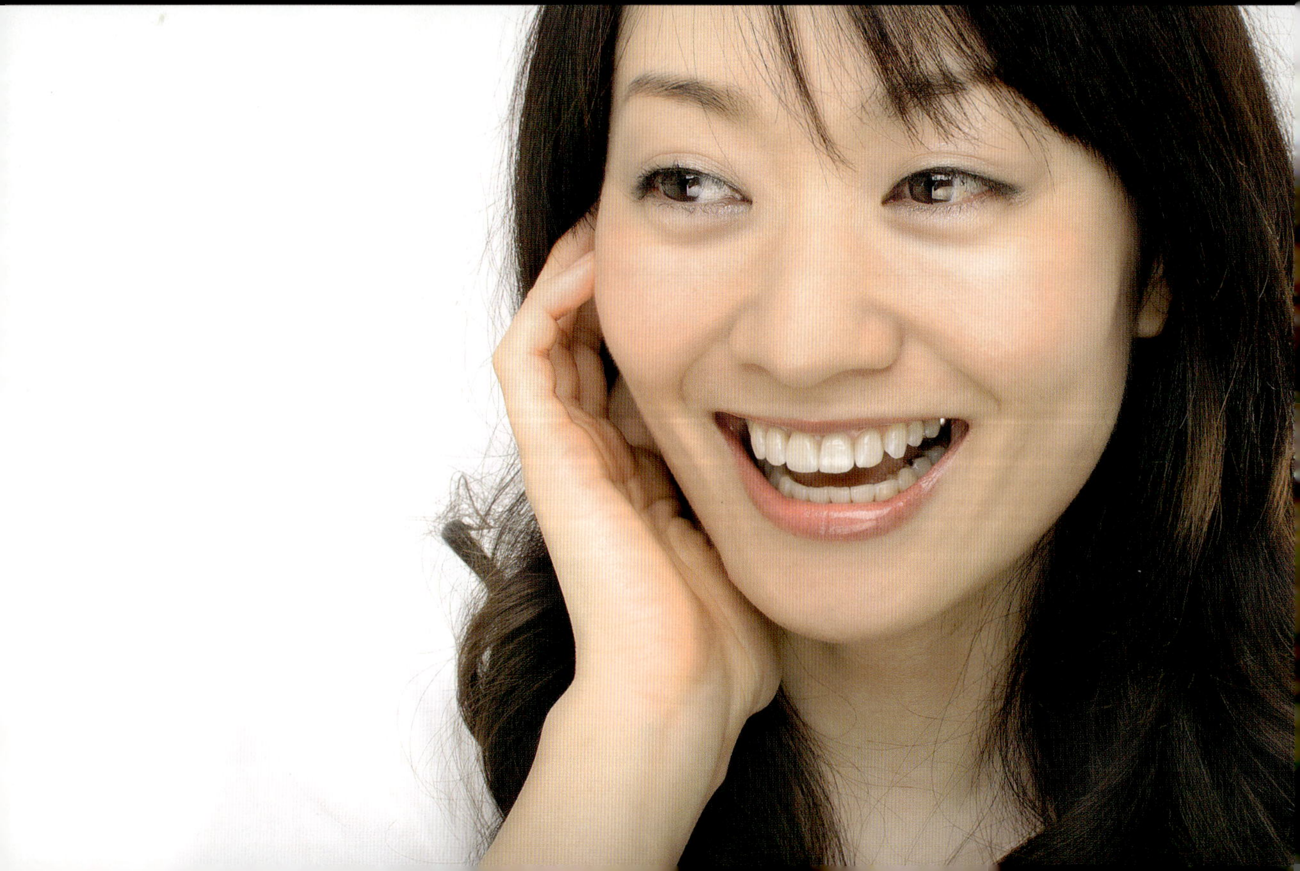

Biologic Esthetics by Gingival Framework Design:

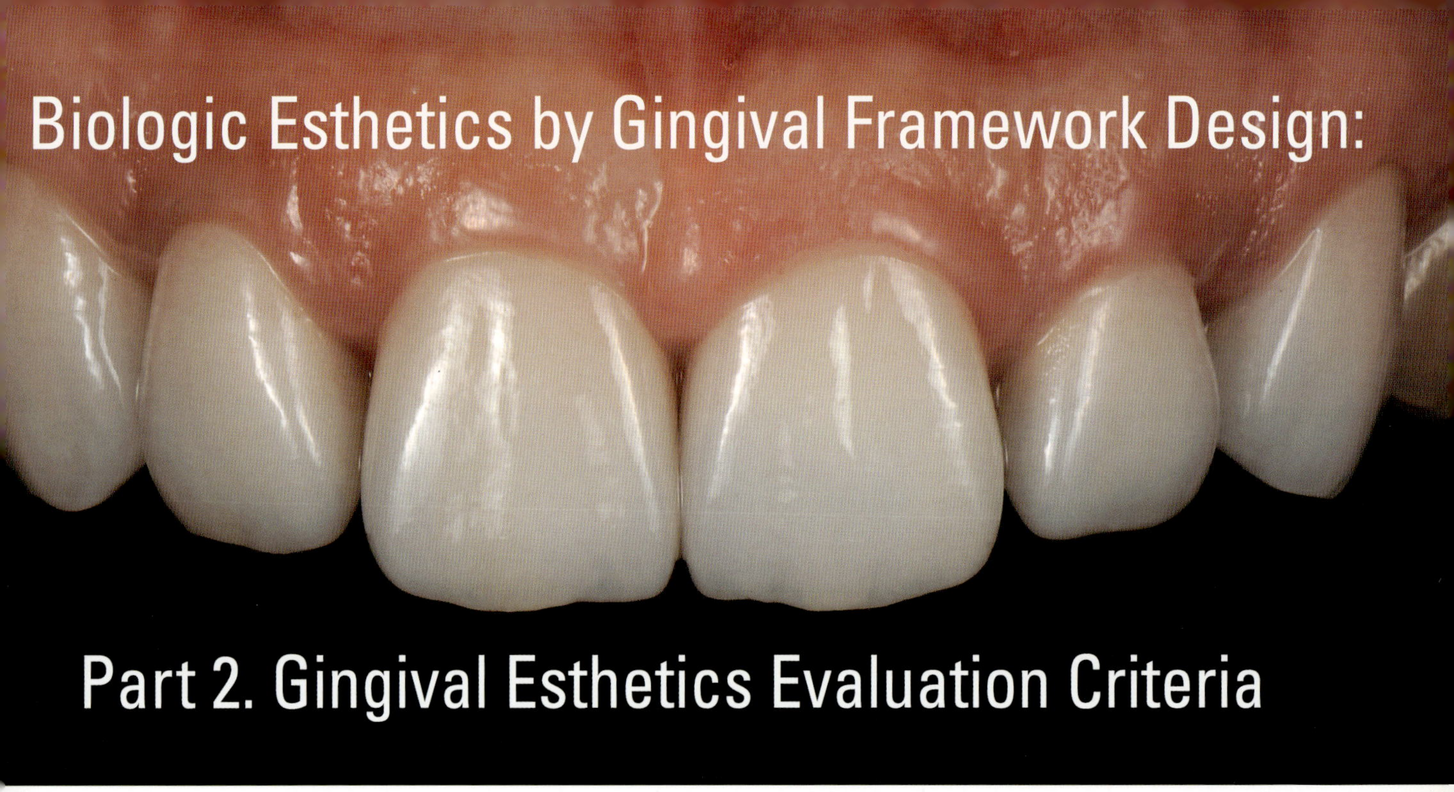

Part 2. Gingival Esthetics Evaluation Criteria

Yuji Tsuzuki, RDT[1]

There are three fundamental components to presenting a beautiful and healthy dentition. The first is tooth morphology, the second is gingival architecture, and the third is the relationship of the lip to all other components. All of these components will create a positive or negative impression depending on color, morphology, and tooth alignment.

Acquiring and maintaining gingival health and oral esthetics is the goal when planning definitive restorations. There are several factors to consider when evaluating gingival health, such as the marginal periodontal condition and tooth alignment. In part 1 of this article, the importance of paying attention to the periodontal condition and constructing a healthy gingival architecture during prosthesis fabrication was discussed in a general manner. In this article, specific techniques to achieve this goal are presented.

GINGIVAL ESTHETICS EVALUATION CRITERIA

It is necessary to pay attention to the gingival framework[1] and to understand the balance between the coronal structure and gingiva (Fig 1). Generally, healthy gingiva has its own features, which vary according to the tooth shape (square, triangle, or ovoid). Moreover, the horizontal alignment of the cementoenamel junction (CEJ), cervical bone crest, and free gingival margin usually appear to be similar to the overlying gingiva[2] (Fig 2). Left-right symmetry is one of the most important factors for a beautiful smile line. To acquire this symmetry, there should be ideal occlusion and the teeth should be in an ideal three-dimensional position. When patients display this ideal oral environment, it is unlikely that they will need major prosthetic work unless they experience an accident or trauma. Usually patients who require major prosthetic treatment have

[1]Dental Technician, Kyoto, Japan.

Correspondence to: Yuji Tsuzuki, Ray Dental Labor, Elitz Yamashina Building 3F, 18-8 Takehanatakenokaidocho Yamashina-ku, Kyoto City, Kyoto, Japan. Email: ray710@camel.plala.or.jp

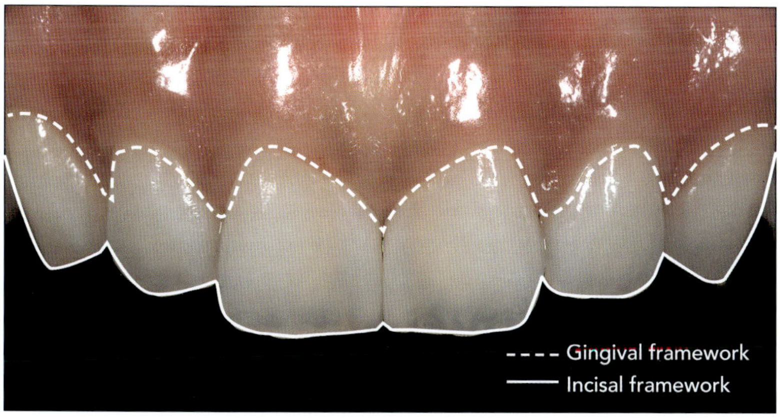

Fig 1 Gingival framework and incisal framework formed by the dentition. Right-left symmetry and continuity toward the posterior teeth determine the esthetic factor of the dentition.

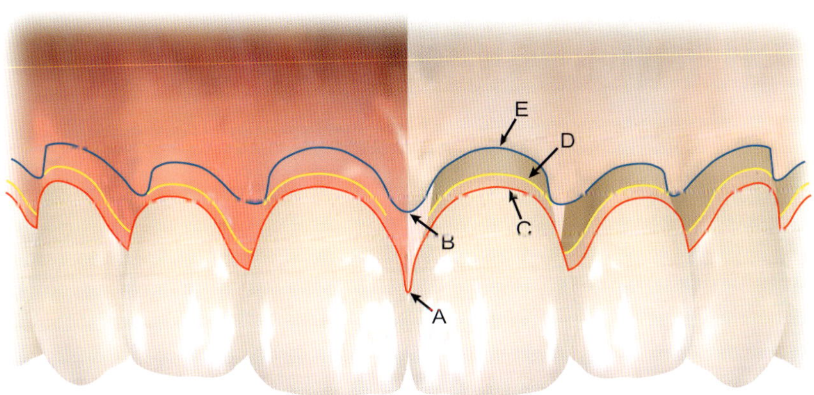

Fig 2 Vertical anatomical index of the anterior teeth, gingiva, and alveolar bone. Generally, a healthy periodontium has its own features that vary according to the tooth shape (square, triangle, ovoid) and that are usually similar to the underlying horizontal alignment of CEJ, cervical bone crest, and free gingival margin. The gingival framework is maintained by the vertical relationship among CEJ, cervical bone crest, and free gingival margin.[3] (Modified from Obama[4] with permission.)

a preexisting intraoral condition such as tooth malalignment. Therefore, it is very important to evaluate the esthetics of the gingiva at the treatment-planning stage. Otherwise, the treatment options will be limited to prosthetics.

Two-Dimensional Considerations

Evaluation items of gingival health and esthetics have been enumerated by Fürhauser et al in the concept he named the "pink esthetic score"[5] (Fig 3). It is vital to have interdental papillae as a landmark for indication of a healthy periodontal condition. Adequate composition of the dentogingival complex[7] (tooth, gingiva, and alveolar bone) (Fig 4) is required for the interdental papilla to fill the interproximal space below the contact point. Two-dimensional (mesiodistal, horizontal, vertical) consideration of the esthetic area is performed based on five evaluation criteria (Fig 5). It is generally considered that a dentition with triangular-shaped teeth creates a more pleasing impression than one with square-shaped teeth in terms of the balance of esthetics of the mouth.

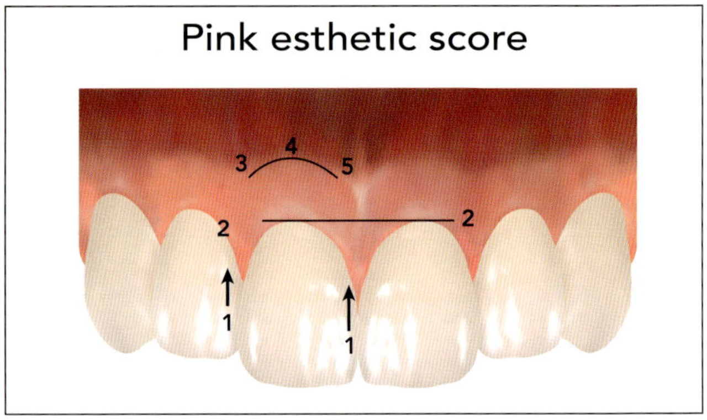

Fig 3 For calculation of the pink esthetic score, there are five esthetic evaluation items for a single implant-supported restoration replacing one missing anterior tooth[5]: *(1)* mesial and distal interdental papillae, *(2)* soft tissue level and contour, *(3)* alveolar process, *(4)* gingival texture, and *(5)* gingival color. A solely prosthetic approach is limited for the fulfillment of all esthetic requirements. Surgical management of hard and soft tissue is required. (Reprinted from Honda et al[6] [modified from Fürhauser et al[5]] with permission.)

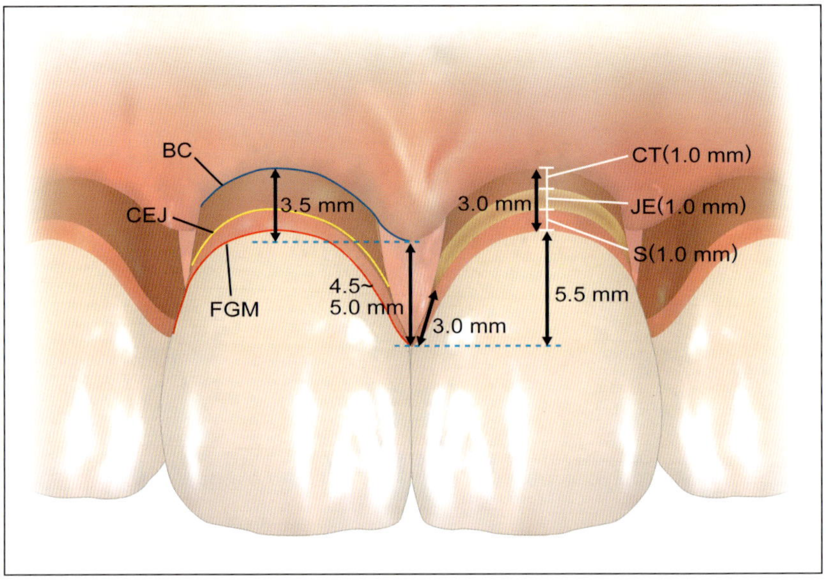

Fig 4 Anatomical composition of the tooth/gingiva/alveolar bone dentogingival complex advocated by Kois.[7] In general, the distance from the highest to the lowest point of the gingival margin is 5.5 mm; for alveolar bone, 3.5 mm. Hence, the distance from alveolar bone crest to gingival margin is 3.0 mm at midfacial and 4.5 to 5.0 mm at the interdental papilla. (Reprinted from Obama[4] [modified from Elian et al[8]] with permission.)

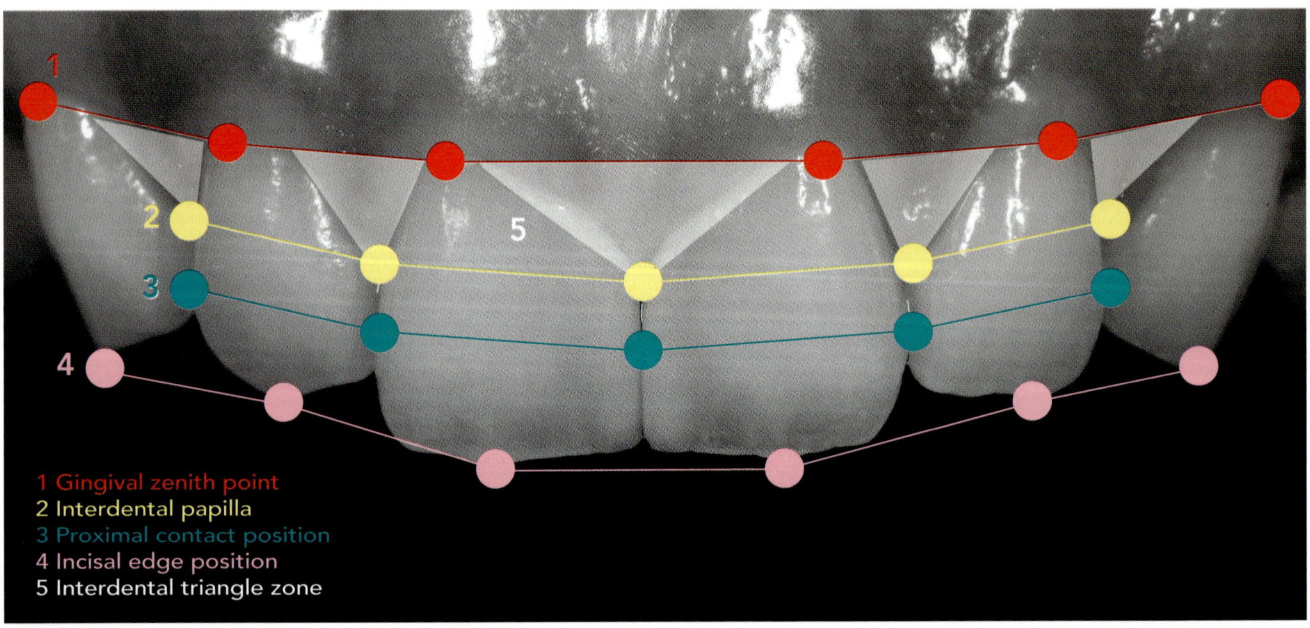

Fig 5 Esthetic evaluation criteria at the dentition level including coronal structures and gingiva. Right-left symmetry and regularity is evaluated two-dimensionally. As long as healthy periodontium and proper tooth positions are maintained, the level of the interdental papillae and proximal contact areas are parallel. The shape of the gingival zenith point and triangle zone changes dramatically according to the shape of the tooth and interdental distance.[9] The existing condition of the interdental papillae is determined by these factors.

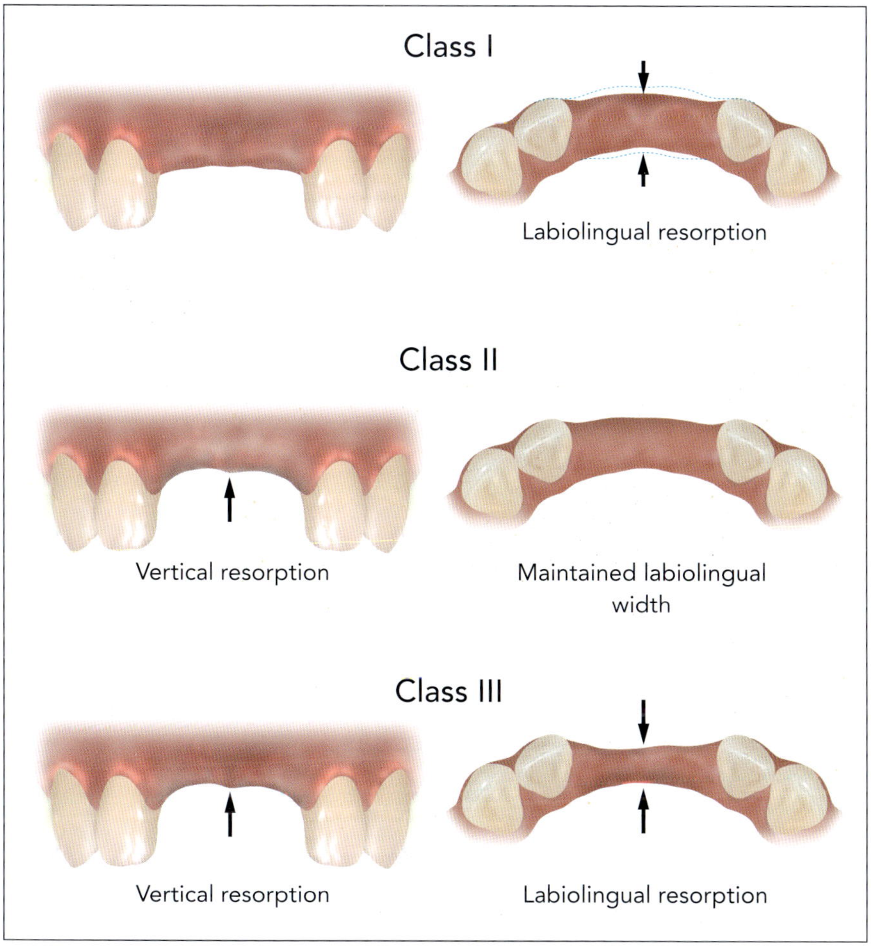

Fig 6 Classification of defect patterns of the alveolar ridge by Seibert and Cohen.[10] Soft tissue or hard tissue grafting is sometimes suggested by the technician at the diagnosis and treatment-planning stage in the presence of such defects. The prosthetic approach may differ according to the condition of the alveolar ridge. It is important to evaluate the condition thoroughly. (Reprinted from Obama[4] [modified from Seibert and Cohen[10]] with permission.)

Three-Dimensional Considerations

The volume of the alveolar ridge is composed of hard tissue (alveolar bone), including teeth, and soft tissue (gingiva). There is much individual variation. Three-dimensional (vertical and horizontal) consideration of the alveolar ridge is required in fixed or implant prosthetic cases. The prosthetic result may often be compromised without surgical reconstruction of hard and soft tissues in patients with a defective alveolar ridge. Moreover, prosthetic treatment is often compromised and limited without orthodontic and surgical treatment to improve three-dimensional esthetics. Seibert and Cohen[10] classified alveolar ridge defects (Fig 6), and soft tissue or hard tissue grafting is sometimes suggested by the technician according to this classification and diagnosis.

Cases 1 and 2 illustrate the use of surgical intervention to improve the prosthetic outcome. In Case 1 (Fig 7), treatment of the patient's maxillary right anterior dentition included ridge augmentation with a connective tissue graft. In Case 2 (Fig 8), horizontal and vertical ridge augmentation improved the treatment outcome of the patient, who presented with a root fracture of the maxillary left central incisor.

CASE 1 *Improvement of the Prosthetic Condition by Surgical Treatment*

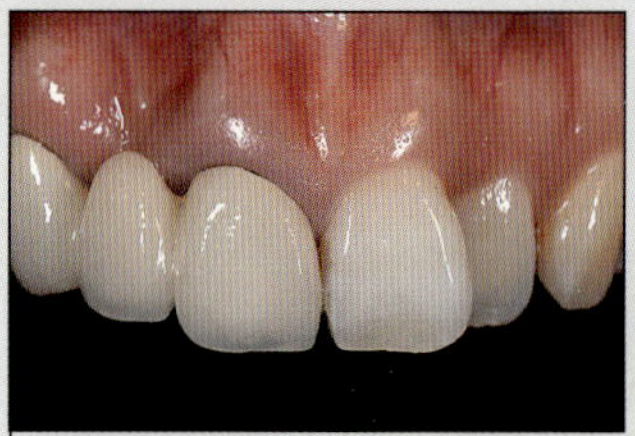
7a
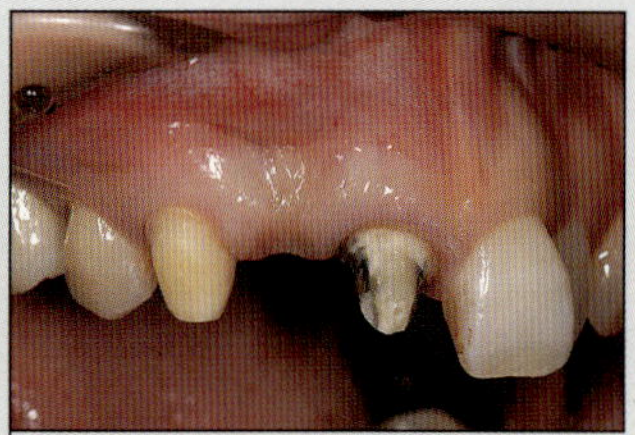
7b
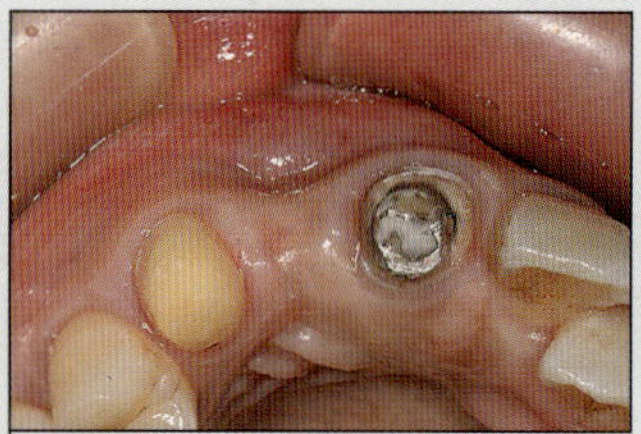
7c
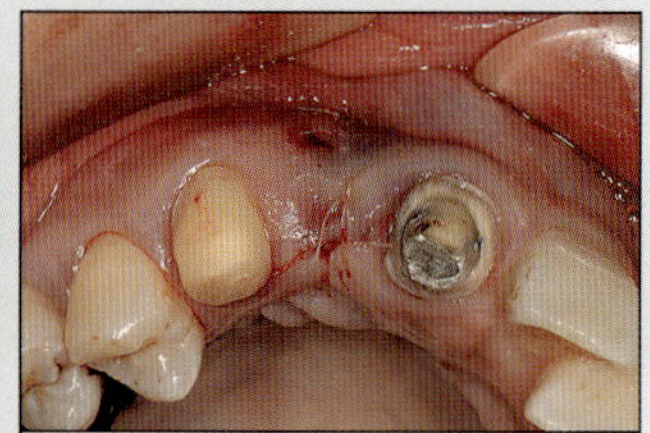
7d
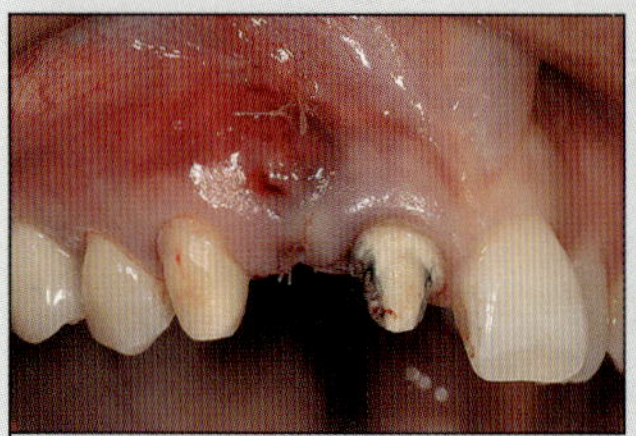
7e
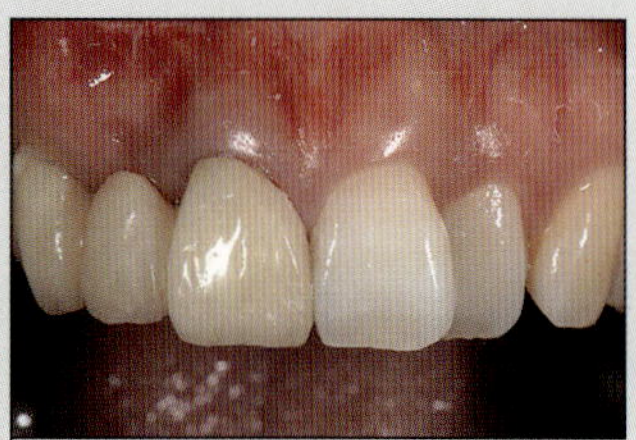
7f
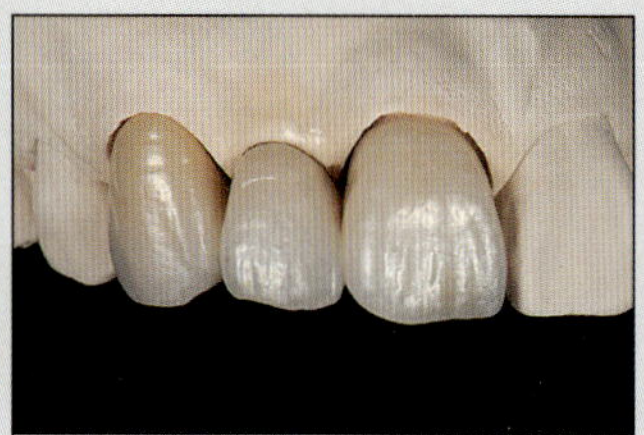
7g
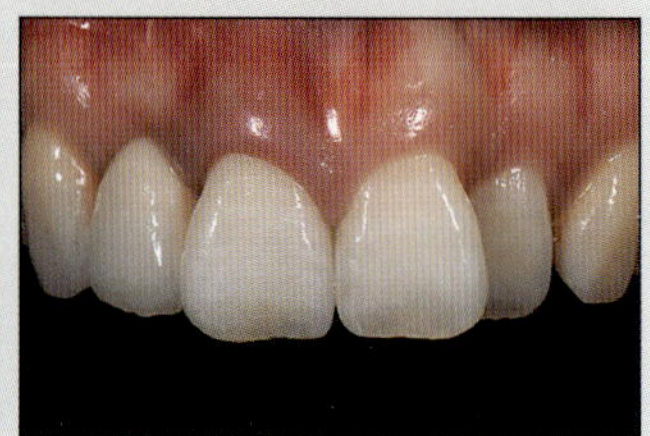
7h

Figs 7a to 7h The patient, a female in her 20s, complained of dissatisfaction with the esthetics of her fixed partial denture. Ridge augmentation was performed in the defective edentulous area of the maxillary right lateral incisor using a connective tissue graft from the palate. The presence of a defect at the pontic site in fixed prosthetic treatment affects not only the alignment but also the shape of the whole prosthesis. Surgical intervention dramatically improved the prosthetic condition and the treatment result. (Courtesy of Dr Hiroyuki Takino, Takino Dental Clinic, Japan.)

CASE 2 *Improvement of the Prosthetic Condition by Surgical Treatment*

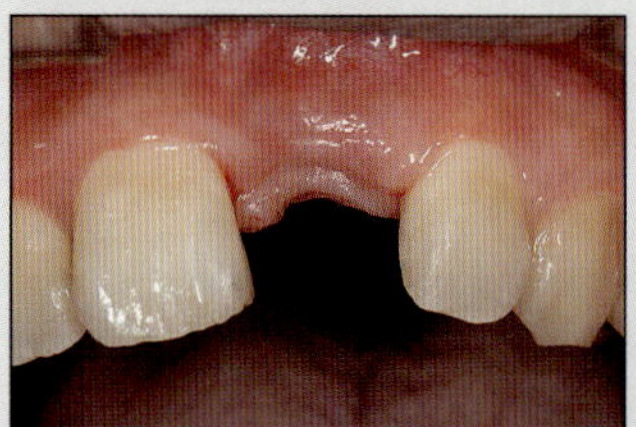
8a
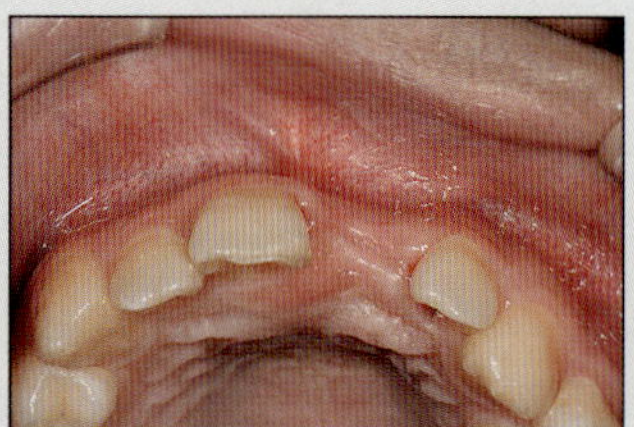
8b
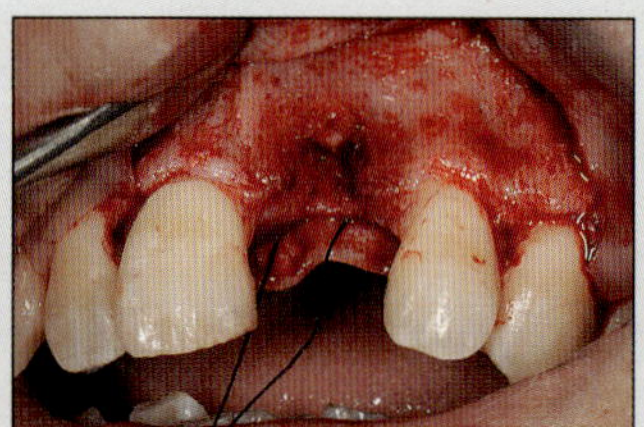
8c
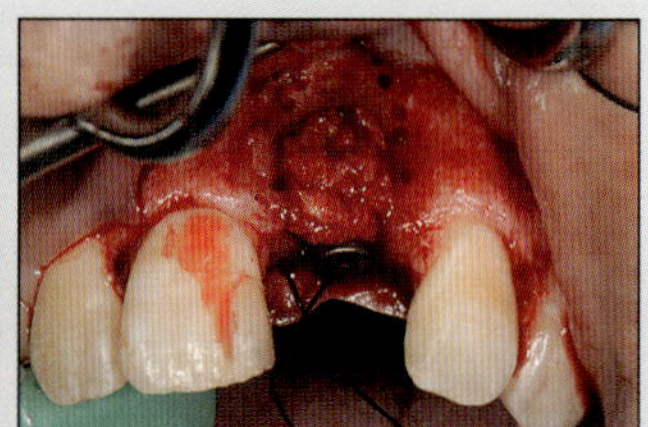
8d
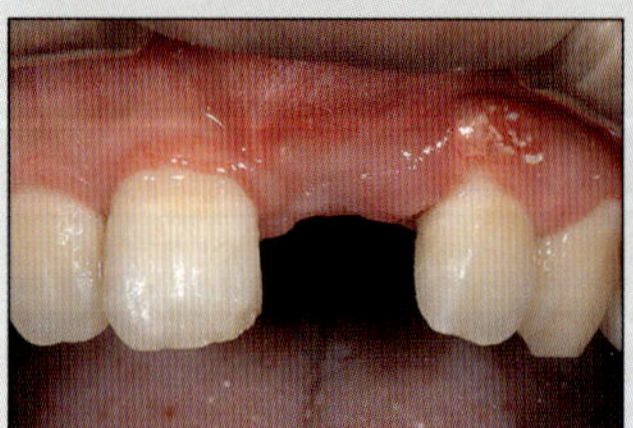
8e
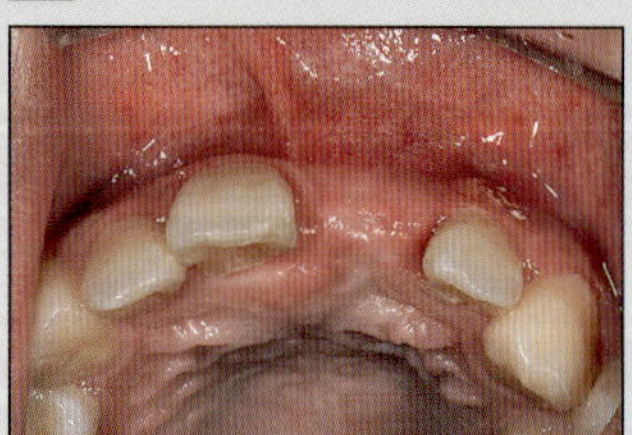
8f
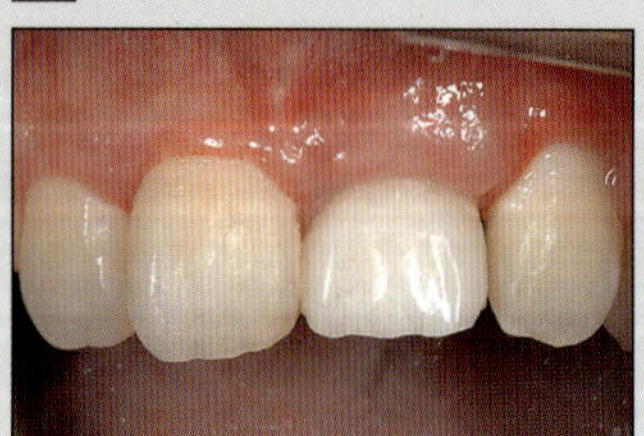
8g
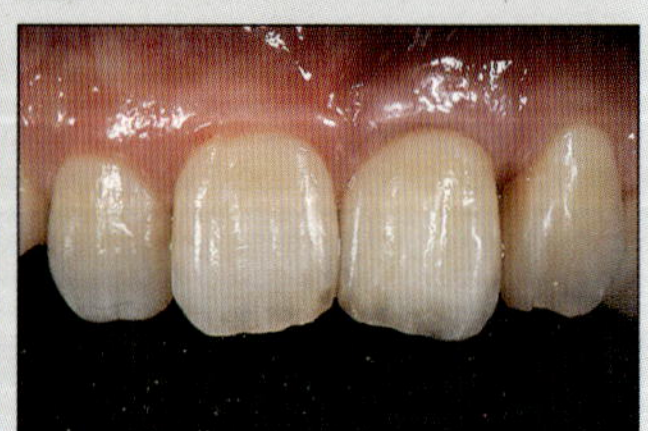
8h

Figs 8a to 8h The patient, a male in his 20s, presented with a root fracture of the maxillary left central incisor. A surgical approach to improve soft and hard tissue defects is inevitable in fixed implant prosthodontics. It improves the treatment result dramatically. The prosthetic condition of this patient was improved by horizontal and vertical ridge augmentation to restore the alveolar ridge defect. (Courtesy of Dr Kotaro Nakata, Nakata Dental Clinic, Japan.)

Table 1 Classification of Various Prosthetic Conditions Considering the Gingival Framework

Type 1: Symmetric	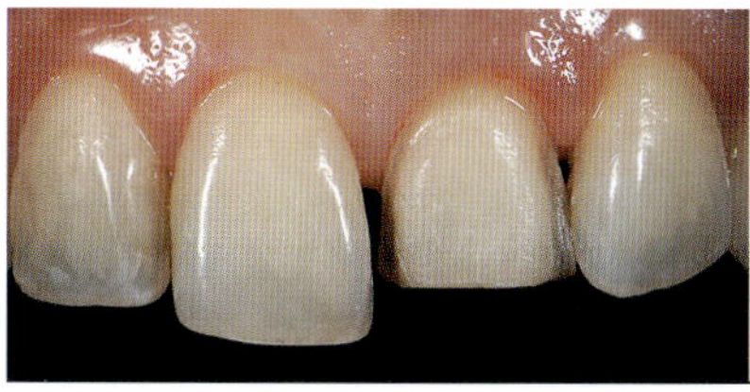	Treatment area does not require particular morphologic consideration of marginal gingiva. There is adequate symmetric marginal gingiva.
Type 2: Alternative	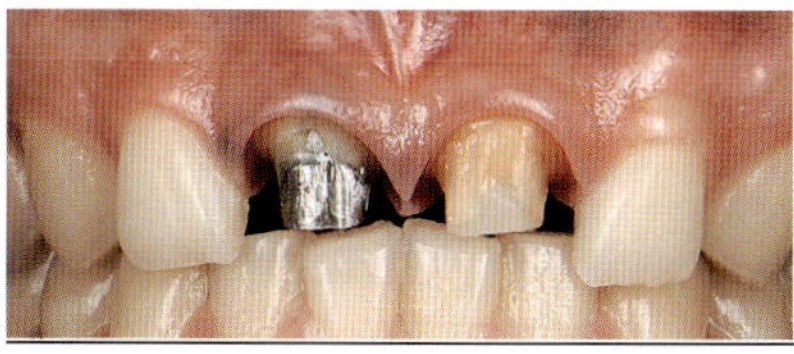	Esthetic disharmony exists at hard and soft tissue level. Adequate improvement can be expected using a surgical and prosthetic approach.
Type 3: Compromised	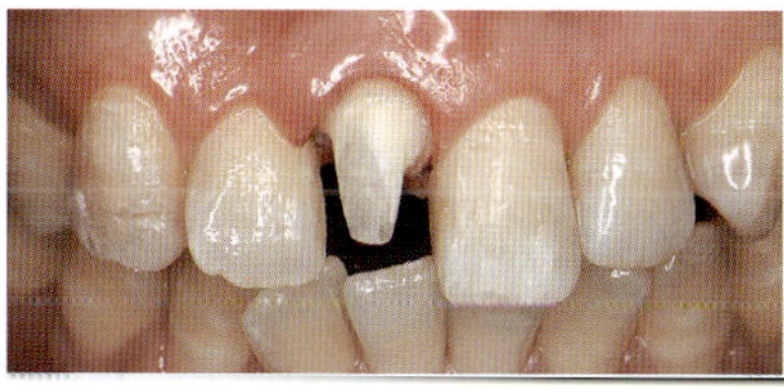	Orthodontic treatment is indicated to improve tooth position. The result will be compromised if prosthodontic treatment is performed alone.
Type 4: Creative	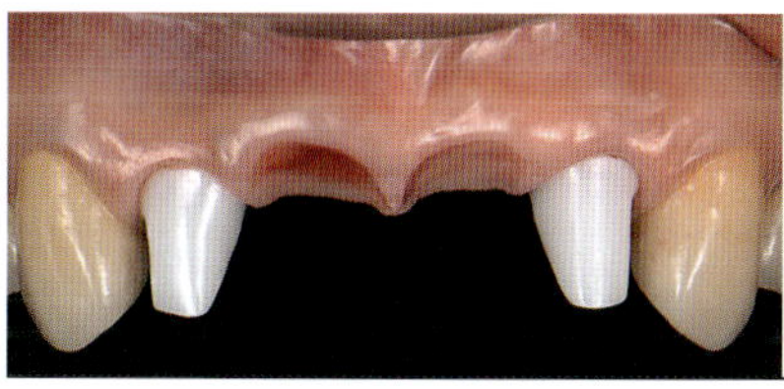	Symmetric edentulous area allows some leeway of the gingival framework design.

CLASSIFICATION OF PROSTHETIC CONDITION

For prosthodontic treatment in esthetic areas, it is necessary to clearly identify the prosthetic condition before setting the appropriate treatment goal by first considering the periodontal health as well as reconstruction of teeth. The author's classification of the prosthetic condition according to the gingival framework is shown in Table 1.

Three of these classifications are illustrated with clinical cases. Case 3 (Fig 9) is a type 2 alternative case. The patient's gingival level was improved by prosthetic treatment. Case 4 (Fig 10) is an example of a type 3 compromised case. In Case 5 (Fig 11), a type 4 creative case, the gingival contours are the result of an implant-supported fixed prosthesis.

CASE 3 *Type 2 (Alternative)—Improvement of the Gingival Level by Prosthetic Treatment*

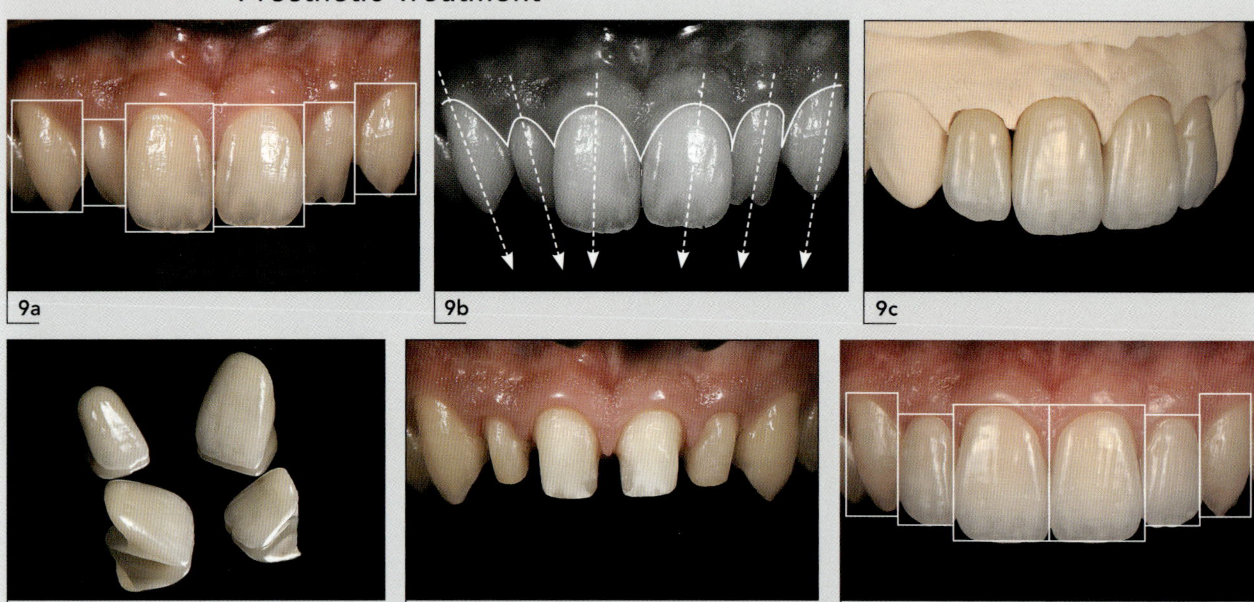

9a 9b 9c 9d 9e 9f

Figs 9a and 9b The patient wanted to improve the esthetics of her anterior teeth. Orthodontic treatment was indicated but was not accepted by the patient. Both central incisors are discolored due to previously placed restorations. The maxillary lateral incisors are peg-shaped. The long axes of these teeth are not in harmony. In particular, the gingival level of the right lateral incisor created disharmony of the gingival framework. Provisional restorations were fabricated from the diagnostic wax-up to rearrange the balance of the dentition (technique previously described by Sulikowski and Yoshida[11]).

Figs 9c and 9d Final restorations on and off of the master cast (IPS e.max Press, Ivoclar Vivadent). The tooth long axes were balanced, and the gingival framework was controlled by the subgingival contours of the restoration.

Fig 9e The gingival levels were altered by the provisional restorations.

Fig 9f Long axes, size, and proportion of teeth are improved and harmonized. Acceptable esthetics was achieved by prosthetic treatment alone in this patient. (Courtesy of Kubota Dental Clinic, Japan.)

CASE 4 *Type 3 (Compromised)—Prosthetic Result Not Optimal Without Orthodontics*

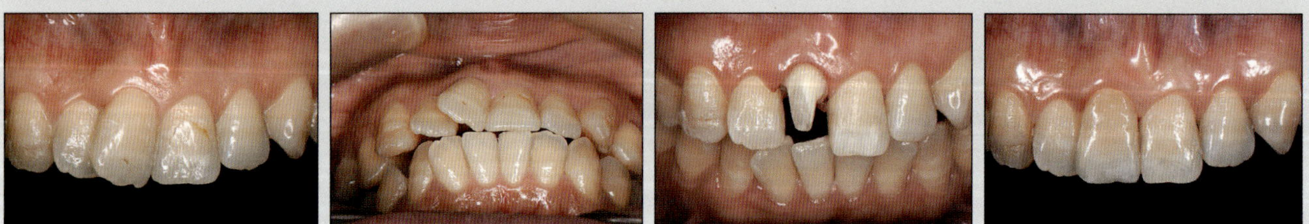

10a 10b 10c 10d

Figs 10a and 10b The patient wanted to improve the esthetics of the anterior teeth because of their malalignment. Orthodontic treatment was indicated and recommended, but the patient refused it. The patient was treated using a prosthetic approach alone. As a result, the maxillary right central incisor underwent root canal therapy, and adjacent teeth were reshaped.

Figs 10c and 10d Posttreatment photographs. The marginal gingiva is harmonized. Although the patient is satisfied with the result, this is not an optimal solution to the chief complaint because the tooth positions were not changed (all-ceramic crown, IPS e.max Press).

CASE 5 *Type 4 (Creative)—Gingival Design by Implant-Supported Prosthesis*

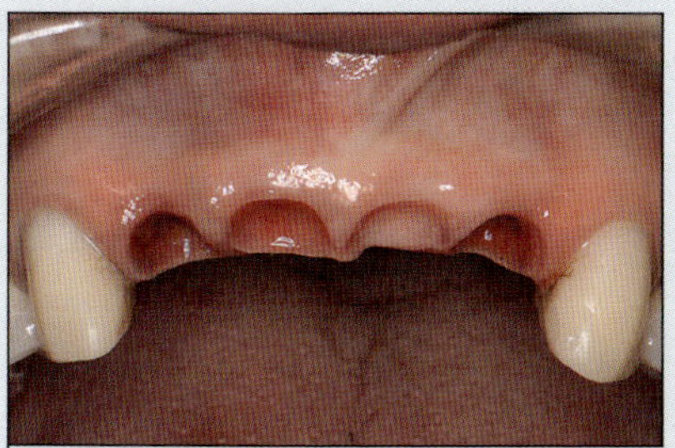
11a

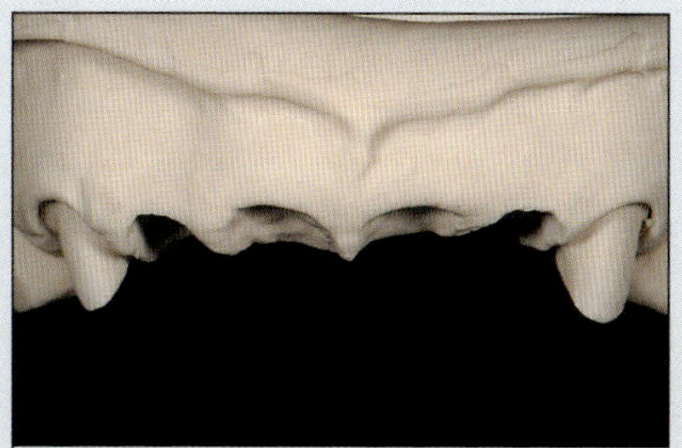
11b

Figs 11a and 11b Implant treatment was indicated for this patient who had fractured anterior teeth. After extraction and socket preservation, the pontic area was designed and contoured by the provisional restoration in consideration of the balance of the gingival framework of the six anterior teeth.

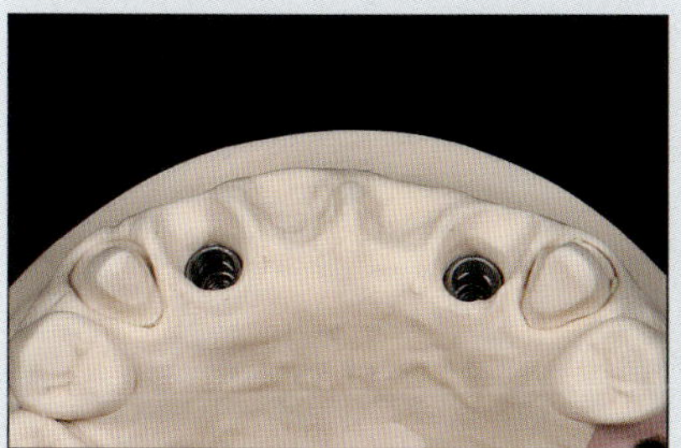
11c

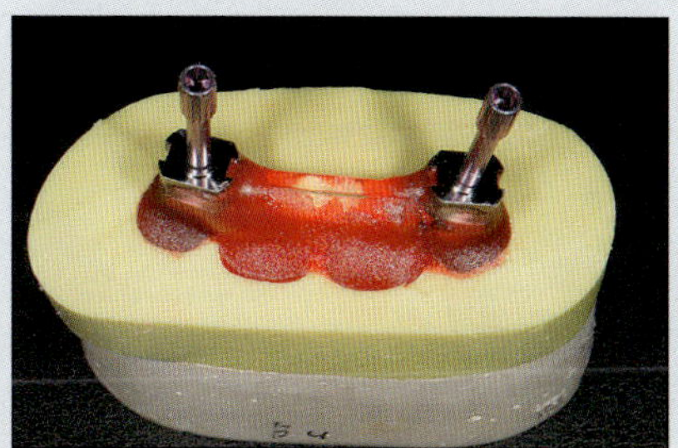
11d

Figs 11c and 11d A custom impression coping was fabricated to transfer the information of reshaped gingiva in the pontic area. Guided surgery was used to place two implants while maintaining parallelism.

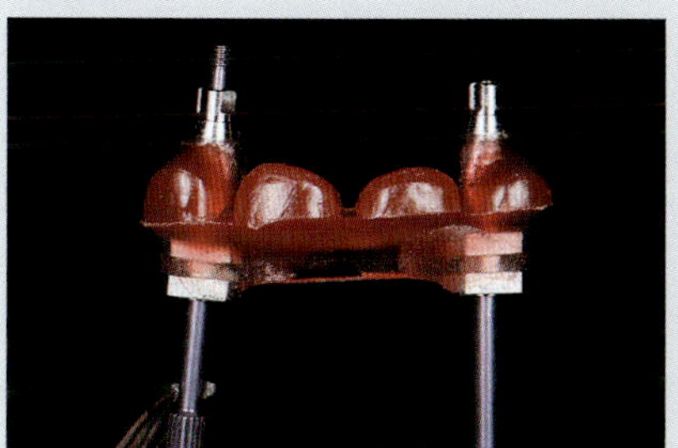
11e

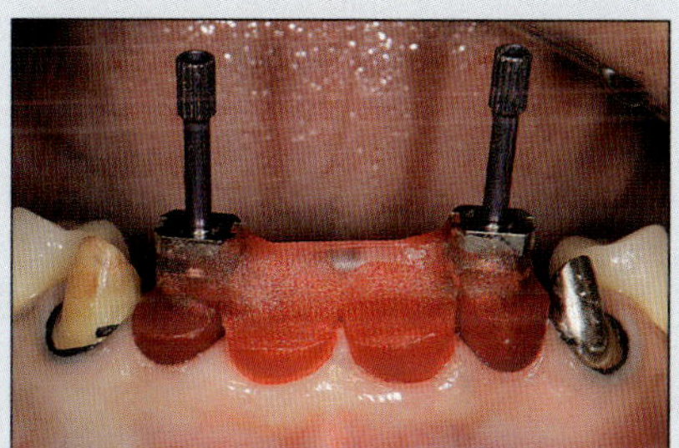
11f

Figs 11e and 11f Custom impression coping. The tissue surface of the implant and pontic area was reproduced with acrylic resin. A plastic bar was used between the two implants to maintain strength.

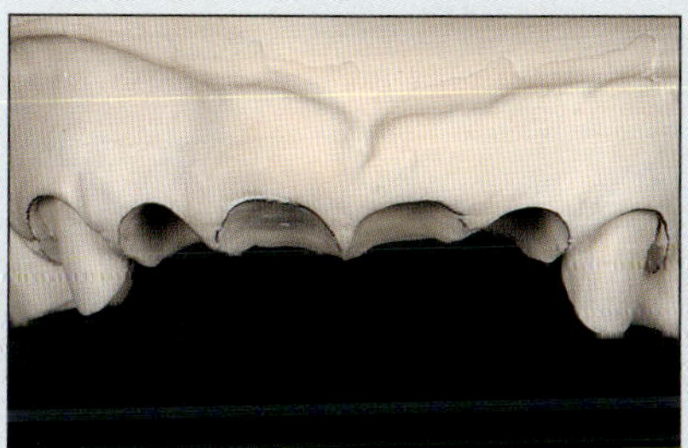
11g

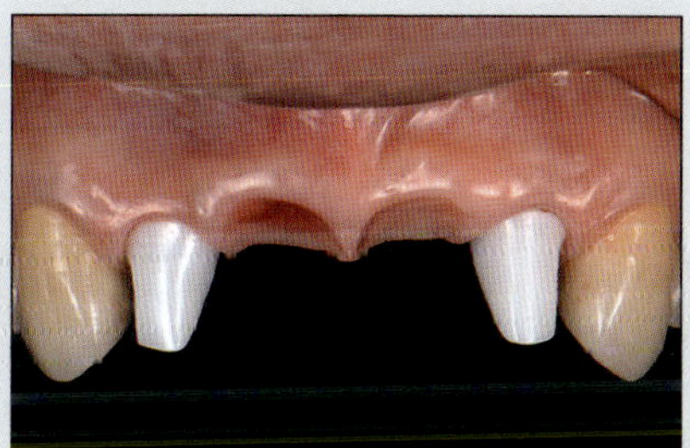
11h

Figs 11g and 11h The cast was sculpted into the contours of the definitive tissue surface of the restoration by grinding. Zirconium abutments were chosen.

Figs 11i to 11m Completed suprastructure of the implant prosthesis. The gingival framework of the six anterior restorations is well balanced (IPS e.max Zirpress, Ivoclar Vivadent).

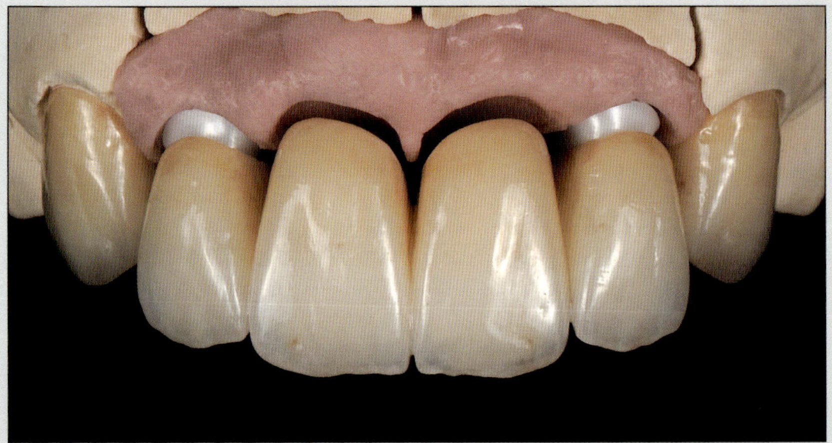

11i

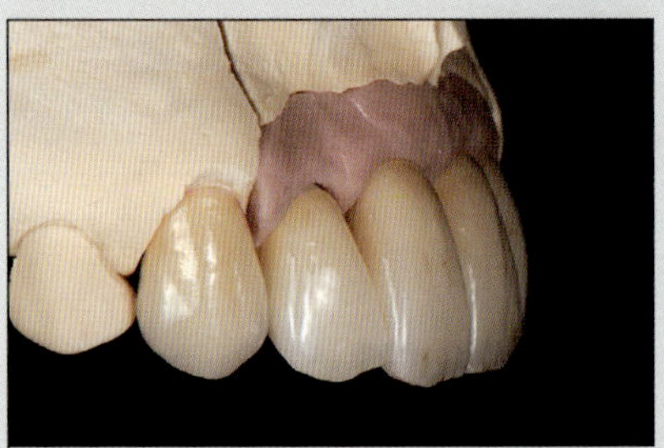

11j

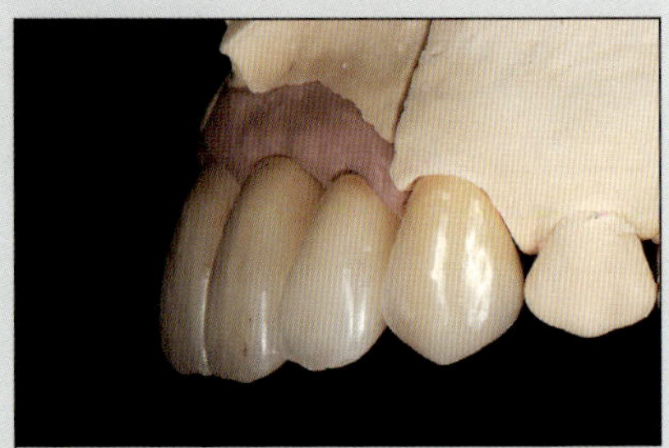

11k

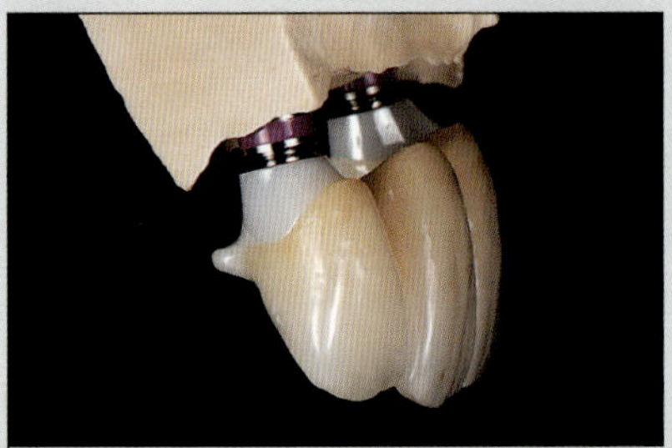

11l

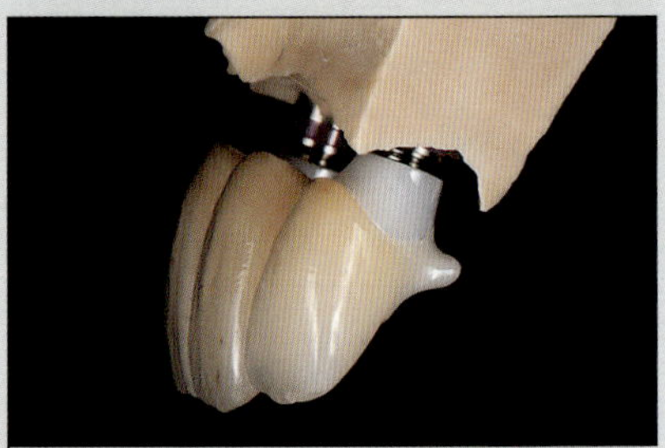

11m

Fig 11n Final prosthesis in place. A favorable gingival framework has been established after well-planned surgical and prosthetic treatment including implant positioning.

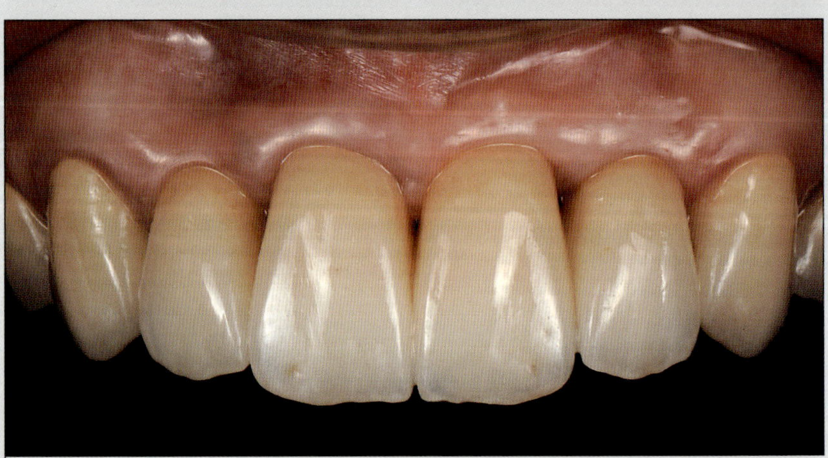

11n

CASE 6 *Prosthetic Treatment with Asymmetric Tooth Positions*

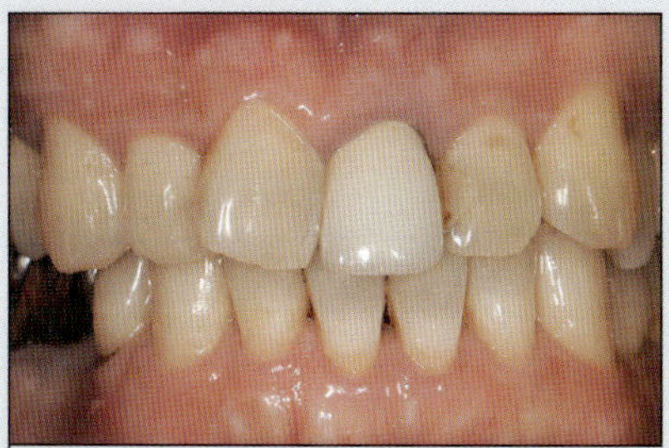
12a

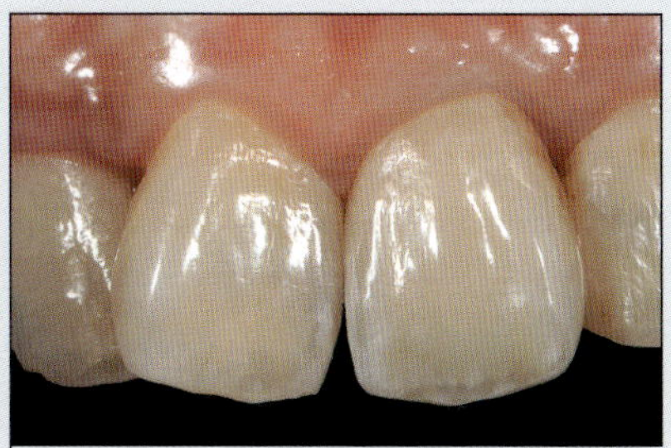
12b

Fig 12a The maxillary left central incisor crown of the patient, a male in his 50s, is esthetically deficient and has a defective marginal fit.

Fig 12b Posttreatment photograph of the all-ceramic crown (IPS e.max Press). Color is reproduced well.

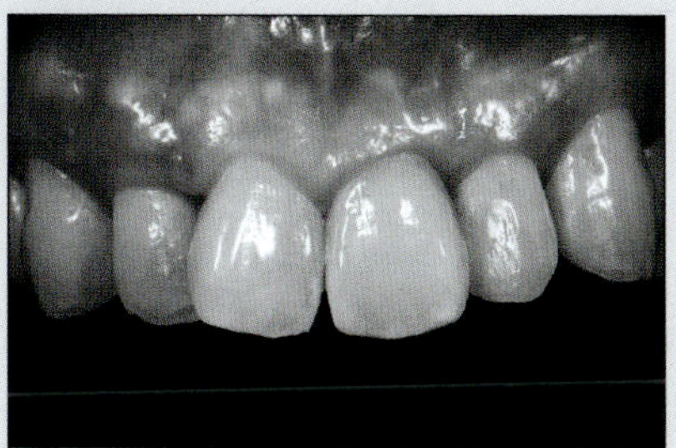
12c

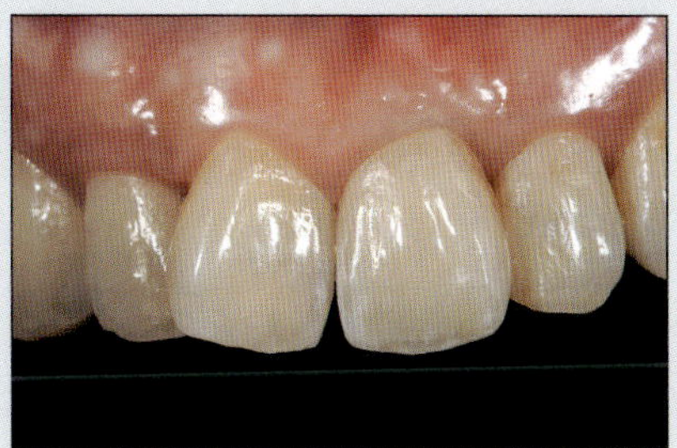
12d

Figs 12c and 12d Consideration was given to the shape and tooth alignment to harmonize with rest of the dentition under the limited prosthetic condition caused by asymmetric tooth positioning and gingival levels. (Courtesy of Takino Dental Clinic, Japan.)

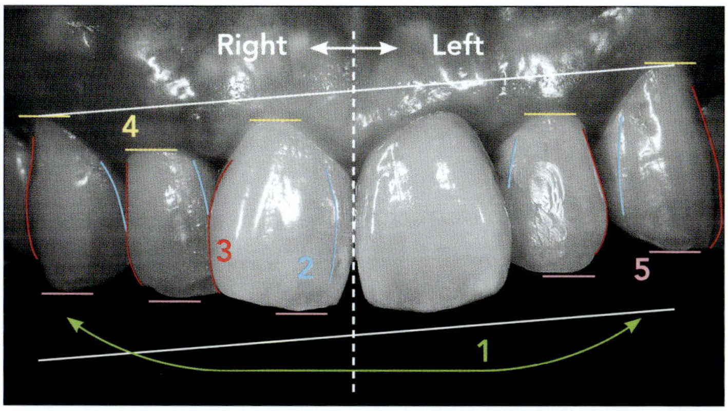

Fig 13 Some balance must be created and maintained in the dentition even when perfect symmetry is not required. Factors that influence the esthetic result of the restored dentition are enumerated and explained.

1: Tooth alignment	Central incisor is the starting point of the dentition. Alignment condition is determined by the size of teeth and alveolar ridge. Shape and alignment of the central incisor influences the impression of the mouth, which represents the personality. Acceptable symmetry of the two central incisors is inevitable.
2: Mesial line angle	Mesial line angle produces regularity of the dentition, which continues toward posterior teeth. Some irregularity is allowed according to the existing dentition and the prosthetic condition.
3: Distal outline	Distal outline produces the contour of the dentition. Harmonized outline of each tooth produces regularity of the dentition.
4: Gingival level	Gingival level affects length of the clinical crown. Symmetry and continuity is required. In this case, gingival level was controlled by subgingival contouring considering the symmetry and continuity toward the canine area (high-low-high gingival level relationship).
5: Incisal edge level	Incisal edge level affects length of the clinical crown as well as the gingival level. In this case, it was designed slightly longer to compensate for the incline of the facial cusp line.

Table 2 **Evaluation of Coronal-Gingival Balance Before and After Treatment Based on the Relationship Between Interdental Papillae and Gingival Zenith Points**

Gingival zenith point and interdental papilla	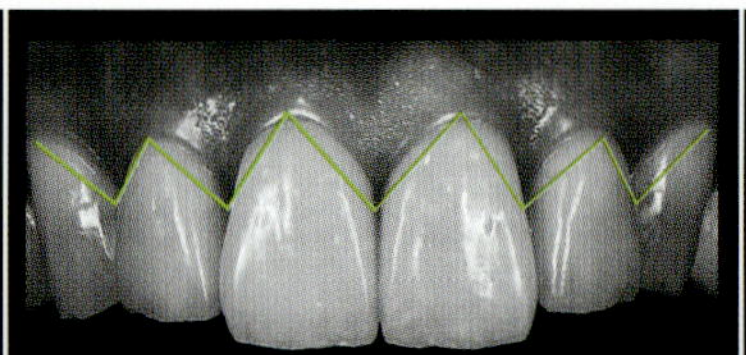 Regular type	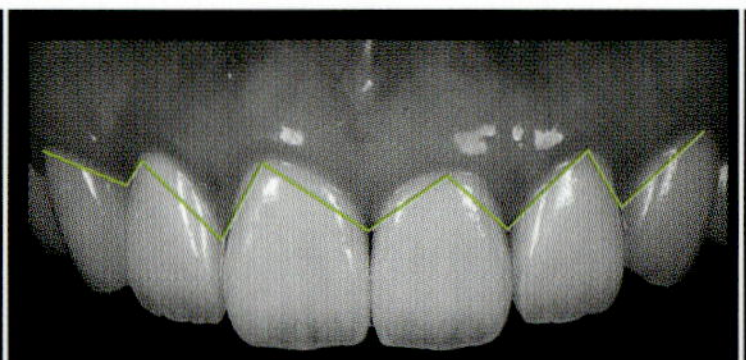 Irregular type	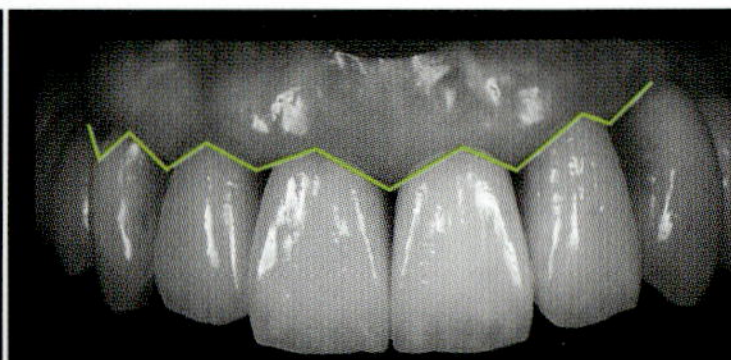 Flat type
Evaluation of coronal-gingival balance	Good symmetry of gingival framework and interdental papillae. Tooth position and periodontium are within normal limits. Well-balanced coronal-gingival relationship.	Asymmetric gingival framework and irregular undulation exists. Tooth positions and periodontium are unfavorable. Unbalanced coronal-gingival relationship.	Symmetry of gingival framework exists to an extent, but undulation is flat due to recession of interdental papillae. This condition is often found with fixed partial denture or implant cases.
Prosthetic approach	If gingival consideration is not required, supragingival prosthetic approach is possible. The dentition can be restored using the anatomical crown shape of the natural teeth.	Set position of finish line of the prosthesis must be carefully considered. Analysis of axial surfaces including subgingival contours using the provisional restoration is required.	Recession of interdental papillae results in black triangles, which must be eliminated using half pontics or the long proximal contact technique. These modifications of the proximal area tend to result in deviation from the natural anatomical tooth shape.
Form arrangement	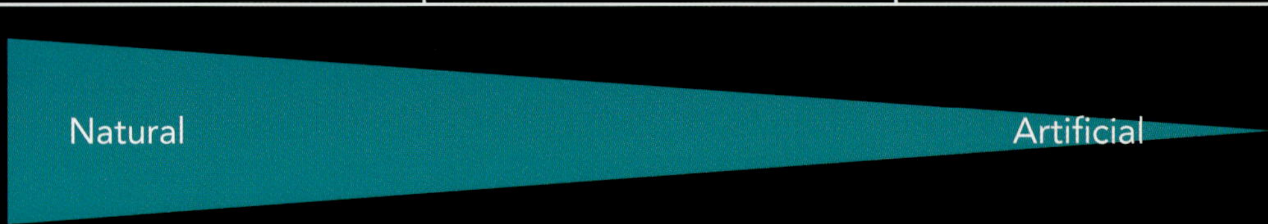		

SOLUTIONS FOR OTHER CASES

Some cases do not fit easily into the classifications described in Table 1. Creativity as well as some compromise considering tooth positions is required to harmonize the total esthetics, as in Case 6 (Fig 12).

Natural Beauty from Asymmetry

Perfect right-left symmetry does not exist in nature, nor does it exist in the mouth. This subtle asymmetry produces natural beauty.

Perfect symmetry is "imaginary beauty," which is created by human desire. Reasonable symmetry produces a more natural, dynamic look (eg, Case 6) than perfect, artificial symmetry. Delicate consideration of the dentition, including the periodontium, leads to the production of a natural-looking prosthesis that will be in harmony with its surrounding environment (Fig 13).

CORONAL-GINGIVAL BALANCE

Symmetry and balance of the crown and gingiva can be evaluated simply by connecting the interdental papillae and gingival zenith points. This relationship can be classified into three types: regular, irregular, and flat. In dentitions with irregular or flat types, prosthetic treatment may require a special arrangement (such as half pontics or long proximal contacts to close the interproximal space; consideration of the axial surface including subgingival contour) in addition to restoring the natural anatomical shape (Table 2).

CONCLUSIONS

Thorough examination and diagnosis of the prosthodontic condition is vital to set the ideal treatment goals for the prosthesis and gingival health. This article has presented gingival esthetics evaluation criteria, with clinical cases showing components of the gingival framework in esthetic areas as well as prosthetic considerations for gingival designs.

REFERENCES

1. Tsuchiya K. Comprehensive Treatment Strategy for Successful Prosthetic Treatment [in Japanese]. Tokyo: Ishiyaku, 2010.
2. Saadoun AP, LeGall M, Touati B. Selection and ideal tridimensional implant position for soft tissue aesthetics. Pract Periodontics Aesthet Dent 1999;11:1163–1072.
3. Obama T. Anterior Esthetic Rehabilitation of Implants: Prosthetic Guidelines and Surgical Treatment Strategy According to the Treatment Purpose [in Japanese]. Tokyo: Quintessence, 2007.
4. Obama T. Esthetic Restoration for Anterior Teeth for Natural Teeth: Differential Diagnosis According to Difficulties and its Treatment Strategy [in Japanese]. Tokyo: Quintessence, 2007.
5. Fürhauser R, Florescu D, Benesch T, Haas R, Mailath G, Watzek G. Evaluation of soft tissue around single-tooth implant crowns: The pink esthetic score. Clin Oral Implants Res 2005;16:639–644.
6. Honda M, Minami M, Yonezawa D, Ito Y. Search for selection criteria of implant prosthesis and conventional fixed prosthesis for maxillary anterior area to fulfill the patient's needs and predictability [in Japanese]. QDT 2007;32(10):18–47.
7. Kois JC. Altering gingival levels: The restorative connection. Part 1: Biologic variables. J Esthet Restor Dent 1994;6:3–7.
8. Elian N, Jalbout ZN, Cho SC, Froum S, Tarnow DP. Realities and limitations in the management of the interdental papilla between implants: Three case reports. Pract Proced Aesthet Dent 2003;15:737–744.
9. Tarnow DP, Magner AW, Fletcher P. The effect of the distance from the contact point to the crest of bone on the presence or absence of the interproximal dental papilla. J Periodontol 1992;63:995–996.
10. Seibert JS, Cohen DW. Periodontal considerations in preparation for fixed and removable prosthodontics. Dent Clin North Am 1987;31:529–555.
11. Sulikowski A, Yoshida A. Management of three-dimensional proportion of anterior crown shape. The coordinates for esthetic restoration [in Japanese]. QDT 2001;26(9):30–40.

BIBLIOGRAPHY

Adolfi D. Natural Esthetics. Chicago: Quintessence, 2002.

Chiche GJ, Aoshima H. Smile Design. Chicago: Quintessence, 2004.

Fradeani M, Yamazaki M (eds). Esthetic Rehabilitation. Vol 1: Esthetic Analysis for Prosthodontic Treatment [in Japanese]. Tokyo, Quintessence, 2006.

Hajto J, Ohata K (eds). Dental Laboratory Supplement. Photo Gallery of Natural Teeth for Esthetic Dental Treatment [in Japanese]. Tokyo: Ishiyaku, 2009.

Hidaka T, Takahashi K. Subgingival contour of implant superstructure. Part I: Decision-making method of the crown shape by team approach [in Japanese]. QDT 2007;32(1):22–44.

Ide Y, Kuwata M, Nishikawa Y. Dental Laboratory Supplement. Biological Crown Contour, Biologically Harmonized Crown Shape [in Japanese]. Tokyo: Ishiyaku, 2008.

Kataoka S, Mutobe Y. Harmony with nature: Part 4 [in Japanese]. In: QDT Supplement Year Book 2000. Tokyo: Quintessence, 2000.

Minami M. Case presentation of missing maxillary single anterior tooth: Periodontal tissue preservation by socket seal surgery [in Japanese]. QDI 2006;13(2):45–53.

Mutobe Y. Basic concept of periodontal tissue and its clinical significance for esthetic prosthodontics of anterior area: Margin placement and crown morphology [in Japanese]. QDT 1999;25(2):28–48.

Nakata K. Periodontal plastic surgery for peri-implant soft tissue to improve predictability [in Japanese]. QDI 2010;17(1):23–42.

Okawa M, Kataoka S. Clinical Prosthodontics Supplement: Anterior 6 White & Pink Esthetics [in Japanese]. Tokyo: Ishiyaku, 2013.

Okawa M, Onishi K, Otake A, et al. Esthetics of dental technology. Part 3: Examination, diagnosis and laboratory steps [in Japanese]. In: QDT Supplement 2004. Tokyo: Quintessence, 2004.

Palacci P, Ericsson I (eds). Implant Esthetic Dentistry: Soft and Hard Tissue Management. Chicago: Quintessence, 2000.

Shigeno K. Periodontal plastic surgery manual for prosthodontic treatment [in Japanese]. Clin Prosthodont 2000;33(1–6):74–82, 190–191, 288–297, 396–405, 526–541, 643–652.

Takahashi K. Clinical guideline of anterior implant prosthesis and labial off-set design concept [in Japanese]. In: Naoki Hayashi N, Takahashi K (eds). Dental Laboratory Supplement. Collaboration Method and Prosthesis Fabrication Technique for Esthetic Restoration [in Japanese]. Tokyo: Ishiyaku, 2012:118–127.

Takahashi K. Subgingival contour of implant suprastructure. Part I/II: Information and discussion points the dental technician should know [in Japanese]. QDT 2007;32(2):15–38.

Takahashi K. Suggestion for team approach in esthetic restorative treatment [in Japanese]. QDT 2008;33(7–8):17–36, 13–42.

Takino H. Art & strategy for tissue management of esthetic area. Surgical treatment strategy for periodontium around anterior natural teeth [in Japanese]. The Quintessence 2011;30(8):90–107.

Tsuzuki Y. Masterpiece: Color reproduction considering emission of natural teeth [in Japanese]. QDT 2013;38(1):86–93.

Tsuzuki Y, Ito Y. Masterpiece/The biological esthetics: Ceramic work with biological harmony and balance [in Japanese]. QDT 2010; 35(6):115–122.

Ubassy G. Analysis: The New Way in Dental Communication. Villa Carcina, Italy: Teamwork Media, 1996.

Yamazaki M. Dental Esthetics. Part 4: Theory and Clinical of Cutting Edge Approach to Esthetic Restoration [in Japanese]. In: Quintessence Year Book 2002. Tokyo: Quintessence, 2002.

Yamazaki M, Minami M. Requirement of a crown contour is support of gingivae [in Japanese]. Clin Prosthodont 2001;34(6):638–657.

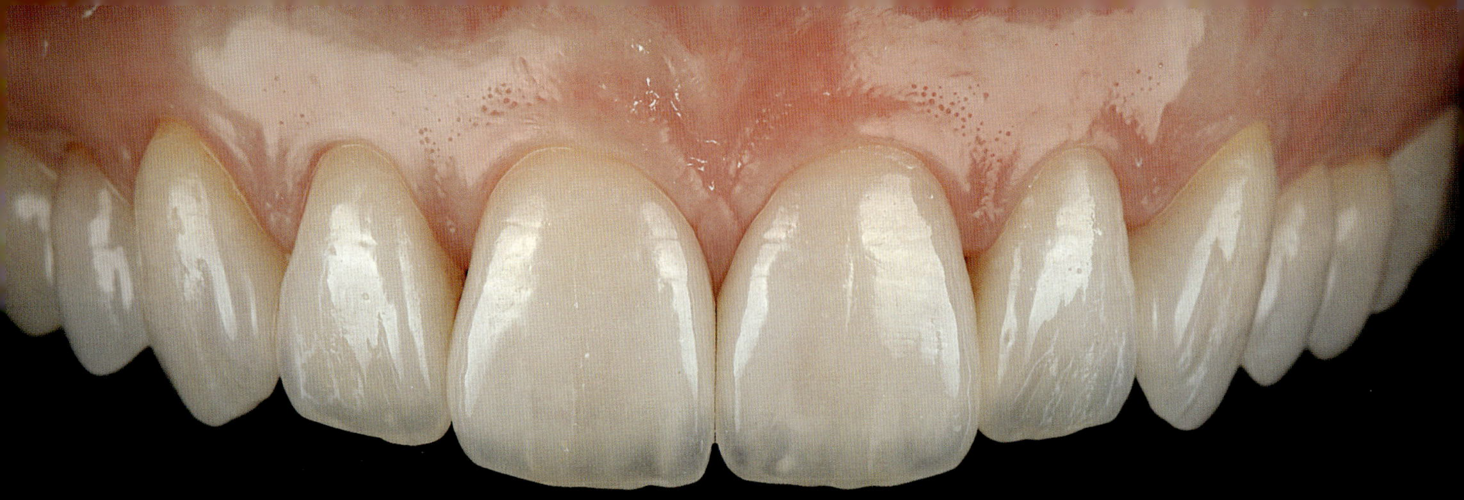

Esthetic Rehabilitation of the Patient with Tetracycline Discoloration and Diastema

Gadzhy Dazhaev, DMD[1]
Thomas Sing, MDT[2]

Providing dental rehabilitation for patients with tetracycline-discolored teeth sets a number of tasks before the clinician, including treatment planning and design and degree of tooth preparation. In addition, there may be a conflict between the desire to conduct minimally invasive dental treatment and the need to achieve the desired esthetic result.

The following case report describes the treatment of a patient with the combined esthetic problems of discolored teeth and presence of significant diastemas between the teeth.

CASE REPORT

A 30-year-old woman came to the dental clinic with a chief complaint of dissatisfaction with the appearance of her teeth and, in particular, their color and shape and the presence of spaces between the teeth. In addition, the patient stated that she did not want orthodontic treatment (Fig 1).

Examination

The examination covered three areas, periodontal, functional, and esthetic, with the use of a risk assessment system in each:

Periodontium

The patient presented with a healthy periodontal condition.

Function

The following functional issues were identified:

- A shift from centric relation (CR) position to maximum intercuspation (MIP) position of ≤ 0.5 mm
- Deep vertical overlap
- Presence of vertical wear facets on the facial surfaces of the mandibular incisors and the palatal surfaces of the maxillary incisors
- Vertical pattern of movement of the mandible
- No problems with masticatory muscles or the temporomandibular joint (TMJ)

[1]Private Practice, Moscow, Russia.

[2]Master Dental Technician, Oral Design New England, Boston, Massachusetts, USA.

Correspondence to: Dr Gadzhy Dazhaev, 2 Novy Pereulok 3-5 17, 107140, Moscow, Russia. Email: gadzhy@gmail.com

Esthetics
The esthetic examination identified several problems:

- Tetracycline discoloration of teeth
- Large diastemas between the maxillary central incisors and between the lateral incisors, canines, and premolars
- Palatal inclination of teeth

During the history-taking and examination of the patient, the sequence of the three areas listed above does not matter; however, when drawing up the treatment plan, the esthetic aspect is crucial.

Treatment Planning

Esthetics
During facial analysis, the midline, commissural, and interpupillary lines were evaluated.

Digital modeling of the teeth helps to analyze the smile and to perform dentoalveolar analysis. In order to measure the desired dimensional changes of the teeth, a digital ruler calibration was performed. The distance between the distal surfaces of the maxillary central incisors was 17 mm (Fig 2). Using this measurement, the digital ruler was calibrated, and a digital mock-up was performed using Keynote software (Apple).

Closure of gaps between teeth inevitably leads to an increase in the width of the teeth and so, to retain their proportions, their length must also be increased. The use of a calibrated ruler allows one to measure the prospective extension of the central incisors, and digital modeling helps to assess whether the proposed changes are esthetically acceptable (Fig 3).

An occlusal photograph of the maxillary dentition helps in planning changes to the facial volume of the maxillary teeth.

To improve the esthetic concerns of the patient, the following was recommended.

1. Teeth whitening
2. Fabrication of 10 bonded porcelain veneers on the maxillary teeth

Function
The proposed treatment also addressed functional concerns:

1. An equilibration of teeth in CR
2. No creation of a constricted envelope of function when modeling the restorations of the maxillary anterior teeth
3. Fabrication of a nightguard at the conclusion of treatment

Digital Simulation and Fabrication of Diagnostic Guides

Digital simulation of the teeth facilitates communication with the ceramist. A presentation of this clinical case was uploaded to a file-hosting service into a folder shared with the ceramist. Photographs and videos of the patient were shared. Video documentation allowed the ceramist to evaluate the dynamics of the smile and face, mobility of the lips, facial expressions, and phonetics. Both the dentist and the dental technician can insert comments directly onto the slides of the presentation, which facilitates communication and exchange of information.

The technician crafted the diagnostic wax-up of the teeth and forwarded it to the clinician (Fig 4). A polyvinyl siloxane index was created, and the wax model was transferred to the patient's teeth using self-curing composite resin (Luxatemp, DMG) (Fig 5). Phonetic tests were conducted, and the patient's appearance and smile were evaluated (Fig 6).

The design and degree of the tooth reduction was thoroughly discussed with the technician beforehand. The volume of the preparation was determined by the following factors: *(1)* the degree of change in tooth color desired, *(2)* the degree of change in the size and position of the teeth, *(3)* the closing of gaps between teeth, and *(4)* the nature of the occlusal relationship with the opposing dentition.

CASE REPORT

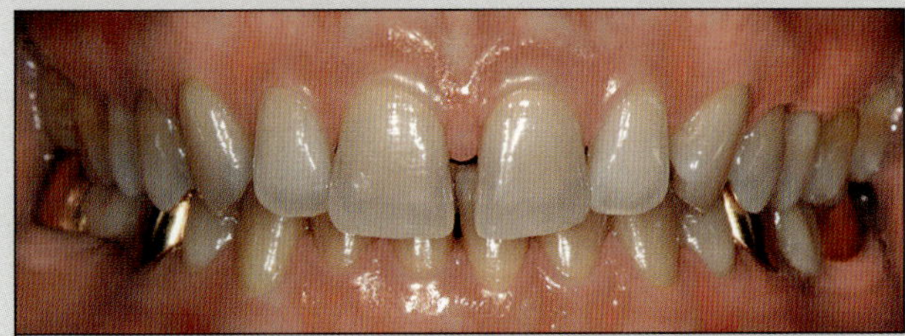

1a

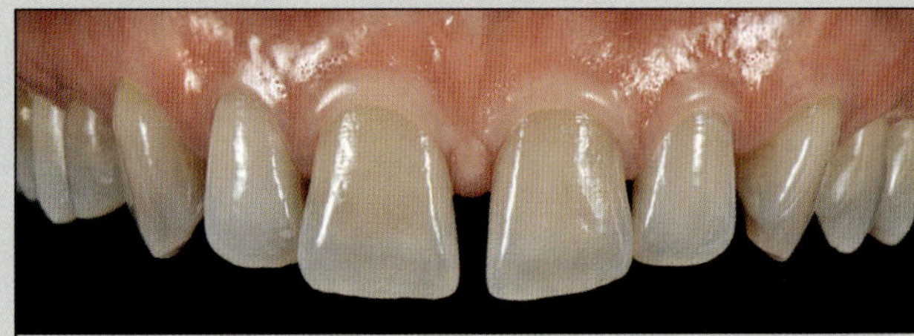

1b

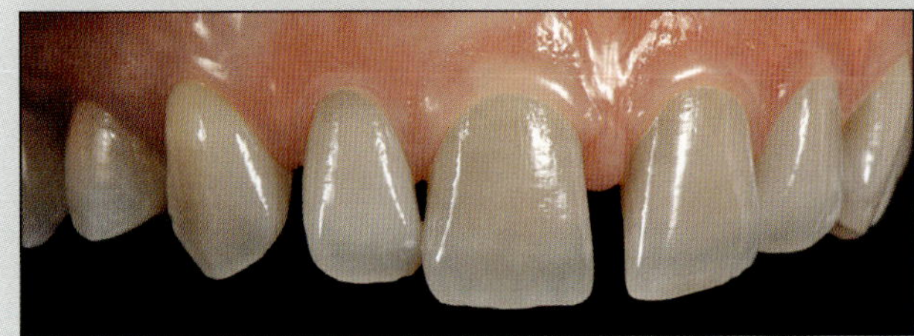

1c

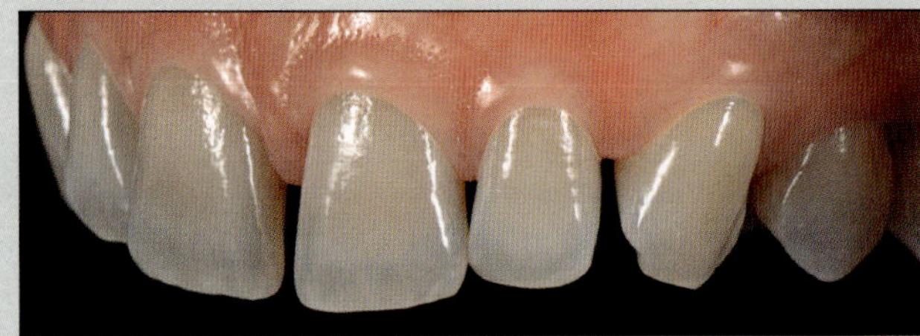

1d

Figs 1a to 1d Initial presentation of a patient with tetracycline-discolored teeth separated by significant diastemas.

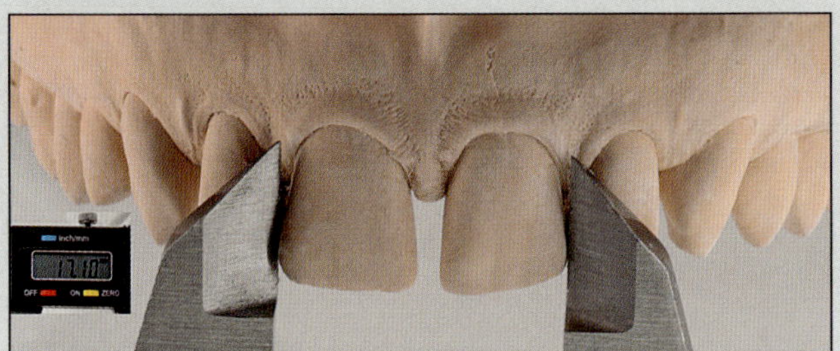

Fig 2 Distance between the distal surfaces of the maxillary central incisors was measured with the use of a caliper.

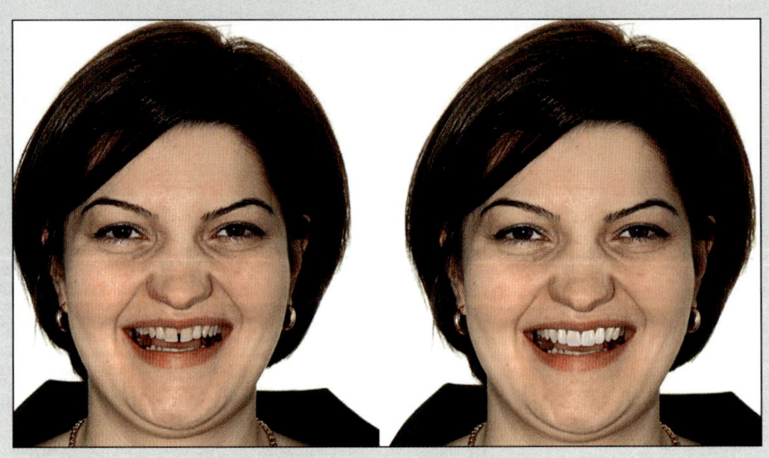

Fig 3 Digital mock-up of the proposed treatment was performed.

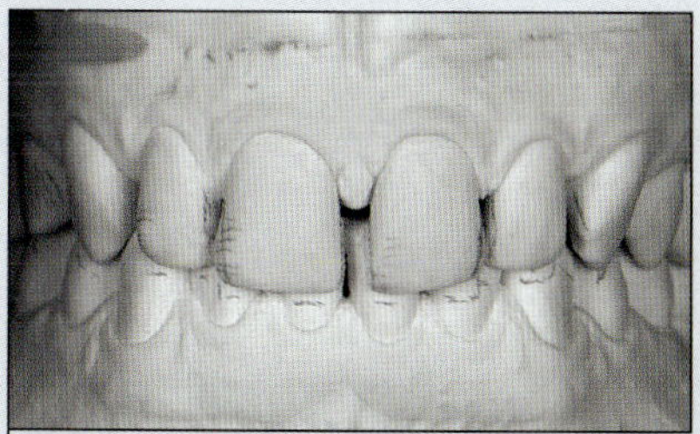
4a

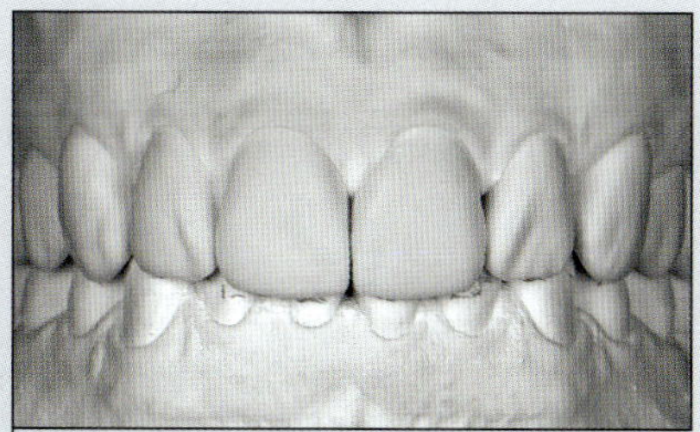
4b

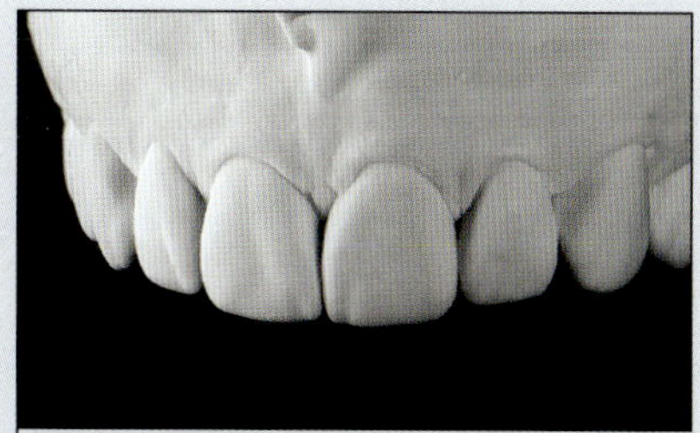
4c

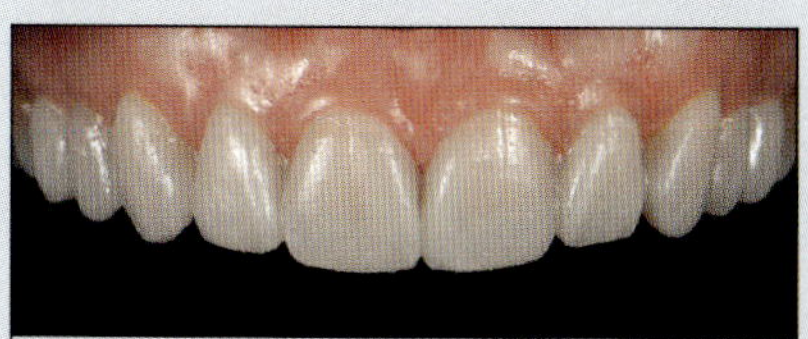
5a

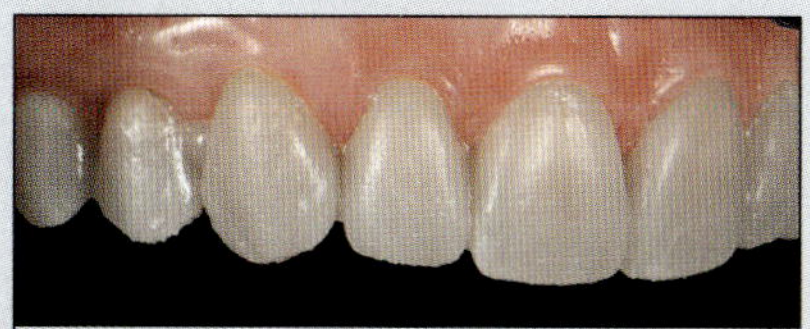
5b

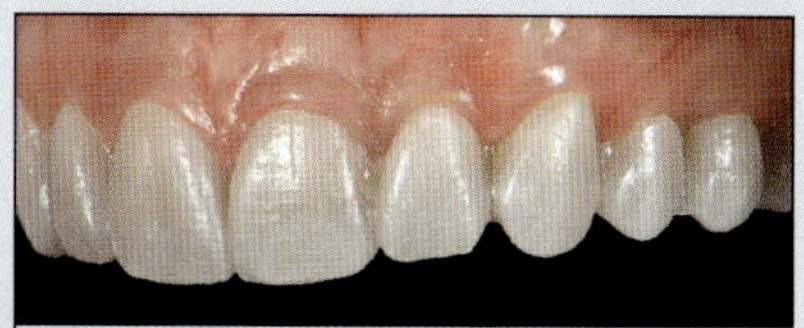
5c

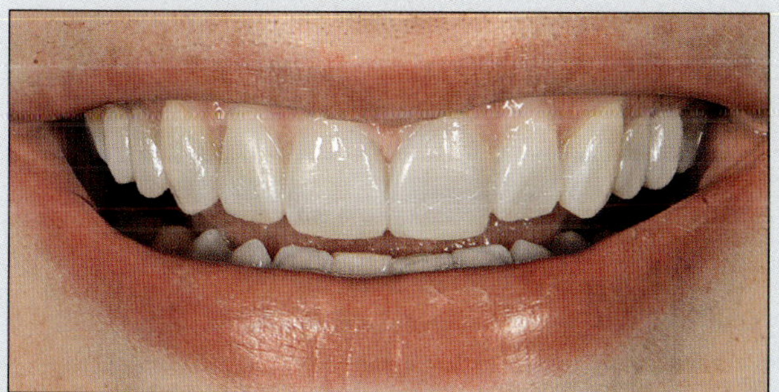
5d

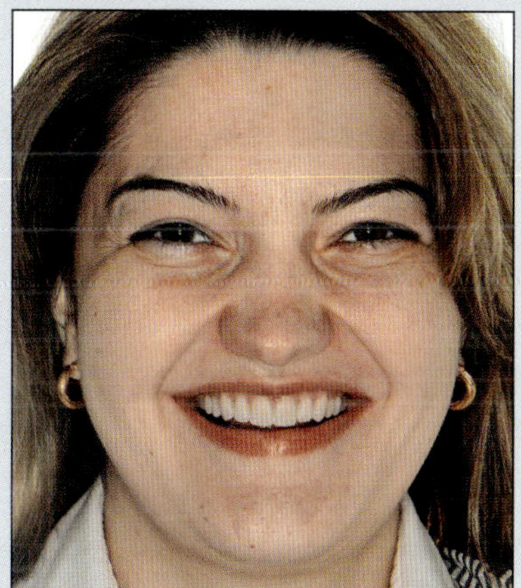
6

Fig 4a Analysis of the casts of initial presentation.

Figs 4b and 4c Casts duplicated from the diagnostic wax-ups.

Figs 5a to 5d Contours of the wax model were transferred to the patient's teeth with the use of a silicone index and self-curing composite resin.

Fig 6 Appearance and smile of patient were evaluated.

Restorative Phase

Treatment of this patient was complicated by two factors: the production of veneers on the mandibular teeth was not planned, and the tetracycline-stained teeth were difficult to whiten. The patient could not fully whiten her teeth because she experienced intense sensitivity during bleaching. Moreover, a significant change in maxillary tooth color by the application of veneers would lead to an unnatural contrast with the mandibular teeth. Thus, it was decided to brighten the maxillary teeth using bonded porcelain veneers so that a subtle difference would remain between the maxillary and mandibular teeth that would be visually imperceptible and simultaneously improve the patient's smile.

This decision was reflected in the degree to which the teeth were prepared. The cervical area was not affected (Fig 7). Nonpreparation veneers were also considered for preservation of tooth structure; however,

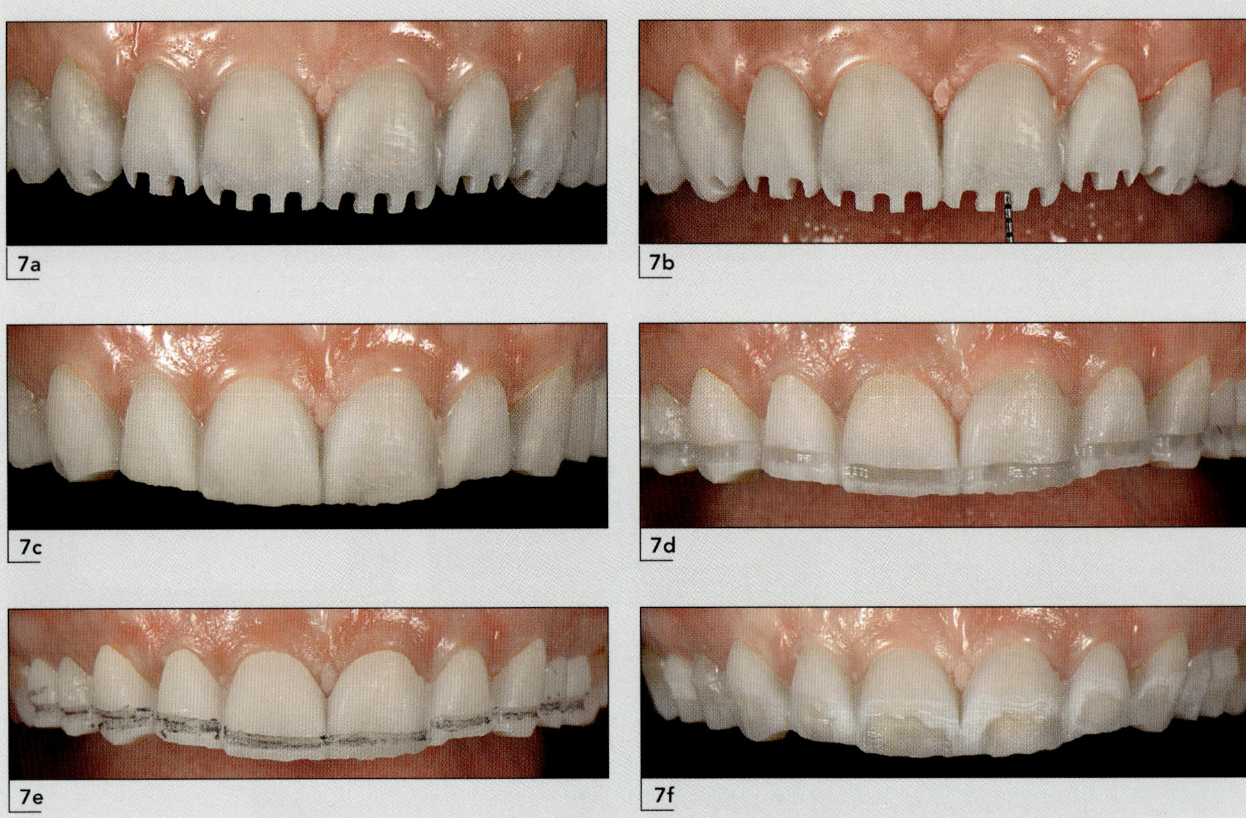

Figs 7a to 7f Preparation of the teeth through the diagnostic mock-up.

an attempt to make nonpreparation veneers in this case would have resulted in the impingement of the overhanging ceramic restoration edges on the gingiva and an unnatural appearance (Figs 8a to 8c). The need to close the gaps between the teeth led to the preparation of interproximal surfaces; otherwise, undercuts would prevent the creation of an accurate marginal fit. The midline papilla was the only area where it was necessary to place the preparation margin below the gingival margin to form a chamfer of 0.1 to 0.2 mm (Figs 8d to 8f; Fig 9). Only in this way was it possible to close such a large diastema between the central incisors and to provide the ceramist the opportunity to create a natural profile of the teeth while at the same time maintaining a healthy condition for the midline papilla. All preparations were performed with the use of a surgical microscope (Carl Zeiss). Facial and palatal silicone keys taken from the wax-up provided an opportunity to assess the degree of tooth reduction (Fig 10).

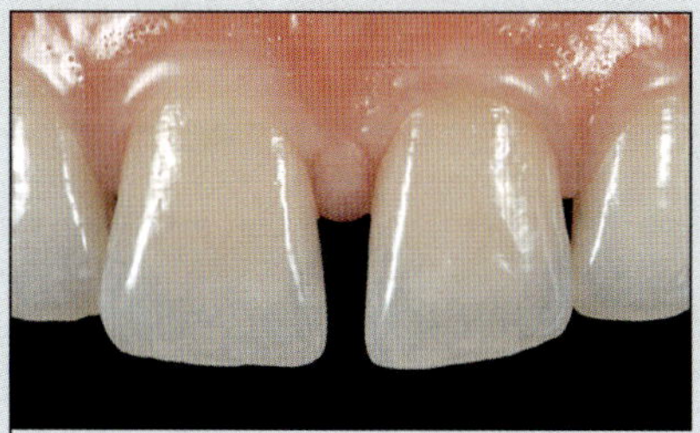

8a

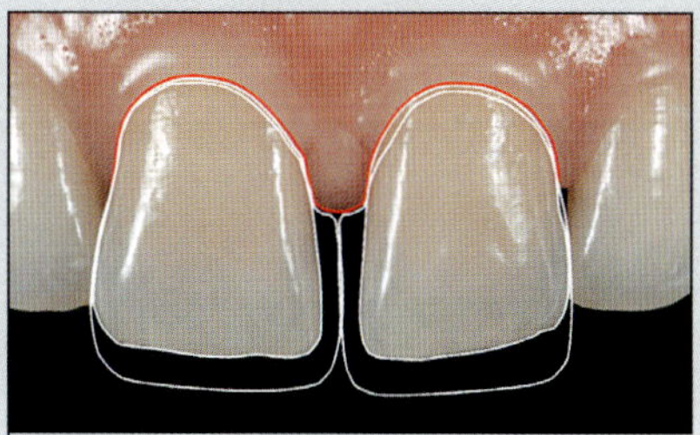

8b

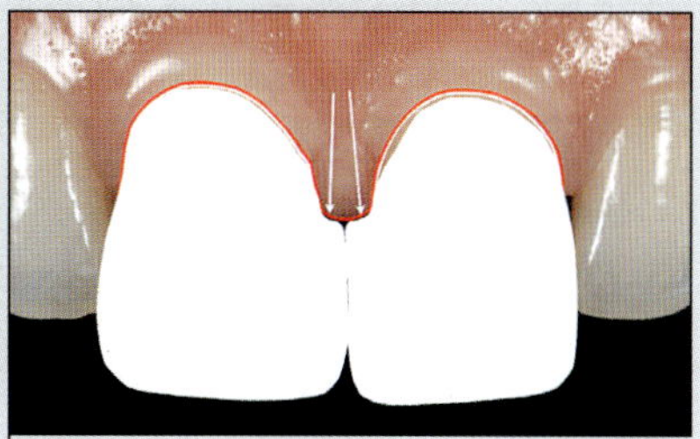

8c

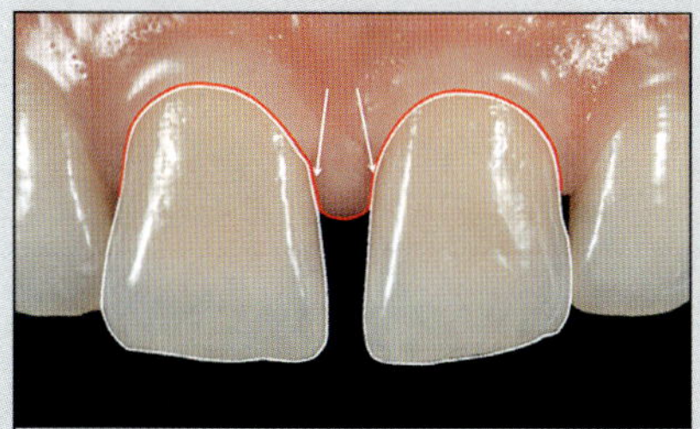

8d

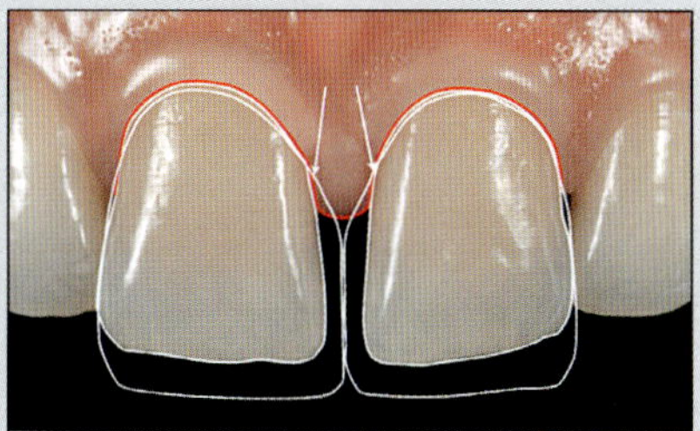

8e

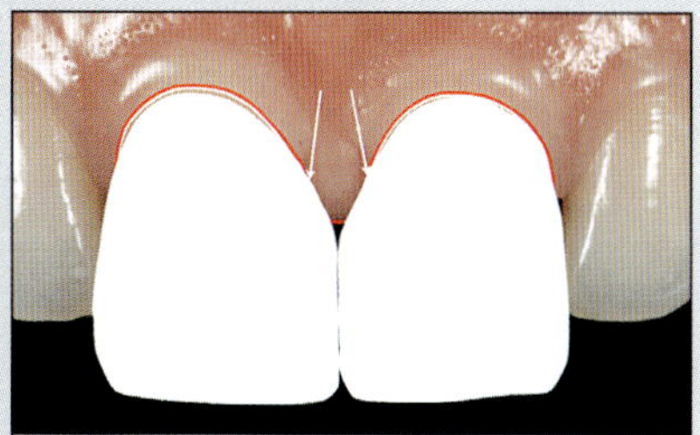

8f

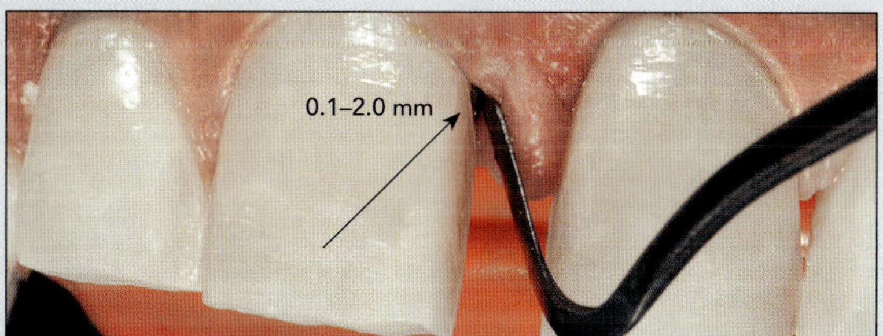

9

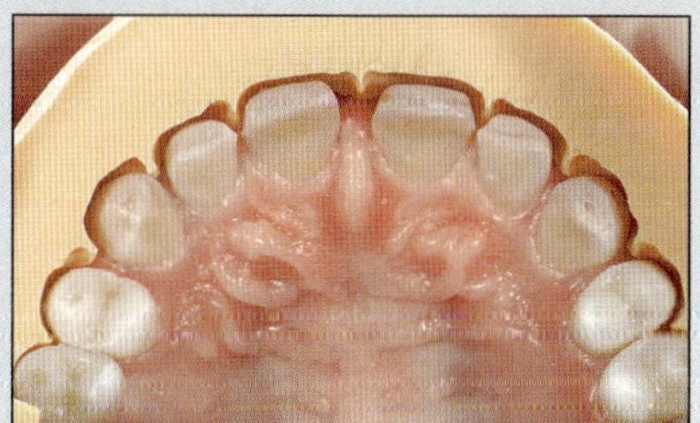

10a

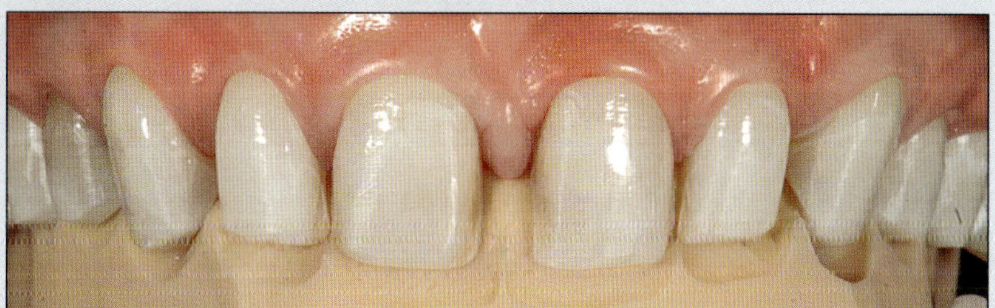

10b

Figs 8a to 8c Nonpreparation veneers would have led to the impingement of the overhanging ceramic restoration edges on the gingiva and an unnatural appearance.

Figs 8d to 8f The midline papilla was the only area where it was necessary to place the preparation margin below the gingival margin.

Fig 9 Small chamfers of 0.1 to 0.2 mm were created below the gingival margin on the mesial surfaces of the central incisors.

Figs 10a and 10b Silicone keys taken from the wax-up helped to assess the degree of tooth reduction.

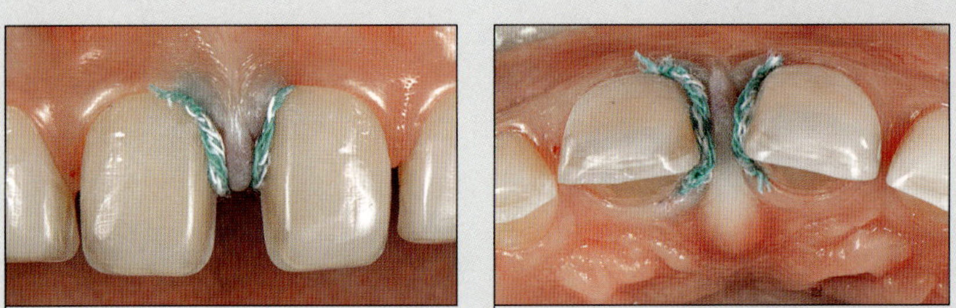

11a 11b

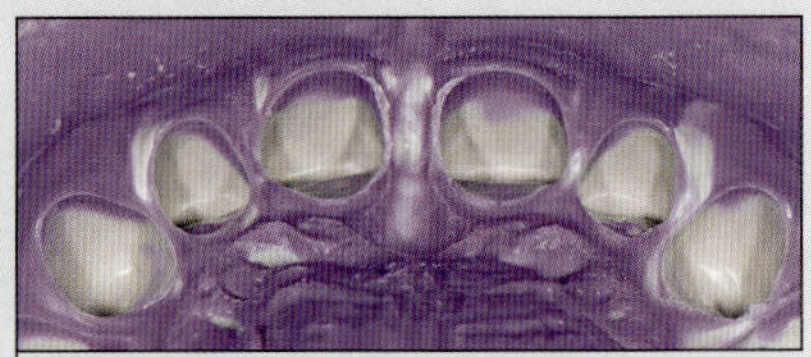

12

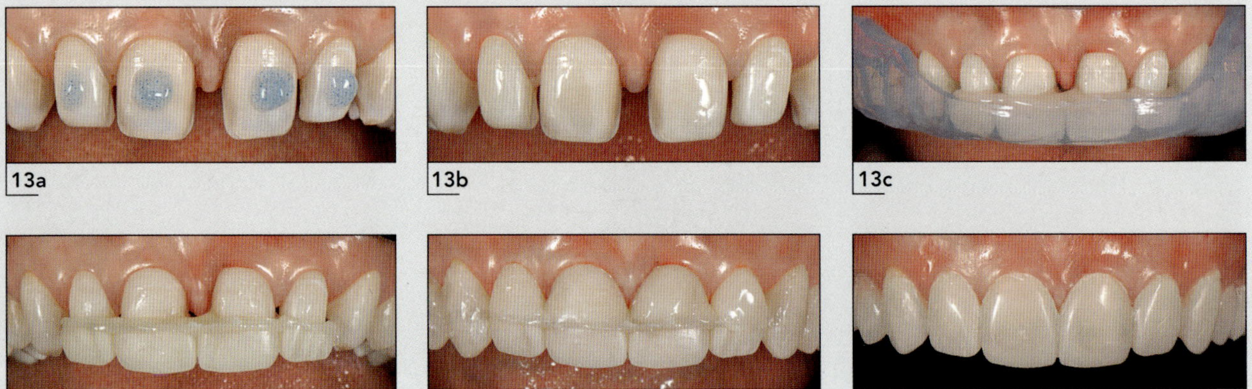

13a 13b 13c 13d 13e 13f

Figs 11a and 11b Gingival retraction cords were required only in the midline papilla area prior to taking impressions.
Fig 12 Impressions were taken with polyvinyl siloxane impression material.
Figs 13a to 13f Fabrication of provisional veneers.

Gingival retraction was only required in the area of the midline papilla prior to taking impressions (Fig 11). Impressions were taken with the polyvinyl siloxane impression material (Express, 3M ESPE) (Fig 12). Provisional veneers were fabricated of composite resin using a spot-etching technique (Fig 13).

In order for the technician to have enough information about the color of the teeth, the maxillary teeth were photographed with shade guide samples before and after the tooth preparation.

After receiving the impressions from the dentist, the technician created three separate casts. The first pour was cut, prepared, and duplicated to make the alveolar cast. After duplication, the first pour was stored and not touched again. The second pour was used for the fabrication of the veneers, and the third pour was needed for final fit tests.

After the technician made the alveolar cast, he poured the same duplication form with refractory die material. One must be aware that the first pour cannot usually be used for the veneer technique because of the presence of impurities. The silicone mold is cleared of the fine layers of residual contaminants by pouring the impression the first time. In addition, one can also check the consistency of the refractory die material. If the first pour looks porous, the refractory die material used might be old and need to be thrown away and a new batch ordered. The technician will use the second pour for layering of the porcelain.

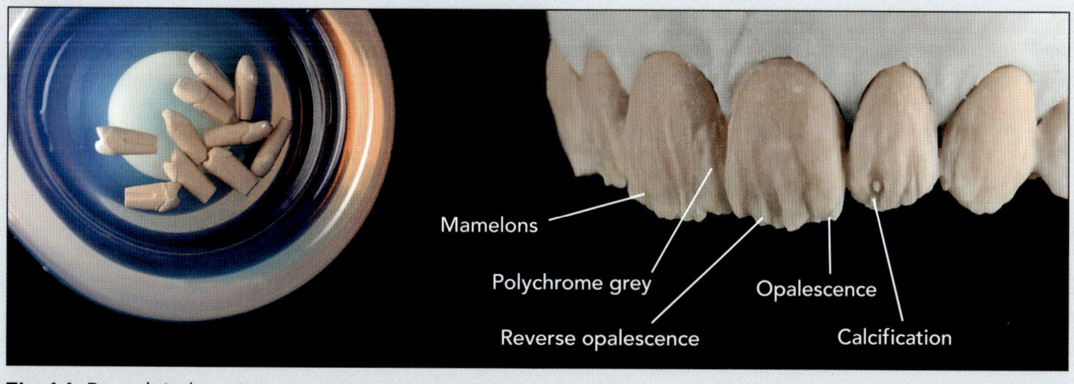

Fig 14 Porcelain layering.

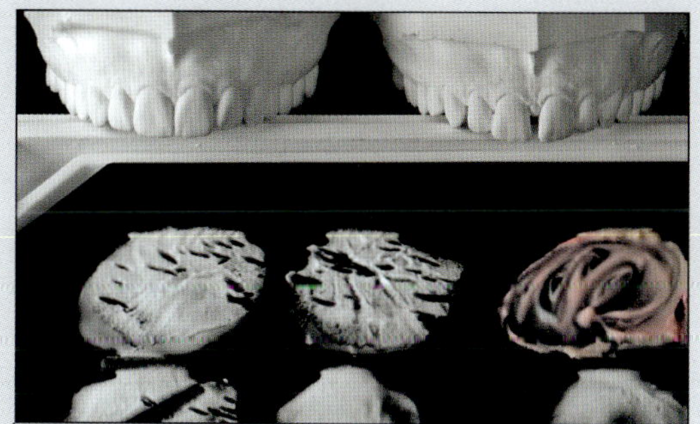

15a

Figs 15a to 15e Laboratory steps of veneer fabrication.

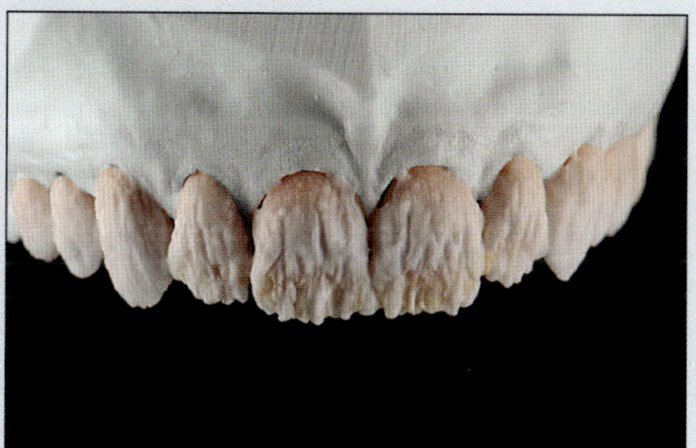

15b

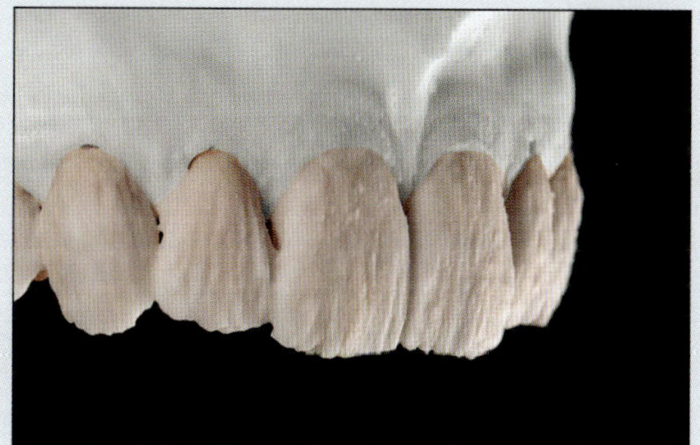

15c

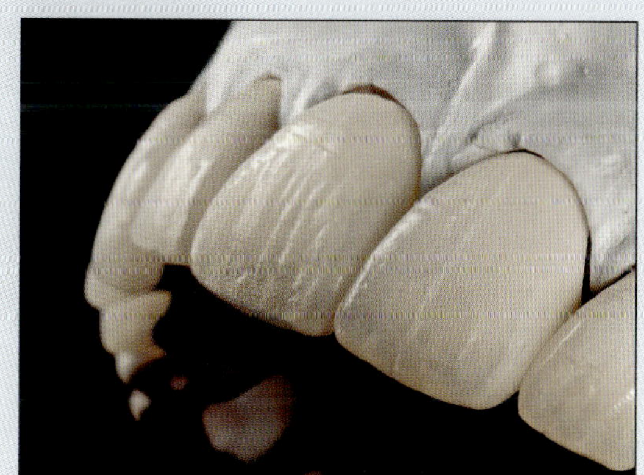

15d

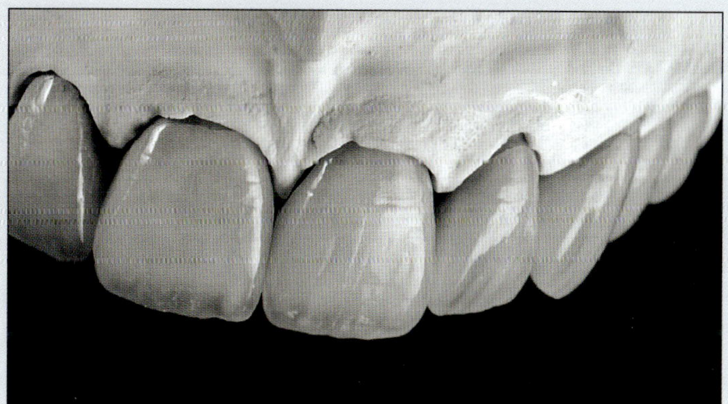

15e

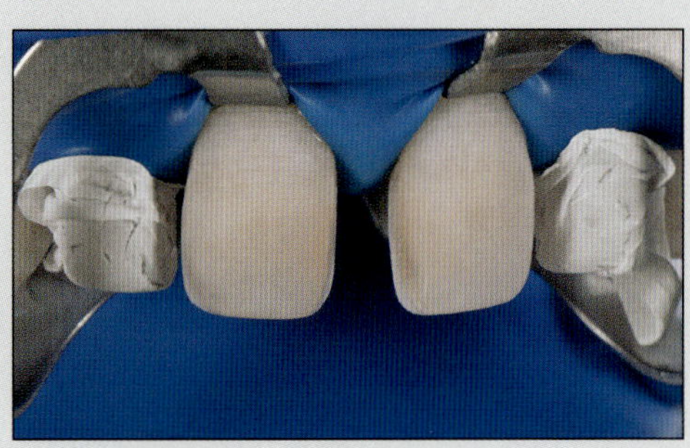

Fig 16a Isolation of the teeth with rubber dam and Teflon tape.

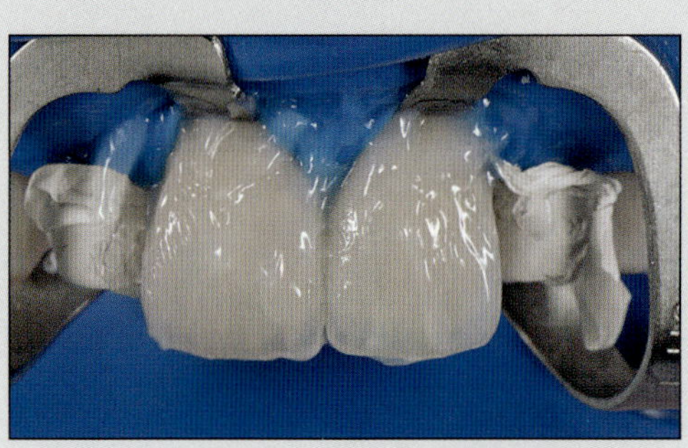

Fig 16b Bonding of the veneers.

The dies were then soaked in distilled water. After at least two connection firings, which close the still minimally porous surface of the refractory die and prevent the ceramic margins from lifting off the die during the firing cycles, the ceramist started the stratification of the feldspathic porcelain (Willi Geller Creation, Klema). Mamelons, opalescence, fluorescence, a balance of opacity and translucency, reverse opalescence, and the use of polychrome grey are needed to create a lifelike natural appearance of the ceramic work (Fig 14).

After the veneers proceeded through the different ceramic firings, surface texture treatment, and glaze firing, as well as high-gloss polishing of the margins and pumice polishing of the labial aspects, they were divested from the refractory die material by using glass beads at the maximum pressure of 1.5 bar. The technician used the two models or die sets he had left to confirm the perfect fit of the hair-thin ceramic shells.

After the fit of the veneers was tested, they were cleaned by immersion in a glass bottle filled with 95% ethanol for 10 minutes. The veneers were not etched before sending them to the dentist (Fig 15).

Once the finalized veneers were received from the lab, they were tried in the patient's mouth with the try-in paste to verify the marginal fit and the overall esthetic composition, and the dentist had the patient evaluated and provided feedback as to the esthetic outcome achieved.

Once approved, the veneers were etched for 90 seconds with 9.5% hydrofluoric acid, rinsed, and cleaned in ethanol in an ultrasonic bath for about 10 minutes. The etched surface was then cleaned manually with a small-tipped instrument.

The teeth were isolated with the help of rubber dam and Teflon tape (Fig 16a). Before the adhesive application, the tooth surface was air abraded intraorally with 27-µm aluminum oxide (Rondoflex, KaVo Dental). The veneers were seated, and large amounts of excess cement (Variolink Veneer, Ivoclar Vivadent) were removed with a dry brush and an explorer. After most of the excess cement was removed, the veneers were tack cured for 2 to 3 seconds, the rest of the excess cement was removed, and then the cement was completely polymerized. Glycerin gel was applied, and the cement margins were postcured through the glycerin gel to avoid contact with atmospheric oxygen to eliminate the air-inhibited layer (Fig 16b). The margins were checked and cleaned with a no. 12 scalpel blade and periodontal microscaler.

The final result completely satisfied the patient (Figs 17 to 19). A systematic approach to history taking, examination, and treatment planning allowed the dentist to avoid functional and esthetic problems during implementation.

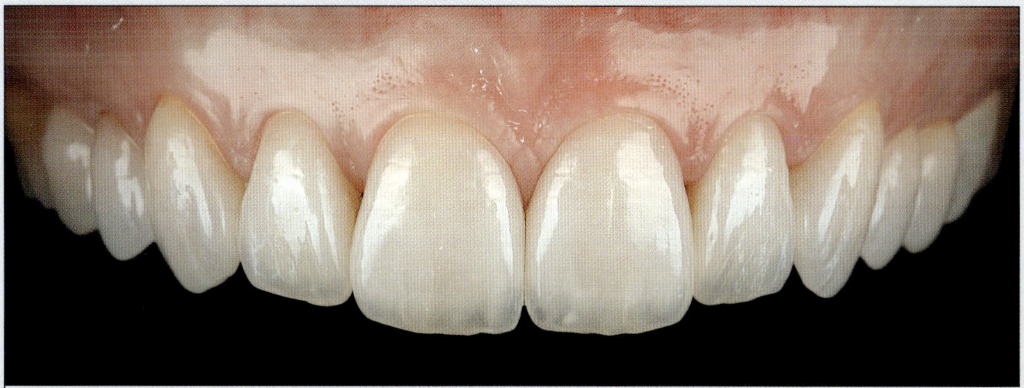

17a

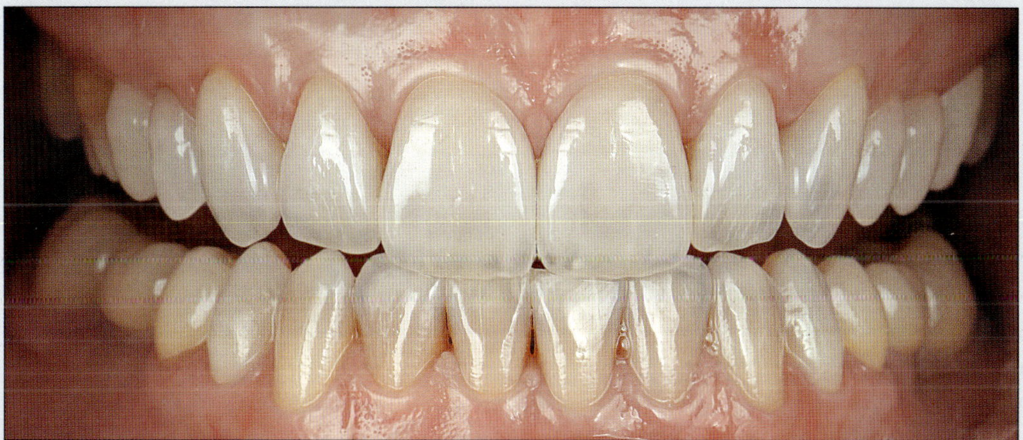

17b

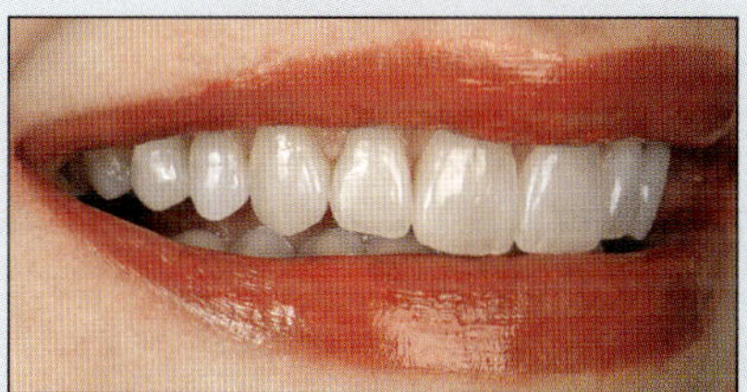

18a

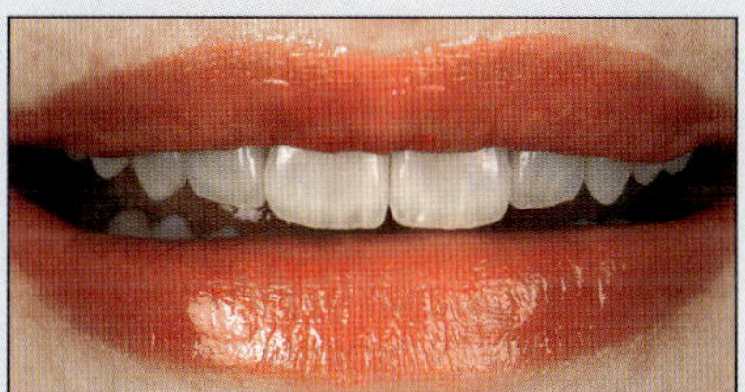

18b

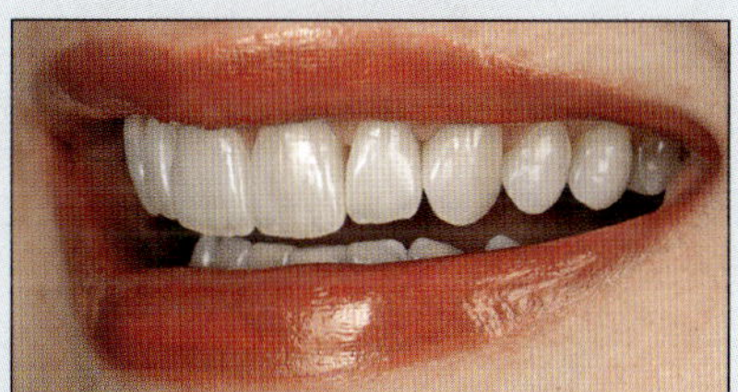

18c

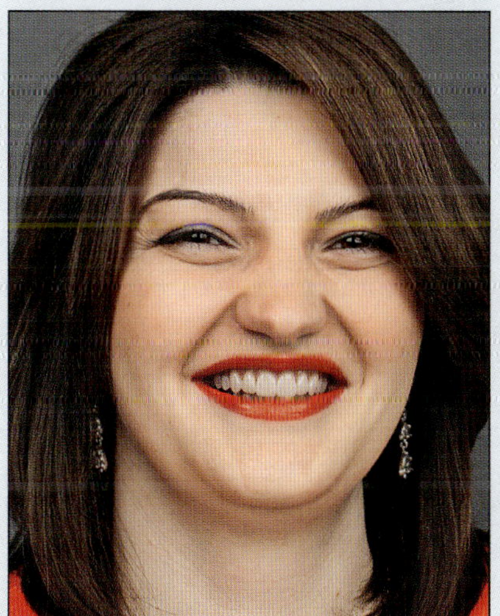

19a

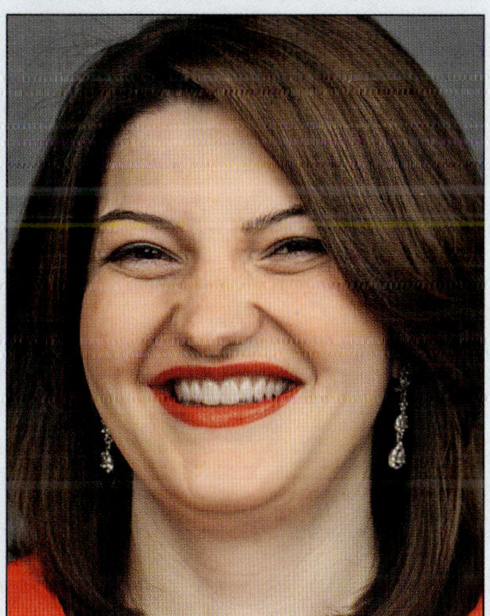

19b

Figs 17a and 17b Intraoral photographs of the final outcome.

Figs 18a to 18c Extraoral photographs of the smile and teeth.

Figs 19a and 19b Patient after completion of treatment.

CONCLUSIONS

With the help of modern means of communication—using the Internet, working with photographic and video documentation, and using presentation software—one can create the correct exchange of information between the clinic and the laboratory, even if they are based on different continents.

Veneers are a very satisfying option for both the patient and the dentist as well as the technician because the transition from "before" to "after" is enormous. With minimal tooth preparation, the patient can be given a big change of smile, appearance, and self-confidence. It requires a great amount of time, knowledge, and skill for the dentist and technician to create very thin porcelain veneers that not only mimic natural enamel but also mask defects and alter the shade and shape of the teeth.

BIBLIOGRAPHY

Coachman C, Calamita MA. Digital smile design: A tool for treatment planning and communication in esthetic dentistry. Quintessence Dent Technol 2012;35:103–111.

Dawson PE. A classification system for occlusions that relate maximal intercuspation to the position and condition of the temporomandibular joints. J Prosthet Dent 1996;75:60–66.

Dawson PE. Functional Occlusion: From TMJ to Smile Design. St Louis: Mosby, 2007.

Dawson PE. Optimum TMJ condyle position in clinical practice. Int J Periodontics Restorative Dent 1985;3:11–31.

Edelhoff D, Sorensen JA. Tooth structure removal associated with various preparation designs for anterior teeth. J Prosthet Dent 2002;87:503–509.

Fradeani M. Esthetic Rehabilitation in Fixed Prosthodontics. Vol 1: Esthetic Analysis: A Systematic Approach to Prosthetic Treatment. Chicago: Quintessence, 2004.

Fradeani M. Evaluation of dentolabial parameters as part of a comprehensive esthetic analysis. Eur J Esthet Dent 2006;1:62–69.

Goldstein MB. No-prep/minimal-prep: The perils of oversimplification. Dent Today 2007;26:10.

Gürel G. Predictable, precise, and repeatable tooth preparation for porcelain laminate veneers. Pract Proced Aesthet Dent 2003;15: 17–24.

Gürel G, Morimoto S, Calamita MA, Coachman C, Sesma N. Clinical performance of porcelain laminate veneers: Outcomes of the aesthetic pre-evaluative temporary (APT) technique. Int J Periodontics Restorative Dent 2012;32:625–635.

Hasanreisoglu U, Berksun S, Aras K, Arslan I. An analysis of maxillary anterior teeth: Facial and dental proportions. J Prosthet Dent 2005;94:530–538.

Kois JC. Diagnostically driven interdisciplinary treatment planning. Seattle Study Club J 2002;6(4):28–34.

Kois JC. "The gingiva is red around my crowns"—A differential diagnosis. Dent Econ 1993;4:101–105.

Kois JC, McGowan S. Diagnostically generated anterior tooth preparation for adhesively retained porcelain restorations: Rationale and technique. J Calif Dent Assoc 2004;32:161–166.

Kokich VO Jr, Kiyak HA, Shapiro PA. Comparing the perception of dentists and lay people to altered dental esthetics. J Esthet Dent 1999;11:311–324.

Magne P, Belser UC. Novel porcelain laminate preparation approach driven by a diagnostic mock-up. J Esthet Restor Dent 2004;16: 7–16.

Magne P, Gallucci GO, Belser UC. Anatomic crown width/length ratios of unworn and worn maxillary teeth in white subjects. J Prosthet Dent 2003;89:453–461.

Magne P, Hanna J, Magne M. The case for moderate "guided prep" indirect porcelain veneers in the anterior dentition. The pendulum of porcelain veneer preparations: From almost no-prep to over-prep to no-prep. Eur J Esthet Dent 2013;8:376–388.

McLaren EA, Garber DA, Figueira J. The Photoshop Smile Design technique (part 1): Digital dental photography. Compend Contin Educ Dent 2013;34:772, 774, 776.

Page R, Martin J, Loeb C. Use of risk assessment in attaining and maintaining oral health. Compendium Contin Educ Dent 2004; 25:657–669.

Schmidt KK, Chiayabutr Y, Phillips KM, Kois JC. Influence of preparation design and existing condition of tooth structure on load to failure of ceramic laminate veneers. J Prosthet Dent 2011;105:374–382.

Spear FM. The maxillary central incisor edge: A key to esthetic and functional treatment planning. Compend Contin Educ Dent 1999; 20:512–516.

Wilkins RG. Using a system of diagnosis and treatment planning to reduce stress. Compend Contin Educ Dent 2000;21:485–492.

State of the Art

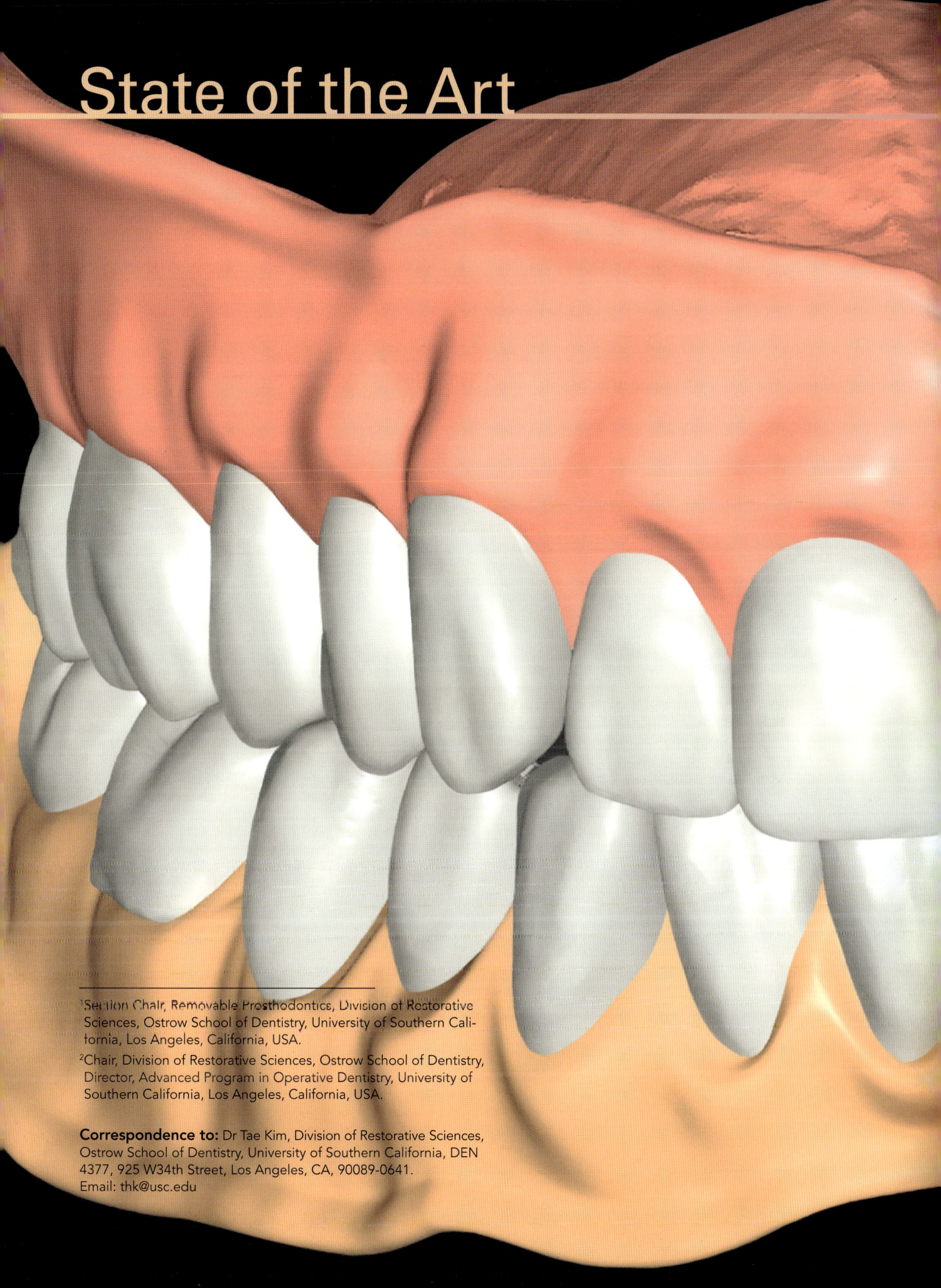

[1]Section Chair, Removable Prosthodontics, Division of Restorative Sciences, Ostrow School of Dentistry, University of Southern California, Los Angeles, California, USA.

[2]Chair, Division of Restorative Sciences, Ostrow School of Dentistry, Director, Advanced Program in Operative Dentistry, University of Southern California, Los Angeles, California, USA.

Correspondence to: Dr Tae Kim, Division of Restorative Sciences, Ostrow School of Dentistry, University of Southern California, DEN 4377, 925 W34th Street, Los Angeles, CA, 90089-0641.
Email: thk@usc.edu

CAD/CAM Technology for Complete Denture Fabrication

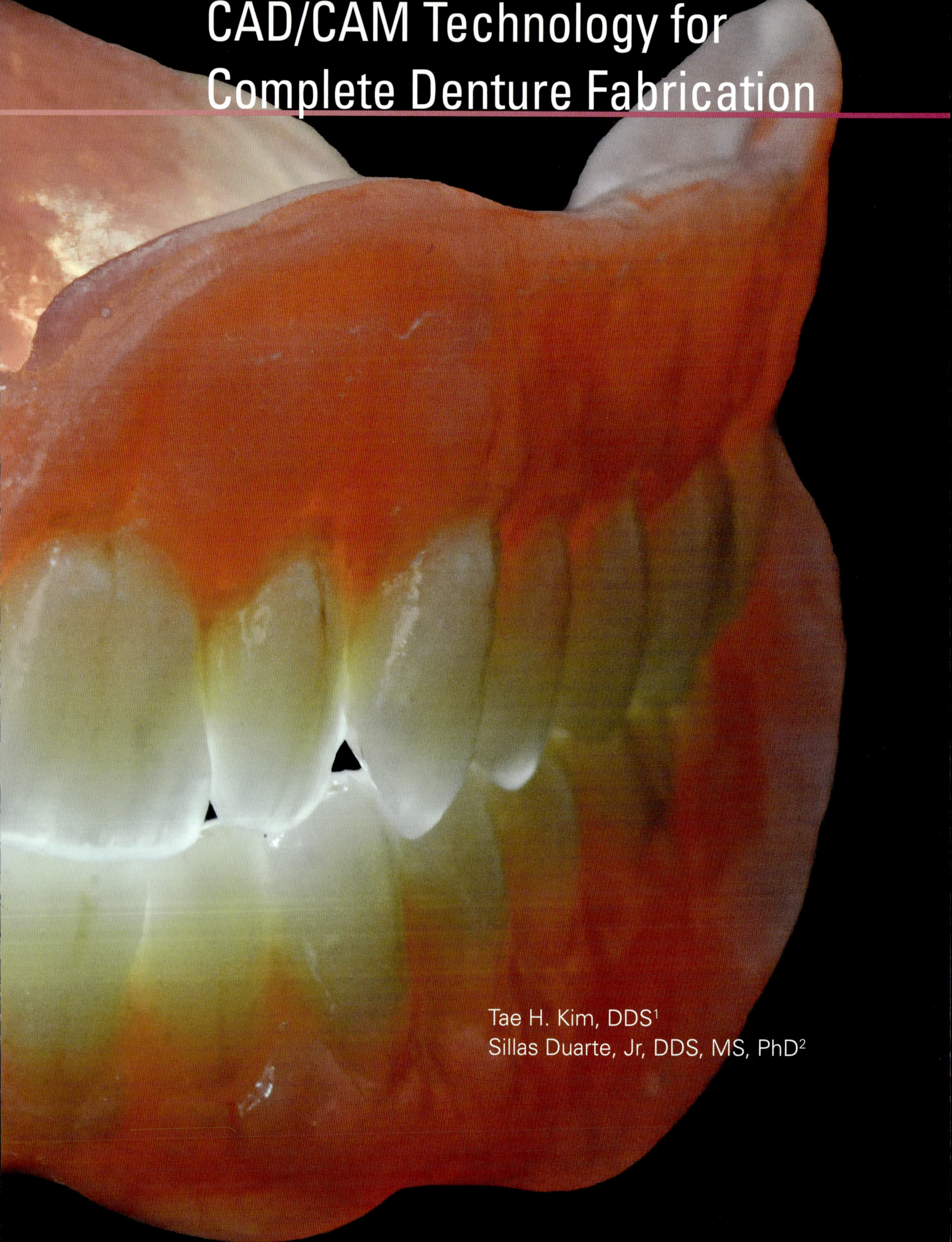

Tae H. Kim, DDS[1]
Sillas Duarte, Jr, DDS, MS, PhD[2]

For decades, the fabrication of complete dentures has involved tedious and time-consuming processes. They include taking the preliminary impressions with stock impression trays, creating a study cast upon which custom trays will be fabricated, taking definitive impressions using the customized trays, constructing occlusal rims with wax, and recording maxillomandibular jaw relations. After these preliminary steps, artificial teeth setup takes place, followed by try-in to ensure proper jaw and occlusal relationships as well as patient comfort and satisfaction.

Undoubtedly, the entire complete denture fabrication process involves a number of visits by the patient, additional time consumed by the dentist, a significant amount of manual labor by the dental technicians, and the possibility of human error and dimensional instability of the dentures. Much effort has been directed toward reducing these processes.[1–4]

In recent years, the use of computer-aided design/computer-assisted manufacture (CAD/CAM) technology (Dentca) has allowed the fabrication of digitally fabricated complete dentures.[5] Dentures created via CAD/CAM software are highly accurate, since there is no manual teeth setup.[6] No plaster model, physical mounting, or wax-up is required.[7] In addition, CAD/CAM dentures are convenient, as only two visits are required. Furthermore, intervention by dental technicians and the subsequent chances for human error are greatly reduced. CAD/CAM dentures remain permanently on record, allowing the digital data to be reused to fabricate duplicate dentures without the need for an additional visit. Lastly, digitally fabricated dentures could make a standardized and controlled study easier to develop and validate scientific data related to removable prostheses.[8]

The following case demonstrates the use of CAD/CAM technology to fabricate a natural-looking complete denture.

PROCEDURES

Maxillary and Mandibular Impressions

The two-piece impression trays provided with the Dentca system are used to take maxillary and mandibular impressions. Each tray has its own separate anterior and posterior components, which can be detached and are provided with a center pin and plate used for jaw relation records. The trays come in various sizes—small, medium, large, and extra large—to best fit the patient's arch (Fig 1).

To record the maxillary impression, fast-setting heavy-body polyvinyl siloxane (PVS) impression material is first loaded onto the tray for the initial customization. The tray is placed in the patient's mouth, seated over the arch, and firm finger pressure is applied on designated finger spots located on the bottom of the tray for 5 seconds, followed by border molding movements. Once the heavy-body PVS is set, any exposed areas of the tray are adjusted with a bur. The tray is then covered with light-body PVS in order to perform the final impression procedure.

The mandibular impression is recorded in exactly the same fashion, with mandibular border molding movements. As before, exposed areas are trimmed and then covered with light-body PVS, and the final impression is taken.

Vertical Dimension and Centric Relation Recording

The posterior segments of both trays are separated along the separation line using a blade (Fig 2). The center pin is attached to the mandibular tray (Fig 3).

Gothic arch tracing is used to record the centric relation (CR) of the jaws, whereby the mandibular stylus draws lines on the maxillary plate to form the shape of an arrow. This requires use of a denture tracing pad (EZ-Tracer, Dentca) on the cameo surface of the maxillary tray (Fig 4). It is inserted with the maxillary tray into the patient's mouth, and the center pin is adjusted clockwise with the fingers or a tweezer until the desired vertical height is reached (Fig 5). If the trays are in contact with each other at any point, those areas can be trimmed with a bur.

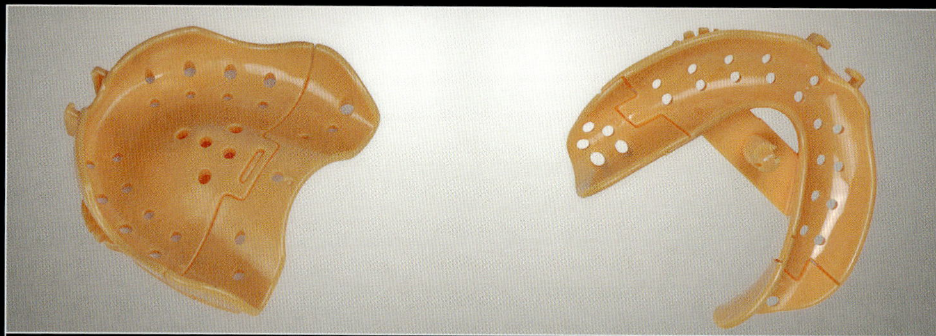

1

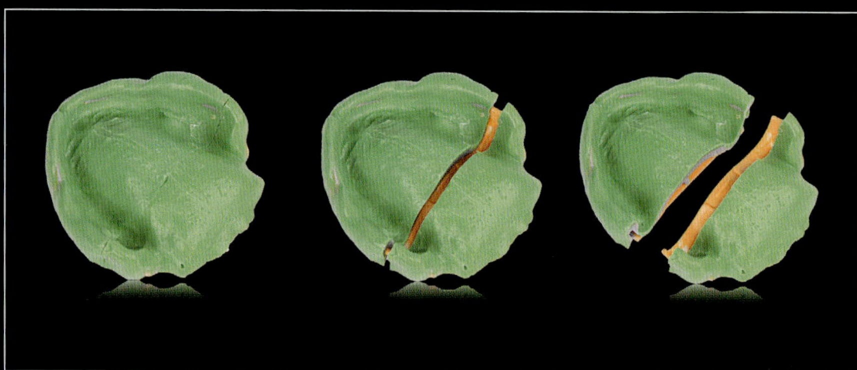

2

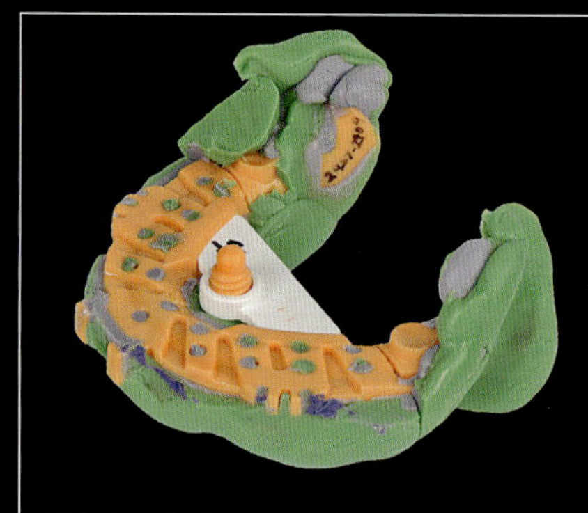

3

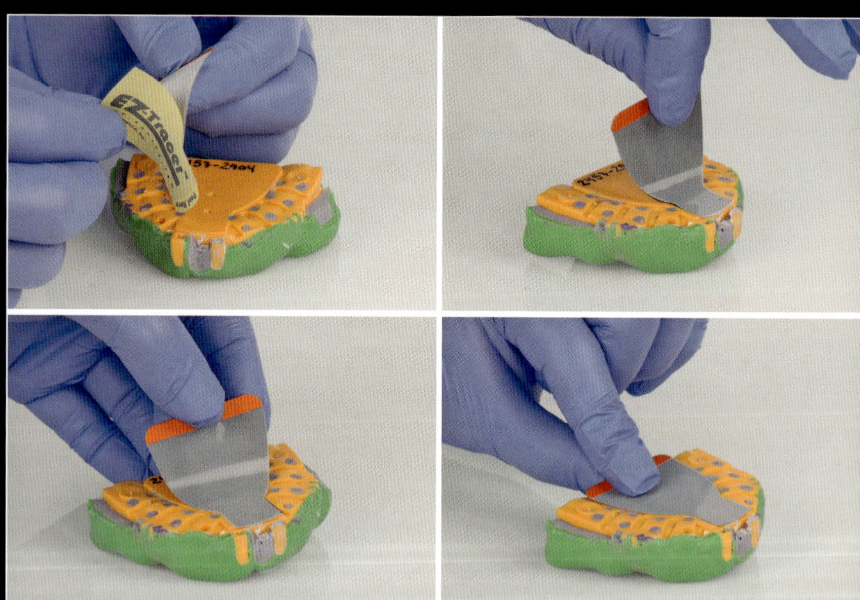

4

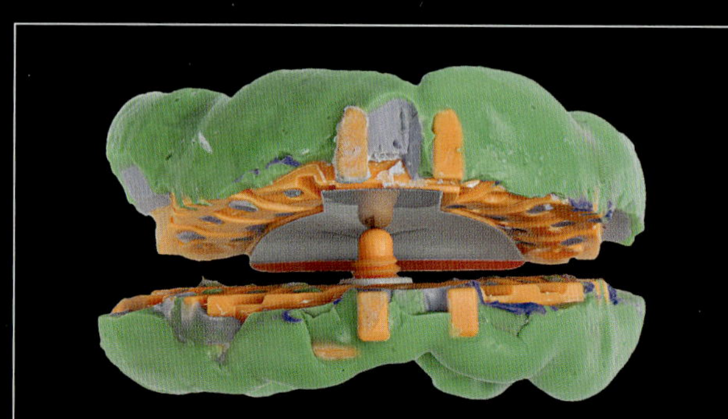

5

Fig 1 Medium-size Dentca impression tray.

Fig 2 Final impression is separated with the use of a blade for CR record.

Fig 3 Intraoral tracing pin is attached to the mandibular impression.

Fig 4 Denture tracing pad is attached on the tray for Gothic arch tracing.

Fig 5 Center pin is adjusted for proper vertical dimension.

The trays are replaced in the patient's mouth with the center pin attached to the mandibular tray. The patient's mandible is guided from the anterior-most to the posterior-most position. The mandible is then moved laterally on each side from its most posterior position and then brought back into its posterior position (Fig 6). The arrow thus formed is the Gothic arch tracing, where the apex of the arrow on the maxillary tray represents CR (Fig 7). A small hole or depression is drilled into the apex to allow the center pin to fit into it during bite registration.

Bite Registration

The trays are seated back in the patient's mouth, and the center pin snaps into the CR hole. Bite registration material is then injected between the trays. When the material sets, the trays are removed and evaluated for accurate positioning of the center pin within the CR hole or recess.

A ruler is used to measure the distance between the incisive papilla and the upper lip border. Once completed, the trays are disinfected and mailed to the Dentca manufacturer along with a printed denture order.

CAD/CAM Process

The maxillary and mandibular impressions are scanned to create virtual images of the edentulous arches using the specialized Dentca CAD software (Figs 8 and 9). Once the CAD process is complete, the virtual images of the dentures are transferred to a 3D printer to create try-in dentures. At this time, two different sets of try-in dentures are generated for the patient's evaluation. The first setup has bold maxillary lateral incisors with minor crowding of the mandibular incisors (Figs 10 to 14). The second setup has soft maxillary lateral incisors with moderate crowding of the mandibular incisors (Fig 15 to 19). After try-in of both sets, the patient decides on the second setup for her final denture (Figs 20 to 23). Now that the decision is made, a converting process is followed to fabricate the definitive complete denture, including internal staining (Fig 24) to create a natural appearance (Figs 25 to 27).

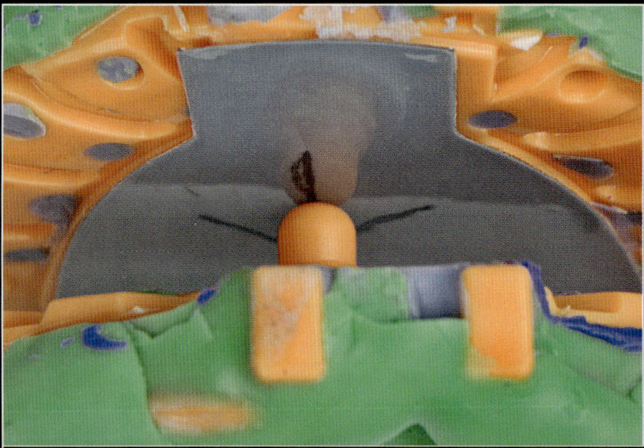

6

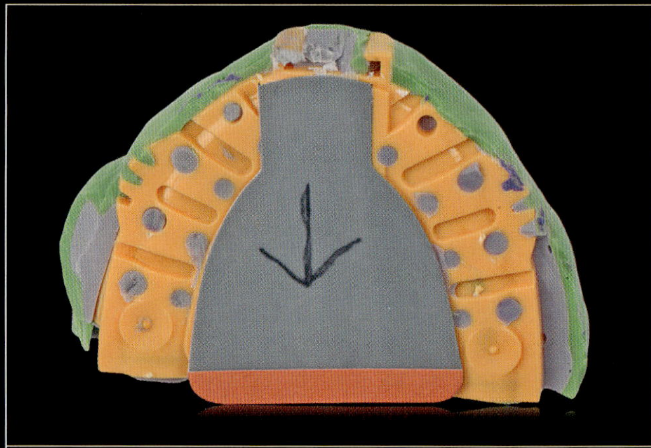

7

Fig 6 Lower tracing pin marks on the denture tracing pad.
Fig 7 Gothic arch tracing on the denture tracing pad.

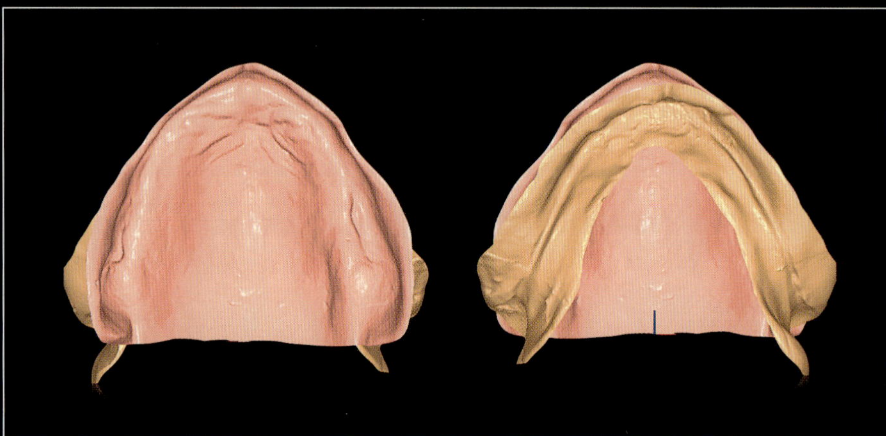

8

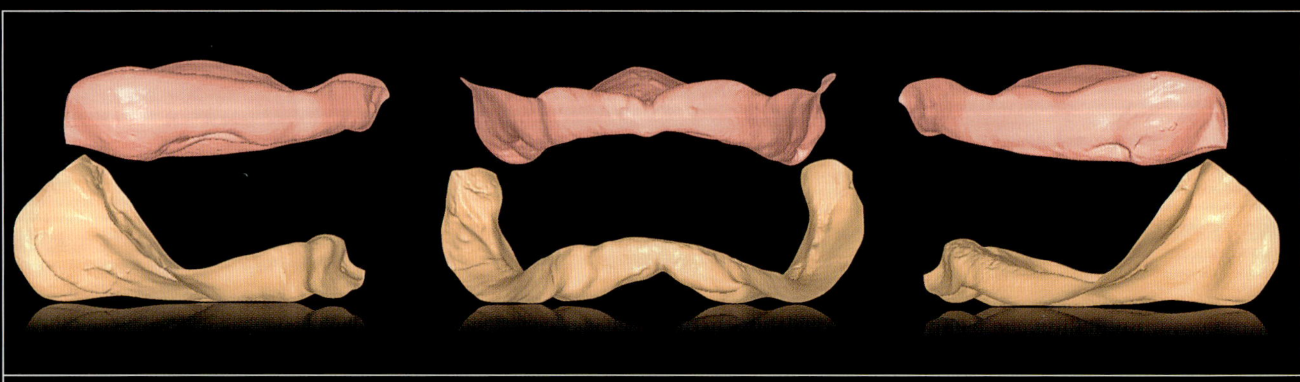

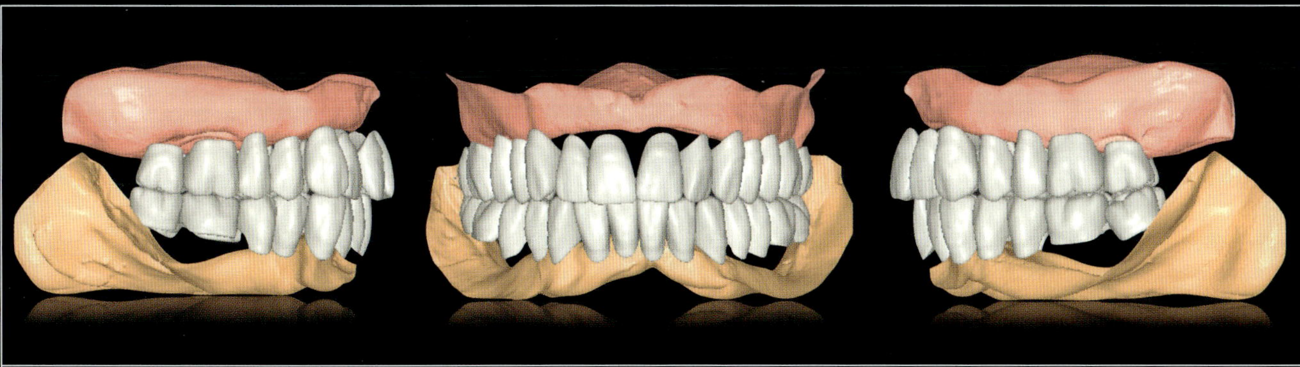

15

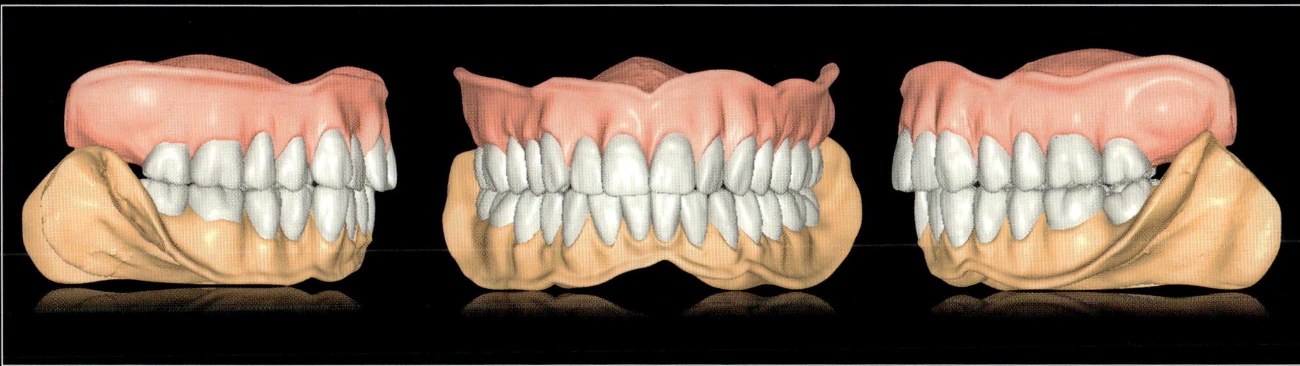

16

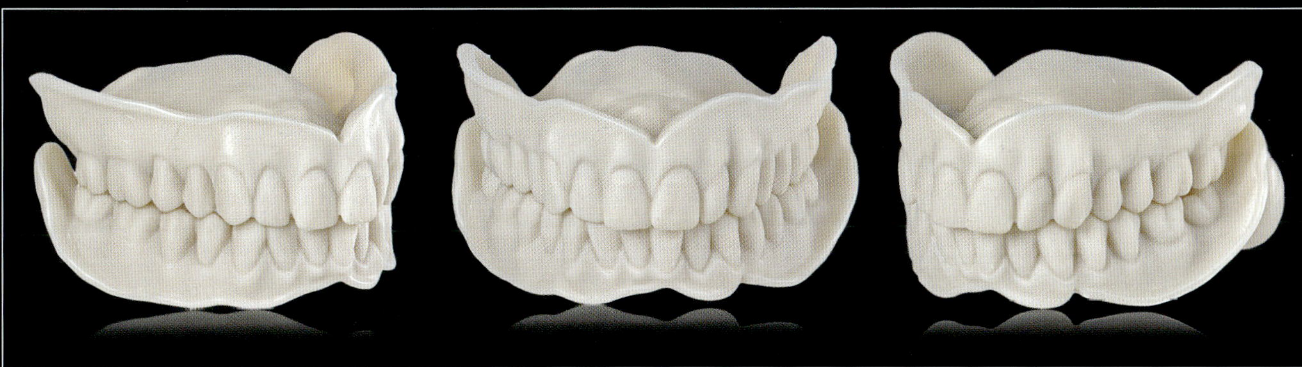

17

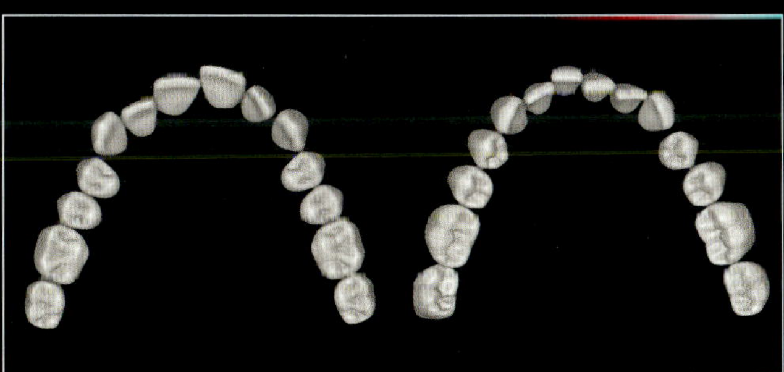

18

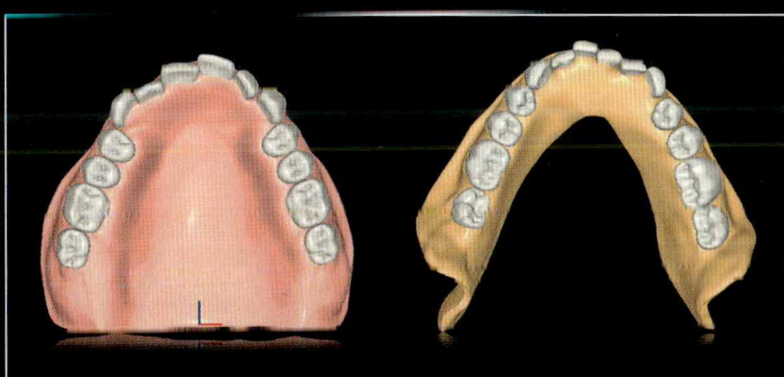

19

Fig 15 Digital image of second teeth setup: soft maxillary lateral incisors and moderate mandibular incisor crowding.
Fig 16 Digital image of completed denture after festooning (second setup).
Fig 17 Try-in denture (second setup).
Fig 18 Teeth alignment (second setup). 3D printed dentures ready for try-in.
Fig 19 Teeth alignment in denture (second setup).

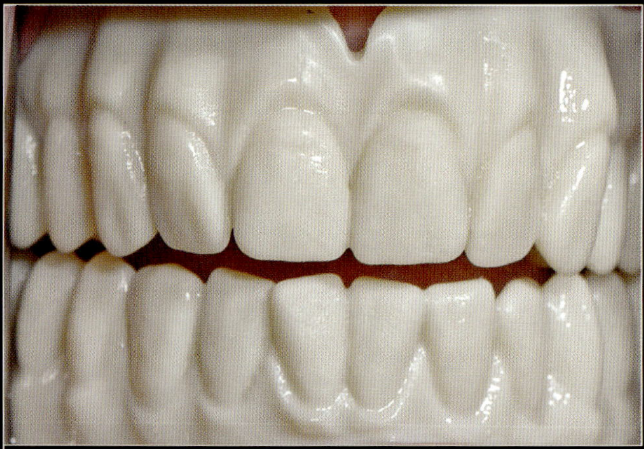

20

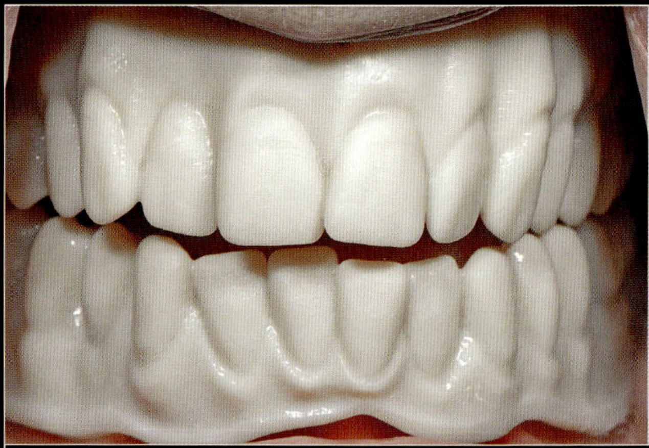

21

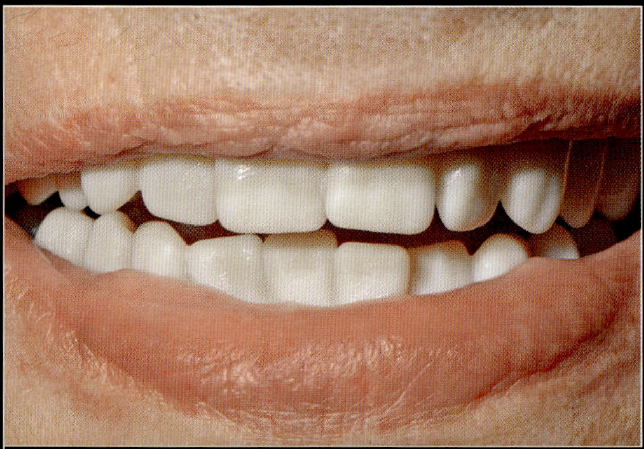

22

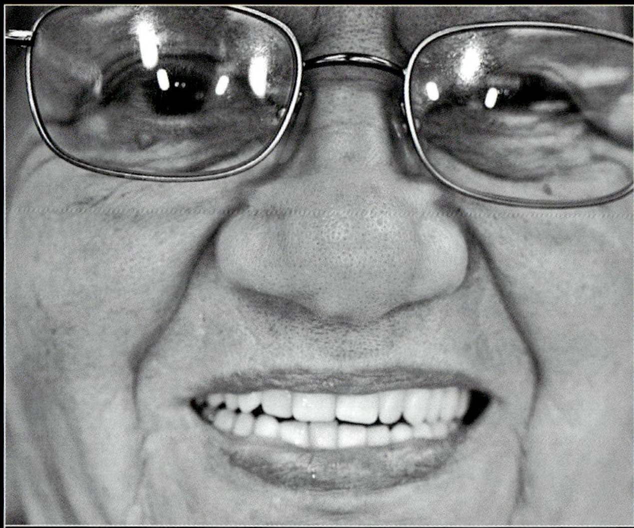

23

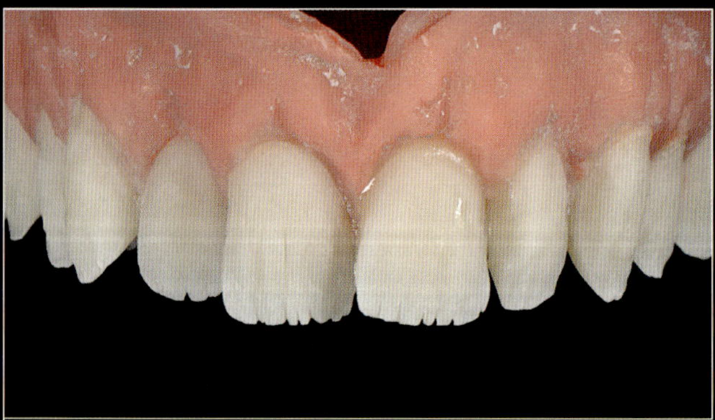

24a

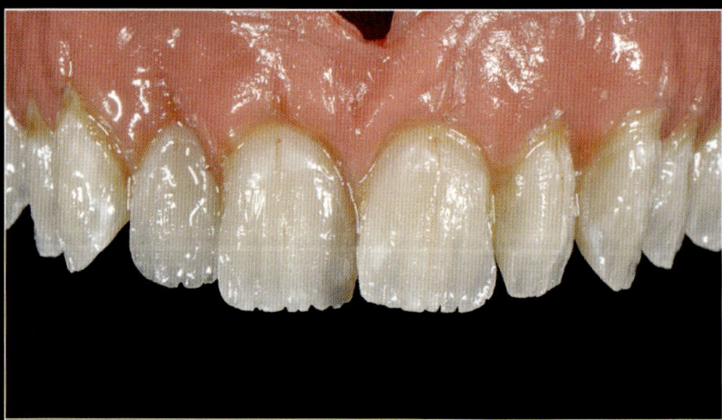

24b

Fig 20 Patient's evaluation of first try-in denture in mouth.
Fig 21 Patient's evaluation of second try-in denture in mouth.
Fig 22 Patient's smile with second try-in denture.
Fig 23 Patient with chosen try-in denture (second setup) in mouth.
Fig 24a Cutback for internal staining and enamel layer.
Fig 24b After application of internal stain.

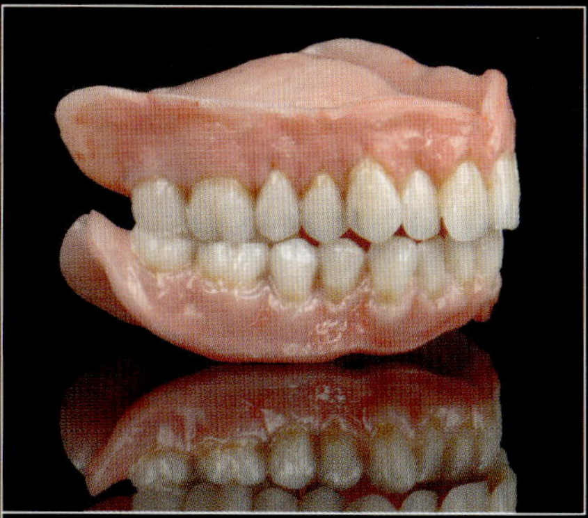

25a

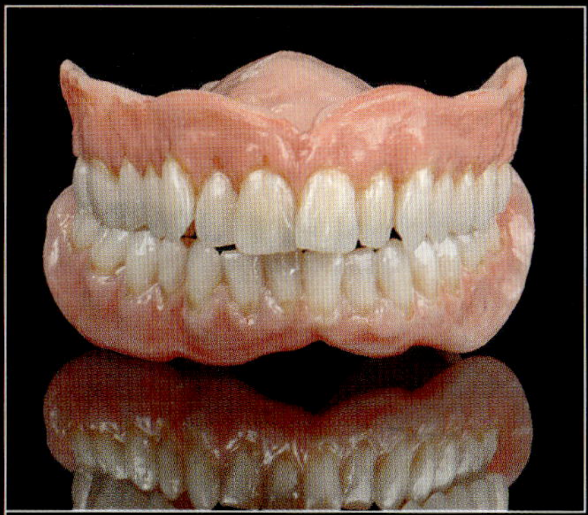

25b

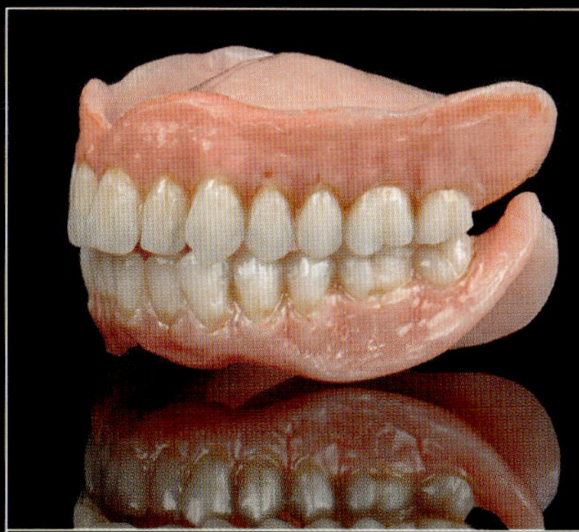

25c

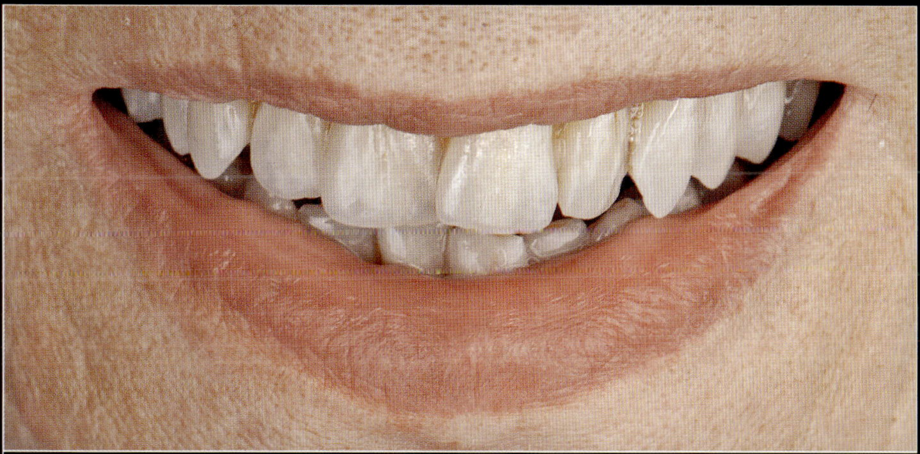

26

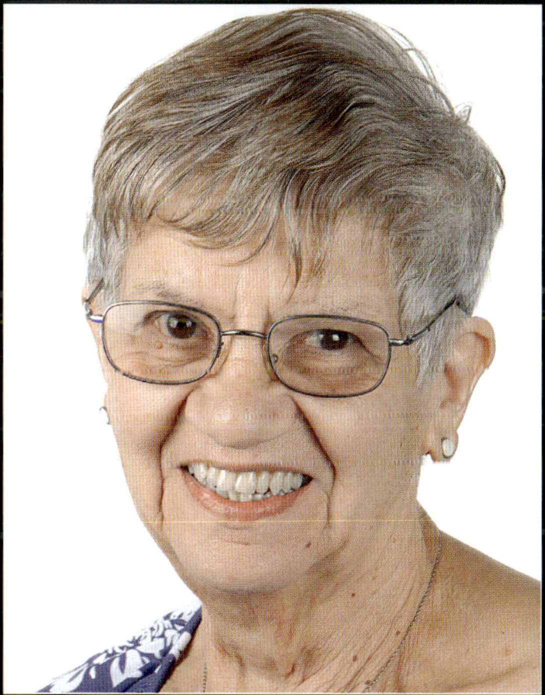

27

Figs 25a to 25c Completed CAD/CAM denture.

Fig 26 Patient's smile with definitive CAD/CAM complete denture.

Fig 27 Patient's natural-looking appearance with the CAD/CAM denture.

CONCLUSIONS

CAD/CAM technology for fabrication of complete dentures represents a new benchmark for the clinician's armamentarium. CAD/CAM dentures provide reliable and predictable oral rehabilitation of edentulous patients with superior performance when compared to traditional methods of denture fabrication.

REFERENCES

1. Maeda Y, Minoura M, Tsutsumi S, Okada M, Nokubi T. A CAD/CAM system for removable denture. Part I: Fabrication of complete dentures. Int J Prosthodont 1994;7:17–21.
2. Kawahata N, Ono H, Nishi Y, Hamano T, Nagaoka E. Trial of duplication procedure for complete dentures by CAD/CAM. J Oral Rehabil 1997;24:540–548.
3. Busch M, Kordass B. Concept and development of a computerized positioning of prosthetic teeth for complete dentures. Int J Comput Dent 2006;9:113–120.
4. Zhang YD, Jiang JG, Liang T, Hu WP. Kinematics modeling and experimentation of the multi-manipulator tooth-arrangement robot for full denture manufacturing. J Med Syst 2011;35:1421–1429.
5. Goodacre CJ, Garbacea A, Naylor WP, Daher T, Marchack CB, Lowry J. CAD/CAM fabricated complete dentures: Concepts and clinical methods of obtaining required morphological data. J Prosthet Dent 2012;107:34–46.
6. Sun Y, Lü P, Wang Y. Study on CAD&RP for removable complete denture. Comput Methods Programs Biomed 20009;93:266–272.
7. Kanazawa M, Inokoshi M, Minakuchi S, Ohbayashi N. Trial of a CAD/CAM system for fabricating complete dentures. Dent Mater J 2011;30:93–96.
8. Inokoshi M, Kanazawa M, Minakuchi S. Evaluation of a complete denture trial method applying rapid prototyping. Dent Mater J 2012;31:40–46.

The Reservoir Technique

Hilal Kuday, CDT[1]
Michel Magne, MDT[2]

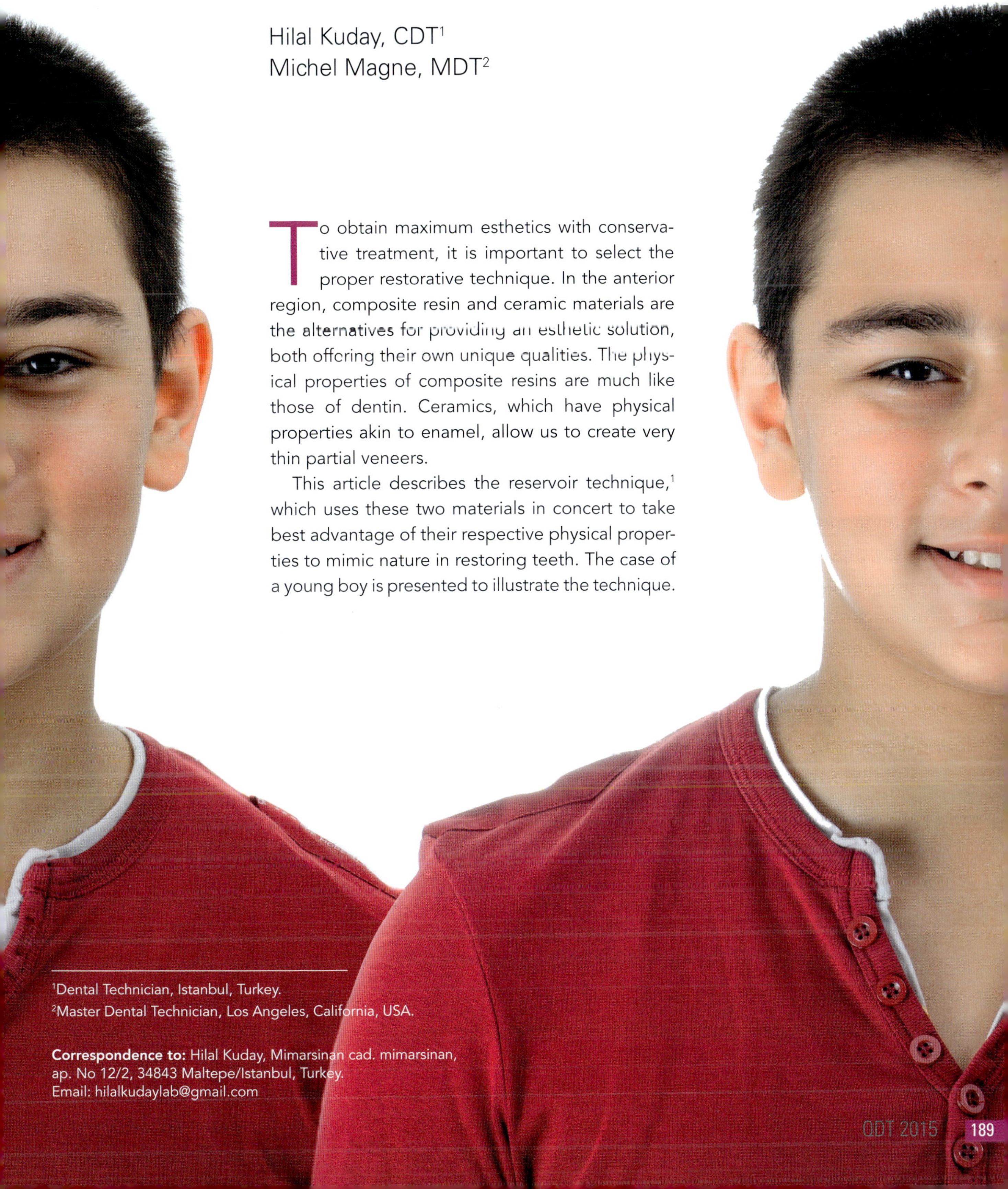

To obtain maximum esthetics with conservative treatment, it is important to select the proper restorative technique. In the anterior region, composite resin and ceramic materials are the alternatives for providing an esthetic solution, both offering their own unique qualities. The physical properties of composite resins are much like those of dentin. Ceramics, which have physical properties akin to enamel, allow us to create very thin partial veneers.

This article describes the reservoir technique,[1] which uses these two materials in concert to take best advantage of their respective physical properties to mimic nature in restoring teeth. The case of a young boy is presented to illustrate the technique.

[1]Dental Technician, Istanbul, Turkey.
[2]Master Dental Technician, Los Angeles, California, USA.

Correspondence to: Hilal Kuday, Mimarsinan cad. mimarsinan, ap. No 12/2, 34843 Maltepe/Istanbul, Turkey.
Email: hilalkudaylab@gmail.com

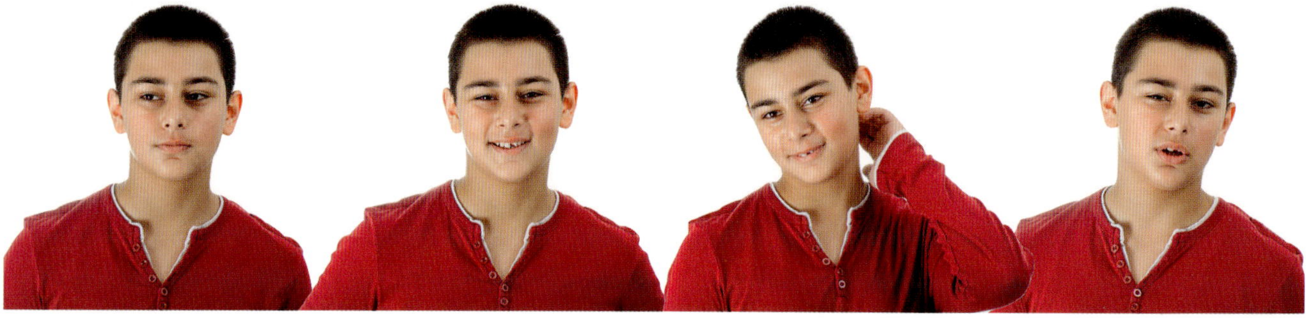

CASE PRESENTATION

A 14-year-old boy, who had broken the incisal edges of the maxillary central incisors and right lateral incisor a few years earlier, presented for treatment. The teeth were tested and confirmed to be vital (Fig 1). Since the patient was still growing, full-coverage ceramic crowns were not considered a restorative option. Using the reservoir technique, the lost enamel on the incisal edges was reproduced by a ceramic shell and the lost dentin with composite resin.

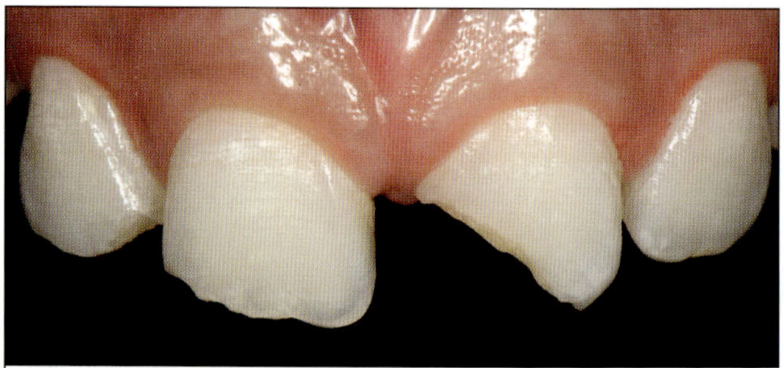

1a

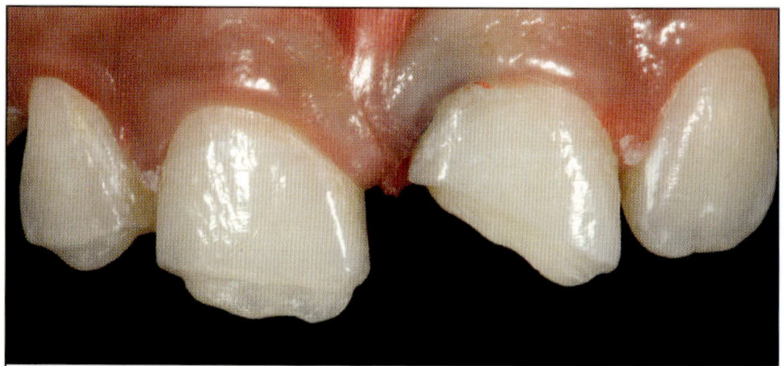

1b

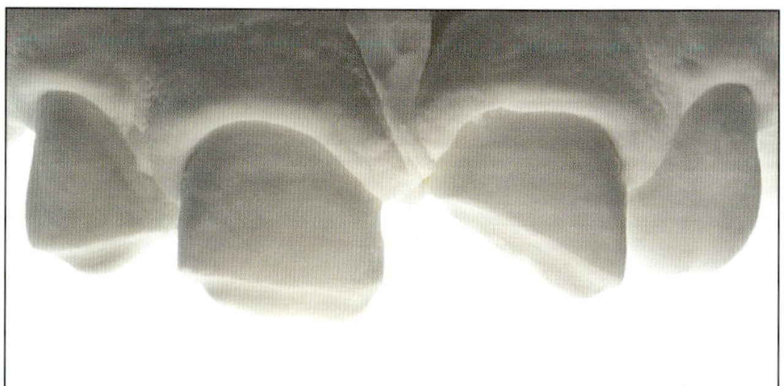

1c

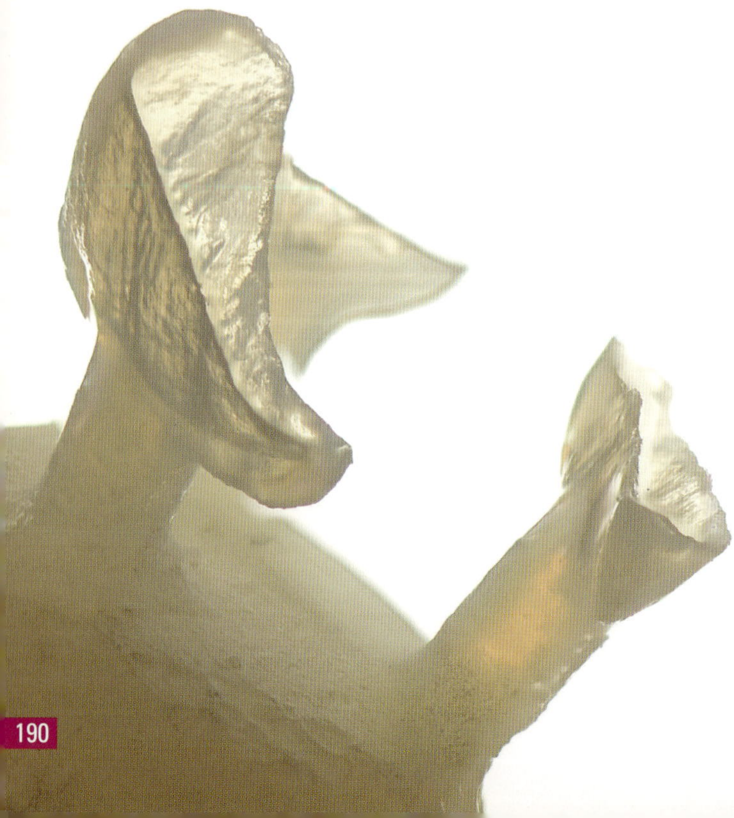

Wax-up

A wax-up was made to analyze the target form. Of course, form needs to be in harmony with occlusion, emergence profile, phonetics, and esthetics (Figs 2a and 2b). The second wax model was designed according to the silicone index. The die space area was limited to 0.5 mm from the marginal borders, which were marked carefully before the second model was made (Fig 2c). Zhermack silicone was used for die duplication and silicone matrices (Figs 2d and 2e) that were made from the wax-up. In this stage, the incisal effects for the appearance of the final image must be considered (Fig 2f).

The positive incisal characterization must be imagined but the spaces waxed as negatives of incisal appearance (Figs 3a and 3b).

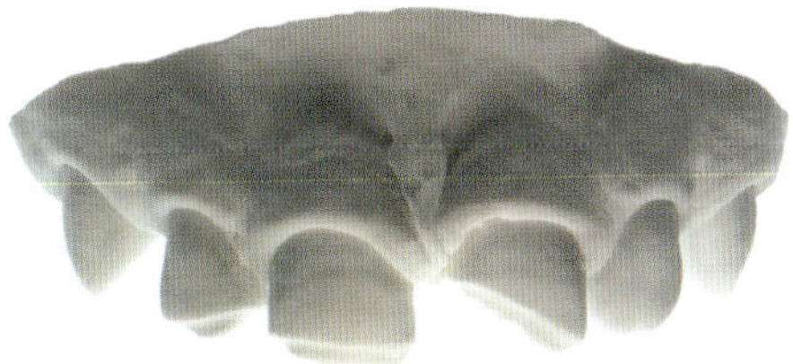

2a

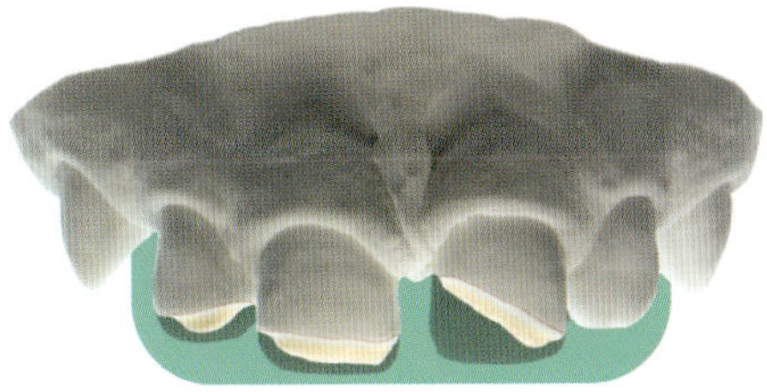

2d

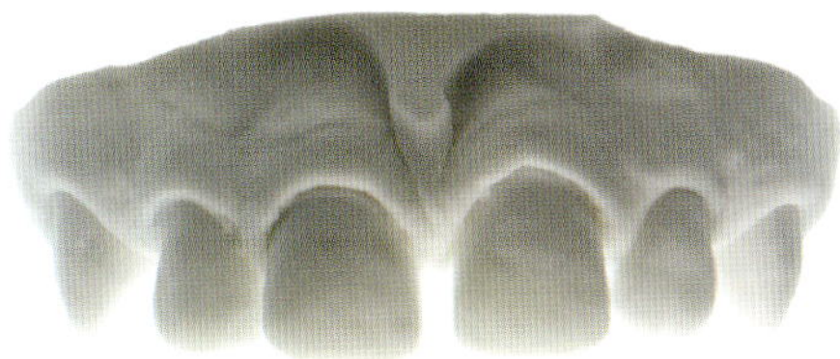

2b

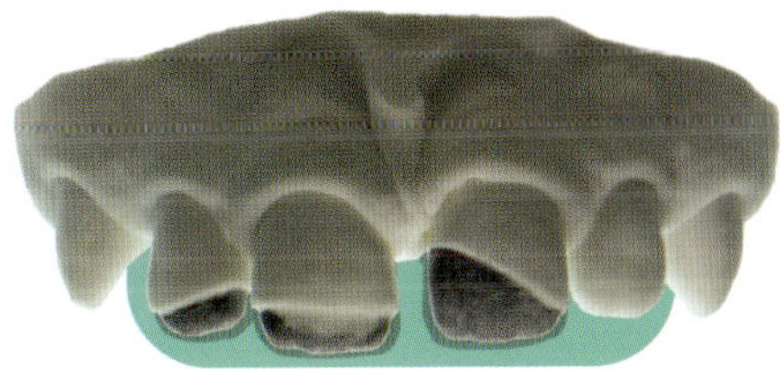

2e

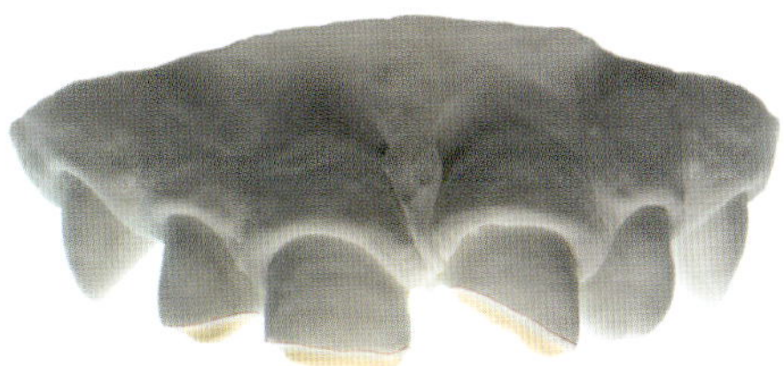

2c

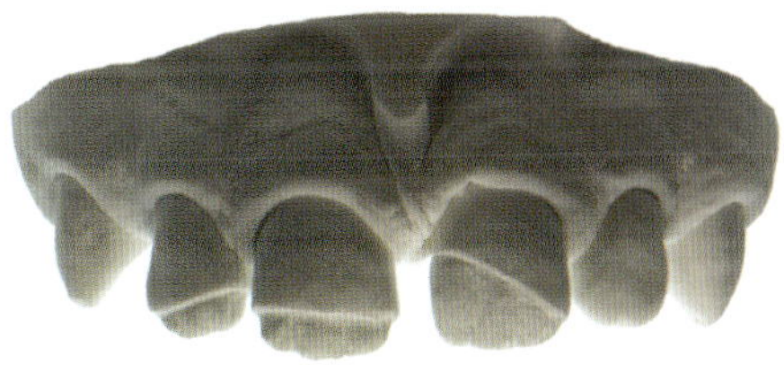

2f

Effect Design

When shaping effects, the chosen ingot's optical behavior must be considered. Each ingot has different effects that are possible based on its thickness. Simply playing with thickness allows us to create internal and external optical effects. Highly detailed microstructural effects can be created in a basic simple manner with grinding tools on the surface of the internal wax structure (see Fig 2e) that would not be possible to create with a brush.

3a

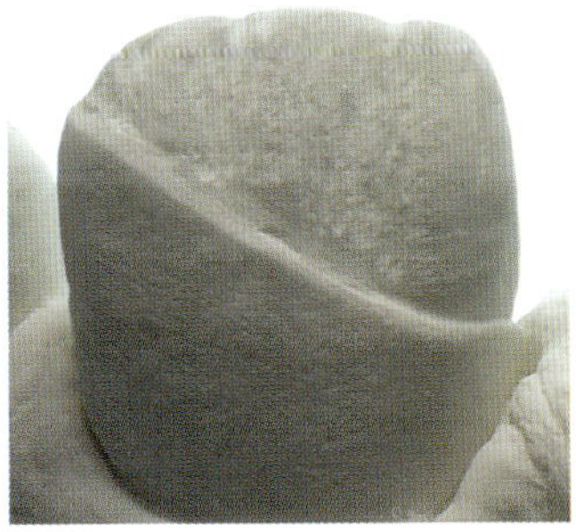

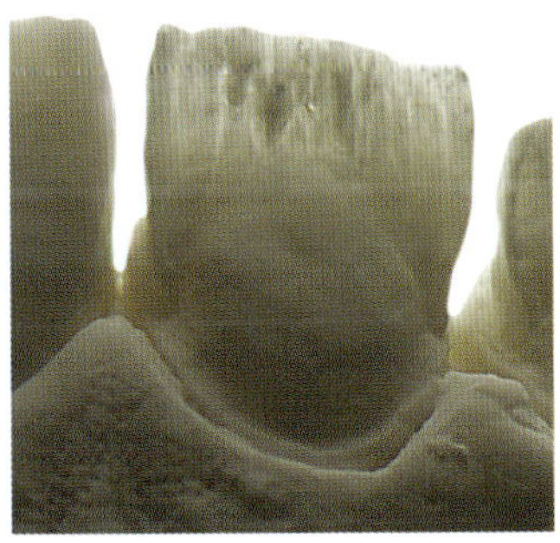

3b

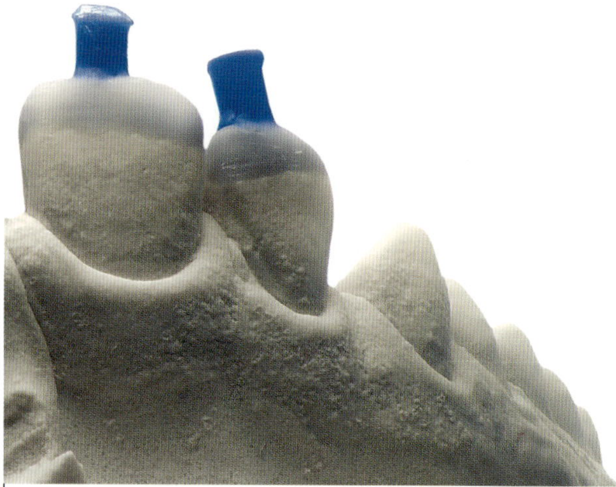

4a

Refractory Cast

The refractory cast[2] is needed because of the naturally angulated structure of the tooth. The wax model must be cut carefully near the margin; standard press procedures can then be followed (Figs 4a and 4b). It must be remembered that the liquid ratio of the mixture may be changed due to absorption while the refractory cast is closed for investment. Alcohol can be used to control absorption so that the concentration at the flask closing procedure is balanced. PressVest speed investment material (Ivoclar Vivadent) was used as closing flask as well as a refractory die material.

The wax model from the silicone index was transformed to a refractory cast. This protects anatomical curvatures of the tooth from breakage when working, since the wax can be less than 0.1 mm thick in some areas. The refractory cast guarantees the marginal fit and controls distortion of the wax form (Fig 4c).

If desired, incredible microstructural effects can be created using basic manipulations under a microscope even on the refractory cast. This can enhance the detail of the optical reflection in the final ceramic.

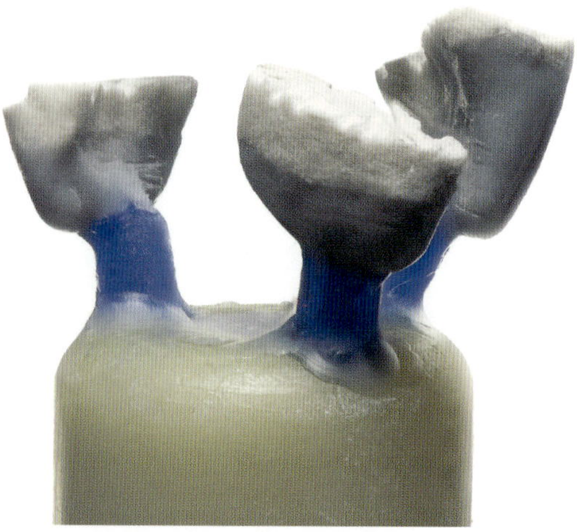

4b

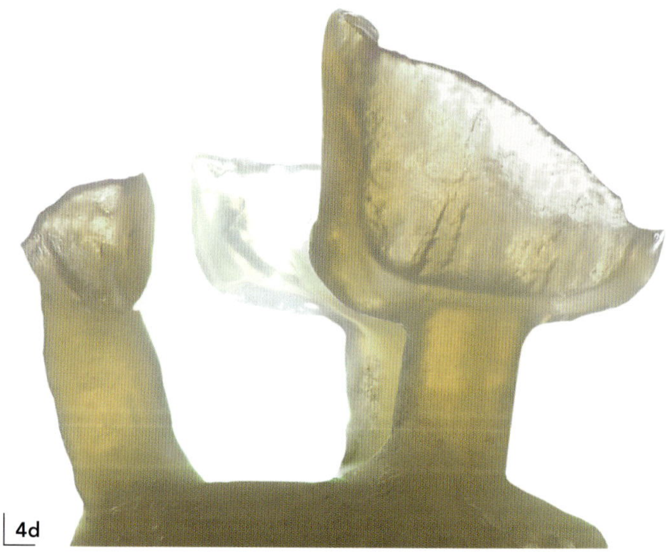

4d

The wax modeling on the refractory cast will be the ceramic shell and it will act as enamel. If the ingot choice is opalescent, eg, e.max Opal 1 or Opal 2, the intensive blue reflection and the halo effect on the incisal border must be controlled (Fig 4d).

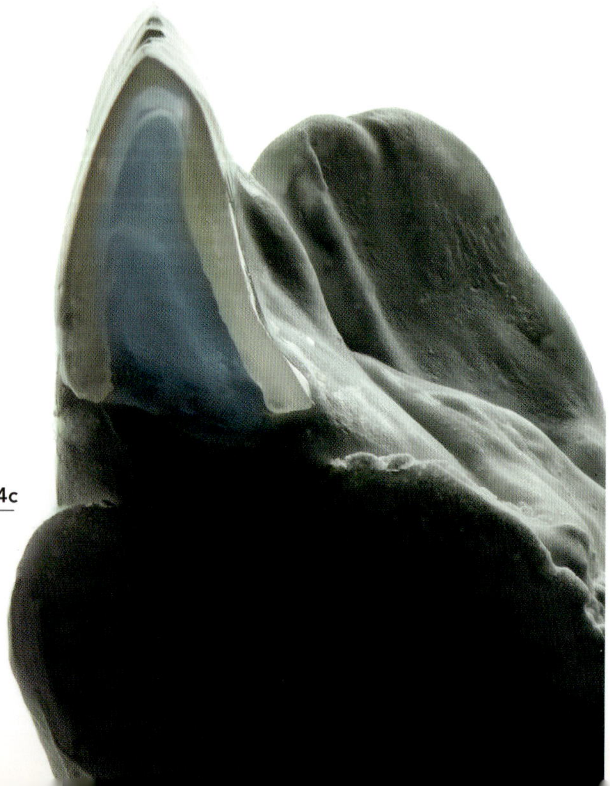

4c

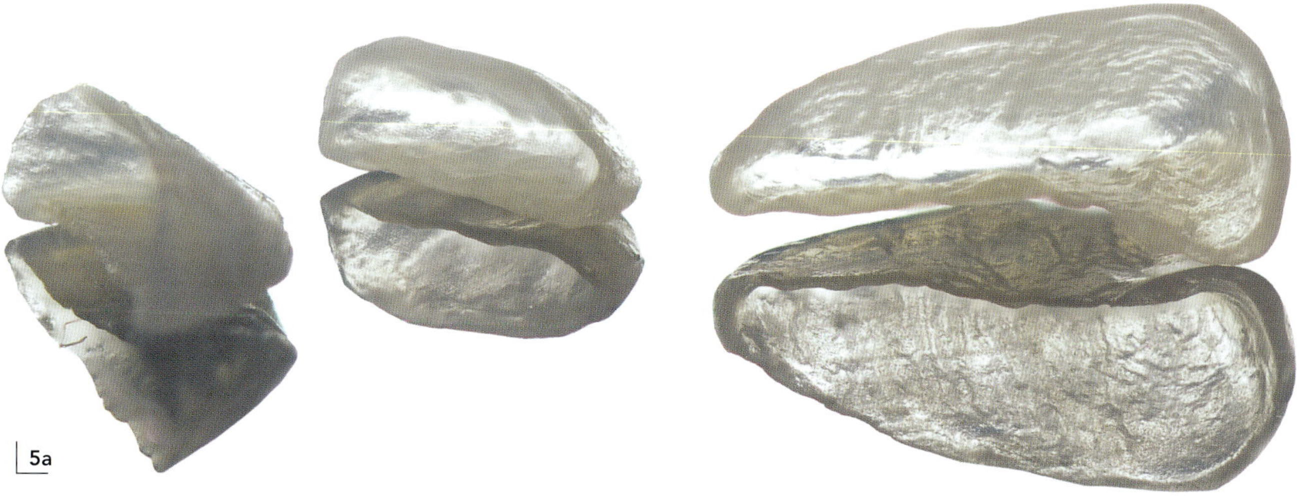

5a

Pressed Monolithic Ceramics

The highly developed textures of the internal and external surfaces of the ceramic (e.max Opal 1, Ivoclar Vivadent) increase the optical quality and afford complex details that cannot be produced with a brush.

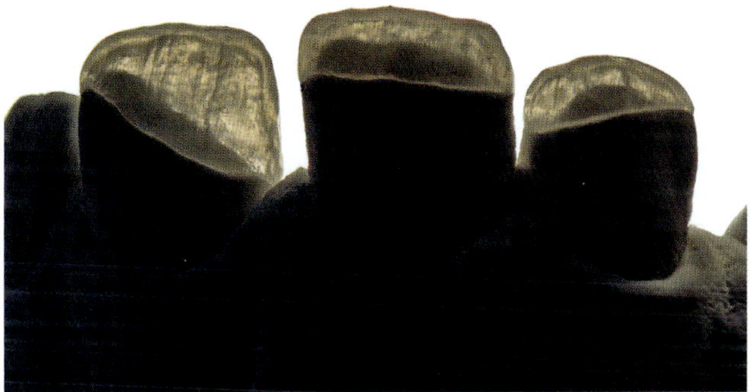

5b

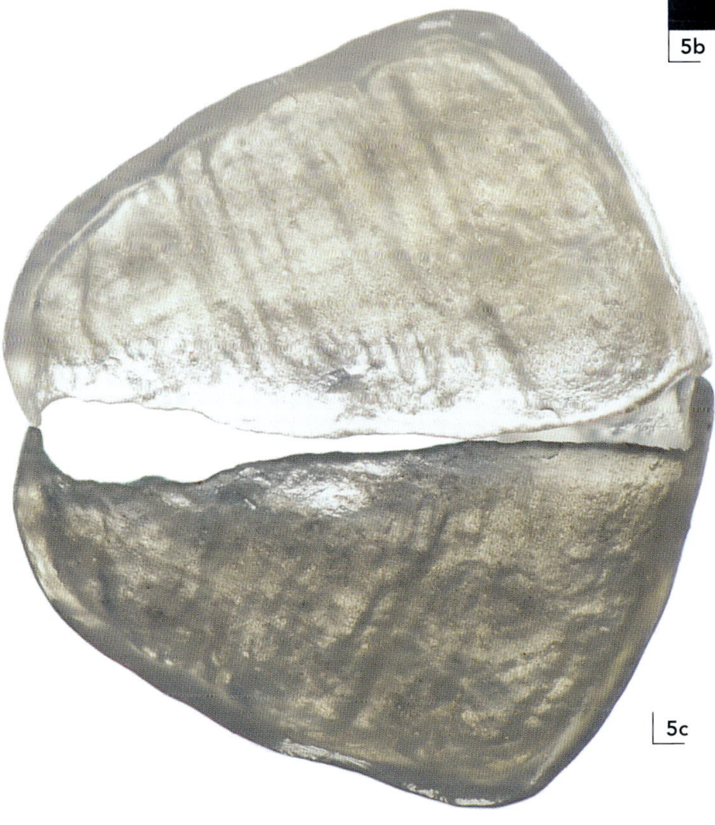

The internal surface of the ceramic shell can be stained with composite-based effect materials before the composite filling procedure. The effects can be highlighted or can be filtered in the desired areas. In this case, internal stains were not used. The effects shown in Figs 5a to 5c were created by internal micro-surface structure.

One must not forget that the effect of the chosen ingot on the final appearance is also related to the thickness. Uncontrolled thickness can cause unwanted grayish color or nonhomogeneous opacity.

5c

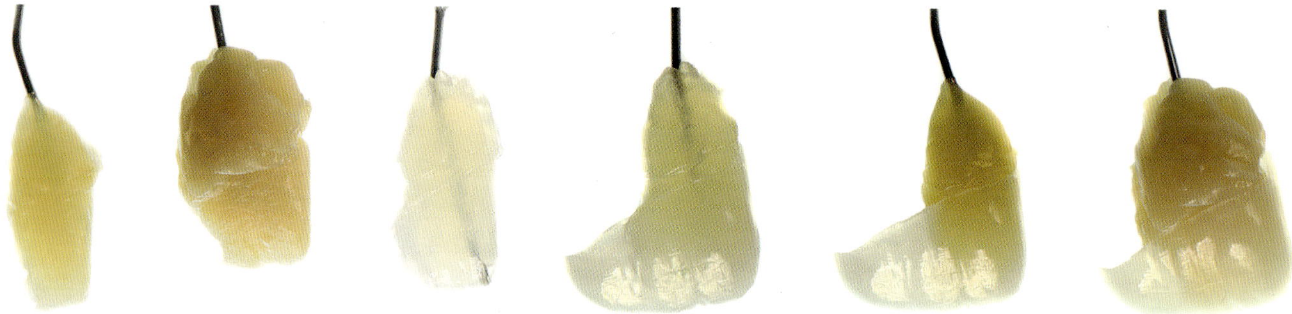

We can easily decide the value and the color of the effects on the ceramic shell, either at the lab or at the clinic. For single crowns or anterior restorations, this procedure provides a great advantage in controlling the value before cementation. In this case, SR Nexco light-curing composite (Ivoclar Vivadent) was used at the lab to fill in shells and then cured in a Lumamat 100 light furnace (Ivoclar Vivadent).

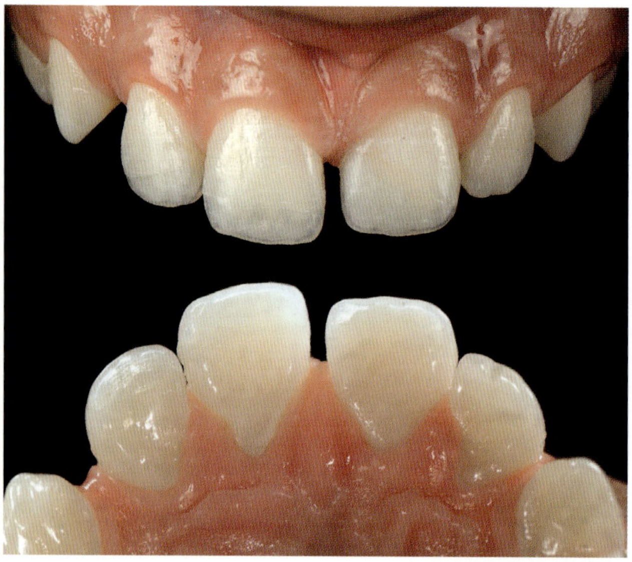

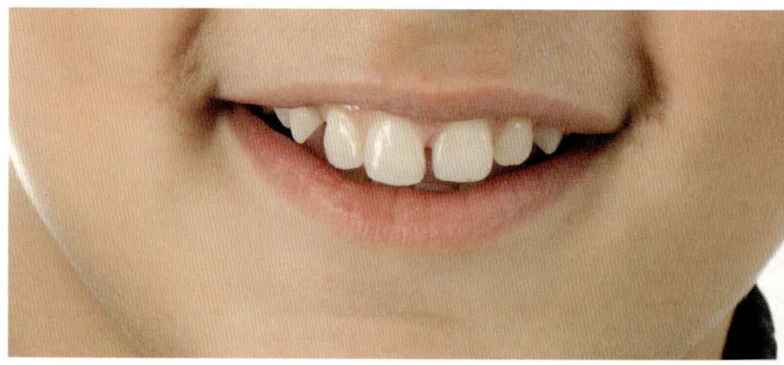

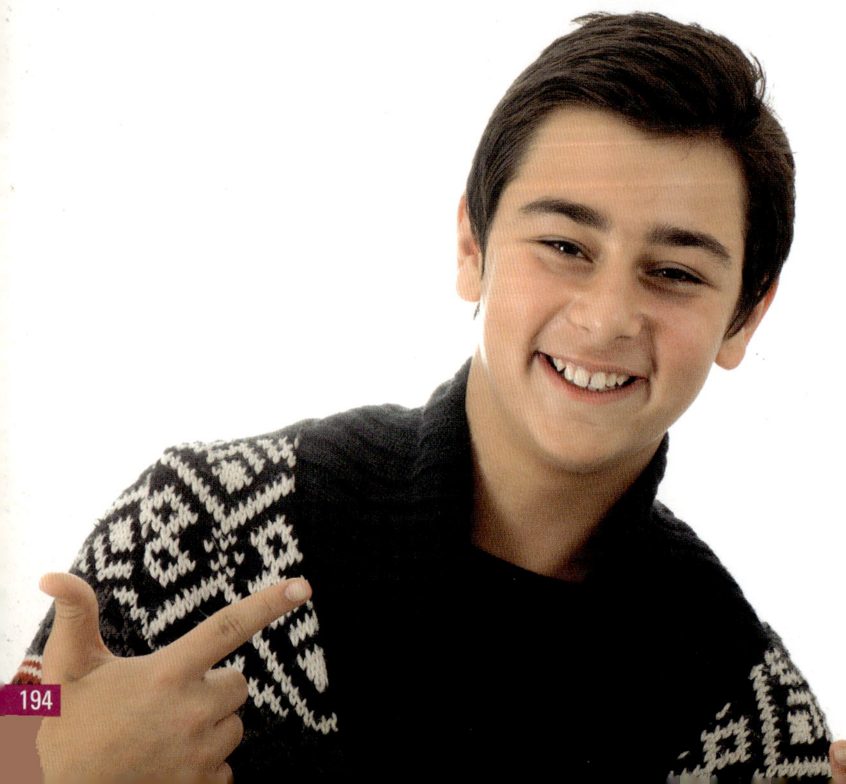

ACKNOWLEDGMENTS

Special thanks to Dr Nihan Özlem Kuday and Dr Ceren Kücük for their wonderful efforts from Dentboutique Clinic in Istanbul.

REFERENCES

1. Magne M, Magne I, Gandolfi Paranhos MP. Bilayer effect with press ceramics—The Reservoir Technique. Spectrum 23/2/2011.
2. Vailati F, Bruguera A, Belser UC. Minimally invasive treatment of initial dental erosion using pressed lithium disilicate glass-ceramic restorations: A case report. Quintessence Dent Technol 2012;35:65–78.

Mental, Visual, and Manual Training: *The MVM Concept*

Ivan Contreras Molina, DDS, MSc, PhD[1]
Panaghiotis Bazos, DDS[2]
Pascal Magne, DMD, MSc, PhD[3]

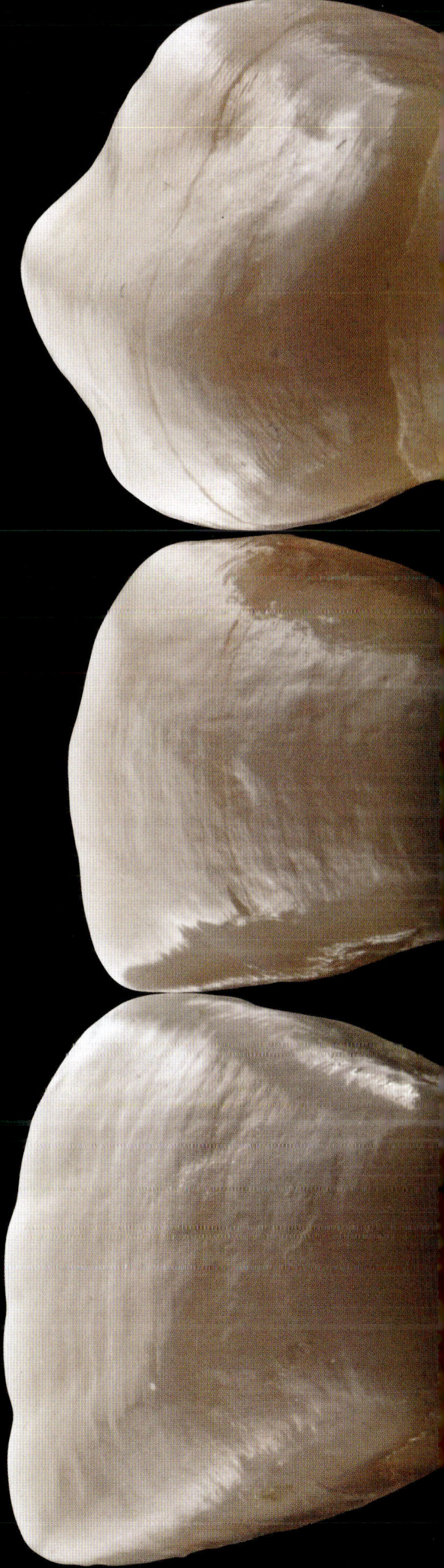

Achieving mastery in high-fidelity dental reproduction is based on the perpetual study of natural teeth by ways of anatomical reproduction via two-dimensional (drawing) and three-dimensional (waxing) training.

Those who endeavor to train further to enhance their education, vocation, and skills need to show considerable individual initiative, discipline, and perseverance. This is particularly true in the evolving disciplines of dentistry, and especially in the areas that require optimized esthetic integration. During the undergraduate training curriculum and in the course of the daily routine in the laboratory, clinicians and technicians have little chance of obtaining improved clinical or technical outcomes due to the lack of time available for continuous training.

[1]Visiting Scholar of Esthetic Dentistry, Division of Restorative Sciences, Ostrow School of Dentistry, University of Southern California, Los Angeles, California, USA.

[2]Private Practice, Athens, Greece.

[3]The Don and Sybil Harrington Professor of Esthetic Dentistry, Division of Restorative Sciences, Ostrow School of Dentistry, University of Southern California, Los Angeles, California, USA.

Correspondence to: Dr Ivan Contreras Molina, Privada Plan de Ayutla #39, Col. Chapultepec sur, Morelia-Mexico.
Email: dr.ivancontreras@gmail.com

The current generation of dental practitioners seek to gain insight and acumen in reproducing the "natural morphology" with greater detail; hence dedication and diligent training of the visual and perceptual abilities must ensue, ultimately forming a harmonious workflow with superior end results. When developing the critical ability of spatial perception with regard to the cognitive process of understanding the static dental morphology, it is necessary to achieve levels of self-paced training to generate the necessary motivation to create autonomy in each of the restorative processes.

This article describes a visceral way to train our brain (mental awareness), eyes (visual perception), and hands (manual dexterity) to achieve higher dental esthetic discernment.

STAGE 1

Observe the natural teeth—study the macro/micro characteristics in terms of shapes, textures, and line angles

There is a principal anatomy among the anterior teeth. This anatomy gradually changes from the central incisor to the canine. Understanding these subtle changes at specific points contributes to the cognition and comprehension of the dental morphology, which will successfully lead to superior esthetic and functional integration.

Labial surface

The labial surface is composed of three primary planes: incisal, middle, and cervical. The middle plane is relatively large and straight, accounting for half of the labial surface. The incisal and cervical planes are accordingly inclined palatally and cervically, and they occupy the greater part of the labial surface (Fig 1).[1]

The surface from the facial marginal ridge to the extension of the interproximal contact is termed the proximal transitional surface. The area between the mesial and distal marginal ridges is termed the flat area or visual area. In the flat area there are two V-shaped groove positions on the labial surface of the tooth, and on the proximal transitional surface there are two points corresponding to the mesial and distal concave lines (Fig 1).[2]

On the central incisor, characteristics are located on virtually the same level, while on the lateral incisor and canine, they have different heights and are located in a lower position than on the central incisor. These points are carved deeper and spread out more mesially on the lateral incisor in the distal interproximal area and are carved primarily on the proximal transitional mesial surfaces. The distal area is located more cervically on the proximal transitional distal surfaces and it must be carved more aggressively farther from the midline (Fig 2).[3,4]

Palatal surface

On the palatal surfaces of the teeth there are two V-shaped grooves. On the central incisor, the two V shapes are located on virtually the same level, while on the lateral incisor and canine, they have different heights and are located in a lower position than on the central incisor. It is important to know these areas when developing the morphology of the lingual surface. Observation of the palatal surface further shows that the central incisor has well-developed marginal ridges and less-developed central and secondary ridges. The central and secondary ridges become gradually more developed and clearly visible at the canine and lateral incisor (Fig 3).

Texture

Irregularities of natural teeth will create unique characteristics on tooth surfaces. These irregularities result from age, tooth position, and enamel hardness. The maturation stage and relative wear are important aspects in the reproduction of teeth. The two types of textures that predominate are horizontal and vertical over the labial tooth surface (Fig 4). The horizontal component is a direct result of the lines of retzius (growth lines), leaving fine parallel stripes on the enamel surface, also called perikymata. The vertical component is defined by the superficial segmentation of the tooth in expressing developmental lobe coalescence.

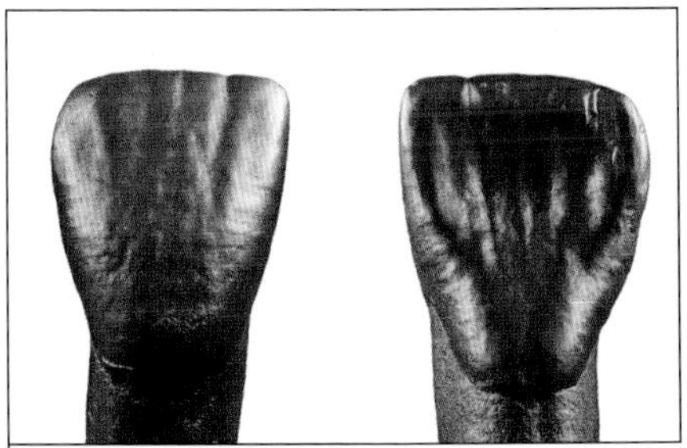

1a

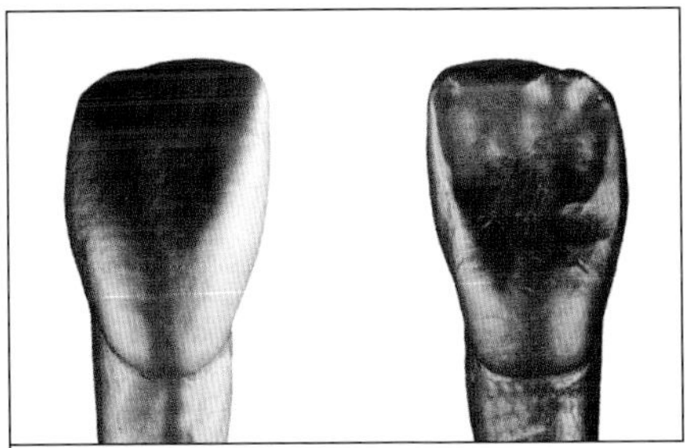

1b

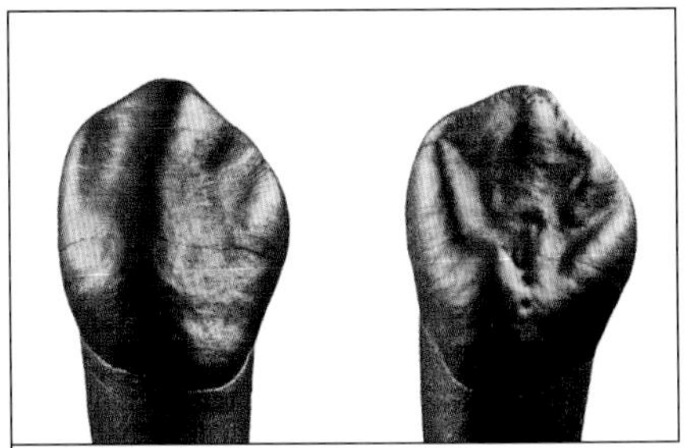

1c

Figs 1a to 1c The model optically highlights the delicate features of the surface structures, enabling improved visualization in order to observe the individualization of the teeth and revealing the facial and palatal morphology (lobes, marginal ridges, concave lines, V shapes) in detail.

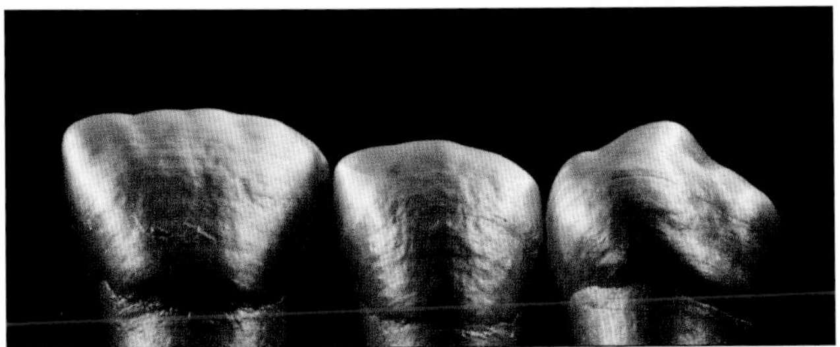

2a

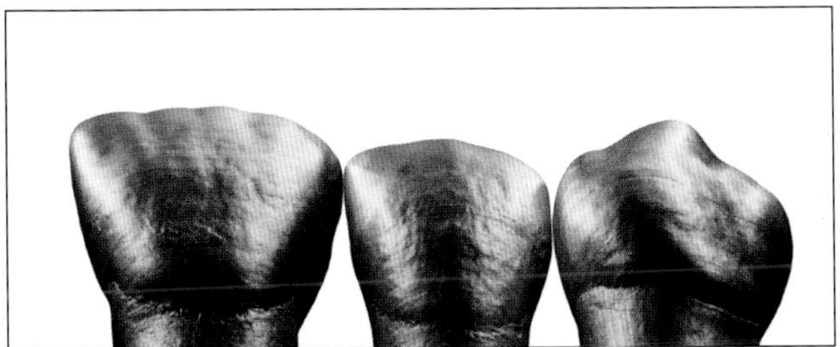

2b

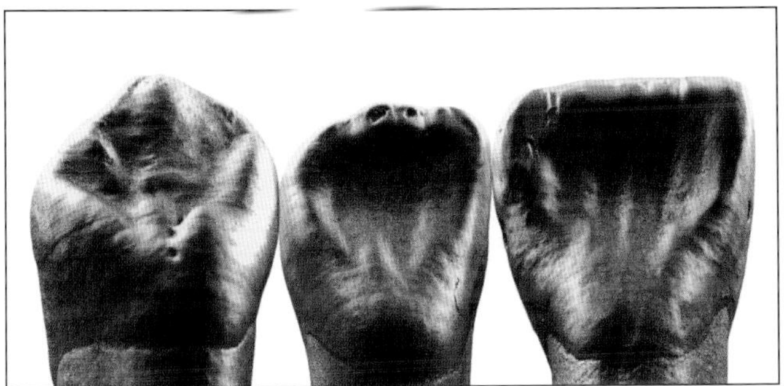

3a

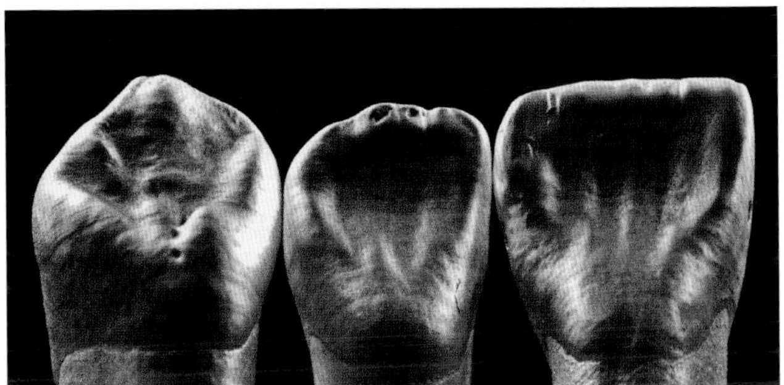

3b

Figs 2a and 2b Observation of the three-dimensional planes (incisal, medium, and cervical) of the anterior teeth by highlighting the facial transitional topography: the proximal transitional surfaces and the central visually dominant area.

Figs 3a and 3b The palatal surface shows the differential development of the marginal ridges, complementary to the morphology of the facial surface with variation of heights.

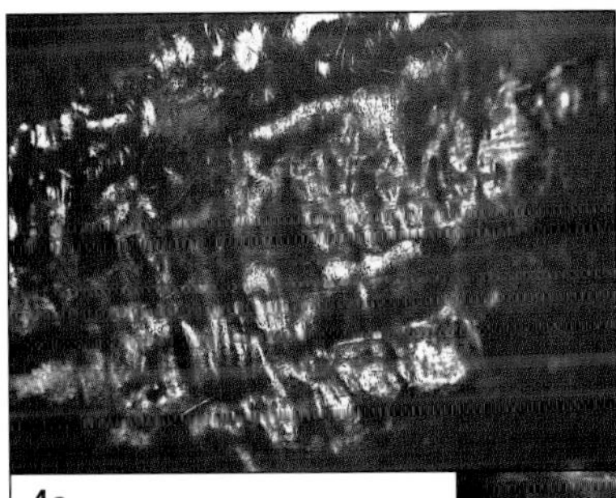

4a

Figs 4a and 4b Horizontal (perikymata and lines of Retzius) and vertical (lobular elevations) components are subtle, with wavelike irregular ridges that surround the tooth circumferentially, being more evident in young teeth and gradually disappearing as the teeth undergo perpetual attrition.

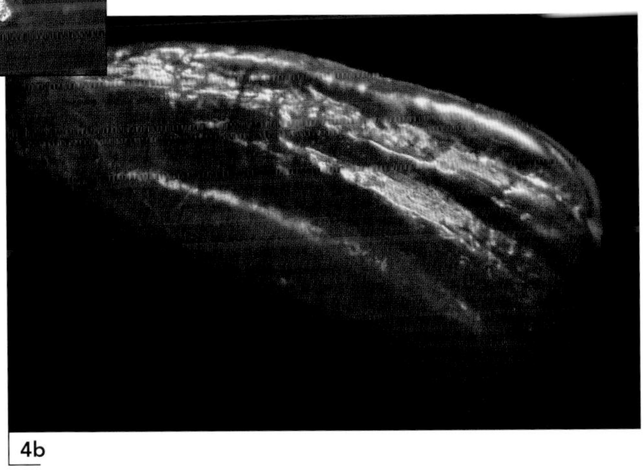

4b

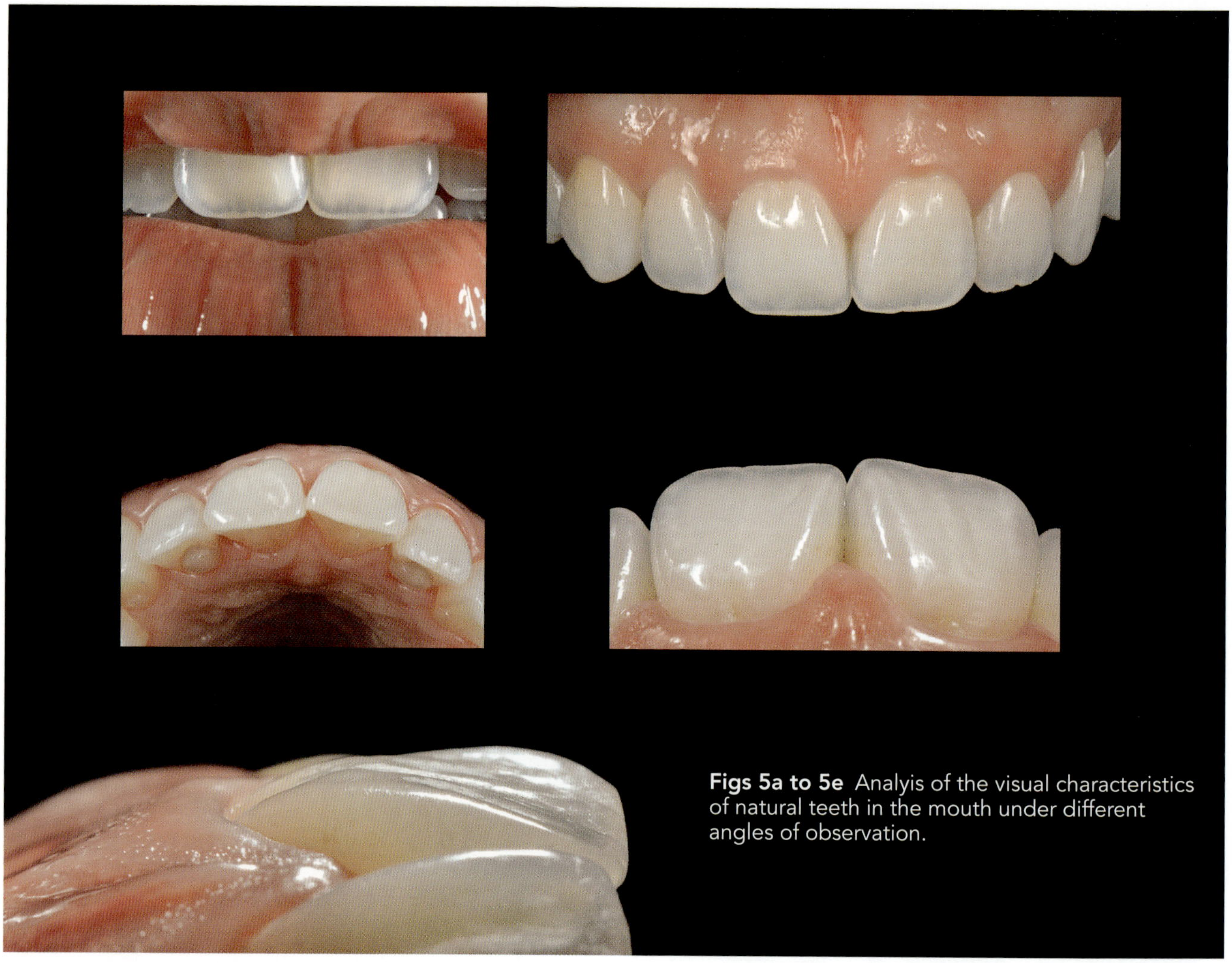

Figs 5a to 5e Analyis of the visual characteristics of natural teeth in the mouth under different angles of observation.

STAGE 2

Observe natural teeth in situ—in the mouth

The morphology and surface characteristics of natural teeth must be used as a basis for restorations. It is imperative that dental students, clinicians, and technicians practice contour techniques based on natural teeth. Natural teeth must be directly observed; therefore, master casts of natural dentitions are more effective during training than using freestanding natural teeth themselves as the model. Successful contour essentially involves training the eye to appreciate natural teeth and training the hands to express what the eyes observe. It is important to highlight that the visual characteristics of the teeth change drastically depending on the angle of observation. A selection of casts of maxillary and mandibular natural teeth with different characteristics and morphology is extremely useful. There are three basic tooth shapes: square, triangular, and oval.[5] The observation of these basic shapes in the mouth from different angles is useful for understanding the morphology and individual characteristics of each tooth (Fig 5). During the design stage, all tooth forms must be evaluated from an incisal, cervical, and frontal view with a right-lateral and left-lateral projection. This evaluation will provide an overall sense of the tooth organization as well as the relationship between the anatomical parts.

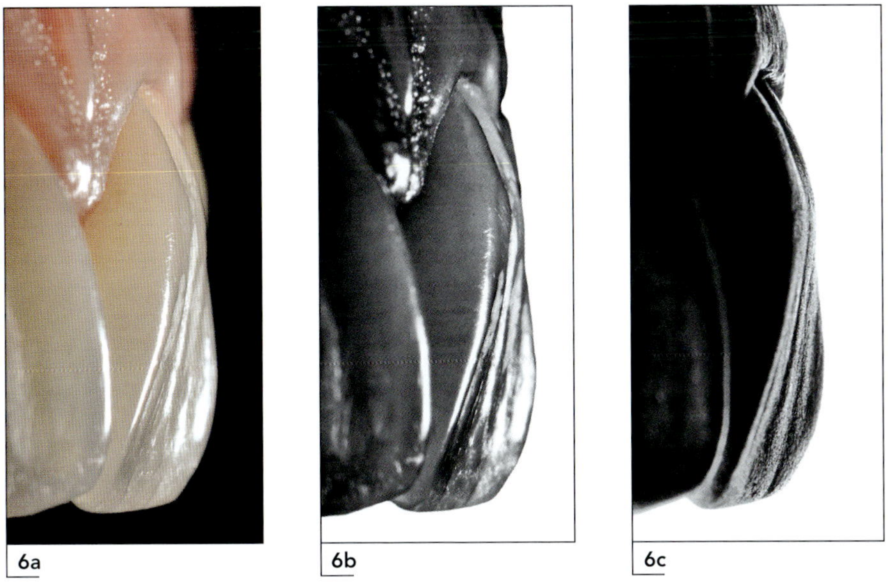

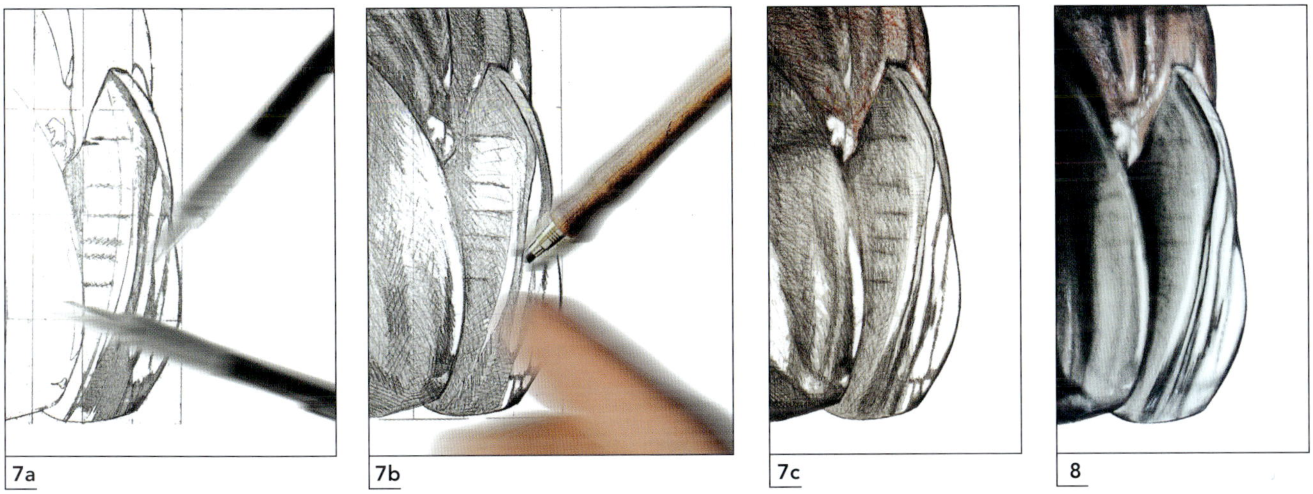

Figs 6 to 8 Skills (edges, spaces, relationships, light and shadows, gestalt) and final result. Drawings by author Pascal Magne.

STAGE 3

Observe a picture and draw it

A conceptual part of training is learning how to draw in 3D using an approach inspired by Betty Edwards[6] and the five perceptual skills of drawing. Those five skills (edges, spaces, relationship, light and shadows, gestalt) were adapted to the situation of a tooth drawing:

1. Frame and dimensions
2. Outline—negative spaces
3. Elements—internal morphology and shadows
4. Shading and highlights—cross-hatching/smudging/eraser
5. Gestalt ("whole")
6. Details (Figs 6 to 8)

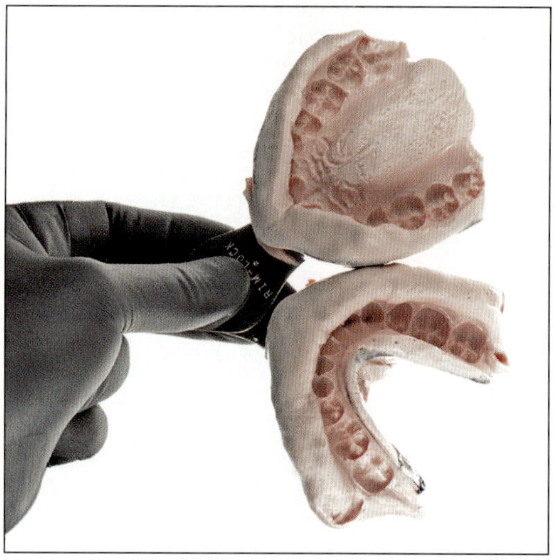

Fig 9 Impression-making for model analysis.

STAGE 4

Make an impression of teeth and analyze the morphology in 3D

The physical form of a tooth is determined by its outline, comprising the incisal border, proximal ridges, and cervical line. These lines dictate the path of the ridges and the shape of the lobes. Thus, the outline of the tooth should be evaluated before analyzing the tooth three-dimensionally (Fig 9).

Surface torsion is another important factor in the design of an artificial tooth. From an incisal view, distal protrusion becomes evident at the level of the cervix. Failure to consider this surface torsion may result in artificial incisors that appear flat or distally protruded. The line of rotation starts from the facial aspect and continues lingually. It is essential to know about the interplay of light and shade to understand form (Figs 10 and 11).

Torsion is common to all teeth, although to varying degrees of intensity. Surface torsion is gentler in the incisors and more pronounced in the canines; however, the dentist may define the extent of torsion based on the desired tooth form. In more facially positioned teeth, surface torsion becomes more evident (Fig 12).[7]

It is important to highlight that the visual characteristics of the teeth change drastically depending on the angle of observation. In this regard, analysis of a selection of casts of maxillary and mandibular natural teeth with different characteristics and morphology is extremely useful.[8] If they are painted with all the features already learned by our brain, their comprehension will be much easier; the use of lines and marks gives us a different perspective of the tooth shape.

Maxillary Central Incisors

Incisors are characterized as follows: The medial outline of the crown can be straight or slightly convex for maxillary incisors, with a more rounded mesioincisal angle for the lateral incisors. The distal of the crown is more convex compared to the mesial outline. Its curvature and inclination can vary significantly according to the typical form of the tooth, and the distal angle is rounded.

The incisal outline of the crown can be irregular or rounded but usually becomes flat due to functional wear. The incisor shape is also related to the anatomy of the interproximal ridges, or transition line angles, which represent strategic light-reflecting areas. These vertical and oblique crests do not influence the crown outline; however, the apparent tooth length and width can be easily modified by the length, position, and direction of the transition line angles.

Maxillary Lateral Incisors

As previously mentioned, the lateral incisors closely resemble the central incisors in their basic outline and transition line angles, which they supplement in function. They differ mainly in terms of their reduced size and more rounded mesioincisal angle.

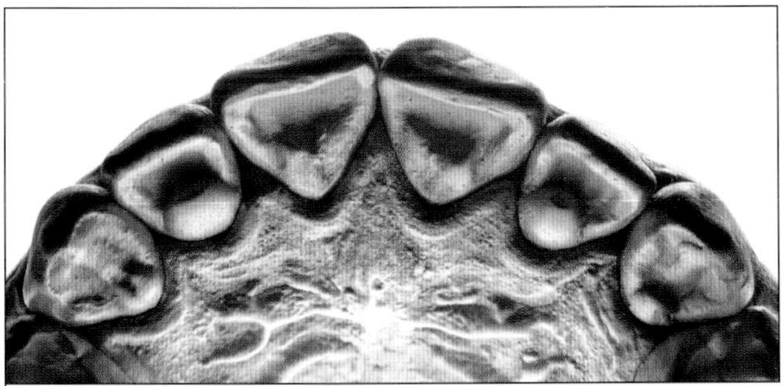

10a

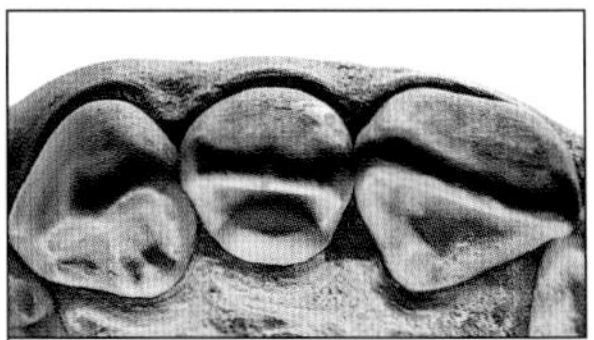

10b

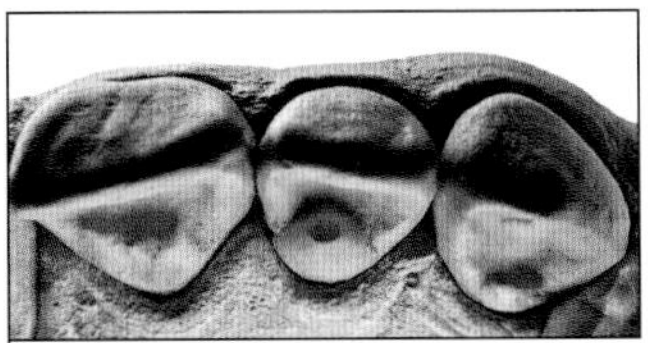

10c

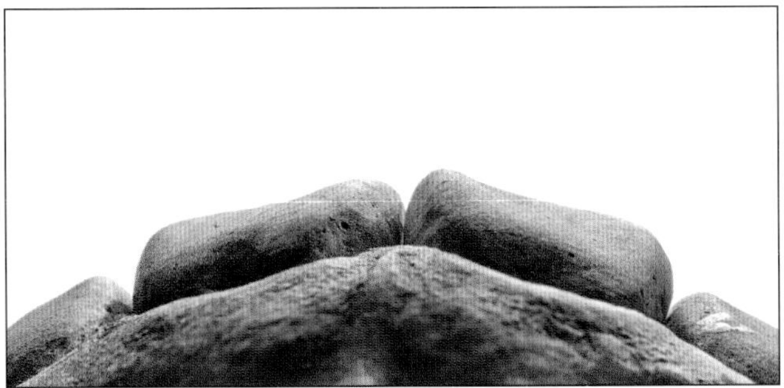

11a

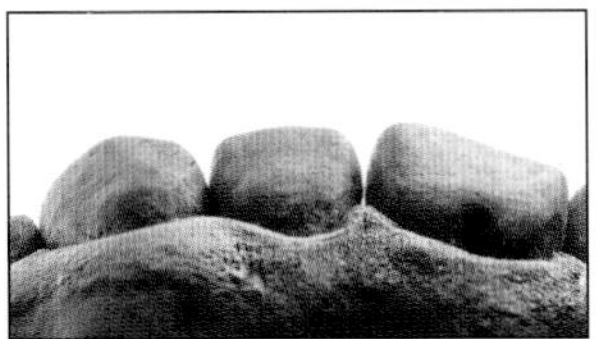

11b

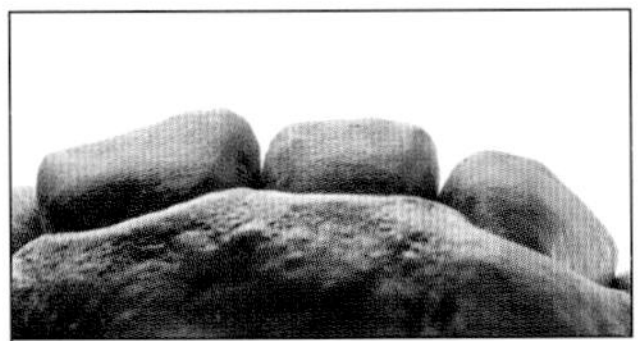

11c

Figs 10 and 11 Observing the model from different angles provides us with valuable functional and esthetic information. It is essential for comprehending the interplay of light, generating high-lights and low lights, which is necessary for a deep understanding of form.

Fig 12 Lateral view of a central incisor makes it possible to observe the effect of morphologic torsion with the flexion expressed distally.

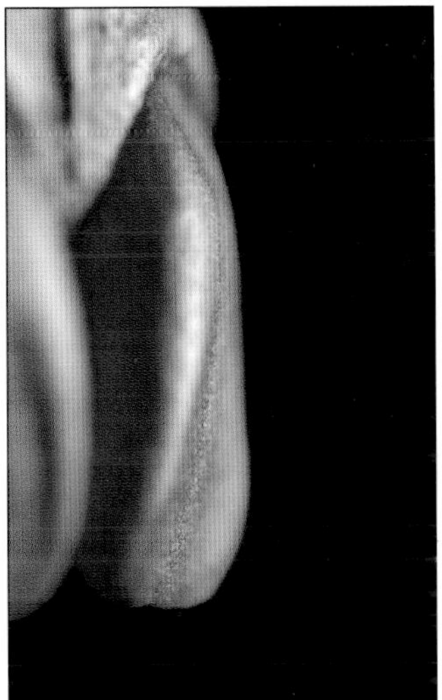

12

Maxillary Canines

The maxillary canines are considered to be the reinforced "cornerstones" within the anterior dentition, characterized by a series of transitional curves and arcs, being thicker labiolingually due to the increased development of the cingulum compared to that of incisors. A distinction is marked by the cusp tip, which is in line with the center of the root.

The mesial outline of the crown of the canine can be slightly convex and resembles that of the lateral incisor, the mesial transition line angle being well developed in the form of a small medial lobe. The distal outline of the crown is flat or concave and resembles that of the premolar (Figs 13 and 14).[9]

The characteristics of tooth form are not separate entities; rather, they combine to create a single feature. In other words, a tooth's topography is characterized by grooves that determine the three-dimensional anatomical areas. A frontal view alone does not provide enough information to reproduce the area around a transition line. Thus, the operator should begin working on each transitional line starting from the lingual surface. In all natural teeth, the ridges and grooves begin at the lingual surface and then connect to the proximal and facial surfaces (Fig 15).[9]

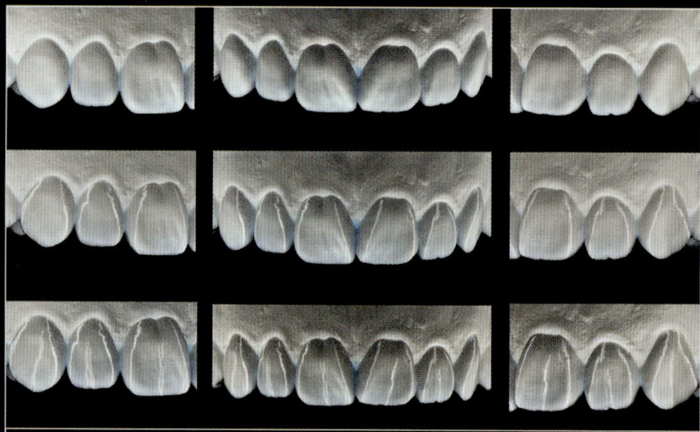

13

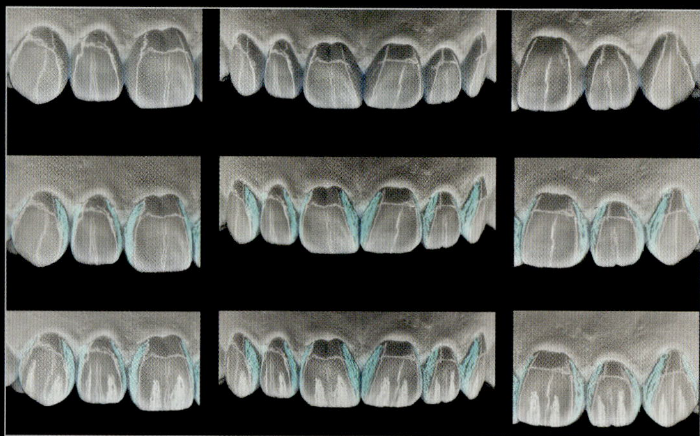

14

Figs 13 and 14 Scribing is essential for the rumination of morphology, as these lines and marks on the model serve as topographic references for morphodifferentiation between the maxillary central incisors, lateral incisors, and canines.

Fig 15 Incisal and palatal views showing the continuum of the proximal and facial morphology.

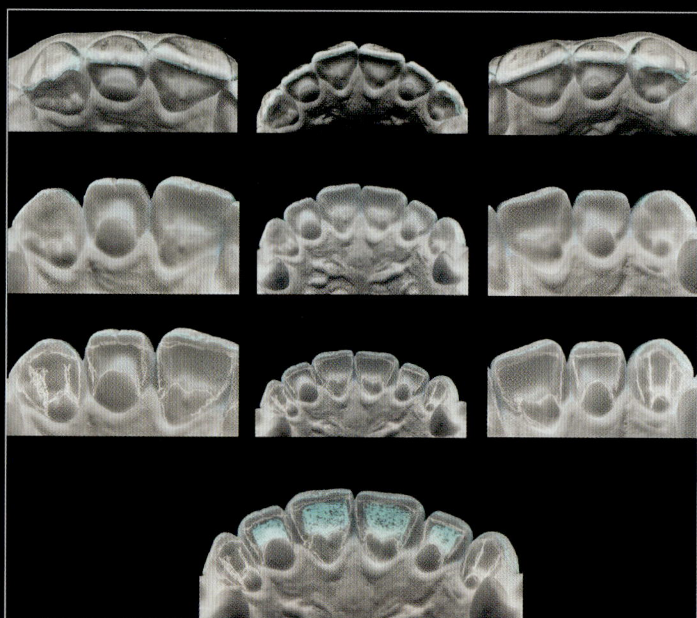

15

Fig 16 Model training involves sequential placement of wax (drop by drop) via the "dip and draw" technique.

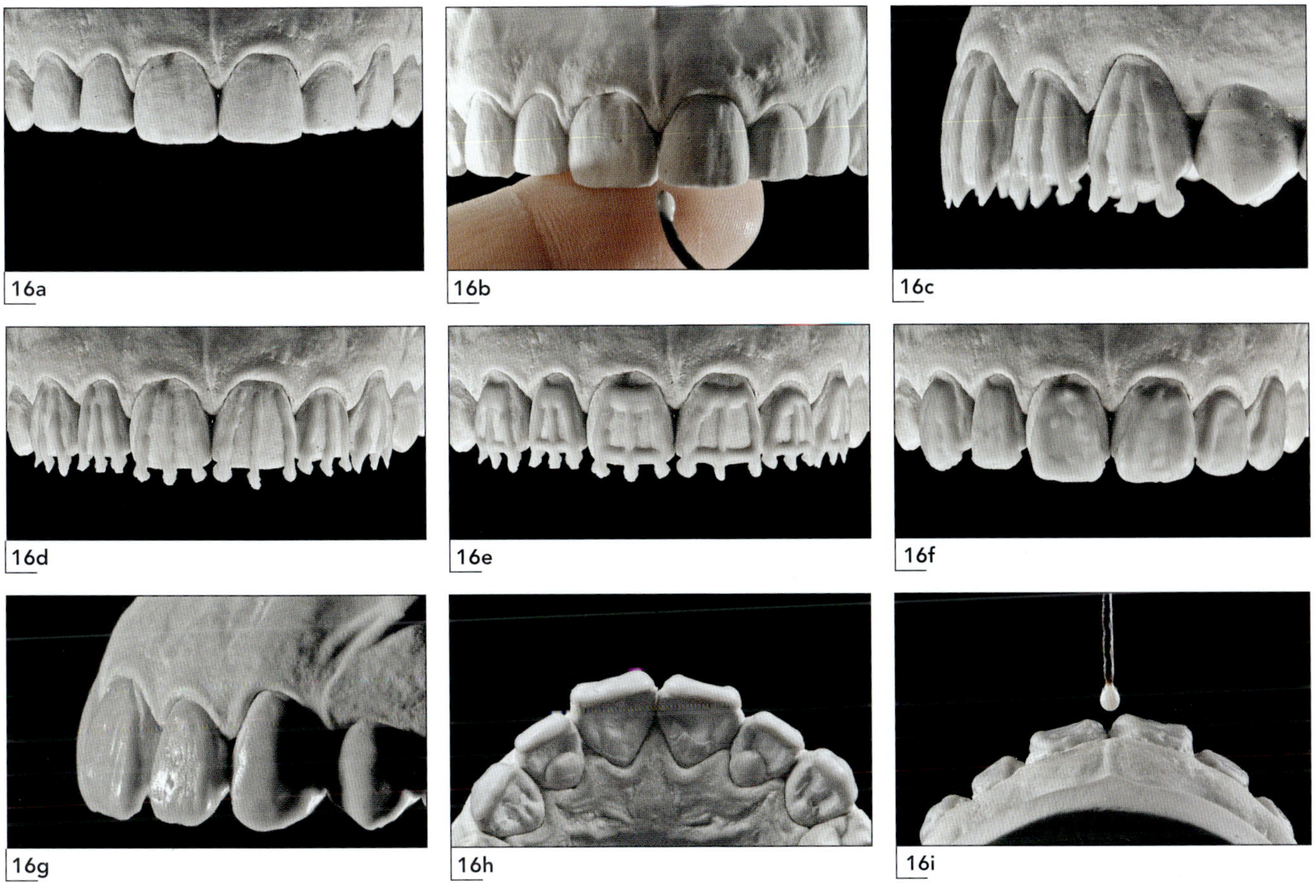

Fig 16a Initial situation.

Figs 16b and 16c Starting at the incisal edge (lobe creation is fingertip assisted), one may establish continuity between the vertical lobes and horizontal sectors for each tooth in the three main planes. One must also keep in mind that the labial curves of the lobes collectively slope toward the distogingival margin (sagittal plane), creating coronal torsion and in the process a convex smile line.

Figs 16d and 16e Incisal and cervical sectors are defined (dip and draw technique), linking the lobes initially with the horizontal incisal sectors and subsequently with cervical sectors.

Fig 16f "Windows" of space between vertical lobes and horizontal sectors are filled in, starting at the incisal edge (use fingertip for incisal part), establishing continuity between the vertical and horizontal topography for each tooth. Thickening of the incisal edge at the lingual aspect, before and after incisal edge thickening and continuity with lingual surfaces. (One's knowledge of natural tooth anatomy is used here, as well as direct comparison with models of natural dentitions.)

Figs 16g and 16h View of windows filled.

Fig 16i To establish continuity with the interdental surfaces, labial interdental surfaces are filled in with hot wax.

STAGE 5

Wax up the same anatomical fidelity within a model

This procedure requires precise knowledge of the strategic elements of tooth anatomy, which can be learned through systematic observation of natural teeth. This stage is defined by intuition, attention to detail, and good visual perception. Rigorous training should allow the dentist to define and attain the end goal of tooth reproduction (Fig 16).

The basic tooth shapes are defined by the vertical proximal crests, representing the transition line angles between the facial and proximal surfaces. The next

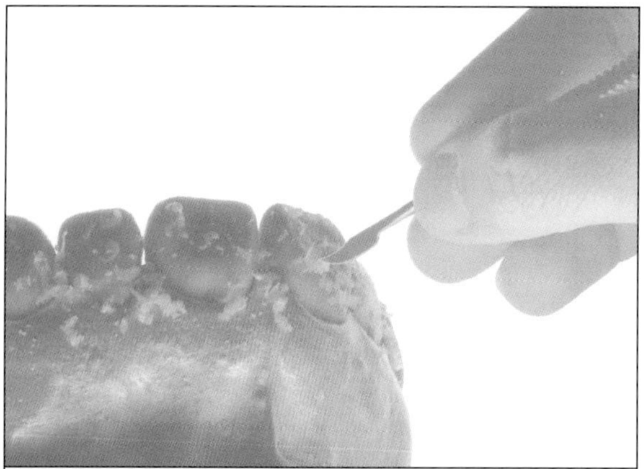

17a

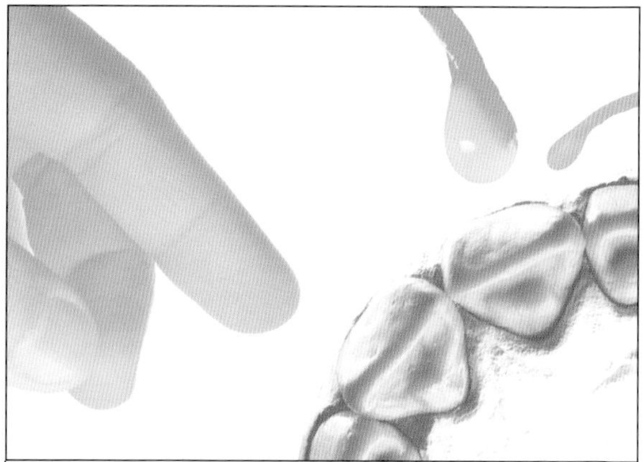

17b

Figs 17a and 17b Final form and surface texture: defining the vertical labial lobes and V shapes between lobes, horizontal texture within the incisal V shapes, horizontal and vertical texture across the labial and palatal surfaces.

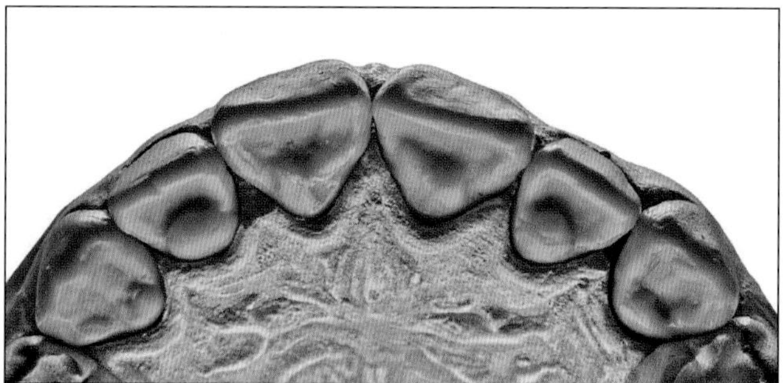

18a

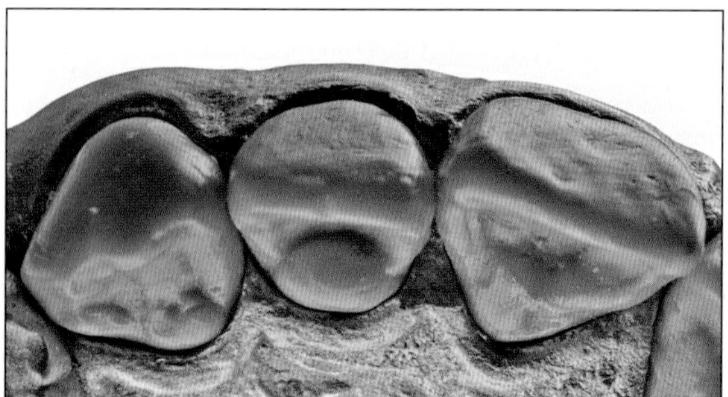

18b

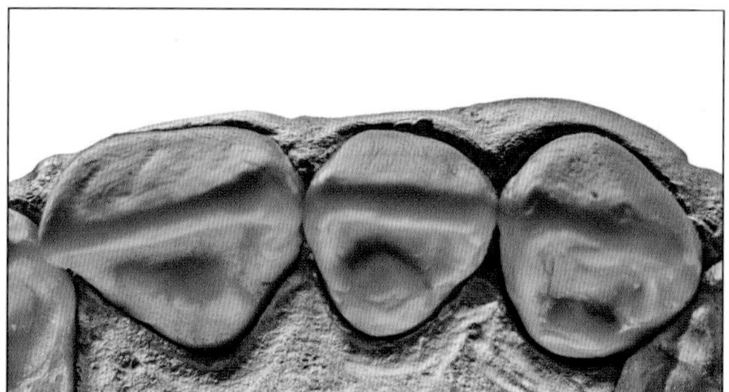

18c

step of the wax-up procedure is to recreate the superficial development lobes and horizontal components of surface topography resulting from the growth lines (Fig 16).[10] Because of their prominence, these ridges are the first to wear off and therefore should be the first elements to be restored by the additive wax-up technique. The position and arrangement of the lobes will influence the tooth form; the differential placement and contouring of the transition line angles can easily generate the illusion of a shorter or wider tooth.[10] The final form and surface texture, vertical labial lobes and V shapes between lobes, horizontal texture within the incisal V shapes, and the horizontal texture across the labial surface (Fig 17) all define the visual replication of natural anatomically formed teeth (Figs 18 to 20).

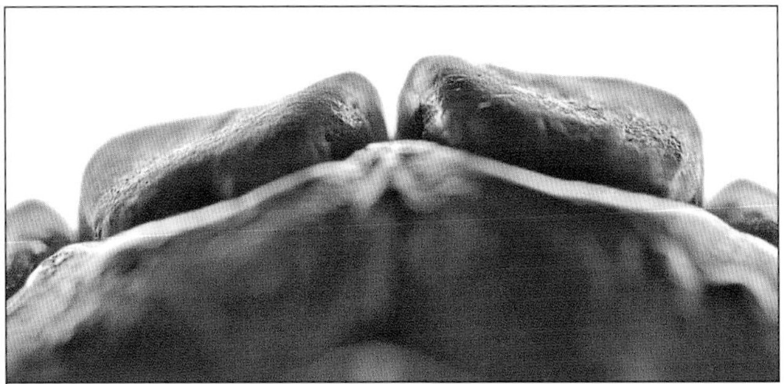

19a

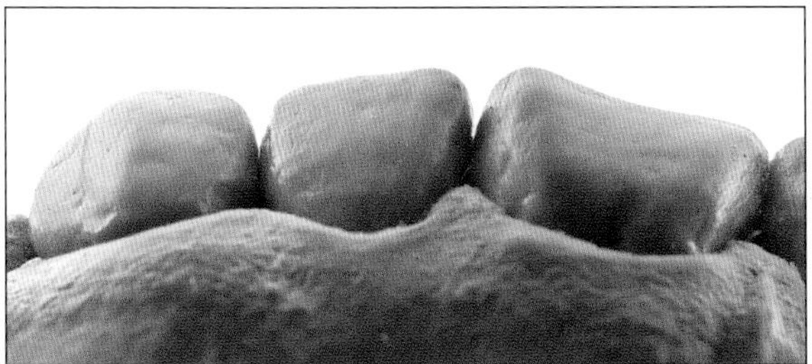

19b

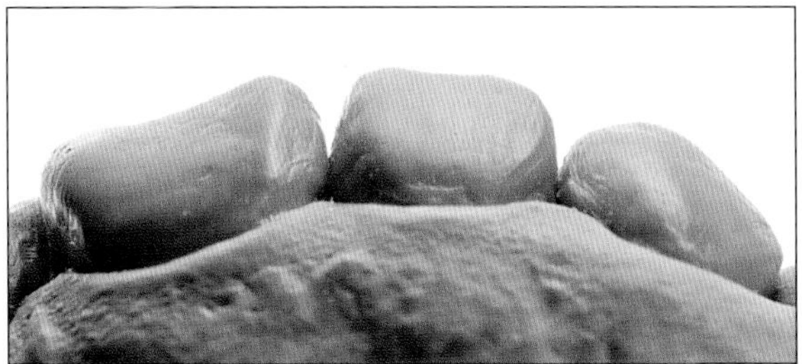

19c

Figs 18 to 20 The final wax-up must be carefully evaluated from all dimensional aspects. Every detail, no matter how miniscule it may be, is considered essential for an exact reproduction of the morphology of the original natural dental archetype, that of the intact tooth.

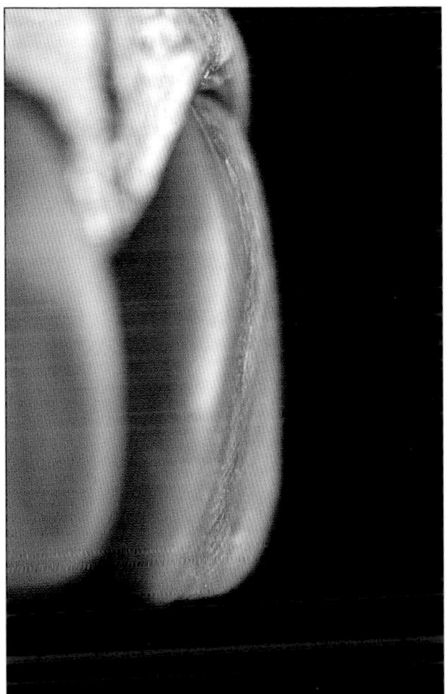

20

CONCLUSIONS

The creative moments between our hands, our eyes, and our brain always must be marked by the fluidity of a single motion. MVM training provides the ultimate path in continuous education and personal training, ensuring gratifying results by the perpetual achievement of higher-fidelity dental reproduction. Study nature and she will reveal her secrets.

ACKNOWLEDGMENTS

The authors would like to express gratitude and appreciation to Bianca Bianco for being the model in this article.

REFERENCES

1. Krishnan IS, Kheur MG. Esthetic considerations for the interdental papilla: Eliminating black triangles around restorations: A literature review. J Indian Prosthodont Soc 2006;6:164–169.
2. Nishimura Y. Reconstruction of coronal anatomy in ceramic restorations of the anterior teeth. Quintessence Dent Technol 1994;17:67–94.
3. Andrews LF. The six keys to normal occlusion. Am J Orthod 1972;62:296–309.
4. Andrews LF. Straight-Wire: The Concept and Appliance. San Diego: LA Wells, 1989.
5. Kataoka S, Yoshimi N. Nature's Morphology—An Atlas of Tooth Shape and Form. Chicago: Quintessence, 2002.
6. Edwards B. Aprender a Dibujar, Un Metodo Garantizado. Madrid: Hermann Blume, 1997.
7. Adolfi D. Natural Esthetics. Chicago: Quintessence, 2002.
8. Adolfi D. Functional, esthetic, and morphologic adjustment procedures for anterior teeth. Quintessence Dent Technol 2009;32: 153–168.
9. Chiche GJ, Pinault A. Esthetics of Anterior Fixed Prosthodontics. Chicago: Quintessence, 1994.
10. Magne P, Belser U. Bonded Porcelain Restorations in the Anterior Dentition: A Biomimetic Approach. Chicago: Quintessence, 2001.

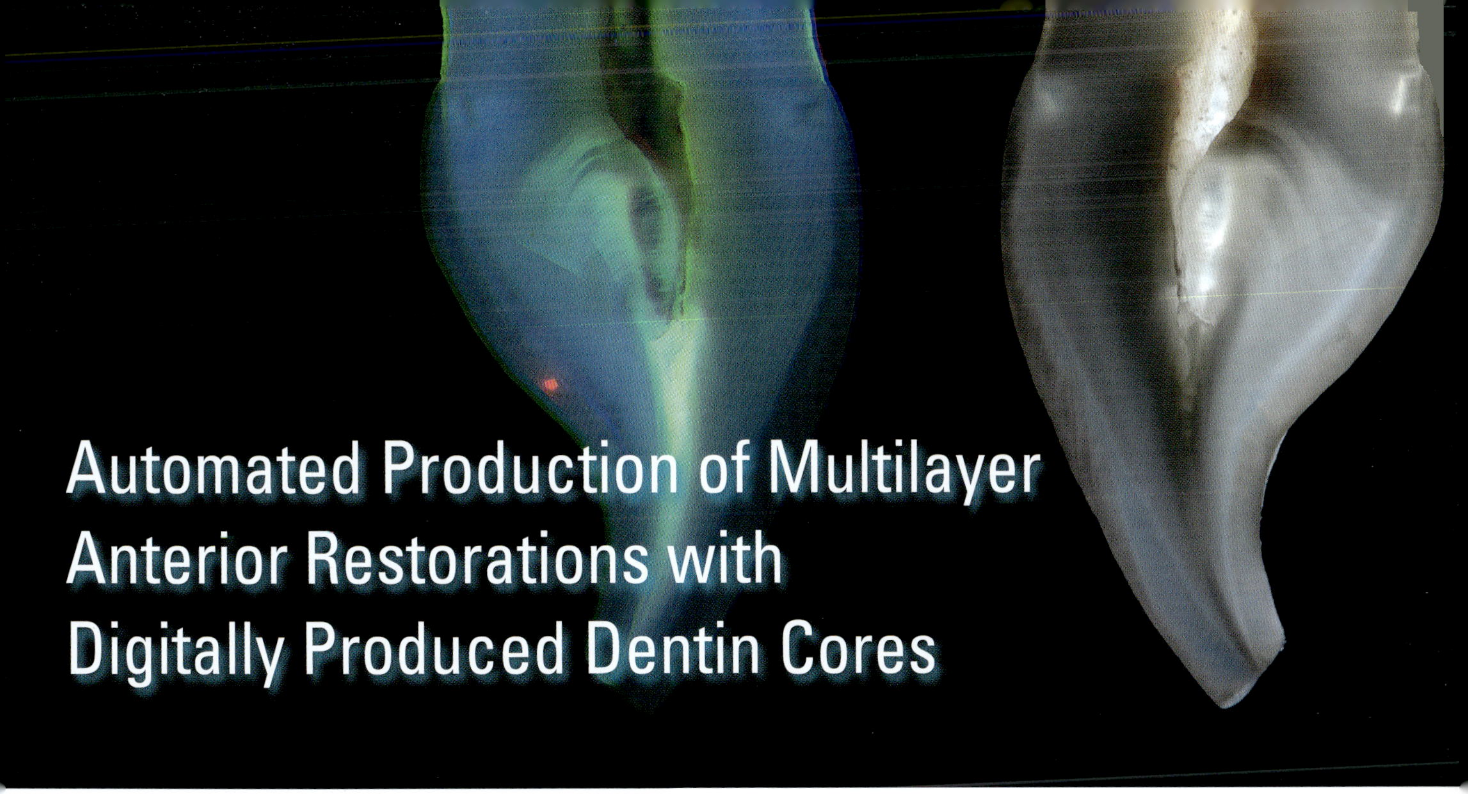

Automated Production of Multilayer Anterior Restorations with Digitally Produced Dentin Cores

Josef Schweiger, CDT[1]
Daniel Edelhoff, CDT, Dr Med Dent, PhD[2]
Michael Stimmelmayr, Dr Med Dent[3]
Jan-Frederik Güth, Dr Med Dent[3]
Florian Beuer, DDS, Dr Med Dent, PhD[3]

When producing digital dental restorations, it is now possible to mirror the geometry of teeth, to output the result as a data record, and to mill the resulting shape monolithically from a tooth-colored blank. The result is acceptable when restoring an entire anterior maxilla or mandible, although the esthetic results achieved with layered tooth build-ups will generally be more natural looking. The identical replication of adjacent teeth creates the illusion of "natural-identical" restorations.

Single maxillary anterior teeth, especially the central incisor, cannot be successfully realized as monolithic crowns, as these cannot adequately mimic the individually layered structure of anterior teeth. Here the craftsmanship of an experienced dental technician will continue to be required. But even the most skillful expert will have to redo maxillary anterior crowns at times, as the desired esthetic result does not always materialize on the first try.

In addition to the correct shape and surface, the shade also plays a significant role. In particular, the correct individual layering—or, in other words, the correct three-dimensional structure—of the crown is crucial for a perfect reproduction of a natural tooth.

The internal structure of the crown—especially the dentin—will determine the esthetics of an anterior restoration to a considerable extent. Experienced dental technicians are able to mimic the dentin in its three-dimensional manifestation but will generally not be

[1]Dental Technician, Department of Prosthodontics, Dental School, Ludwig-Maxmilians University, Munich, Germany.
[2]Director and Chair, Department of Prosthodontics, Dental School, Ludwig-Maxmilians University, Munich, Germany.
[3]Assistant Professor, Department of Prosthodontics, Dental School, Ludwig-Maxmilians University, Munich, Germany.

Correspondence to: Josef Schweiger, Department of Prosthodontics, Ludwig-Maxmilians University, Goethestrasse 70, 80336 Munich, Germany. Email: Josef.Schweiger@med.uni-muenchen.de

able to provide any precise spatial definitions. The design of the dentin core is therefore based mainly on the training and the experience of the dental technician and often follows a "traditional" approach. Thus, almost all dental technicians leave a clearly discernible "signature" as they prepare their restorations, a restorative artefact that does not, strictly speaking, have any connection with the case at hand.

STATE OF THE ART

Ingots with Plane-Parallel Layers

Various approaches have been used to imitate the layered structure of natural teeth using digital methods. For example, various manufacturers offer ingots for computer-aided design/computer-assisted manufacture (CAD/CAM) processing that consist of several plane-parallel layers, with the individual layers having different shades. Examples include the Vitablocs TriLuxe forte ingot (Vita Zahnfabrik), the CEREC Bloc C PC (Sirona), and the Noritake Katana Zirconia ML disc (Kuraray Noritake). These ingots attempt to mimic the shade gradient of the natural tooth, from cementum and dentin to enamel, by presenting differently colored layers within the material. The software can modify the vertical alignment of the restoration within the ingot, allowing the chroma of the restoration to be modified. The esthetic results of restorations from these polychromatic blocks are certainly better than the esthetics of restorations made from monochromatic blanks. Nevertheless, they cannot be used to create customized, patient-specific layers.

Three-Dimensional Ingot Structure with Dentin Core and Enamel Coating

A second approach to imitating the layered structure of natural teeth is a millable ingot that has a three-dimensional block structure with dentin core and enamel coating and an arched gradient between the dentin and incisal (VITA RealLife Block, Sirona CEREC Blocs C In). The software can relocate the virtual design within the ingot such that the proportion of dentin and enamel is modified. This is supposed to give users the opportunity to imitate the appearance of natural teeth as closely as possible. But even these ingots cannot be used to produce customized, patient-specific layers.

Semi-finished Crowns

A third approach is that of the so-called semi-finished crowns, such as the priti crown (pritidenta), which already features the anatomical outer geometry of the clinical crown and a standardized layered structure of the dentin and incisal areas. The only thing left to do is use the CAD/CAM system to remove a volume corresponding to the prepared tooth in shape and form of the basal aspect of the crown. The disadvantage is that only subtractive processing is possible, so that slightly larger blanks are generally used that are reduced by milling to match the CAD design. Milling can never add material!

Tooth Databases

Systems for computer-aided manufacturing of dental restorations include tooth databases based on data from scanned natural teeth, scanned prefabricated teeth, or scanned manually waxed-up tooth shapes. However, these databases invariably refer only to the external tooth geometry.

Biogeneric Occlusal Surfaces

Sirona's CEREC system uses so-called "biogenic occlusal surfaces" (developed by Professor Dr Albert Mehl of the University of Zürich, Switzerland), which operates on the basis of several thousand scanned natural teeth. The system determines the closest match in the tooth database to the remaining tooth structure, "adds" the missing portions, and thereby obtains a very natural partial-crown (or inlay, or onlay) geometry. But even the "biogeneric tooth model" is confined exclusively to the external tooth geometry.[1] In the biogeneric tooth model, missing parts of the external tooth surface are added in by adapting a generic record of the desired tooth to the residual tooth structures and/or antagonists and/or adjacent teeth

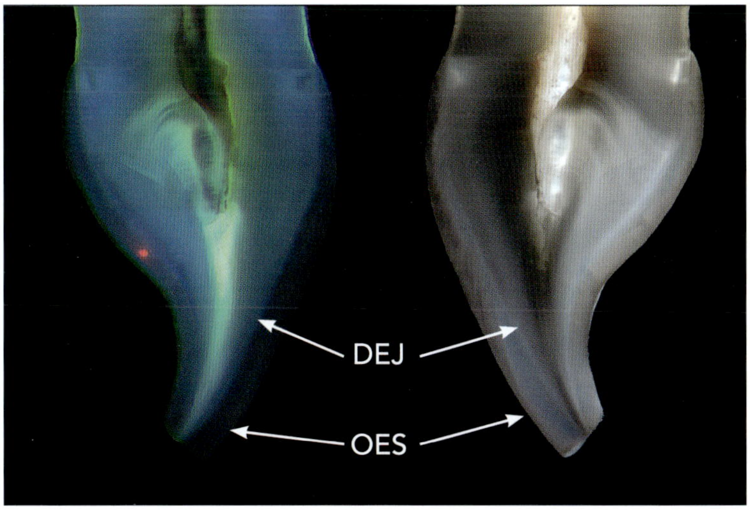

Fig 1 Sagittal sections of anterior crowns. The dentinoenamel junction (DEJ) and the outer enamel surface (OES) are clearly discernible.

situation and/or bite registration. Furthermore, Sirona provides a database for the CEREC system in which the user is presented with a static mamelon structure, generated according to geometric design guidelines, which is then customized by CAD and produced by CAM in the milling unit.

In his doctoral thesis, Probst[2] described the morphology of maxillary anterior teeth and the determination of similarity metrics of identical anterior tooth types in the left and right maxilla. However, he did not address the layered internal three-dimensional structure of anterior teeth.

Looking at the current state of the art as just presented, it can be summarized that no database is currently available for the layered internal three-dimensional tooth structures in the anterior and posterior regions. The term "tooth-structure database" as used below denotes a database/library that includes internal three-dimensional tooth structures and the corresponding surfaces of the respective specific teeth in digital and/or physical form. Neither has a method been described for the automated generation of the layered internal tooth structure, especially the dentin.

DEJ AND OES

By far the largest part of the human tooth consists of dentin, which forms the inner "protective coating" for the pulp cavity in its center. The pulp consists mainly of loosely packed connective tissue with numerous cells, intercellular basic substance, reticular and collagen fibers, and—not least—nerves and blood vessels.[3] The dentin in turn is covered by enamel in the clinical crown area and by cementum in the root area. Together, enamel, dentin, and cementum represent the hard tissue of the human tooth. The enamel is the hardest substance in the human body, with a Vickers hardness of 250 to 550 and a compressive strength of 300 to 450 MPa. Its modulus of elasticity is 50,000 to 85,000 MPa.[4] The dentin, by contrast, is much more elastic (Young's modulus of 15,000 to 20,000 MPa), because it contains a significantly higher percentage of organic matter. The Vickers hardness of the dentin is 60 to 70, and its compressive strength is 200 to 350 MPa.[4] The cementum is similar to human bone in both structure and hardness but differs from bone in that it is not vascularized. The cementum is already considered part of the attachment apparatus, or periodontium. This is where the periodontal fibers are attached that keep the teeth in their bony sockets, or alveoli.[3]

The dentinoenamel junction (DEJ) and the outer enamel surface (OES) (Fig 1) are essential features of the three-dimensional structure of the tooth and significantly affect its visual appearance. Some study results indicate that the DEJ provides considerable information about the OES.[5–25] It is known that the shape of the DEJ closely resembles the shape that the OES reflects[6,7,26] and that, unlike the OES, the DEJ is preserved intact in abraded teeth.

There are different ways to represent the DEJ in three dimensions, as described as follows.

Chemical Removal of the Enamel Layer

Chemical removal of the enamel layer is a destructive method for preparing the DEJ. The entire enamel layer can be removed with 37% phosphoric acid.[5,15–18] Since the enamel layer is destroyed in the process, it is necessary to preserve the OES. This can be done in an analog manner, by taking an impression of the tooth crown and subsequent pouring of a cast, or digitally, by scanning the tooth crown. The scan operation can be performed mechanically (eg, Procera Forte, Nobel Biocare) or by means of an optical scanner (eg, BEGO 3Shape D 700, Bego Medical).

Computed Tomography

The three-dimensional geometry of the OES and DEJ can be acquired by standard computed tomography (CT) or cone beam computed tomography (CBCT). The resolution and accuracy of the data vary greatly depending on the manufacturer. Therefore, it is often difficult to obtain 3D data sufficiently accurate for further processing from CT or CBCT data. The InVesalius software (CTI Renato Archer) can convert two-dimensional data from CT scans to three-dimensional DICOM (Digital Imaging and Communications in Medicine) data. These DICOM data are then converted to STL (Standard Tessellation Language) data.[27–29]

Microcomputed Tomography

The best way to acquire three-dimensional OES and DEJ data is by microcomputed tomography (microCT). In the study presented here, the extracted teeth were scanned with the exaCT S S60 HRE desktop CT unit (Wenzel Volumetrik). The voxel size was 45 µm. The exaCT Analysis software (Wenzel) was used for data acquisition and output. The data for the enamel (with the OES on the outside and the DEJ on the inside) and the root with dentin core (DEJ) and pulp chamber were converted to the STL format and output.

PRINCIPLE OF THE DENTIN-CORE CROWN

As early as 1945, Weidenreich had noted that the surface relief of the dentin (the DEJ) could not be a purely accidental feature without any morphologic importance.[19,30] The basic principle of the digital dentin-core crown/digital dentin-core bridge according to Schweiger[31] is as follows: "There is a clear correlation between the three-dimensional tooth surface (OES) and the layered internal structure of a tooth (the dentin core and DEJ)" (Fig 2). As used here, the term "correlation" signifies the association of a record describing the structure of the internal layer (ie, the DEJ) with a record defining the external geometry of the tooth (ie, the OES).

Based on this axiom,[32] a tooth-structure database can be compiled that allows, for the first time, crown or bridge restorations to be produced accurately and with an esthetic appearance that replicates the natural model (Fig 2).

Tooth-Structure Database

The idea on which the invention is based calls for acquiring not only the outer structures of the tooth but also the layered internal tooth geometry and to use it in conjunction with the external geometry, for example by storing them in a database (Figs 3 to 9).[31,33,34] If the external and layered internal tooth structures can be connected with each other dynamically, this is a particular advantage, as a virtual modification of the external geometry of the tooth can then be reflected by corresponding changes in the internal structure. Another advantage is that the digital acquisition of a large number of three-dimensional external and internal tooth geometries allows the establishment of a well-defined relationship between the layered structure of the inner tooth and its outer shape. Furthermore, once a suitable external geometry has been selected, the database can propose an internal tooth geometry that, with great probability, will correspond to the internal geometry of the natural tooth.

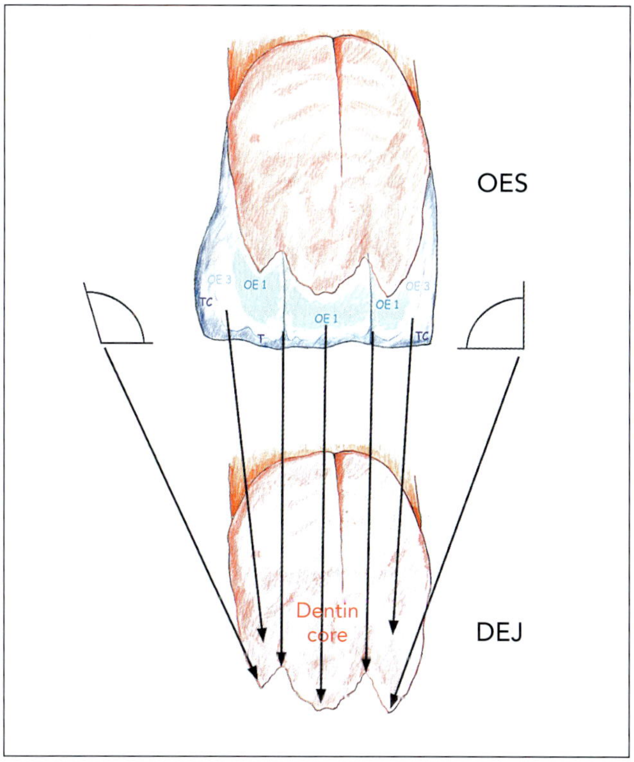

Fig 2 Principle of the digital dentin-core crown according to Schweiger ("inward biogenerics"). OES = outer enamel surface. DEJ = dentinoenamel junction.

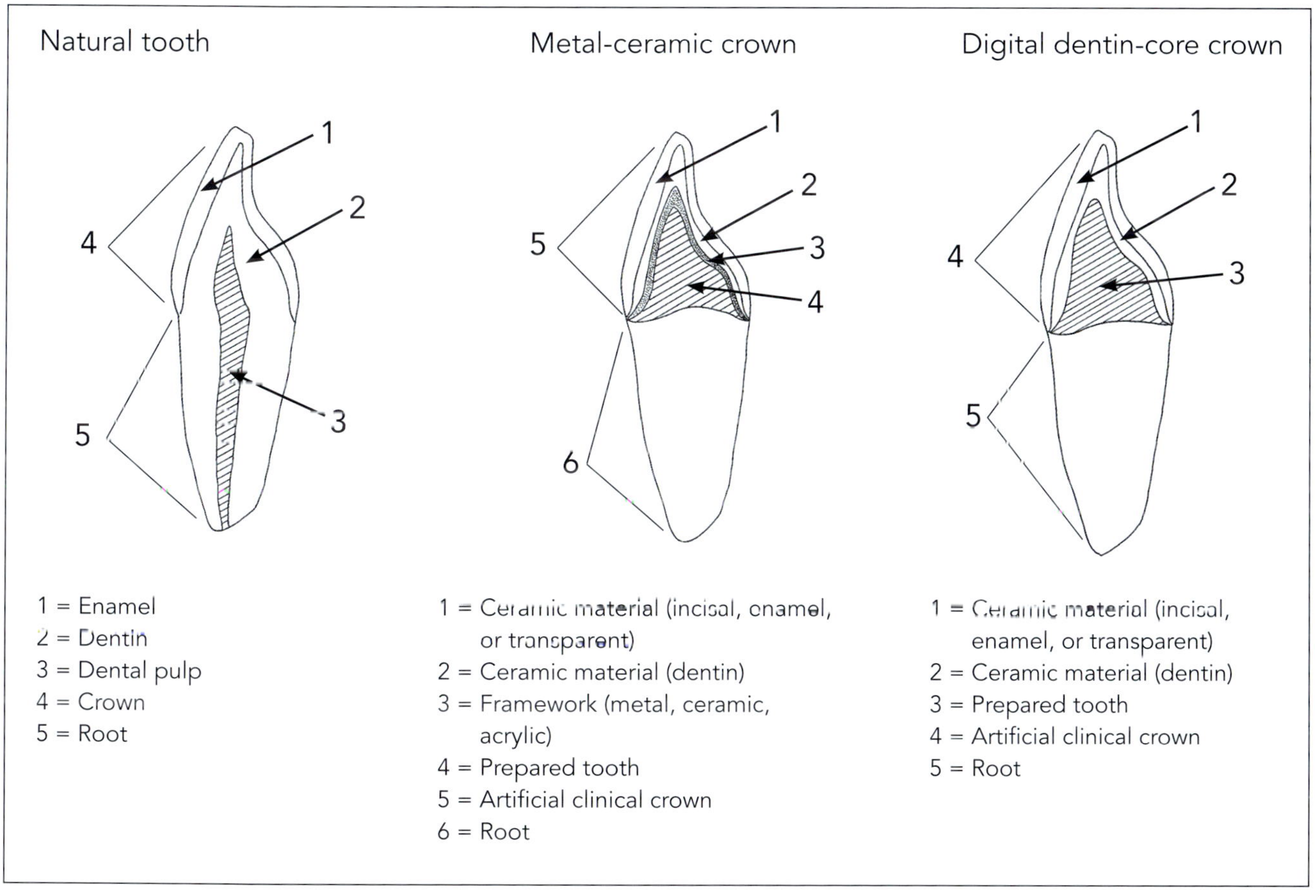

Fig 3 Natural tooth, metal-ceramic crown, and dentin-core crown (longitudinal sections).

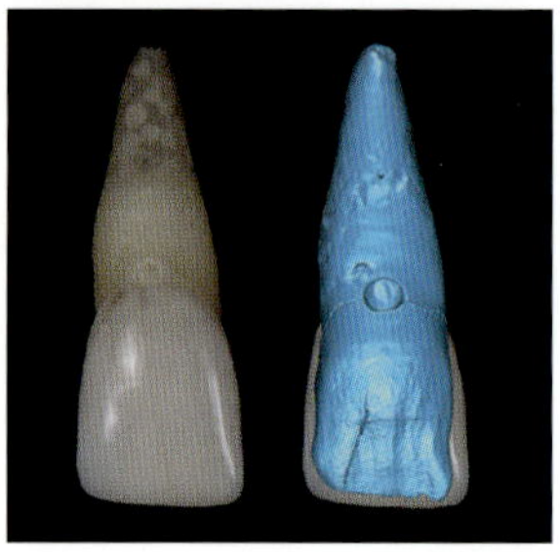

Fig 4 Natural tooth with corresponding dentin core.

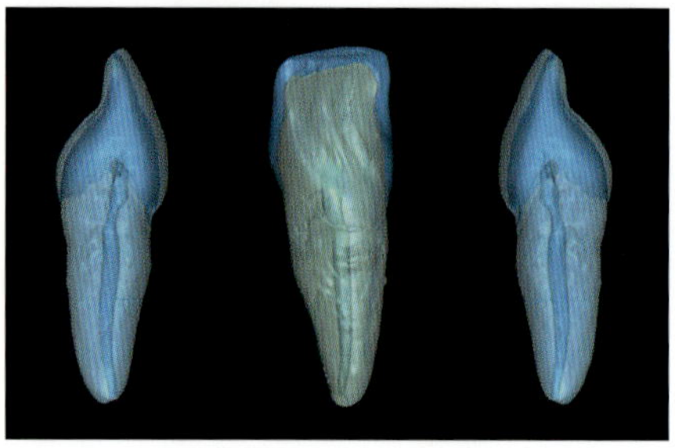

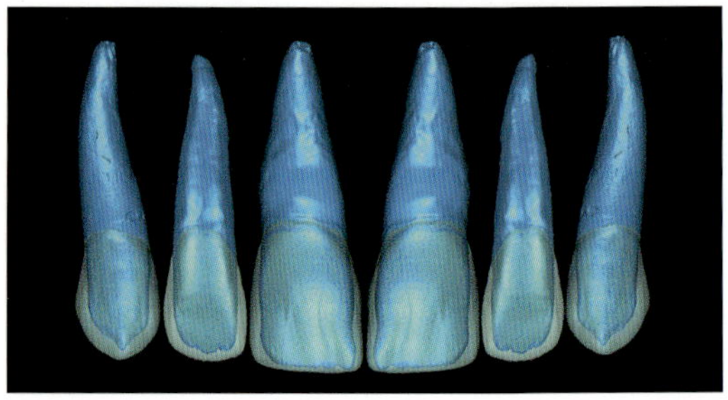

Figs 5a and 5b STL records from a tooth structure database of the outer enamel surface and the dentinoenamel junction.

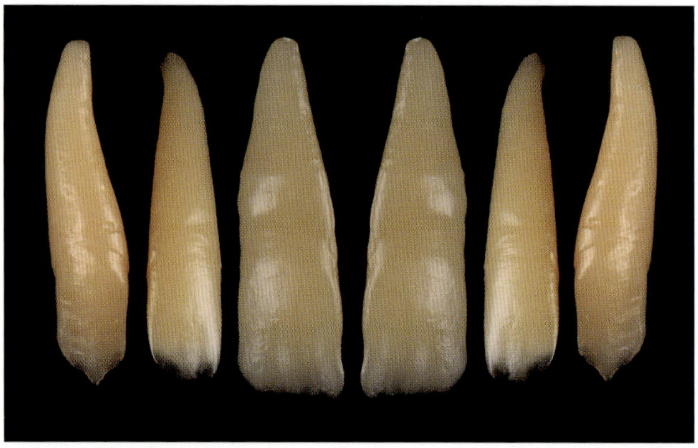

Fig 6 CAD/CAM dentin cores, manufactured based on STL data of the dentinoenamel junction.

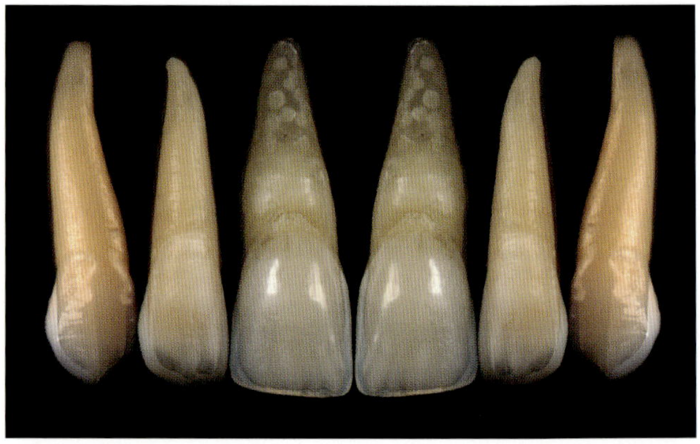

Fig 7 Virtual rendering of the outer enamel surface and the CAD/CAM dentin cores.

Correlations between the external and internal tooth geometries are recognized, for instance when certain types of tooth shapes (eg, oval, square, triangular) are associated with characteristic internal tooth structures (eg, pronounced mamelons in the case of projecting triangular teeth). Tooth types can be further subdivided into different shape groups by looking at tooth-specific surface and shape characteristics, including:

- Mesiodistal curvature
- Incisocervical curvature
- Rounding of the distal incisal edge
- Rounding of the mesial incisal edge
- Angle characteristics
- Incisal edge contours
- Surface-structure components such as longitudinal grooves or elevations

Data records of scans can be assigned to shape groups either by visual inspection or digitally using the best-fit alignment method. Either way, the result will be a database of teeth that subdivides the different tooth types into multiple shape groups.

Similarly, it is possible to assign the acquired internal tooth structures (especially the dentin cores) of the various tooth types (central incisors, lateral incisors, canines, first and second premolars, first to third molars) to different shape groups by using the same method. Here, again, the assignment can be made by visual inspection or using the best-fit alignment method. The result is a database of internal tooth structures, again subdivided into multiple shape groups. In addition, it is possible to establish a correlation between the internal and external tooth geometries. Using the database data, an internal tooth geometry is proposed for a given external tooth shape. It is highly probable that this proposal corresponds to the "real" internal tooth geometry (Figs 8 and 9)—the more so, the more records are included in the tooth database. BEGO Medical already realized this in its Dentaldesigner software from 3Shape. This software stored, for the first time, tooth geometries that are created on the basis of the real tooth.

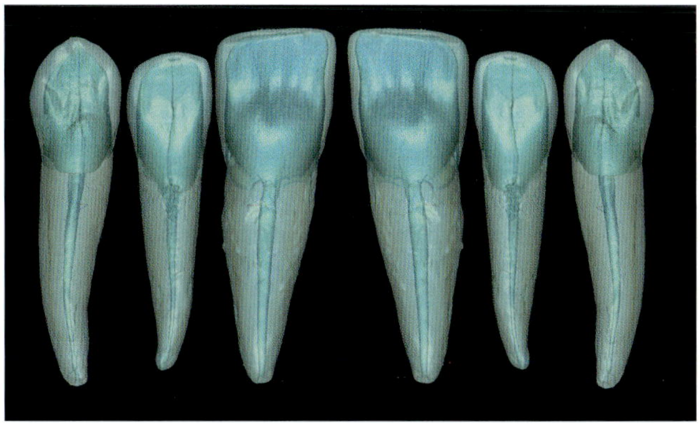

Fig 8 Palatal view of tooth structure data of maxillary anterior teeth, showing the dental pulp, the dentinoenamel junction, and the outer enamel surface.

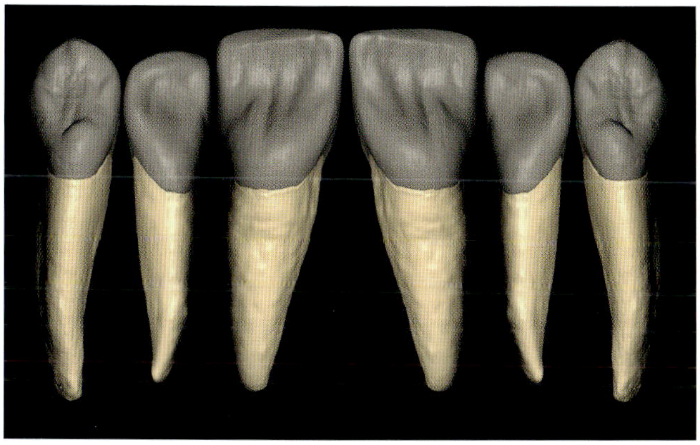

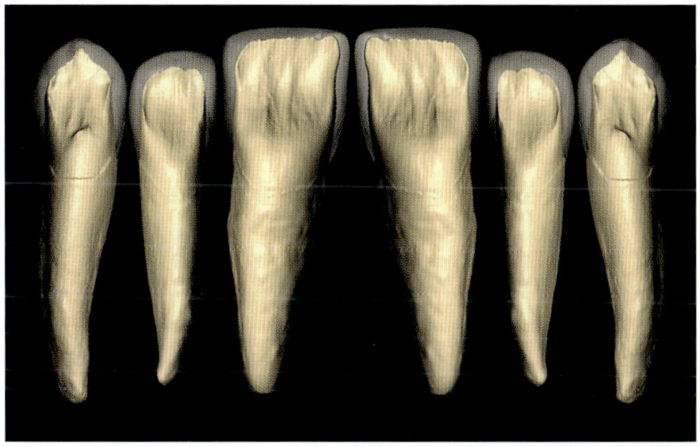

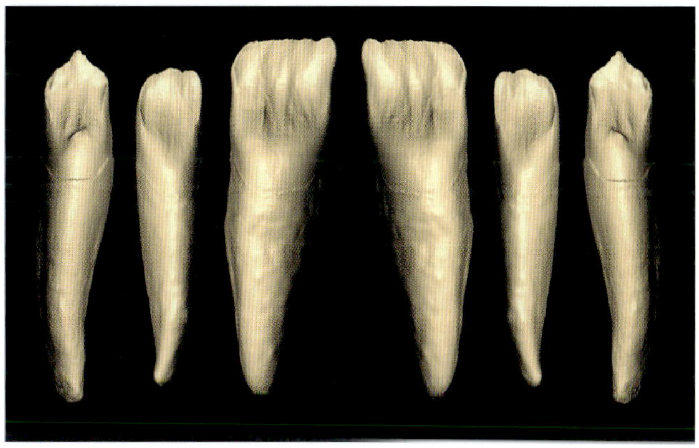

Figs 9a to 9c STL records of dentin cores and enamel coatings of maxillary anterior teeth.

A novel application—the biogeneric tooth model—is also supported. This model calculates, based on the vast number of different tooth records in the database, an internal tooth geometry (eg, a dentin core) that has all the features characteristic of the respective tooth type. This is not achieved by merely averaging or superimposing the individual data points (x_n, y_n, z_n) that describe the internal tooth geometry, as this would result in noisy, unstructured data that do not correspond in any way to the typical geometry. Rather, the dentin core is segmented into individual building blocks (mamelons, incisal grooves, incisal contours of the dentin, etc) to uncover correspondences and to compare like with like. This prevents essential structures of the dentin core from being averaged out in calculating the geometry, as happens, for example, with mamelons during conventional alignment calculations, for example with regard to mamelons. This method produces an average internal tooth geometry with averaged values for the characteristic building blocks, such as mamelons, incisal grooves, incisal edges, etc.

In the next step, the deviation of the individual internal geometries from the respective average geometry is calculated by a principal-axis transformation. If the goal is to reconstruct a layered internal tooth structure, the biogeneric tooth model must be correlated with the external tooth geometry. Here, the layered internal tooth structure—especially the dentin core—corresponds to the missing hard tissue of the tooth substance in a biogeneric inlay reconstruction. A certain spatial distribution of a few design points on the external tooth surface requires a certain morphology of the dentin core. The combination of an average dentin core with the biogeneric model of the external tooth geometry makes it possible to assign the most probable dentin core to a given external tooth geometry. The morphologic relationship between the external tooth geometry and the layered internal tooth structure is essentially based on a genetic blueprint. The probability is high that a specific external tooth geometry can be correlated with a specific layered internal tooth structure, especially with regard to the dentin core, and vice versa. It should be pointed out in this context that one of the lead structures during odontogenesis is the preformative membrane, which eventually forms the DEJ.

This membrane is an anatomical structure that forms during tooth development. As a basement membrane, it constitutes the interface between the mesenchymal connective tissue (the mesodermal papilla) and the ectodermal enamel organ. Shortly before the dentin begins to form, this basement membrane thickens and henceforth separates the dentin from the enamel. Here, odontoblasts and ameloblasts are initially located back-to-back as the pre-dentin/pre-enamel is converted, gradually moving away from each other while the hard tissues of the tooth they have formed are left behind.

Once the external tooth geometry has been digitally linked to the internal tooth geometry, a correlation is formed between the two records, a correlation that can be either dynamic or static. In a static correlation, the internal geometry is not changed by a modification of the outer geometry, which among other things implies that the dentin core always retains its shape. In a dynamic correlation, however, the internal tooth structure is modified in response to any modifications of the external tooth surface. On modifying the external tooth geometry, all X/Y/Z values of the internal tooth geometry change proportionately to the X/Y/Z values of the external tooth geometry (scaling). Rotations will be performed with the same angle, and translations with the same X/Y/Z values will be performed by adding the translation values.

This database with correlations between the internal and external tooth geometries (correlations database) can be used in different ways in the production of dental restorations. Using computer-assisted output devices (computer numerical control [CNC]; rapid prototyping [RP]), restorations can be produced that mimic the layered internal structure of a natural tooth. The internal structure of the restoration is produced based on a record from the database, where the external surface corresponds exactly to the internal tooth structure of a record selected from the database. Suitable materials for creating the internal core include materials with a toothlike esthetic appearance in terms of shade and translucency, especially resin, glass ceramics, feldspar ceramics, lithium disilicate ceramics, and oxidic high-performance ceramics such as zirconia and alumina. Once this computer-generated internal aspect of the restoration has been produced, the incisal aspects can be added. This can be performed manually using a ceramic layering technique or a wax-up technique with subsequent overpressing. Alternatively, this incisal area can be designed by subtracting the internal tooth structure from the external tooth surface, creating a differential record that can be transformed into a real-world object using a CAM procedure. In a subsequent additive step, this incisal area is then connected to the dentin core by sintering (using a ceramic connector mass), by a polymerization process, or adhesively.

In the context of the method described here, there are several ways to design and manufacture dental restorations digitally (Fig 10), as shown below.

Best-fit alignment

The arch situation comprising the teeth to be replaced as well as the adjacent teeth is acquired by three-dimensional scanning (intraoral or extraoral). If a "mirror tooth" is present, its three-dimensional structure is mirrored. A study[2] has shown that mirror-image replacements of anterior teeth are satisfactory with respect to interproximal, occlusal, and esthetic aspects. Using an iterative procedure, the external structure of the mirror-image tooth is compared to and correlated

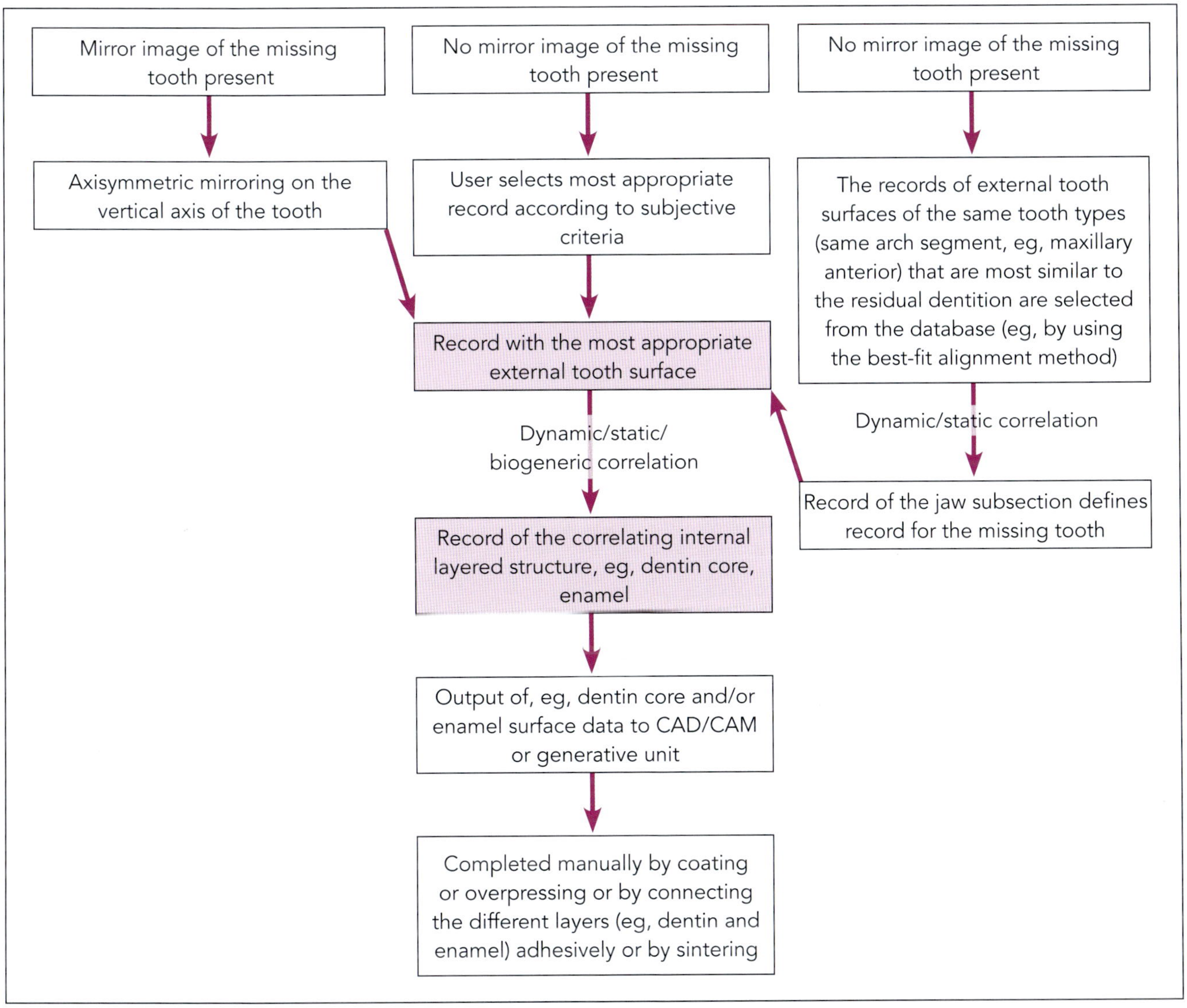

Fig 10 Schematic representation of the fabrication of dental restorations with the aid of a tooth-structure database.

with the natural or manually designed teeth in the correlations database until the most appropriate record is found. To determine the appropriate record by way of an iterative procedure, it is possible to devise a similarity metric based on the standard deviation of the smallest distances of points on the surface of the mirrored tooth from the respective closest points of each tooth record in the database.

$$SD = \sqrt{\frac{\sum_{i,j}^{n} [(X_{1i} - x_{2j}) + (y_{1i} - y_{2j}) + (z_{1i} - z_{2j})]^2}{n}}$$

(SD = standard deviation over the shortest distance = similarity metric)

This method is also called "best-fit alignment." To achieve a best-fit alignment, the tooth is mirrored and then superimposed on a reference tooth from the database in the optimal position by rotation, translation, and possibly also scaling. Image analysis software (eg, Geomagic Qualify, Geomagic GmbH) can be used for this. As a layered internal tooth structure exists for the best-fitting record, this structure can be used for designing the restoration, and specifically its dentin core, using computer-assisted methods. Once the dentin core has been created, the incisal aspect can be built up manually; alternatively, a CAM-created incisal segment can be connected to the dentin core by sintering or adhesively.

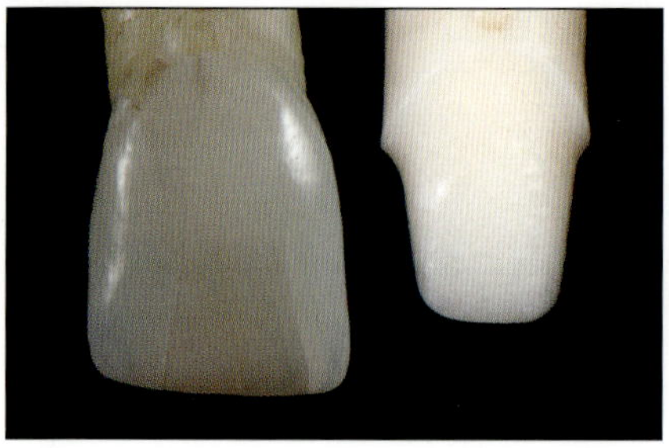

Fig 11 Maxillary right central incisor and the corresponding die of the left central to be restored.

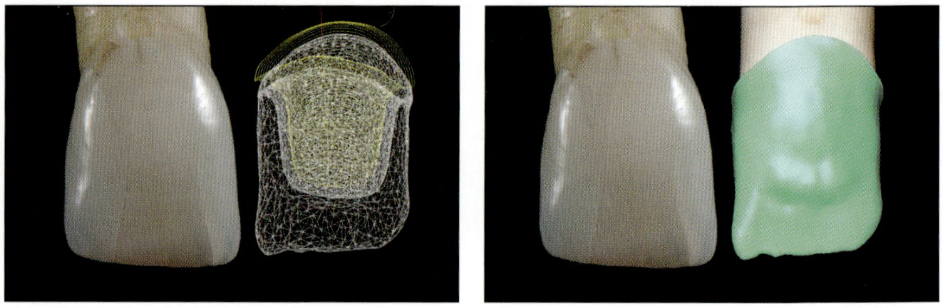

Figs 12a and 12b STL data of the mirrored dentinoenamel junction of the maxillary right central.

Customizing the data according to user preferences

The arch situation comprising the teeth to be replaced as well as the adjacent teeth is acquired by three-dimensional scanning (intraoral or extraoral). If no mirror-image tooth is present, a record presumed to be appropriate is selected from the database and can be three-dimensionally adapted to the actual situation by rotation, translation, and scaling. Due to the dynamic correlation of the record of the three-dimensional external tooth geometry with the record of the three-dimensional layered internal tooth structure, a design for a layered core, eg, a dentin core, will be suggested. The suggested dentin core can then be customized as required. The three-dimensional record is implemented physically on a computer-assisted output device such as a CNC or RP unit.

Best-fit alignment after customizing the data according to user preferences

The arch situation comprising the teeth to be replaced as well as the adjacent teeth is acquired by three-dimensional scanning (intraoral or extraoral). If no mirror-image tooth is present, the software compares the residual dentition with the records from the database of arch segments, and the record presumed to be the most appropriate is selected using the best-fit alignment method. Since this record is assigned to exactly one record of the missing tooth, it can serve as a basis for the tooth to be replaced. Due to the dynamic correlation of the three-dimensional external tooth geometry with the three-dimensional layered internal tooth structure, a design for a layered core, eg, a dentin core, will be suggested. The suggested dentin core can then be customized as required. The three-dimensional record is implemented physically on a computer-assisted output device such as a CNC or RP unit (eg, Bego Medical).

Automated Manufacturing Process for Individual Anterior Crowns

Using tooth-structure databases it is possible to produce—using a partially or fully automated process—highly esthetic restorations, especially for the anterior region.

Let us assume a single anterior crown is to be provided for the maxillary left central incisor using a digital process, where the natural right central incisor is used as a template. Producing a single crown for a maxillary central incisor is considered one of the most difficult challenges in prosthodontics. The procedure consists of the following steps:

1. Acquiring the external tooth surface
2. Identifying the matching dentin core
3. Mirroring the external tooth surface and dentin core data
4. Digital manufacturing of the dentin core
5. Adding the incisal region
6. Digital finishing of the tooth surface
7. Finalizing the crown (glaze firing, polishing, etc)

Acquiring the external tooth surface

The external surface of the natural right central incisor can be acquired by three-dimensional digital scanning (Fig 11) with a mechanical or optical scanner or using a sonographic or radiologic procedure such as CT, CBCT, or micro-CT.

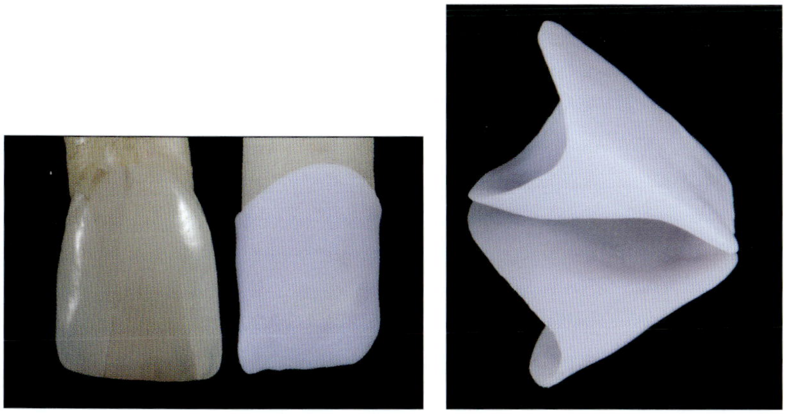

Figs 13a and 13b CNC-milled dentin core made of lithium metasilicate to restore the maxillary left central.

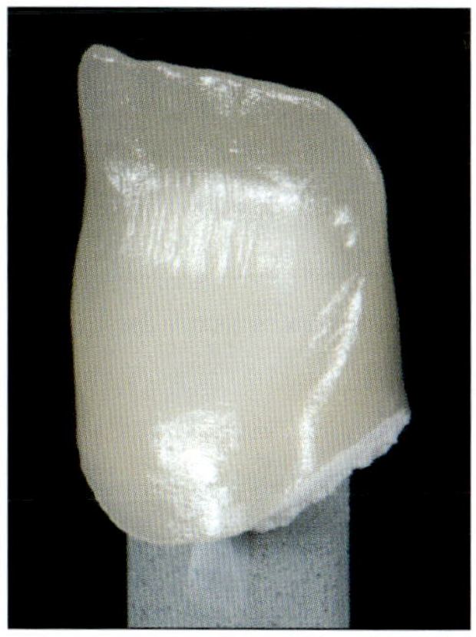

Fig 14 Dentin core from lithium disilicate after crystallization at 840°C.

Identifying the matching dentin core

The dentin core matching the external surface of the tooth dentin can be determined based on the tooth structure database. The acquired surface data are compared with the records of tooth surfaces in the tooth-structure database, and the record that is in closest agreement with the newly acquired data is selected. In the tooth-structure database, each external tooth surface is associated with a unique dentin core. Consequently, it is possible, on the basis of the acquired data, to identify the matching dentin core.

Mirroring the external tooth surface and dentin core data

Next, the two records are mirrored (Fig 12) to produce the crown based on the mirrored external tooth surface and dentin core data.

Digital manufacturing of the dentin core

Using dental CAD software, the record of the digital dentin core can be placed on the prepared tooth. The three-dimensional orientation of the dentin core data set is determined by the external tooth surface data. Next, the CAM software calculates the milling paths and corresponding NC file based on the CAD record of the dentin core. In the example shown, the dentin core was produced using the Everest unit (KaVo) and was prepared using the "counter-bed" procedure. In this procedure, once the cavity side has been milled, the cavity is filled with polyurethane resin. Once the resin has hardened, the surface of the dentin core (the DEJ) is milled. The material used was lithium disilicate (IPS e.max CAD LT, Ivoclar Vivadent). A side benefit of the counter-bed procedure is that it produces a copy of the die in polyurethane that is precisely positioned within the CNC unit in relation to the machine zero and workpiece zero points, facilitating precise repositioning of the crown within the CNC unit. The CAM process uses diamond grinding points. The IPS e.max CAD material is present in the metasilicate phase because it is easier to mill in this phase. After milling, the dentin core is crystallized at 840°C; then the lithium metasilicate is converted into lithium disilicate, attaining the target tooth shade and the final strength of 360 MPa (Figs 13 and 14).

Adding the incisal region

The ceramic veneer was made of IPS e.max Ceram (Ivoclar Vivadent). Before the actual application of the ceramic in the incisal area, a wash firing was performed at 760°C. Experience has shown that a mixture of Transpa Incisal and Opal Effect 1 at a ratio of 1:1 achieves a good result when using the incisal single-layer technique. Material is applied generously to the incisal area to provide enough bulk for the subsequent subtractive process. Once applied, the ceramic material is fired at 750°C (Figs 15 and 16).

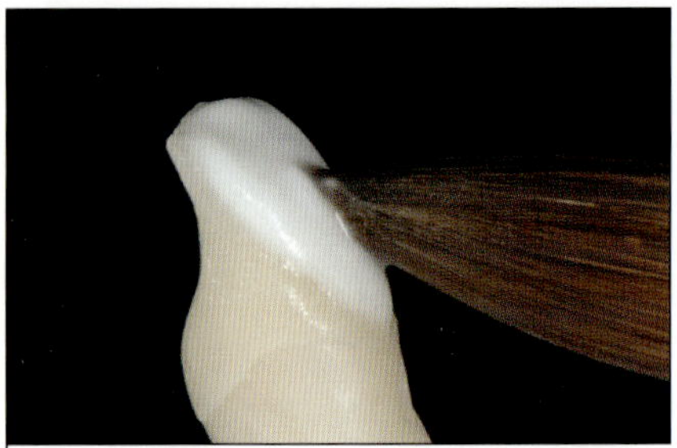
15

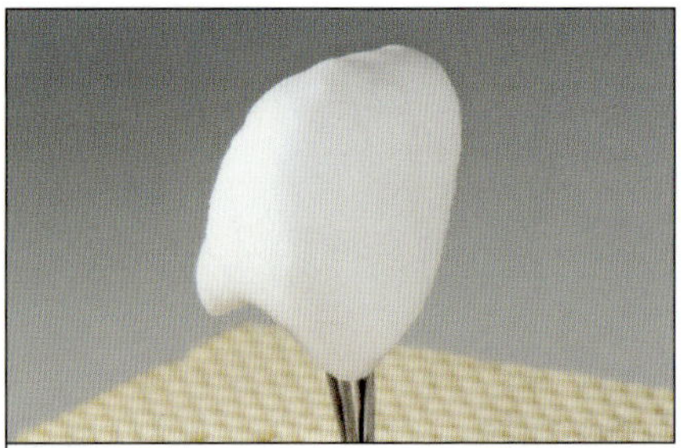
16a

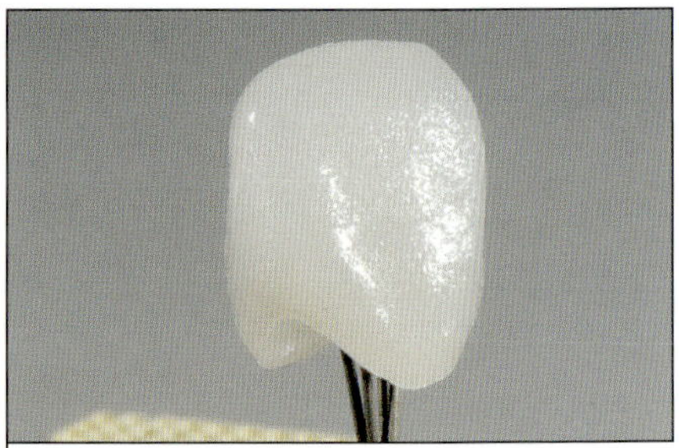
16b

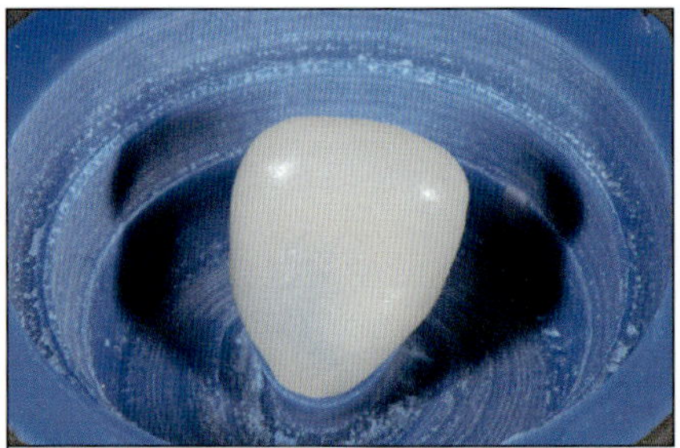
17a

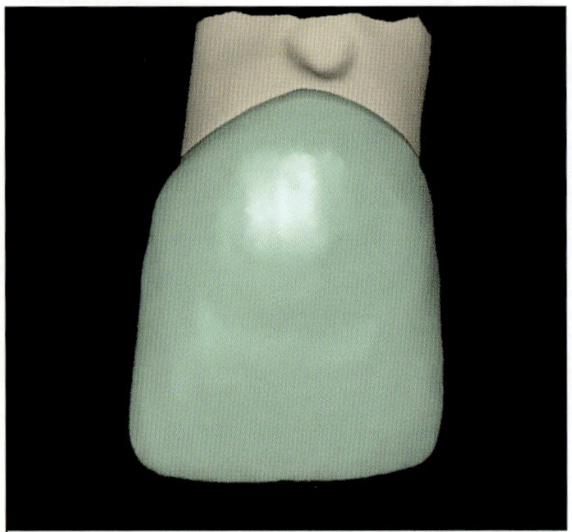
17b

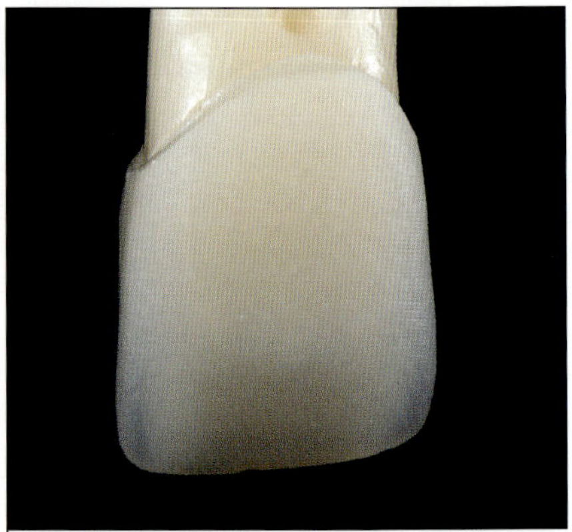
17c

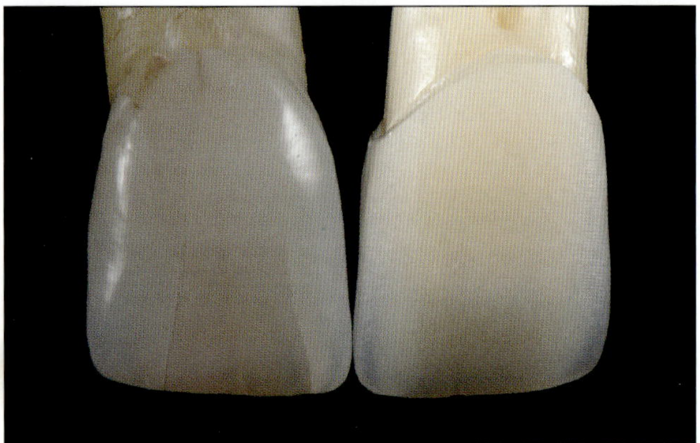
17d

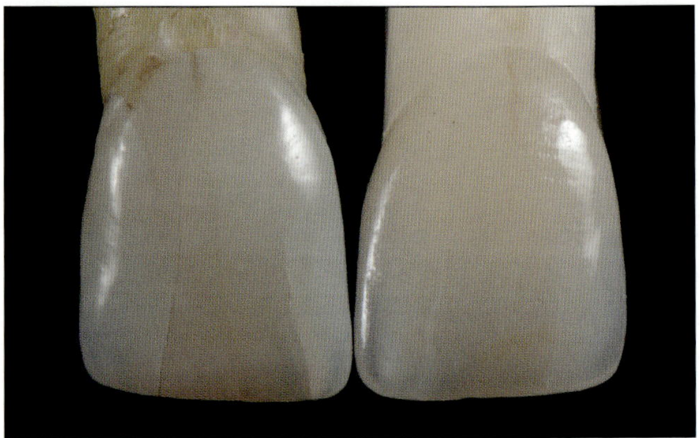
18

Fig 15 Application of incisal veneering material (IPS e.max Ceram, 50% Transpa Incisal 2, 50% Opal Effect 1).

Figs 16a and 16b The ceramic material is fired at 750°C.

Figs 17a to 17d The tooth surface is machined based on the three-dimensional record of the outer enamel surface. Repositioning is done with the aid of the polyurethane "copy."

Fig 18 The restoration is completed with a stain and glaze firing.

Digital finishing of the tooth surface

After ceramic firing, the entire crown is repositioned on the polyurethane die that was produced by the counter-bed process. Next, the tooth surface is machined based on the three-dimensional record of the outer enamel surface (Fig 17). The result is a two-layer restoration in which both the inner dentin core and the outer enamel surface were obtained in a digital procedure.

Finalizing the crown (glaze firing, polishing, etc)

The manufacturing process is finalized with a stain-and-glaze firing and final polishing of the restoration (Fig 18).

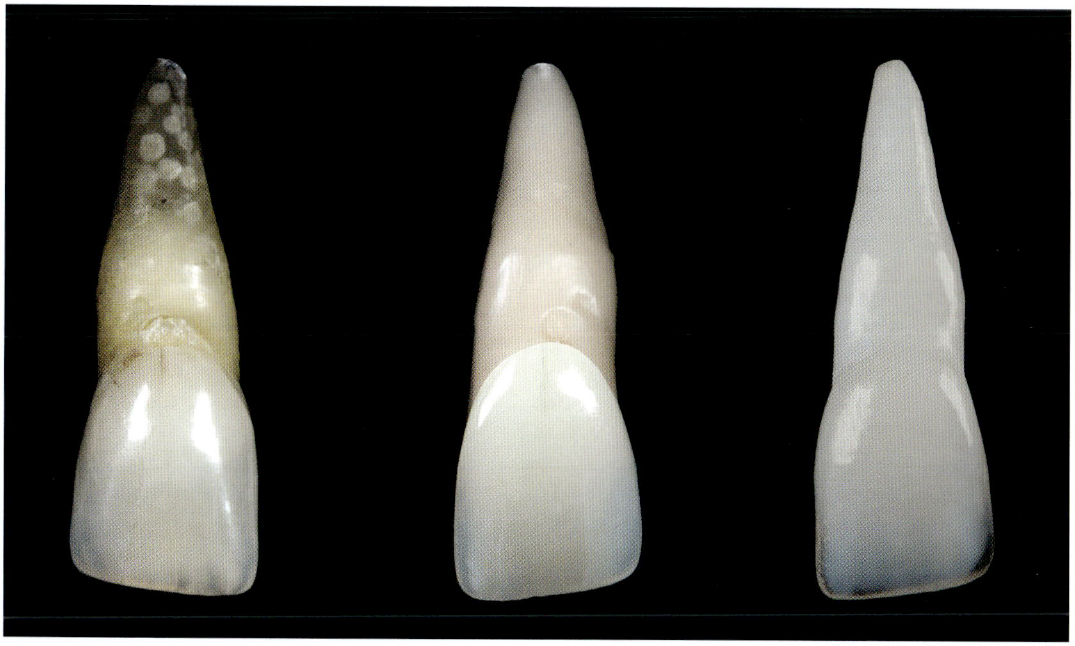

Fig 19 *(Left to right)* Natural tooth, CAD/CAM-fabricated anterior crown on tooth, 3D-printed (RP) tooth.

CONCLUSIONS

The process described in this article allows, for the first time, fabrication of highly esthetic anterior restorations based on tooth structure records in a digital, and therefore reproducible, procedure. The result is predictable, and good outcomes can be achieved even by users who are experienced in these technical matters. The digital dentin core is the key to digital anterior esthetics. It is important to create tooth structure databases that contain data both for the external geometry of the teeth and the corresponding dentin cores. The data for natural teeth especially will open up an entire new dimension of natural anterior esthetics. Production options include both subtractive and additive manufacturing processes (Fig 19).

Users have the ability to access a wide variety of tooth shapes and their structural designs to achieve reproducible results. Ultimately, it should be possible to use the digitally acquired external geometry of a tooth to identify the corresponding dentin core from a database in a highly predictable manner. Future research projects will have to demonstrate the statistical relationship between the external tooth shapes and dentin cores.

REFERENCES

1. Mehl A. Verfahren zur Herstellung von Zahnersatzteilen oder Zahnrestaurationen unter Verwendung elektronischer Zahndarstellungen. German patent no. 102 52 298 B3, 2002.
2. Probst F. Dreidimensionale Untersuchungen zur Morphologie der oberen Frontzähne [thesis]. Munich: Ludwig-Maximilians University, 2009.
3. Hellwig E, Klimek J, Attin T. Einführung in die Zahnerhaltung, ed 2. Munich-Jena: Urban & Fischer, 1999: 3–11.
4. Körber K. Funktionslehre. In: Zahnärztliche Prothetik. Stuttgart: Georg Thieme, 1995:3–7.
5. Kraus BS. Morphologic relationships between enamel and dentin surfaces of lower first molar teeth. J Dent Res 1952;31:248–256.
6. Korenhof CAW. Morphogenetical Aspects of the Human Upper Molar. Utrecht, The Netherlands: Uitgeversmaatschappij, 1960.
7. Korenhof CAW. The enamel-dentine border: A new morphological factor in the study of the (human) molar pattern. Proc Koninkl Nederl Acad Wetensch 1961;64B:639–664.
8. Korenhof CAW. De evolutie van het ondermolaarpatroon en overblijfselen van het trigonid bij de mens (I). Ned Tijdschr Tandheelkd 1978;85:456–495.
9. Korenhof CAW. Evolutionary trends of the inner enamel anatomy of deciduous molars from Sangiran (Java, Indonesia). In: Kurtén B (ed). Teeth: Form, Function and Evolution. New York: Columbia University Press, 1982:350–365.
10. Nager G. Der Vergleich zwischen dem räumlichen Verhalten des Dentinkronenreliefs und dem Schmelzrelief der Zahnkrone. Acta Anat 1960;42:226–250.

11. Schwartz GT, Thackeray JF, Reid C, van Reenan JF. Enamel thickness and the topography of the enamel-dentine junction in South African Plio-Pleistocene hominids with special reference to the Carabelli trait. J Hum Evol 1998;35:523–542.
12. Sakai T, Hanamura H. A morphology study of enamel-dentin border on the Japanese dentition. Part V. Maxillary molar. J Anthropol Soc Nippon 1971;79:297–322.
13. Sakai T, Hanamura H. A morphology study of enamel-dentin border on the Japanese dentition. Part VI. Mandibular molar. J Anthropol Soc Nippon 1973a;81:25–45.
14. Sakai T, Hanamura H. A morphology study of enamel-dentin border on the Japanese dentition. Part VII. General conclusion. J Anthropol Soc Nippon 1973b;81:87–102.
15. Sakai T, Sasaki I, Hanamura H. A morphology study of enamel-dentin border on the Japanese dentition. Part I. Maxillary median incisor. J Anthropol Soc Nippon 1965;73:91–109.
16. Sakai T, Sasaki I, Hanamura H. A morphology study of enamel-dentin border on the Japanese dentition. Part II. Maxillary canine. J Anthropol Soc Nippon 1967a;75:155–172.
17. Sakai T, Sasaki I, Hanamura H. A morphology study of enamel-dentin border on the Japanese dentition. Part III. Maxillary premolar. J Anthropol Soc Nippon 1967b;75:207–223.
18. Sakai T, Sasaki I, Hanamura H. A morphology study of enamel-dentin border on the Japanese dentition. Part IV. Mandibular premolar. J Anthropol Soc Nippon 1969;77:71–98.
19. Skinner M. Enamel-dentine junction morphology of extant hominoid and fossil hominin lower molars. J Hum Evol 2008;54: 173–186.
20. Corruccini RS. The dentinoenamel junction in primates. Int J Primatol 1987;8:99–114.
21. Corruccini RS. Relative growth from the dentino-enamel junction in primate maxillary molars. J Hum Evol 1987;2:263–269.
22. Corruccini RS. The dentino-enamel junction in primate mandibular molars. In: Lukacs JR (ed). Human Dental Development, Morphology, and Pathology: A Tribute to Albert A. Dahlberg. Portland: University of Oregon Anthropological Papers, 1998: 1–16.
23. Corruccini RS, Holt BM. The dentinoenamel junction and the hypocone in primates. Hum Evol 1989;4:253–262.
24. Sasaki K, Kanazawa E. Morphological traits on the dentino-enamel junction of lower deciduous molar series. In: Mayhall JT, Heikkinen T (eds), Proceedings of the 11th International Symposium on Dental Morphology, Oulu, Finland, 1998. Oulu, Finland: Oulu University Press, 1999:167–178.
25. Gallagher RR, Demos SG, Balooch M, Marshall GW Jr, Marshall SJ. Optical spectroscopy and imaging of the dentin-enamel junction in human third molars. J Biomed Mater Res A 2003;64:372–377.
26. Butler PM. The ontogeny of molar pattern. Biological Reviews 1956;31:30–70.
27. Conroy GC. Enamel thickness in South African australopithecines: Noninvasive evaluation by computed tomography. Palaeont Afr 1991;28:53–58.
28. Conroy GC, Lichtman JW, Martin LB. Brief communication: Some observations on enamel thickness and enamel prism packing in the Miocene hominoid Otavipithecus namibiensis. Am J Phys Anthropol 1995;98:595–600.
29. Grine FE. Computed tomography and the measurement of enamel thickness in extant hominoids: Implications for its palaeontological application. Palaeont Afr 1991;28:61–69.
30. Weidenreich F. Giant early man from Java and South China. Anthropol Pap Am Mus Nat Hist 1945;40:1–134.
31. Schweiger J. Verfahren, Vorrichtung und Computerprogramm zur Herstellung eines Zahnersatzes. German patent, DE 10 2010 002 484 A1 (2010).
32. Hilbert D, Ackermann W. Grundzüge der theoretischen Logik. Berlin, Göttingen, Heidelberg: Springer, 1972:24.
33. Schweiger J. Method, Device and Computer Program for Producing a Dental Prosthesis. European patent, EP 000002363094 A2 (2011).
34. Schweiger J. Method, Apparatus and Computer Program for Producing a Dental Prosthesis. US patent 8, 775, 131, B2 (2011).